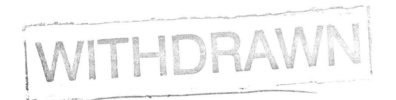

Pharmaceutical Process Scale-Up

Pharmaceutical Process Scale-Up

Third Edition

Edited by

Michael Levin
Milev Pharmaceutical Technology Consulting,
West Orange, New Jersey, USA.

informa
healthcare

New York   London

Published in 2011 by Informa Healthcare, Telephone House, 69-77 Paul Street, London EC2A 4LQ, UK. Simultaneously published in the USA by Informa Healthcare, 52 Vanderbilt Avenue, 7th floor, New York, NY 10017, USA.

A CIP record for this book is available from the British Library.

ISBN-13: 978-1-6163-1001-1

Orders may be sent to: Informa Healthcare, Sheepen Place, Colchester, Essex CO3 3LP, UK
Telephone: +44 (0)20 7017 5540
Email: CSDhealthcarebooks@informa.com
Website: http://informahealthcarebooks.com/

For corporate sales please contact: CorporateBooksIHC@informa.com
For foreign rights please contact: RightsIHC@informa.com
For reprint permissions please contact: PermissionsIHC@informa.com
Printed in United Kingdom

To my wife, Sonia,
my children Hanna, Daniela, Ilan, Emanuel, and Maya,
and to the memory of my parents

Preface

This book deals with a subject that is both fascinating and vitally important for the pharmaceutical industry—the procedures of transferring the results of R&D obtained on laboratory scale to the pilot plant and finally to production scale.

Although some theory and history of process scale-up are presented in several chapters, no special knowledge of physics or engineering is required of the general reader since all theoretical considerations are fully explained.

The primary objective of this volume, however, is to provide an insight into the practical aspects of the process scale-up. As a source of information on batch enlargement techniques, this book will be of practical interest to formulators, process engineers, validation specialists, and quality assurance personnel, as well as production managers. It will also provide an interesting reading material for anyone involved in Process Analytical Technology, technology transfer, and product globalization.

The regulatory aspects of scale-up and postapproval changes are addressed in detail throughout the book and in a separate chapter. A diligent attempt was made to keep all references to FDA regulations as complete and current as possible.

The process of scale-up in pharmaceutical industry involves, in general, moving a product from research and development into production. Numerous pitfalls could be met on this path. It is a well-known fact that oftentimes the production process cannot achieve the same quality of the product as was envisioned in the development and preapproval stages. Losses in terms of effort and money can be enormous. That is why scale-up and postapproval changes are so important and so strictly regulated.

This volume is designed to provide some answers that can facilitate the scale-up process. The main underlying theme that can be detected in almost every chapter of the book is a reference to dimensional analysis, a theoretical approach that makes it possible to describe any unit operation (in fact, any process) in terms of dimensionless variables. Once this mathematical model is achieved, the process becomes "scale invariable," that is, independent of scale. In other words, the key to successful scale-up is to eliminate the scale (linear dimensions, time, etc.) from your process description.

What sounds good in theory may be very difficult to achieve in practice, of course. Not only because theoretical modeling is just a model, an approximation of reality. There are always some practical "trade secrets" that are known to experienced operators and the experts in the field and that do not necessarily emerge from any academic discussion. These hands-on recommendations and advices are given a prominent place in this book along with theoretical considerations.

Since the publication of very successful first and second editions of *Pharmaceutical Process Scale-Up*, several crucial related FDA documents have been revised. Also, Quality by Design (QbD), Question-Based Review (QbR), and Process Analytical Technology (PAT) initiatives have been applied throughout the pharmaceutical industry, with a limited success.

PAT guidance published by FDA in September 2004 contained nonbinding recommendations with clear implications for scientific approach to scale-up. To quote:

Structured product and process development on a small scale, using experimental design and on- or in-line process analyzers to collect data in real time, can provide increased insight and understanding for process development, optimization, scale-up, technology transfer, and control. Process understanding then continues in the production phase when other variables (e.g., environmental and supplier changes) may possibly be encountered (1).

Scale-up studies are referred to as one of the primary sources of data and information needed to understand the "multi-factorial relationships among various critical formulation and process factors and for developing effective risk mitigation strategies (e.g., product specifications, process controls)" (1). Using small-scale equipment (to eliminate certain scale-up issues) in continuous processing is considered to be one of the ways to achieve the declared PAT goal "to design and develop processes that can consistently ensure a predefined quality at the end of the manufacturing process" (1). Experts in the field (both from FDA and the industry) started talking about "Make Your Own SUPAC" concept (alternatively called PAT-SUPAC or SUPAC-C). Indeed, if the new technology can provide a better process understanding and risk management, then, perhaps, the resulting better quality assurance during postapproval changes should provide some regulatory relief (2).

In 2006, FDA has published the "Quality Systems Approach to Pharmaceutical Current Good Manufacturing Practice Regulations," where the notion of product design is discussed in the framework of product development and robust manufacturing process (3). FDA recommends "that scale-up studies be used to help demonstrate that a fundamentally sound design has been fully realized."

In addition to readjusting the focus of this book to show the importance of the PAT and QbD initiatives for pharmaceutical process scale-up, there have been several major revisions and additions.

Most of the chapters have been updated to reflect the increased body of knowledge in the respective areas of unit operations. The sections on scale-up of tableting and on pilot plants have been completely revised. New sections have been added, namely, on the scale-up risk analysis and evaluation, robust process design and design of experiments for scale-up, and process validation issues during scale-up. A new chapter on scale-up of pan-coating process has also been added.

If you are familiar with the first and second editions of this book, you are encouraged to peruse this third edition because

- the book makes a special emphasis on "connecting the dots" between SUPAC, PAT, and QbD guidances (reflecting the new direction that FDA and the industry are now taking);
- many chapters underwent a thorough revision based on the rapid change in the state of the art and/or reader's practical suggestions;
- the chapter on compaction and tableting is completely rewritten to reflect the more comprehensive perspective, in both theoretical and practical aspects; and
- new chapters on risk evaluation, DOE, validation, and pan-coating unit operation have been added.

All in all, this new edition should be a welcome addition to the libraries of pharmaceutical scientists, process engineers, and educators.

REFERENCES

1. FDA. Guidance for Industry: PAT—A Framework for Innovative Pharmaceutical Development, Manufacturing, and Quality Assurance. Rockville, MD: U.S. Department of Health and Human Services, Food and Drug Administration, September 2004. http://www.fda.gov/downloads/Drugs/GuidanceComplianceRegulatoryInformation/Guidances/ucm070305.pdf.
2. Hussain A. FDA's Initiative on a Drug Quality System for the 21st Century: A Once in a Lifetime Opportunity. AAPS Meeting Presentation, October 2003.
3. FDA. Guidance for Industry. Quality Systems Approach to Pharmaceutical Current Good Manufacturing Practice Regulations. Rockville, MD: U.S. Department of Health and Human Services, Food and Drug Administration, September 2006. http://www.fda.gov/downloads/Drugs/GuidanceComplianceRegulatoryInformation/Guidances/ucm070337.pdf.

Michael Levin
milev@comcast.net

Contents

Contributors

Albert W. Alexander   Department of Chemical and Biochemical Engineering, Rutgers University, Piscataway, New Jersey, U.S.A.

Larry L. Augsburger   University of Maryland School of Pharmacy, Baltimore, Maryland, U.S.A.

Gabriele Betz   Industrial Pharmacy Laboratory, Institute of Pharmaceutical Technology of the Univbersity of Basel, Basel, Switzerland

Lawrence H. Block   Duquesne University, Pittsburgh, Pennsylvania, U.S.A.

Marco Cacciuttolo   Percivia LLC, Cambridge, Massachusetts, U.S.A.

John Chon (deceased)   Percivia LLC, Cambridge, Massachusetts, U.S.A.

Marc Allen S. Donsmark   Donsmark Process Technology A/S, Copenhagen, Denmark

Atul Dubey   Department of Chemical and Biochemical Engineering, Rutgers University, Piscataway, New Jersey, U.S.A.

Yijie Gao   Department of Chemical and Biochemical Engineering, Rutgers University, Piscataway, New Jersey, U.S.A.

Igor Gorsky   Global Pharmaceutical Technology, Shire, Wayne, Pennsylvania, U.S.A.

Kathryn A. Gray   Chemical Sciences Team Manager, AstraZeneca, Macclesfield, United Kingdom

Marianthi G. Ierapetritou   Department of Chemical and Biochemical Engineering, Rutgers University, Piscataway, New Jersey, U.S.A.

Raman M. Iyer   Pharmaceutical and Analytical Research and Development, Hoffmann–La Roche, Nutley, New Jersey, U.S.A.

David M. Jones   OWI-Consulting Inc., Ramsey, New Jersey, U.S.A.

Hans Leuenberger   Institute for Innovation in Industrial Pharmacy (IFIIP), Basel, Switzerland

Michael N. Leuenberger   American Institute for Innovative Computer-Aided Solutions (AMIFICAS Inc.), Oviedo, Florida, U.S.A.

Michael Levin   Milev Pharmaceutical Technology Consulting, West Orange, New Jersey, U.S.A.

Ronald W. Miller   President, Miller Pharmaceutical Technology Consulting, Travelers Rest, South Carolina, U.S.A.

Jeffrey Moriarty   Pfizer Inc, Eastern Point Road, Groton, Connecticut, U.S.A.

Matthew P. Mullarney   Pfizer Inc, Eastern Point Road, Groton, Connecticut, U.S.A.

Frans L. Muller Associate Principal Scientist, AstraZeneca, Macclesfield, United Kingdom

Fernando J. Muzzio Department of Chemical and Biochemical Engineering, Rutgers University, Piscataway, New Jersey, U.S.A.

Steven Ostrove Ostrove Associates, Inc., Elizabeth, New Jersey, U.S.A.

Dilip M. Parikh DPharma Group Inc., Ellicott City, Maryland, U.S.A.

Stuart C. Porter Senior Director, Global Pharmaceutical Applications R&D, International Specialty Products, Wayne, New Jersey, U.S.A.

James K. Prescott Jenike & Johanson, Inc., Tyngsboro, Massachusetts, U.S.A.

Maxim Puchkov Center for Innovation in Computer-Aided Pharmaceutics (CINCAP GmbH), Basel, Switzerland

Graham E. Robinson Process Chemistry Team Manager, AstraZeneca, Macclesfield, United Kingdom

Harpreet K. Sandhu Pharmaceutical and Analytical Research and Development, Hoffmann–La Roche, Nutley, New Jersey, U.S.A.

Navnit H. Shah Pharmaceutical and Analytical Research and Development, Hoffmann–La Roche, Nutley, New Jersey, U.S.A.

Aditya U. Vanarase Department of Chemical and Biochemical Engineering, Rutgers University, Piscataway, New Jersey, U.S.A.

Greg Zarbis-Papastoitsis Eleven Biotherapeutics, Cambridge, Massachusetts, U.S.A.

Marko Zlokarnik University of Cologne, Cologne, Germany

Introduction

Scale-up is generally defined as the process of increasing the batch size. Scale-up of a process can also be viewed as a procedure for applying the same process to different output volumes. There is a subtle difference between these two definitions: batch size enlargement does not always translate into a size increase of the processing volume.

In mixing applications, scale-up is indeed concerned with increasing the linear dimensions from the laboratory to the plant size. On the other hand, processes exist (e.g., tableting) where the term "scale-up" simply means enlarging the output by increasing the speed. To complete the picture, one should point out special procedures (especially in biotechnology) where an increase of the scale is counterproductive and "scale-down" is required to improve the quality of the product.

In moving from R&D to production scale, it is sometimes essential to have an intermediate batch scale. This is achieved at the so-called pilot scale, which is defined as the manufacturing of drug product by a procedure fully representative of and simulating that used for full manufacturing scale. This scale makes it possible also to produce enough product for clinical testing and to manufacture samples for marketing. However, inserting an intermediate step between R&D and production scales does not, in itself, guarantee a smooth transition. A well-defined process may generate a perfect product both in the laboratory and in the pilot plant and then fail quality assurance tests in production.

Imagine that you have successfully scaled up a mixing or a granulating process from a 10-L batch to 75-L and then to 300-L batch. What exactly happened? You may say: "I got lucky." Apart from luck, there had to be some physical similarity in the processing of the batches. Once you understand what makes these processes similar, you can eliminate many scale-up problems.

A rational approach to scale-up has been used in physical sciences, viz. fluid dynamics and chemical engineering, for quite some time. This approach is based on process similarities between different scales and is employing dimensional analysis that was developed a century ago and has since gained wide recognition in many industries, especially in chemical engineering (1).

Dimensional analysis is a method for producing dimensionless numbers that completely characterize the process. The analysis can be applied even when the equations governing the process are not known. According to the theory of models, two processes may be considered completely similar if they take place in similar geometrical space and if all the dimensionless numbers necessary to describe the process have the same numerical value (2).

The scale-up procedure, then, is simple: express the process using a complete set of dimensionless numbers, and try to match them at different scales. This dimensionless space in which the measurements are presented or measured will make the process scale invariant.

Dimensionless numbers, such as Reynolds and Froude numbers, are frequently used to describe mixing processes. Chemical engineers are routinely concerned with problems of water-air or fluid mixing in vessels equipped with turbine stirrers where scale-up factors can be up to 1:70 (3). This approach is being applied to pharmaceutical granulation since the early work of Hans Leuenberger in 1982 (4).

One way to eliminate potential scale-up problems is to develop formulations that are very robust with respect to processing conditions. A comprehensive database of excipients detailing their material properties may be indispensable for this purpose. However, in practical terms, this cannot be achieved without some means of testing in the production environment, and, since the initial drug substance is usually available in small quantities, some form of simulation is required on a small scale.

In tableting applications, the process scale-up involves different speeds of production in what is essentially the same unit volume (die cavity in which the compaction takes place). Thus, one of the conditions of the theory of models (similar geometric space) is met. However, there are still kinematic and dynamic parameters that need to be investigated and matched for any process transfer. One of the main practical questions facing tablet formulators during development and scale-up is this: Will a particular formulation sustain the required high rate of compression force application in a production press without lamination or capping? Usually, such questions are never answered with sufficient credibility, especially when only a small amount of material is available and any trial and error approach may result in costly mistakes along the scale-up path.

As tablet formulations are moved from small-scale research presses to high-speed machines, potential scale-up problems can be eliminated by simulation of production conditions in the formulation development lab. In any process transfer from one tablet press to another, one may aim to preserve mechanical properties of a tablet (density and, by extension, energy used to obtain it) as well as its bioavailability (e.g., dissolution that may be affected by porosity). Scientifically sound approach would be to use the results of the dimensional analysis to model a particular production environment. Studies done on a class of equipment generally known as compaction simulators or tablet press replicators can be designed to facilitate the scale-up of tableting process, by matching several major factors, such as compression force and rate of its application (punch velocity and displacement) in their dimensionless equivalent form.

Any significant change in a process of making a pharmaceutical dosage form is a subject of a regulatory concern. Scale-up and postapproval changes (SUPAC) are of a special interest to FDA as is evidenced by a growing number of regulatory documents released in the last several years by the Center for Drug Evaluation and Research (CDER), including Immediate Release Solid Oral Dosage Forms (SUPAC-IR), Modified Release Solid Oral Dosage Forms (SUPAC-MR), and Semi-solid Dosage Forms (SUPAC-SS). Additional SUPAC guidance documents being developed include Transdermal Delivery Systems (SUPAC-TDS), Bulk Actives (BACPAC), and Sterile Aqueous Solutions (PAC-SAS). Collaboration between FDA, pharmaceutical industry, and academia in this and other areas has recently been launched under the framework of the Product Quality Research Institute (PQRI).

In Europe, scale-up issues are indirectly addressed in several directives, but there seems to be no coherent framework except a referral to International Conference on Harmonisation (ICH) Harmonised Tripartite Guidelines. ICH Topic Q8 Annex (Pharmaceutical Development) deals with design space and potential risks involved in the scale-up process. This topic is further clarified in a Q&A dated June 2009. ICH Q10 (Pharmaceutical Quality System) discusses, among other things, the importance of scale-up process in technology transfer.

Scale-up problems may require postapproval changes that affect formulation composition, site change, and manufacturing process or equipment changes (by the way, from the regulatory standpoint, scale-up and scale-down are treated with the same degree of scrutiny). In a typical drug development cycle, once a set of clinical studies have been completed or NDA/ANDA has been approved, it becomes very difficult to change the product or the process to accommodate specific production needs. Such needs may include changes in batch size and manufacturing equipment or process.

Postapproval changes in the size of a batch from the pilot scale to larger or smaller production scales call for submission of additional information in the application, with a specific requirement that the new batches are to be produced using similar test equipment and in full compliance with current good manufacturing processes and the existing standard operating procedures. Manufacturing changes may require new stability, dissolution, and in vivo bioequivalence testing. This is especially true for level 2 equipment changes (change in equipment to a different design and different operating principles) and the process changes of level 2 (process changes including changes such as mixing times and operating speeds within application/validation ranges) and level 3 (changes in the type of process used in the manufacture of the product, such as a change from wet granulation to direct compression of dry powder).

Any such testing and accompanying documentation are subject to FDA approval and can be very costly. In 1977, FDA's Office of Planning and Evaluation (OPE) undertook a study of the impact on and cost savings to industry of the SUPAC guidance. The findings indicated that the guidance generated substantial savings to the industry because it permitted, among other factors, shorter waiting times for site transfers, more rapid implementation of process and equipment changes, as well as batch size increases and reduction of quality control costs.

In early development stages of a new drug substance, relatively little information is available regarding its polymorphic forms, solubility, etc. As the final formulation is developed, changes to the manufacturing process may change the purity profile or physical characteristics of the drug substance and thus cause batch failures and other problems with the finished dosage form.

FDA inspectors are instructed to look for any differences between the process filed in the application and the process used to manufacture the bio/clinical batch. Furthermore, one of the main requirements of a manufacturing process is that the process will yield a product that is equivalent to the substance on which the biostudy or pivotal clinical study was conducted. Validation of the process development and scale-up should include sufficient documentation so that a link between the bio/clinical batches and the commercial process can be established. If the process is different after scale-up, the company has to demonstrate that the product produced by a modified process will be equivalent, using data such as granulation studies, finished product test results, and dissolution profiles.

Many of the FDA's postapproval, premarketing inspections result in citations because validation (and consistency) of the full-scale batches could not be established owing to problems with product dissolution, content uniformity, and potency. Validation reports on batch scale-ups may also reflect selective reporting of data.

Of practical importance are the issues associated with a technology transfer in a global market. Equipment standardization will inevitably cause a variety of engineering and process optimization concerns that, generally speaking, can be classified as SUPAC.

To summarize, the significant aspects of pharmaceutical scale-up are presented in this book to illustrate potential concerns, theoretical considerations, and practical solutions based on the experience of the contributing authors. In no way do we claim a comprehensive treatment of the subject. A prudent reader may use this handbook as a reference and an initial resource for further study of the scale-up issues.

REFERENCES

1. Zlokarnik M. Dimensional Analysis and Scale-Up in Chemical Engineering. Berlin: Springer-Verlag, 1991.
2. Buckingham E. On physically similar systems; Illustrations of the use of dimensional equations. Phys Rev NY 1914; 4:345–376.
3. Zlokarnik M. Problems in the application of dimensional analysis and scale-up of mixing operations. Chem Eng Sci 1998; 53(17):3023–3030.
4. Leuenberger H. Scale-up of granulation processes with reference to process monitoring. Acta Pharm Technol 1983; 29(4):274–280.

1 Dimensional analysis and scale-up in theory and industrial application

Marko Zlokarnik

INTNODUOTION

A chemical engineer is generally concerned with the industrial implementation of processes in which chemical or microbiological conversion of material takes place in conjunction with the transfer of mass, heat, and momentum. These processes are scale-dependent, that is, they behave differently on a small scale (in laboratories or pilot plants) and a large scale (in production). They include heterogeneous chemical reactions and most unit operations. Understandably, chemical engineers have always wanted to find ways of simulating these processes in models to gain insights that will assist them in designing new industrial plants. Occasionally, they are faced with the same problem for another reason: an industrial facility already exists but will not function properly, if at all, and suitable measurements have to be carried out to discover the cause of the difficulties and provide a solution.

Irrespective of whether the model involved represents a "scale-up" or a "scale-down," certain important questions always apply:

1. How small can the model be? Is one model sufficient or should tests be carried out in models of different sizes?
2. When must or when can physical properties differ? When must the measurements be carried out on the model with the original system of materials?
3. Which rules govern the adaptation of the process parameters in the model measurements to those of the full-scale plant?
4. Is it possible to achieve complete similarity between the processes in the model and those in its full-scale counterpart? If not, how should one proceed?

These questions touch on the fundamentals of the theory of models, which are based on dimensional analysis. Although they have been used in the field of fluid dynamics and heat transfer for more than a century—cars, aircraft, vessels and heat exchangers were scaled up according to these principles—these methods have gained only a modest acceptance in chemical engineering. University graduates are usually not skilled enough to deal with such problems at all. On the other hand, there is no motivation for this type of research at universities, since, as a rule, they are not confronted with scale-up tasks and are not equipped with the necessary apparatus on the bench-scale. All this gives a totally wrong impression that these methods are, at most, of marginal importance in practical chemical engineering, otherwise they would have been taught and dealt with in greater depth.

DIMENSIONAL ANALYSIS
The Fundamental Principle
The dimensional analysis is based on the recognition that a mathematical formulation of a physicotechnological problem can be of general validity only when the process equation is *dimensionally homogenous*, which means that it must be valid in any system of dimensions.

What Is a Dimension?
A dimension is a purely *qualitative* description of a perception of a physical entity or a natural appearance. A length can be experienced as a height, a depth, and a breadth. A mass presents itself as a light or heavy body, and time as a short moment or a long period. The dimension of a length is length (L), the dimension of a mass is mass (M), etc.

What Is a Physical Quantity?
Unlike dimension, a physical quantity represents a *quantitative* description of a physical quality (e.g., a mass of 5 kg). It consists of a measuring unit and a numerical value. The measuring unit of length can be a meter, a foot, a cubit, a yardstick, a nautical mile, a light year, etc. The measuring units of energy are, for example, Joule, calorie, electron volt, etc. (It is therefore necessary to establish the measuring units in an appropriate measuring system.)

Base and Derived Quantities, Dimensional Constants
A distinction is being made between base and secondary quantities, the latter being often referred to as derived quantities. The base quantities are based on standards and are quantified by comparison with these standards.

The secondary units are derived from the primary ones according to physical laws, for example, velocity = length/time. (The borderline separating both types of quantities is largely arbitrary: for example, 50 years ago a measuring system was used in which force was a base dimension instead of mass.)

All secondary units must be coherent with the base units (Table 1), for example, the measuring unit of velocity must not be miles/hr or km/hr but m/sec.

If a secondary unit has been established by a physical law, it can happen that it contradicts another one. For example, according to the Newton's second law of motion, force F is expressed as a product of mass m and acceleration a, $F = ma$, having the measuring unit of (kg m/sec^2 $\equiv$ N). According to the Newton's law of gravitation, force is defined by $F \propto m_1 m_2 / r^2$, thus leading to

TABLE 1   Base Quantities, Their Dimensions and Units According to SI

Base quantity	Base dimension	Base unit
Length	L	m (meter)
Mass	M	kg (kilogram)
Time	T	s (second)
Thermodynamic temperature	Θ	K (Kelvin)
Amount of substance	N	mol (mole)
Electric current	I	A (ampère)
Luminous intensity	I_v	cd (Candela)

completely different measuring unit (kg^2/m^2). To remedy this, the gravitational constant **G**—a dimensional constant—had to be introduced to ensure the dimensional homogeneity of the latter equation: $F = \mathbf{G}m_1m_2/r^2$. Another example affects the universal gas constant **R**, the introduction of which ensures that in the perfect gas equation of state $pV = n\mathbf{R}T$, the secondary unit for work $W = PV$ [$M\ L^2\ T^{-2}$] is not offended.

Another class of derived quantities is represented by the coefficients in diverse physical equations, for example, transfer equations. They are established by the respective equations and determined via measurement of their constituents, for example, heat and mass transfer coefficients.

Dimensional Systems

A dimensional system consists of all the primary and secondary dimensions and corresponding measuring units. The currently used International System of Dimensions (Système International d'unités, SI) is based on seven base dimensions. They are presented in Table 1 together with their corresponding base units. For some of them a few explanatory remarks may be necessary:

Temperature expresses the thermal level of a system and not its energy content. (A fivefold mass of a matter has the fivefold thermal energy at the same temperature.). The thermal energy of a system can indeed be converted into mechanical energy (unit Joule).

Mole is the amount of matter and must not be confused with the quantity of mass. Molecules react as individual entities regardless of their mass: One mole of hydrogen (2 g/mol) reacts with one mole of chlorine (71 g/mol) to produce two moles of hydrochloric acid, HCl (73 g/mol).

Table 2 shows the most important secondary dimensions. Table 3 refers to some very frequently used secondary units that have been named after famous researchers.

TABLE 2   Often Used Physical Quantities and Their Dimensions According to the Currently Used SI in Mechanical and Thermal Problems

Physical quantity	Dimension
Angular velocity, shear rate, frequency mass transfer coefficient $k_L a$	T^{-1}
Velocity	$L\,T^{-1}$
Acceleration	$L\,T^{-2}$
Kinematic viscosity, diffusion coefficient, thermal diffusivity	$L^2\,T^{-1}$
Density	$M\,L^{-3}$
Surface tension	$M\,T^{-2}$
Dynamic viscosity	$M\,L^{-1}\,T^{-1}$
Momentum	$M\,L\,T^{-1}$
Force	$M\,L\,T^{-2}$
Pressure, stress	$M\,L^{-1}\,T^{-2}$
Angular momentum	$M\,L^2\,T^{-1}$
Energy, work, torque	$M\,L^2\,T^{-2}$
Power	$M\,L^2\,T^{-3}$
Heat capacity	$L^2\,T^{-2}\,\Theta^{-1}$
Thermal conductivity	$M\,L\,T^{-3}\,\Theta^{-1}$
Heat transfer coefficient	$M\,T^{-3}\,\Theta^{-1}$

TABLE 3 Important Secondary Measuring Units in the Mechanics, Named After Famous Researchers

Secondary quantity	Dimension	Measuring unit	Abbreviation
Force	$M\,L\,T^{-2}$	$kg\,m/sec^2 \equiv N$	Newton
Pressure	$M\,L^{-1}\,T^{-2}$	$kg/m/sec^2 \equiv Pa$	Pascal
Energy	$M\,L^2\,T^{-2}$	$kg\,m^2/sec^2 \equiv J$	Joule
Power	$M\,L^2\,T^{-3}$	$kg\,m^2/sec^3 \equiv W$	Watt

Dimensional Homogeneity of a Physical Content

The aim of dimensional analysis is to check whether the physical content under examination can be formulated in a dimensionally homogeneous manner or not. The procedure necessary to accomplish this consists of two parts:

1. First, all physical parameters necessary to describe the problem are listed. This so-called "relevance list" of the problem consists of the quantity in question and of all the parameters that influence it. In each case only *one* target quantity must be considered; it is the only dependent variable. On the other hand, all the influencing parameters must be primarily independent of each other.

2. In the second step, the dimensional homogeneity of the physical content is checked by transferring it in a dimensionless form. *Note*: A physical content that can be transformed into dimensionless expressions is dimensionally homogeneous.

The information given to this point will be made clear by following instructive example:

Example 1: Which is the correlation between the baking time and the weight of the Christmas turkey?

We first recall the physical situation. To facilitate this we draw a sketch (Fig. 1). At high oven temperatures the heat is transferred from the heating elements to the meat surface by both radiation and heat convection. From there it is

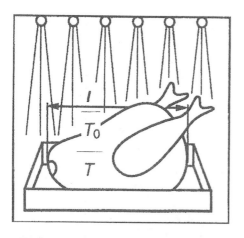

FIGURE 1 Oven with the piece of poultry.

transferred solely by the unsteady state heat conduction that surely represents the rate-limiting step of the whole heating process.

The higher the thermal conductivity k of the body, the faster the heat spreads out. The higher its volume-related heat capacity ρC_p, the slower the heats transfer. Therefore, the unsteady state heat conduction is characterized by *only one* material property, the thermal diffusivity $a \equiv k/\rho C_p$ of the body.

Physical quantity	Symbol	Dim
Baking time	θ	T
Surface of meat	A	L^2
Thermal diffusivity	a	$L^2\,T^{-1}$
Temperature on the surface	T_0	Θ
Temperature distribution	T	Θ

Baking is an endothermal process. The meat is cooked when a certain temperature distribution (T) is reached. It is about the time θ necessary to achieve this temperature field.

After these considerations we are able to precisely construct the relevance list:

$$\{\theta, A, a, T_0, T\} \tag{1}$$

The base dimension of temperature Θ appears only in two parameters. They can, therefore, produce only one dimensionless quantity:

$$\textstyle\prod_1 \equiv \frac{T}{T_0} \text{ or } \frac{T_0 - T}{T_0} \tag{2}$$

The residual three quantities form one additional dimensionless number:

$$\textstyle\prod_2 \equiv \frac{a\theta}{A} \equiv \text{Fo} \tag{3}$$

In the theory of heat transfer, $\prod_2$ is known as the Fourier number Fo. Therefore, the baking procedure can be presented in a two-dimensional frame:

$$\frac{T}{T_0} = f(\text{Fo}) \tag{4}$$

Here, five dimensional quantities (Eq. 1) produce two dimensionless numbers (Eq. 4). This had to be expected because the dimensions in question are compressed up of three base dimensions: $5 - 3 = 2$ (see the discussion on pi theorem later in this chapter).

We can now easily answer the question concerning the correlation between the baking time and the weight of the Christmas turkey, without explicitly knowing the function f, which connects both numbers (Eq. 4). To achieve the same temperature distribution T/T_0 or $(T_0 - T)/T_0$ in differently sized bodies, the dimensionless quantity $a\theta/A \equiv$ Fo must have the same (= idem) numerical value. Because of the fact that the thermal diffusivity a remains unaltered in the meat of the same kind ($a =$ idem), this demand leads to

$$T/T_0 = \text{idem} \rightarrow Fo \equiv a\theta/A = \text{idem} \rightarrow \frac{\theta}{A} = \text{idem} \rightarrow \theta \propto A \tag{5}$$

This statement is obviously useless as a scale-up rule because meat is bought according to weight and not surface. We can remedy this simply.

In geometrically similar bodies, the following correlation between mass m, surface A, and volume V exists:

$$m = \rho V \propto \rho L^3 \propto \rho A^{3/2} \; (A \propto L^2) \qquad (6)$$

Therefore, from $\rho =$ idem, it follows

$$A \propto m^{2/3}$$

and by this

$$\theta \propto A \propto m^{2/3} \rightarrow \theta_2/\theta_1 \propto (m_2/m_1)^{2/3} \qquad (7)$$

This is the scale-up rule for baking or cooking time in case of meat of the same kind (a, $\rho =$ idem). It states that when the mass of meat is doubled, the cooking time will increase by $2^{2/3} = 1.58$.

West (1) refers to "inferior" cookbooks that simply say something like "20 minutes per pound," implying a linear relationship with weight. However, there exist "superior" cookbooks, such as the *Better Homes and Gardens Cookbook* (Des Moines Meredith Corp., 1962), that recognize the nonlinear nature of this relationship. The graphical representation of measurements in this book confirms the relationship

$$\theta \propto m^{0.6} \qquad (8)$$

which is very close to the theoretical evaluation giving $\theta \propto m^{2/3} = m^{0.67}$.

The elegant solution of this first example should not tempt the reader to believe that dimensional analysis can solve every problem solely by a theoretical consideration. To treat this example by dimensional analysis, the physics of unsteady state heat conduction had to be understood.

Bridgman's (2) comment on this situation is particularly appropriate:

> The problem cannot be solved by the philosopher in his armchair, but the knowledge involved was gathered only by someone at some time soiling his hands with direct contact.

This transparent and easy example clearly shows how dimensional analysis deals with specific problems and what conclusions it allows. It should now be easier to understand Lord Rayleigh's sarcastic comment with which he began his short essay on "The Principle of Similitude" (3):

> I have often been impressed by the scanty attention paid even by original workers in physics to the great principle of similitude. It happens not infrequently that results in the form of "laws" are put forward as novelties on the basis of elaborate experiments, which might have been predicted *a priori* after a few minutes' consideration.

From the above examples we also learn that a transformation of a physical dependence from a dimensional into a dimensionless form is automatically accompanied by an essential *compression* of the statement: The set of the dimensionless numbers is smaller than the set of the quantities contained in them, but it describes the problem equally comprehensively. In the above example, the dependency between five dimensional parameters is reduced to a dependency between only two dimensionless numbers. This is the proof of the so-called pi theorem (pi after $\prod$, the sign used for products), which states:

> Every physical relationship between n physical quantities can be reduced to a relationship between $m = n - r$ mutually independent dimensionless groups, whereby r stands for the rank of the dimensional matrix, made up of the physical quantities in question and generally equal to the number of the base quantities contained in them.

(The pi theorem is often associated with the name of *Buckingham*, because he introduced this term in 1914. But the proof of it had already been accomplished in the course of a mathematical analysis of partial differential equations by *Federmann* in 1911, see Ref. 4, chap. 16.1).

DETERMINATION OF A PI SET BY MATRIX CALCULATION
Establishment of a Relevance List of a Problem
As a rule, more than two dimensionless numbers will be necessary to describe a physicotechnological problem and therefore they cannot be derived by the method described above. In this case, the easy and transparent matrix calculation introduced by Pawlowski (5) is increasingly used. It will be demonstrated by the following example. It treats an important problem in industrial chemistry and biotechnology because gas-liquid contacting ("gassing") in mixing vessels belongs to very frequent mixing operations.

Example 2: The determination of the pi set for the stirrer power in gas-liquid contacting

We examine the power consumption of a turbine stirrer, the so-called "Rushton turbine" (Fig. 2 and the inset in Fig. 3) installed in a baffled vessel and supplied by gas from below.

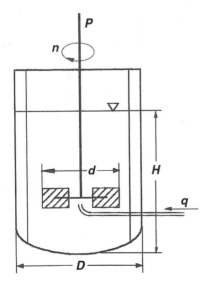

FIGURE 2 Sketch of the mixing vessel.

Dimensional Analysis

We facilitate the procedure by systematically listing the target quantity and all the parameters influencing it:

1. Target quantity: mixing power P
2. Influencing parameters
   a. Geometrical: stirrer diameter d
   b. Physical properties:
      Fluid density ρ
      Kinematic viscosity ν
   c. Process related:
      Stirrer speed n
      Gas throughput q
      Gravitational acceleration g

The relevance list reads:

$$\{P; d; \rho, \nu; n, q, g\} \tag{9}$$

We interrupt the procedure by asking some important questions concerning

1. The determination of the characteristic geometric parameter
2. The setting of all relevant material properties
3. The taking into account of the gravitational acceleration

Determination of the Characteristic Geometric Parameter

It is obvious that we could name all the geometric parameters indicated in the sketch. They were all the geometric parameters of the stirrer and of the vessel, especially its diameter D and the liquid height H. In case of complex geometry, such a procedure would compulsorily deflect from the problem. It is therefore advisable to introduce only one characteristic geometric parameter, knowing that all the others can be transformed into dimensionless geometric numbers by division with this one.

The stirrer diameter, d, was introduced as the characteristic geometric parameter in the above case. This is reasonable. One can imagine how the mixing power would react to an increase in the vessel diameter D: It is obvious that from a certain D onward there would be no influence of it, but a small change of the stirrer diameter d would always have an impact.

Setting of All Relevant Material Properties

In the above relevance list only the density and the viscosity of the liquid were introduced. The material properties of the gas are of no importance as compared with the physical properties of the liquid. It was also ascertained by measurements (6) that the interfacial tension σ does not affect the stirrer power. Furthermore, these measurements revealed that the coalescence behavior of the material system is not affected if aqueous glycerol or cane syrup mixtures are used to increase viscosity in model experiments.

The Importance of the Gravitational Constant

Because of the extreme density difference between gas and liquid ($\sim 1{:}1{,}000$), it must be expected that the gravitational acceleration g will exert big influence.

(One should actually write $g\Delta\rho$, but—since $\Delta\rho = \rho_L - \rho_G \approx \rho_L$—the dimension-less number would contain $g\Delta\rho/\rho_L \approx g\rho_L/\rho_L = g$.

Constructing and Solving of a Dimensional Matrix

In transforming the relevance list (Eq. 9) of the above seven physical quantities into a dimensional matrix, the following should be kept in mind in order to minimize the calculations required:

1. The dimensional matrix consists of a square core matrix and a residual matrix.
2. The rows of the matrix are formed of base dimensions, contained in the dimensions of the quantities, and they determine the rank r of the matrix. The columns of the matrix are presented by the physical quantities or parameters.
3. Quantities of the square core matrix may eventually appear in all of the dimensionless numbers as "fillers," whereas each element of the residual matrix will appear only in one dimensionless number. For this reason the residual matrix should be loaded with essential variables like the target quantity and the most important physical properties and process-related parameters.
4. By this extremely easy matrix rearrangement (linear transformations), the core matrix is transformed into a matrix of unity. The main diagonal consists only of ones and the remaining elements are all zero. One should therefore arrange the quantities in the core matrix in a way to facilitate this procedure.
5. After the generation of the matrix of unity, the dimensionless numbers are created as follows: Each element of the residual matrix forms the numerator of a fraction while its denominator consists of the fillers from the matrix of unity with the exponents indicated in the residual matrix.

Let us now return to Example 2. The dimensional matrix reads:

	ρ	d	n	P	ν	q	g
Mass M	1	0	0	1	0	0	0
Length L	−3	1	0	2	2	3	1
Time T	0	0	−1	−3	−1	−1	−2
	Core matrix			Residual matrix			

Only one linear transformation is necessary to transform −3 in L-row/ρ-column into zero. The subsequent multiplication of the T-row by −1 transfers −1 to 1:

	ρ	d	n	P	ν	q	g
M	1	0	0	1	0	0	0
3M + L	0	1	0	5	2	3	1
−T	0	0	1	3	1	1	2
	Unity matrix			Residual matrix			

The residual matrix contains four parameters, therefore four $\prod$ numbers result:

$$\prod_1 \equiv \frac{P}{\rho^1 n^3 d^5} = \frac{P}{\rho n^3 d^5} \equiv \text{Ne (Newton number)}$$

$$\prod_2 \equiv \frac{\nu}{\rho^0 n^1 d^2} = \frac{\nu}{nd^2} \equiv \text{Re}^{-1} \text{(Reynolds number)}$$

$$\prod_3 \equiv \frac{q}{d^3 n} \equiv \text{Q (Gas throughput number)}$$

$$\prod_4 \equiv \frac{g}{d\,n^2} \equiv \text{Fr}^{-1} \text{ (Froude number)}$$

The interdependence of seven dimensional quantities of the relevance list (Eq. 9) reduces to a set of only $7 - 3 = 4$ dimensionless numbers:

$$\{\text{Ne}, \text{Re}, \text{Q}, \text{Fr}\} \quad \text{or} \quad f(\text{Ne}, \text{Re}, \text{Q}, \text{Fr}) = 0 \qquad (10)$$

Thus, again confirming the pi theorem.

Determination of the Process Characteristics

The functional dependence (Eq. 10) is the maximum that dimensional analysis can offer here. It cannot provide any information about the form of the function f. This can be accomplished solely by experiments.

The first question we must ask is: Are laboratory tests performed in one single piece of laboratory apparatus—that is, on one single scale—capable of providing binding information on the decisive process number? The answer here is affirmative. We can change Fr by means of the stirrer speed, Q by means of the gas throughput, and Re by means of the liquid viscosity, independently of each other.

The results of these model experiments are described in detail in Ref. 6. For our consideration, it is sufficient to present only the main result here. This states that in the industrially interesting range (Re $\geq 10^4$ and Fr ≥ 0.65), the power number Ne is dependent only on the gas throughput number Q (Fig. 3). By

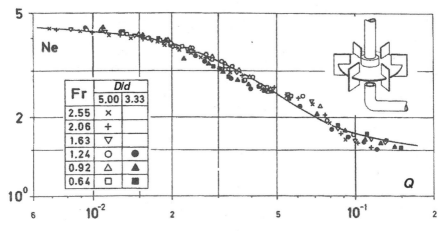

FIGURE 3 Power characteristics of a turbine stirrer (Rushton turbine) in the range Re $\geq 10^4$ and Fr ≥ 0.65 for two D/d values. Material system: water/air. *Source*: From Refs. 6,7.

raising the gas throughput number Q and thus enhancing gas hold-up in the liquid, liquid density diminishes and the Newton number Ne decreases to only one-third of its value in a nongassed liquid.

This power characteristic, the analytical expression for which is

$$Ne = 1.5 + (0.5Q^{0.075} + 1600Q^{2.6})^{-1} \qquad (Q \leq 0.15) \qquad (11)$$

can be used to reliably design a stirrer drive for the performance of material conversions in the gas/liquid system (e.g., oxidations with O_2 or air, fermentations) as long as the physical, geometric, and process-related boundary conditions (Re, Fr, and Q) comply with those of the model measurement.

FUNDAMENTALS OF THE THEORY OF MODELS AND OF SCALE-UP
Theory of Models Based on the Scale Invariance of the Dimensionless Representation of the Measurements

The results in Figure 3 have been acquired by changing the stirrer speed and the gas throughput whereas the liquid properties and the characteristic length (stirrer diameter d) remained constant. But these results could have also been acquired by changing the stirrer diameter: It does not matter, by which means a relevant number (here Q) is changed because it is dimensionless and therefore independent of scale ("scale-invariant"). This fact presents the basis for a reliable scale-up:

> Two processes may be considered completely similar if they take place in similar geometrical space and if all the dimensionless numbers necessary to describe them have the same numerical value ($\prod_i$ = identical or "idem").

Clearly, the scale-up of a desired process condition from a model to industrial scale can be accomplished reliably only if the problem was formulated and dealt with according to the dimensional analysis.

Model Experiments and Scale-up

In the above example, the process characteristics (here: power characteristics) presenting a comprehensive description of the process were evaluated. This often expensive and time-consuming method is certainly not necessary if one has to only scale-up a given process condition from the model to the industrial plant (or vice versa). With the last example and assuming that the Ne(Q) characteristics like that in Figure 3 is *not* explicitly known, the task is to predict the power consumption of a Rushton turbine of $d = 0.8$ m, installed in a baffled vessel of $D = 4$ m ($V = 50$ m^3, $D/d = 5$) and rotating with $n = 200$/min. The air throughput is $q = 500$ m^3/hr and the material system is water/air.

One only needs to know—and this is *essential*—that the hydrodynamics in this case is governed *solely* by the gas throughput number and that the process is described by an unknown dependency Ne(Q). Then one can calculate the Q number of the industrial plant:

$$Q \equiv \frac{q}{nd^3} = 8.14 \times 10^{-2}$$

What will the power consumption of the turbine be?

Let us assume that we have a geometrically similar laboratory device of $D = 0.4$ m ($V \approx 0.050$ m^3 = 50 L) with the turbine stirrer of $d = 0.08$ m and that the stirrer speed is $n = 750/\text{min}$. What must the gas throughput be to obtain $Q = $ idem in the laboratory device? The answer is

$$\frac{q}{nd^3} = 8.14 \times 10^{-2} \rightarrow q \approx 1.88\,\text{m}^3/\text{hr}$$

Under these conditions the stirrer power must be measured and the power number $\text{Ne} \equiv P/(\rho n^3 d^5)$ calculated.

We find $\text{Ne} = 1.75$. Because of the fact that $Q = $ idem results in $\text{Ne} = $ idem, the power consumption P_T of the industrial stirrer can be obtained:

$$\text{Ne} = \text{idem} \rightarrow \text{Ne}_T = \text{Ne}_M \rightarrow \left(\frac{P}{n^3\,d^5}\right)_T = \left(\frac{P}{n^3\,d^5}\right)_M \tag{12}$$

From $\text{Ne} = 1.75$ found in laboratory measurement, the power P of the industrial turbine stirrer of $d = 0.8$ m and a stirrer speed of $n = 200/\text{min}$ is calculated as follows:

$$P = \text{Ne}\rho n^3 d^5 = 1.75 \times 1 \times 10^3 \times \left(\frac{200}{60}\right)^3 \times 0.8^5 = 21.200\,\text{W} \cong 21\,\text{kW}$$

This results in $21/50$ kW/m^3 ≈ 0.42 kW/m^3, which is a fair volume-related power input for many conversions in the gas/liquid system.

We realize that in scale-up, comprehensive knowledge of the functional dependency $f(\prod_i) = 0$—like that in Figure 3—is not necessary. All we need is to know which pi space describes the process.

FURTHER PROCEDURES TO ESTABLISH A RELEVANCE LIST
Consideration of the Acceleration Due to Gravity *g*

If a natural or universal physical constant has an impact on the process, it has to be incorporated into the relevant list, whether it will be altered or not. In this context, the greatest mistakes are made with regard to the gravitational constant *g*. Lord Rayleigh (3) complained bitterly, saying:

> I refer to the manner in which gravity is treated. When the question under consideration depends essentially upon gravity, the symbol of gravity (*g*) makes no appearance, but when gravity does not enter the question at all, *g* obtrudes itself conspicuously.

This is all the more surprising in view of the fact that the relevance of this quantity is easy enough to recognize if one asks the following question:

Would the process function differently if it took place on the moon instead of on Earth?

If the answer to this question is affirmative, *g* is a relevant variable.

The gravitational acceleration *g* can be effective solely in connection with the density as gravity $g\rho$. When inertial forces play a role, the density ρ has to be listed additionally. Thus, it follows that:

1. In cases involving the ballistic movement of bodies, the formation of vortices in stirring, the bow wave of a ship, the movement of a pendulum, and other processes affected by the Earth's gravity, the relevance list comprises $g\rho$ and ρ.
2. Creeping flow in a gravitational field is governed by the gravity $g\rho$ alone.
3. In heterogeneous physical systems with density differences (sedimentation or buoyancy), the difference in gravity $g\Delta\rho$ and ρ play a decisive role.

In Example 2, we have already treated a problem where the gravitational constant is of prime importance due to extreme difference in densities in the gas/liquid system, provided that the Froude number is low: Fr < 0.65 (6,7).

Introduction of Intermediate Quantities

Many engineering problems involve several parameters that impede the elaboration of the pi space. Fortunately, in some cases, a closer look at a problem (or previous experience) facilitates reduction of the number of physical quantities in the relevance list. This is the case when some relevant variables affect the process by way of a so-called "intermediate" quantity. Assuming that this intermediate variable can be measured experimentally, it should be included in the problem relevance list if this facilitates the removal of more than one variable from the list.

The impact, which the introduction of intermediate quantities can have on the relevance list, will be demonstrated in the following by one elegant example.

Example 3: Mixing time characteristics for liquid mixtures with differences in density and viscosity

Mixing time θ necessary to achieve a molecular homogeneity of a liquid mixture—normally measured by decolorization methods (7)—depends in material systems *without* differences in density and viscosity on only four parameters: stirrer diameter d, density ρ, kinematic viscosity ν, stirrer speed n:

$$\{\theta; d; \rho, \nu; n\} \tag{13}$$

From this, the mixing time characteristic results to

$$n\theta = f(\text{Re}) \quad \text{where Re} = \frac{nd^2}{\nu} \tag{14}$$

(See Example 7.2 and Fig. 15.)

In material systems *with* differences in density and viscosity, the relevance list (Eq. 13) enlarges by the physical properties of the second mixing component by the volume ratio of both phases $\varphi = V_2/V_1$ and, due to the density differences, inevitably by the gravity difference $g\Delta\rho$ to nine parameters:

$$\{\theta; d; \rho_1, \nu_1, \rho_2, \nu_2, \varphi; g\Delta\rho, n\} \tag{15}$$

This results in a mixing time characteristics incorporating six numbers:

$$n\theta = f(\text{Re, Ar, } \rho_2/\rho_1, \nu_2/\nu_1, \varphi) \tag{16}$$

(Re $\equiv nd^2/\nu_1$—Reynolds number; Ar $\equiv g\Delta\rho d^3/(\rho_1\nu_1^2)$—Archimedes number)

Meticulous observation of this mixing process (the slow disappearance of the Schlieren patterns as a result of the disappearance of density differences) reveals that macromixing is quickly accomplished compared to the micromixing. This time-consuming process already takes place in a material system that can be fully described by the physical properties of the mixture:

$$\nu* = f(\nu_1, \nu_2, \varphi) \quad \text{and} \quad \rho* = f(\rho_1, \rho_2, \varphi) \tag{17}$$

By introducing these intermediate quantities ν^* and ρ^*, the nine-parametric relevance list (Eq. 15) reduces by three parameters to a six-parametric one:

$$\{\theta; d; \rho^*, \nu^*; g\Delta\rho, n\} \tag{18}$$

and gives a mixing characteristics of only three numbers:

$$n\theta = f(\text{Re}, \text{Ar}) \tag{19}$$

(In this case, Re and Ar have to be formed by ρ^* and ν^*.)

The process characteristics of a cross-beam stirrer was established in this pi space by evaluation of corresponding measurements in two different-sized mixing vessels ($D = 0.3$ and 0.6 m) using different liquid mixtures ($\Delta\rho/\rho^* = 0.01$–0.29 and $\nu_2/\nu_1 = 1$–$5{,}300$). It reads (see Ref. 7, pp. 110–112):

$$\sqrt{n\theta} = 51.6\,\text{Re}^{-1}(\text{Ar}^{1/3} + 3) \quad \text{where} \quad \text{Re} = 10^1 - 10^5; \text{Ar} = 10^2 - 10^{11} \tag{20}$$

This example clearly shows the big advantages achieved by the introduction of intermediate quantities.

Note: The fluid velocity v in pipes—or the superficial gas velocity v_G in mixing vessels or in bubble columns—presents a well-known process parameter that combines the fluid throughput q and the diameter of the device D: $v \approx q/D^2$. Nevertheless, this parameter is not an intermediate quantity. It cannot replace the diameter of the device; it is simply another expression for the liquid throughput. *Reference*: The kinematic process numbers like the Reynolds and Froude numbers, which govern the hydrodynamics, necessarily contain the linear dimension of the device. They are extremely scale-dependent.

Material Systems of Unknown Physical Properties

With foams, sludges, and slimes often encountered in biotechnology, we are confronted with the problem of not being able to list the physical properties because they are still unknown and therefore cannot be quantified. This situation often leads to the opinion that the dimensional analysis would fail in such cases.

It is obvious that this conclusion is wrong: The dimensional analysis is a *method* based on logical and mathematical fundamentals (2,5). If relevant parameters cannot be listed because they are unknown, one cannot blame the method! The only solution is to perform the model measurements with the *same* material system and to *change* the model scales.

Example 4: Scale-up of a mechanical foam breaker

The question is posed about the mode of performing and evaluating model measurements with a given type of mechanical foam breaker (foam centrifuge, see Fig. 4) to obtain reliable information on dimensioning and scale-up of these devices. Preliminary experiments have shown that for each foam emergence—proportional to the gas throughput q_G—for each foam breaker of diameter d a minimum rotational speed n_{min} exists that is necessary to control it. The dynamic properties of the foam (e.g., density and viscosity, elasticity of the foam lamella) cannot be fully named or measured. We will have to content ourselves with listing them wholesale as material properties S_i. In our model experiments we will of course be able to replace S_i by the known type of surfactant (foamer) and its concentration c_f (ppm).

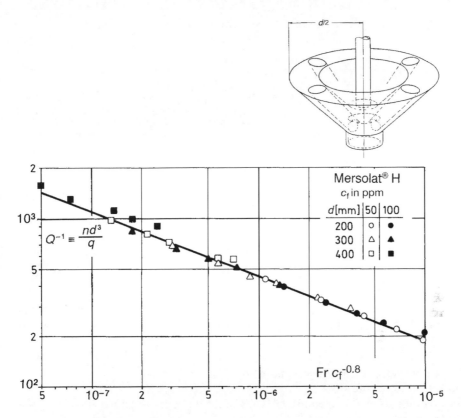

FIGURE 4 Process characteristics of the foam centrifuge (sketch) for a particular foamer (Mersolat H of Bayer AG, Germany). *Source*: From Ref. 8.

In discerning the process parameters, we realize that the gravitational acceleration g has no impact on the foam breaking *within* the foam centrifuge: The centrifugal acceleration n^2d exceeds the gravitational one (g) by far. However, we have to recognize that the water content of the foam entering the centrifuge depends very much on the gravitational acceleration: On the moon, the water drainage would be by far less effective. In contrast to the dimensional analysis presented in Ref. 8, we are well advised to add g to the relevance list:

$$\{n_{min}; d; \text{type of foamer}, c_f; q_G, g\} \qquad (21)$$

For the sake of simplicity, in the following, n_{min} will be replaced by n and q_G by q. For each type of foamer, we obtain the following pi space:

$$\left\{\frac{nd^3}{q}, \frac{n^2d}{g}, c_f\right\} \quad \text{or, abbreviated,} \quad \{Q^{-1}, Fr, c_f\} \qquad (22)$$

To prove this pi space, measurements in differently sized model equipment are necessary to produce reliable process characteristics. For a particular foamer (Mersolat H of Bayer AG, Germany), the results are given in Figure 4. They fully confirm the pi space Eq. (22).

The fitting line in Figure 4 corresponds to the analytic expression:

$$Q^{-1} = \text{Fr}^{-0.4} c_f^{0.32} \tag{23}$$

which reduces in dimensional terms to

$$nd = \text{const}\, q^{0.2} f(c_f) \tag{24}$$

Here, the foam breaker will be scaled up according to its tip speed $u - \pi nd$ in model experiments, which will also depend moderately on the foam yield (q).

In all other foamers examined (8), the correspondence $Q^{-1} \propto \text{Fr}^{-0.45}$ was found. If the correlation

$$Q^{-1} \propto \text{Fr}^{-0.5} f(c_f) \tag{25}$$

proves to be true, then it can be reduced to

$$\frac{n^2 d}{g} = \text{const}\, f(c_f) \tag{26}$$

In this case, the centrifugal acceleration ($n^2 d$) would present the scale-up criterion and would depend only on the foamer concentration and not on foam yield (q).

Short summary of the Essentials of the Dimensional Analysis and Scale-Up

The advantages made possible by correct and timely use of dimensional analysis are as follows:

1. *Reduction of the number of parameters required to define the problem (compression of the physicotechnological statement)*: The pi theorem states that a physical problem can always be described in dimensionless terms. This has the advantage that the number of dimension*less* groups that fully describe it is much smaller than the number of dimensional physical quantities. It is generally equal to the number of physical quantities minus the number of basic units contained in them.

2. *Reliable scale-up of the desired operating conditions from the model to the full-scale plant (due to the scale invariance of the dimensionless representation of the measurements)*: According to the theory of models, two processes may be considered similar to one another if they take place under geometrically similar conditions and all dimensionless numbers that describe the process have the same numerical value.

3. *A deeper insight into the physical nature of the process*: By presenting experimental data in a dimensionless form, one distinct physical state can be isolated from the other (e.g., turbulent or laminar flow region) and the effect of individual physical variables can be identified.

4. *Flexibility in the choice of parameters and their reliable extrapolation within the range covered by the dimensionless numbers*: These advantages become clear if one considers the well-known Reynolds number, $\text{Re} = vL/\nu$, which can be varied by altering the characteristic velocity v, or a characteristic length L, or

the kinematic viscosity ν. By choosing appropriate model fluids, the viscosity can very easily be altered by several orders of magnitude. Once the effect of the Reynolds number is known, extrapolation of both v and L is allowed within the examined range of Re.

Area of Applicability of the Dimensional Analysis

The application of dimensional analysis is indeed heavily dependent on the available knowledge. The following five steps (Fig. 5) can be outlined as:

1. The physics of the basic phenomenon is unknown.
    → Dimensional analysis cannot be applied.
2. Enough is known about the physics of the basic phenomenon to compile a first, tentative relevance list.
    → The resultant pi set is unreliable.
3. All the relevant physical variables describing the problem are known.
    → The application of dimensional analysis is unproblematic.
4. The problem can be expressed in terms of a mathematical equation.
    → A closer insight into the pi relationship is feasible and may facilitate a reduction of the set of dimensionless numbers.
5. A mathematical solution of the problem exists.
    → The application of dimensional analysis is superfluous.

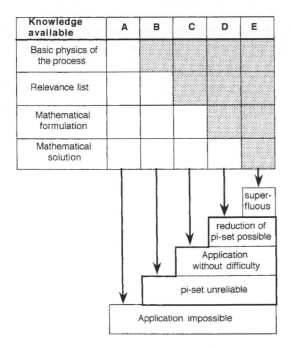

FIGURE 5 Graphical representation of the four levels of knowledge and their impact on the treatment of the problem by the dimensional analysis. *Source*: Courtesy of J. Pawlowski, personal communication, 1984.

It must, of course, be said that approaching a problem from the point of view of dimensional analysis also remains useful even if all the variables relevant to the problem are not yet known: The timely application of dimensional analysis may often lead to the discovery of forgotten variables or the exclusion of artifacts.

Experimental Methods for Scale-Up

In the Introduction, a number of questions were posed that are often asked in connection with model experiments.

How small can a model be? The size of a model depends on the scale factor L_T/L_M, and on the experimental precision of measurement. Where $L_T/L_M = 10$, a ±10% margin of error may already be excessive. A larger scale for the model will therefore have to be chosen to reduce the error.

Is one model scale sufficient or should tests be carried out in models of different sizes? One model scale is sufficient if the relevant numerical values of the dimensionless numbers necessary to describe the problem (the so-called "process point" in the pi space describing the operational condition of the industrial plant) can be adjusted by choosing the appropriate process parameters or physical properties of the model material system. If this is not possible, the process characteristics must be determined in models of different sizes, or the process point must be extrapolated from experiments in technical plants of different sizes.

When must model experiments be carried out exclusively with the original material system? Where the material model system is unavailable (e.g., in the case of non-Newtonian fluids) or where the relevant physical properties are unknown (e.g., foams, sludges, slimes), the model experiments must be carried out with the original material system. In this case, measurements must be performed in models of various sizes (cf. Example 4).

Partial Similarity

The theory of models requires that in the scale-up from a model (index M) to the technological scale (index T) not only the geometric similarity be ensured but also all dimensionless numbers describing the problem retain the same numerical values ($\prod_i$ = idem). This means that in scale-up of boats or ships, for example, the dimensionless numbers governing the hydrodynamics here

$$\text{Fr} \equiv \frac{v^2}{Lg} \quad \text{and} \quad \text{Re} \equiv \frac{vL}{\nu}$$

must retain their numerical values: $\text{Fr}_T = \text{Fr}_M$ and $\text{Re}_T = \text{Re}_M$. It can easily be shown that this requirement cannot be fulfilled here.

Because of the fact that the gravitational acceleration g cannot be varied on Earth, the Froude number Fr of the model can be adjusted to that of the full-scale vessel only by its velocity v_M. Subsequently, Re = idem can be achieved only by adjusting the viscosity of the model fluid. In case where the model size is only 10% of the full size (scale factor $L_T/L_M = 10$), Fr = idem is achieved in the model at $v_M = 0.32v_T$. To fulfill Re = idem, for the kinematic viscosity of the model fluid ν_M, it follows:

$$\frac{\nu_M}{\nu_T} = \frac{v_M L_M}{v_T L_T} = 0.32 \times 0.1 = 0.032$$

No liquid exists, whose viscosity would be only 3% of that of water.

We have to realize that sometimes requirements concerning physical properties of model materials exist that cannot be implemented. In such cases only a partial similarity can be realized. For this, essentially only two procedures are available (for details see Ref. 4). One consists of a well-planned experimental strategy, in which the process is divided into parts that are then investigated separately under conditions of complete similarity. This approach was first applied by *William Froude* (1810–1879) in his efforts to scale up the drag resistance of the ship's hull.

The second approach consists in deliberately abandoning certain similarity criteria and checking the effect on the entire process. This technique was used by *Gerhard Damköhler* (1908–1944) in his trials to treat a chemical reaction in a catalytic fixed-bed reactor by means of dimensional analysis. Here the problem of a simultaneous mass and heat transfer arises—they are two processes that obey completely different fundamental principles.

It is seldom realized that many "rules of thumb" utilized for scale-up of different types of equipment are represented by quantities that fulfill only a partial similarity. As examples, only the volume-related mixing power, P/V— widely used for scaling up mixing vessels—and the gas superficial velocity, v_G, which is normally used for scale-up of bubble columns, should be mentioned here.

The volume-related mixing power P/V presents an adequate scale-up criterion only in liquid/liquid dispersion processes and can be deduced from the pertinent process characteristics $d_p/d \propto We^{-0.6}$ (d_p is the particle or droplet diameter and We is the Weber number). In the most common mixing operation, the homogenization of miscible liquids, where a macro- and back-mixing is required, this criterion fails completely (see Ref. 7, chap. 3.4).

Similarly, the superficial velocity of the gas throughput v_G as an intensity quantity is a reliable scale-up criterion only in mass transfer in gas/liquid systems in bubble columns. In mixing operations in bubble columns, requiring that the whole liquid content be back-mixed (e.g., in homogenization), this criterion completely loses its validity (see Ref. 4, Example 35).

We must draw the following conclusion: A particular scale-up criterion that is valid in a given type of apparatus for a particular process is not necessarily applicable to other processes occurring in the same device.

TREATMENT OF VARIABLE PHYSICAL PROPERTIES BY DIMENSIONAL ANALYSIS
Why Is This Consideration Important?

A complete similarity between the model and the technical realization implies geometric, material, and process-related similarity. The geometric similarity can be realized without problems in most cases. The same is true for the process-related similarity, as it can be seen in the examples later on. Material similarity can cause difficulties if in model experiments different materials must be used than in the technical plant.

The scale invariance of the pi space allows working with different material systems in the model compared to the industrial scale. This presents one of the essential advantages, offered by the Theory of Models. A lot of conditions of flow in the technical plant can only be scaled down to the model scale when an appropriate model material system has been chosen.

Example: The Reynolds number for a mixing vessel is given by $Re \equiv nd^2/\nu$. Because of the fact that the scale of length (here, stirrer diameter d) enters Re with its square, in an essential scale-down it will also be necessary to diminish the kinematic viscosity of the liquid ν essentially in order to work with a reasonable stirrer speed.

The process point of the technical plant is given by

$$d = 1\,\text{m};\ n = 1/\text{sec}\ (= 60/\text{min});\ \nu = 1 \times 10^{-4} \rightarrow Re = 10^4$$

In a laboratory device that is scaled down by the scale factor of $L_T{:}L_M = 10{:}1$ and that applies the same fluid ($\nu = 1 \times 10^{-4}\,\text{m}^2/\text{sec}$), stirrer speed must amount to $n = 100/\text{sec}\ (= 6000/\text{min})$ in order to sustain the same flow condition ($Re = 10^4$). At this extreme stirrer speed, reasonable mixing is absolutely impossible. If on the other hand measurements are performed with water ($\nu = 1 \times 10^{-6}\,\text{m}^2/\text{sec}$), the experiment can be carried out with a reasonable stirrer speed of $n = 1/\text{sec}\ (= 60/\text{min})$.

In this example, it has been assumed that the liquid is a Newtonian one and the temperature is constant. So the physical properties of the fluid (dynamic viscosity μ and density ρ) remained constant.

There are, however, processes in which the constancy of the physical properties cannot be expected. For example, a temperature field in a considered material system will often produce a viscosity and possibly also a density field. In case of non-Newtonian (pseudoplastic or/and viscoelastic) fluids, a viscosity field will also be caused by the shear stress.

Of some other problems of this kind, three of them will be shortly mentioned:

Hydrocracking, thermocracking, etc. will be performed at temperatures of 270 to 500°C and pressures of 50 to 200 bar. Which model fluid may be used to investigate the hydrodynamics in a model plant at room temperature to assure that this fluid behaves similarly to the petrol fraction with respect to the temperature dependence of their material parameters?

May breakers and grinding mills be dimensioned for grinding quartz on the basis of measurements with limestone?

May absorption measurements be performed with pure water/air system to obtain dimensioning rules for biological wastewater treatment plants? Is pure water similar to the civil or industrial wastewater with respect to the oxygen absorption process?

Similarity in physical properties between different materials can only be recognized if the variability of each of them is presented in dimensionless form by a standard representation of the material function.

Dimensionless Representation of a Material Function

The dimensional-analytical treatment of variable material properties will be presented in the following by two examples, for example, on the standard representation of the temperature dependence of the viscosity of Newtonian fluids and on the dependence of particle strength of solids on particle diameter. The same procedure is obvious for every changeable material parameter (e.g., surface tension) and every influencing parameter (e.g., pressure, concentration, etc.).

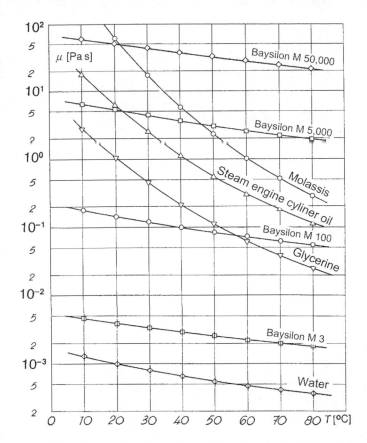

FIGURE 6 Temperature dependency of the viscosity $\mu(T)$. *Source*: From Ref. 4.

Example 5: Standard representation of the temperature dependence of the viscosity

Figure 6 presents the dependence of the dynamic viscosity μ on the temperature for eight different fluids, which differ in viscosity at room temperature for five decades. Five of them show a relatively small temperature dependence on the viscosity (water, 4 Baysilone, silicone oils of the Bayer AG), the remaining three (glycerin, steam engine cylinder oil, molasses) show a pronounced one.

From the representation $\mu(T)$, a similarity between the eight fluids cannot be concluded. To decide this, the dimensional space $\mu(T)$ must be transformed into a dimensionless one. This is possible through standardization (normalization) of this dependence.

For this purpose we choose a reference temperature T_0 (preferably the middle temperature of the measuring range), to which a reference viscosity μ_0 is related. Further on, we determine at the point T_0 the gradient $\Delta\mu/\Delta T$, with which the "temperature coefficient of the viscosity"

$$\gamma_0 \equiv \left(\frac{1}{\mu_0}\frac{\partial\mu}{\partial T}\right)_{T_0} < 0 \tag{27}$$

is calculated.

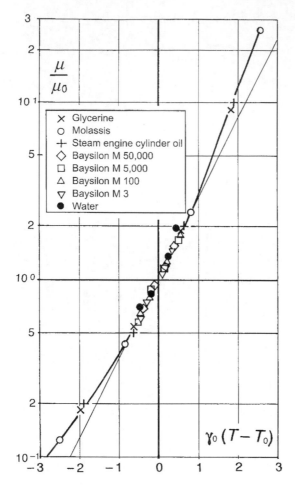

FIGURE 7 Standard representation of the measurements in Figure 6, which leads to the reference-invariant (T/T_0 is irrelevant) approximation of the material function.

By doing this, the dimensional space $\mu(T)$ is widened by three parameters. Now the relevance list

$$\{\mu, \mu_0, T, T_0, \gamma_0\} \tag{28}$$

delivers three dimensionless numbers without problems

$$\{\mu/\mu_0, T/T_0, \gamma_0\Delta T\} \tag{29}$$

From Figure 7, following facts can be realized:

1. With respect to the temperature dependence $\mu(T)$ all investigated fluids behave similarly to each other; they correspond to the same standard representation $\mu/\mu_0 = f(\gamma_0\Delta T)$.

2. The standard representation proves to be invariant to the reference temperature T_0: The dimensionless number T/T_0 has no influence.
3. Water is obviously a special stuff. Its μ/μ_0 values coincide with the other values only in the range near to the reference point (i.e., at $\gamma_0 \Delta T \approx 0 \pm 1$). Outside this range they deviate strongly.
4. The thinly plotted straight line is a very good approximation of this dependence in the range near the reference point (at $\gamma_0 \Delta T \approx 0 \pm 1$). It represents the engineering representation of the temperature dependence of the viscosity of a liquid

$$\ln\left(\frac{\mu}{\mu_0}\right) = \exp(\gamma_0 \Delta T) \tag{30}$$

Because of the equivalence between μ/μ_0 and $\gamma_0 \Delta T$, the quotient μ/μ_0 is preferably used in the engineering literature as the viscosity number $Vis \equiv \mu_w/\mu$ (μ_w, wall viscosity; μ, bulk viscosity).

Example 6: Standard representation of particle strength of different materials in dependence on particle diameter

The particle strength $\sigma \equiv F/A$ of solids plays an important role in the comminution. It is defined as force F, which is exerted in breaking point, whereas nominal cross-sectional area $A = (\pi/4)d_V^2$ is related to the diameter d_V of a sphere of equal volume. It depends strongly on the particle diameter, because due to the progression of comminution, the defects in the solid decrease and thus become more homogeneous and therefore stronger.

Figure 8 shows the dependence between particle strength σ and particle diameter d_p for a series of solids. The diversities in the dependencies are pronounced in a way that one cannot conclude any similarity with regard to particle strength between different solids. On the basis of this fact, for example, one cannot decide whether the measurements of the comminution of limestone are suitable for dimensioning a grinder for quartz or not.

Figure 9 shows the standard representation of this fact in the pi space:

$$\sigma/\sigma_0 = f\{-\Phi(d_p - d_{p,0})\} \tag{31}$$

where the coefficient Φ of the particle strength has been gained in a similar way as the coefficient γ_0 was gained before (Eq. 27):

$$\Phi \equiv \left(\frac{1}{\sigma_0}\frac{\partial\sigma}{\partial d_p}\right)_{d_{p,0}} \tag{32}$$

The curves in Figure 9 represent the reference-invariant approximations of individual point collectives. The thickly drawn curve describes most of the examined materials with a relative variance of 3.13×10^{-2}; these are similar to each other. The thinly drawn curves apply to quartz and boron carbide. They deviate strongly than the other solids in respect to the particle strength in the range $\sigma/\sigma_0 < 1$.

It must be left to experts to decide what importance these findings have for their experiments.

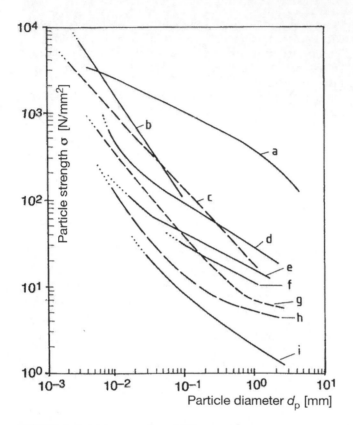

FIGURE 8 Particle strength σ of different materials in dependence on particle diameter d_p. a, glass beads; b, boron carbide (B_4C); c, crystallized boron; d, cement clinker; e, marble; f, cane sugar; g, quartz; h, limestone; i, coal. *Source*: From Ref. 4.

The third number, resulting from the relevance list of five parameters

$$\{\sigma, \sigma_0, d_p, d_{p,0}, \Phi\} \tag{33}$$

namely $\Phi \times d_{p,0}$, is obviously irrelevant, as the measuring data can be described by the reference-invariant approximations.

NON-NEWTONIAN LIQUIDS

The main characteristics of Newtonian liquids is that simple shear flow (e.g., Couette flow) generates shear stress τ that is proportional to the shear rate $\dot{\gamma} \equiv dv/dy[\sec^{-1}]$. The proportionality constant, the dynamic viscosity μ, is the only material constant in the Newton's law of motion:

$$\tau = \mu\dot{\gamma} \tag{34}$$

where μ depends only on pressure and temperature.

In the case of non-Newtonian liquids, μ depends on $\dot{\gamma}$ as well. These liquids can be classified into various categories of materials depending on their flow behavior: $\mu(\dot{\gamma})$ is the flow curve and $\mu(\tau)$ is the viscosity curve.

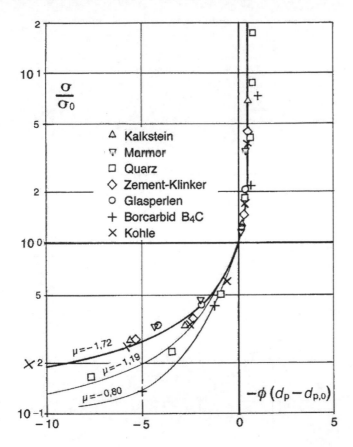

FIGURE 9 Standard representation of particle strength σ of different materials in dependence on particle diameter d_p. As reference parameter without exception $d_{p,0} = 0.1$ mm was applied. *Source*: From Ref. 4.

Pseudoplastic Fluids

An extensive class of non-Newtonian fluids is formed by pseudoplastic fluids whose flow curves obey the so-called "power law"

$$\tau = K\dot{\gamma}^m \rightarrow \mu_{eff} = K\dot{\gamma}^{(m-1)} \tag{35}$$

These liquids are known as *Ostwald-de Waele* fluids. Figure 10 depicts a typical course of such a flow curve.

Figure 11 shows a dimensionless standardized material function of two pseudoplastic fluids often used in biotechnology. It proves that the examined polymers [carboxymethyl-cellulose (CMC), a chemical polymer, and Xanthan, a biopolymer] are not completely similar to each other; if they were, the exponent m must not have been different by a factor of 2 (see insert in Fig. 11).

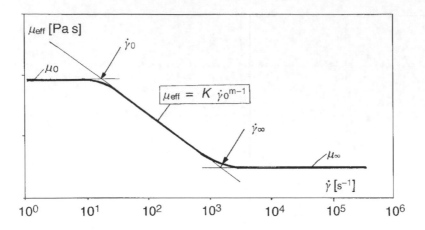

FIGURE 10 Typical course of the flow curve of an *Ostwald-de Waele* fluid obeying the so-called "power law" behavior.

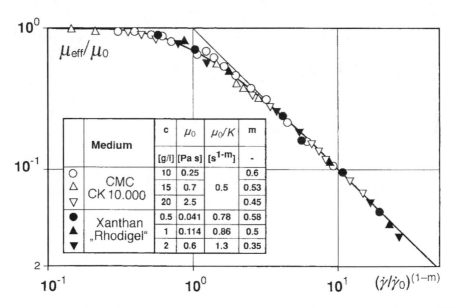

FIGURE 11 Dimensionless standardized material function of two pseudoplastic fluids (CMC and Xanthan) often used in biotechnology. *Abbreviation*: CMC, carboxymethyl-cellulose. *Source*: From Ref. 11.

Viscoelastic Liquids

Almost every biological solution of low viscosity [but also viscous biopolymers such as Xanthane and dilute solutions of long-chain polymers, for example, CMC, polyacrylamide (PAA), polyacrylnitrile (PAN), etc.] displays not only viscous but also viscoelastic flow behavior. These liquids are capable of storing a part of the deformation energy elastically and reversibly. They evade mechanical stress by contracting like rubber bands. This behavior causes a secondary

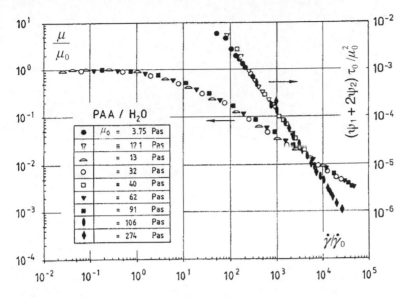

FIGURE 12 Flow curves of a family of PAA/water solutions of different concentrations and viscosities. Left side: Normalized viscosity curves $\mu/\mu_0 = f_1(\dot{\gamma}/\dot{\gamma}_0)$, right side: Normalized stress coefficients $(\Psi_1 + 2\Psi_2)\tau_0/\mu_0^2 = f_2(\dot{\gamma}/\dot{\gamma}_0)$. *Abbreviation*: PAA, polyacrylamide. *Source*: From Ref. 12.

flow that often runs contrary to the flow produced by mass forces (e.g., the liquid "climbs" the shaft of a stirrer, the so-called Weissenberg effect).

Elastic behavior of liquids is characterized mainly by the ratio of first differences in normal stress, N_1, to the shear stress, τ. This ratio, the Weissenberg number $\text{Wi} = N_1/\tau$, is usually represented as a function of the rate of shear $\dot{\gamma}$.

Another often used representation of the viscoelastic flow behavior utilizes normal stress coefficients $\Psi_i = N_i/\gamma^2$. Figure 12 depicts flow curves of a family of PAA/water solutions differing in concentrations and therefore in their viscosities. Normalized by the zero-shear viscosity μ_0 and by a constant shear rate $\dot{\gamma}_0$ at a shear stress value of $\tau_0 = 1 \text{ N/m}^2$, they produce master curves for viscosity and the normal stress coefficient. The preparation of appropriate rheological substances as a set of liquids with similar rheological properties is indispensable if scale-up measurements have to be performed in differently scaled vessels. This will be demonstrated by the following example concerning the power consumption of a stirrer in a PAA/water solution.

PI SET AND THE POWER CHARACTERISTIC OF A STIRRER IN A VISCOELASTIC FLUID

In the next chapter, the working out of a power characteristics of a stirrer in a Newtonian fluid is presented in detail. It is shown, how a relevance list containing five parameters: stirrer power P, stirrer diameter d, density ρ, viscosity μ of the liquid, and the stirrer speed n:

$$\{P, d, \rho, \mu, n\}$$

is condensed to only two dimensionless numbers

$$\prod_1 = \frac{P}{\rho n^3 d^5} \equiv \text{Ne(Newton number)}$$

$$\prod_2 = \frac{nd^2\rho}{\mu} \equiv \text{Re(Reynolds number)}$$

and therefore the process characteristics is given by the dependency

$$\text{Ne} = f(\text{Re}) \tag{36}$$

In a viscoelastic liquid, the relevance list has to be extended by two rheological parameters being known *in advance*: shear rate $\dot{\gamma}_0$ and the first difference in normal stress $N_{1,0}$. Besides this, the viscosity μ has to be replaced by the zero viscosity μ_0, which is also known in advance (Figs. 10 and 11). The relevance list reads:

$$\{P, d, \rho, \mu_0, N_{1,0}, \dot{\gamma}_0; n\} \tag{37}$$

resulting in $7 - 3 = 4$ dimensionless numbers

$$\frac{P}{\rho n^3 d^5} \equiv \text{Ne}, \quad \frac{nd^2\rho}{\mu_0} \equiv \text{Re}_0, \quad \frac{N_{1,0}}{\mu_0\dot{\gamma}_0} \equiv \frac{N_{1,0}}{\tau_0} \equiv \text{Wi}, \quad \frac{\dot{\gamma}_0}{n} \tag{38}$$

Three dimensionless numbers contain the stirrer speed n. By combining two of them we obtain a new number that will be called B:

$$B = \text{Re}_0 \frac{\dot{\gamma}_0}{n} = \frac{d^2\rho\dot{\gamma}_0}{\mu_0} = \frac{d^2\rho\tau_0}{\mu_0^2} \tag{39}$$

We immediately discover that in scaling up or down, the quotient d/μ_0 has to remain constant: halving d requires halving μ_0. Therefore, in model measurements with non-Newtonian liquids, a family of liquids with similar rheological behavior (Fig. 12) is required.

By keeping the Weissenberg number Wi (a pure material number) and the B number constant, measurements are performed and presented in a dimensionless frame

$$\text{Ne} = f(\text{Re}_0) \quad \text{at} \quad \text{Wi}, B = \text{const} \tag{40}$$

Figure 13 depicts the power characteristics of a Rushton turbine stirrer in geometrically similar cylindrical vessels ($H/D = 1$; $D/d = 2$) without baffles. To keep the B number constant at different scales, viscosity of the PAA solutions had to be fitted as discussed above.

This correlation contains an essential error. It respects the effective viscosity μ_{eff} according to Metzner–Otto (13) as an applicable description of the pertinent viscosity in pseudoplastic fluids. Although this approach is still prevailing in the Anglo-Saxon literature (14), there are meanwhile convincing proofs for its failure (15,16). Particularly the measurements presented in Ref. 16, performed in bubble columns of industrial size (up to 50 m^3 volume), verify this convincingly.

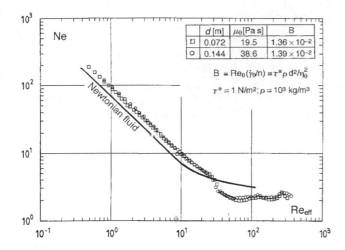

FIGURE 13 Power characteristics of a Rushton turbine stirrer under given geometric conditions, measured in two differently scaled vessels (scale 1:2) and fitting the flow behavior of the viscoelastic fluid (PAA solutions) by changing their viscosity. *Abbreviation*: PAA, polyacrylamide. *Source*: From Ref. 12.

From the viewpoint of the dimensional analysis, it was always clear that the process characteristic of a stirrer in a non-Newtonian fluid cannot be described by a Ne(Re) frame but by only a Ne(Re, B) frame. Therefore, measurements of stirrer power in non-Newtonian fluids cannot be adjusted in the Ne(Re) frame.

DETERMINATION OF OPTIMUM PROCESS CONDITIONS BY COMBINING PROCESS CHARACTERISTICS

The example presented in this chapter shows how a meaningful combining of appropriate process characteristics makes it possible to gain the information necessary for the optimization of the process in question.

Example 7: Optimum conditions for the homogenization of liquid mixtures

The homogenization of miscible liquids is one of the most frequent mixing operations. It can be executed properly if the power characteristics and the mixing time characteristics of the stirrer in question are known. If these characteristics are known for a series of common stirrer types under favorable installation conditions, one can go on to consider optimum operating conditions by asking the question: Which type of stirrer operates within the requested mixing time θ with the lowest power consumption P and hence the minimum mixing work ($P\theta = \min$) in a given material system and a given vessel (vessel diameter D)?

Example 7.1: Power characteristics of a stirrer

The relevance list of this task consists of the target quantity (mixing power P) and the following influencing parameters: stirrer diameter d, density ρ, kinematic viscosity ν of the liquid, and stirrer speed n:

$$\{P; d; \rho, \nu, n\} \tag{41}$$

By choosing the dimensional matrix

	ρ	d	n	P	ν
Mass M	1	0	0	1	0
Length L	−3	1	0	2	2
Time T	0	0	−1	−3	−1
	Core matrix			Residual matrix	

only one linear transformation is necessary to obtain the unity matrix:

	ρ	d	n	P	ν
M	1	0	0	1	0
3 M + L	0	1	0	5	2
−T	0	0	1	3	1
	Unity matrix			Residual matrix	

The residual matrix consists of only two parameters, therefore only two pi numbers result:

$$\Pi_1 \equiv \frac{P}{\rho^1 n^3 d^5} = \frac{P}{\rho n^3 d^5} \equiv \mathrm{Ne} \text{ (Newton number)}$$

$$\Pi_2 \equiv \frac{\nu}{\rho^0 n^1 d^2} = \frac{\nu}{n d^2} \equiv \mathrm{Re}^{-1} \text{(Reynolds number)}$$

The process characteristics

$$\mathrm{Ne} = f(\mathrm{Re}) \tag{42}$$

for three well-known slowly rotating stirrers (leaf, frame, and cross-beam stirrer) are presented in Figure 14.

From Figure 14, we learn the following:

1. In the range Re < 20, the proportionality Ne $\propto$ Re^{-1} is found, thus resulting in the expression NeRe $\equiv P/(\eta n^2 d^3)$ = const. Density is irrelevant here because we are dealing with the *creeping* flow region.
2. In the range Re > 50 (vessel with baffles) or Re > 5 × 10^4 (unbaffled vessel), the Newton number Ne $\equiv P/(\rho n^3 d^5)$ remains constant. In this case, viscosity is irrelevant because we are dealing with a *turbulent* flow region.
3. Understandably, the baffles do not influence the power characteristics within the laminar flow region where viscosity forces prevent rotation of the liquid. However, their influence is extremely strong at Re > 5 × 10^4. Here, the installation of baffles under otherwise unchanged operating conditions increases the power consumption of the stirrer by a factor of 20.

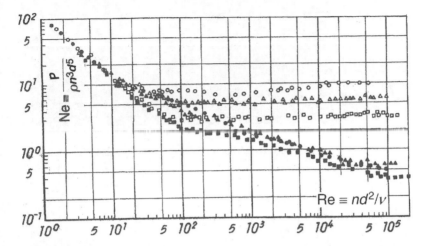

FIGURE 14 Power characteristics of three slowly rotating stirrers (leaf, frame, cross-beam stirrer) installed in a vessel with and without baffles. Stirrer geometry and the installation conditions are given in Figure 15. *Source*: From Ref. 10.

4. The power characteristics of these three stirrers do not differ much from each other. This is understandable because their mixing patterns are very much similar.

Example 7.2: Mixing time characteristics of a stirrer

Mixing time θ is the time necessary to completely homogenize an admixture with its contents of the vessel. It can easily be determined visually by a decolorization reaction (neutralization or a redox reaction in the presence of a color indicator). The relevance list of this task consists of the target quantity (mixing time θ) and of the same parameters as in the case of mixing power—on condition that both liquids have similar physical properties:

$$\{\theta; d; \rho, \nu; n\} \tag{43}$$

This relevance list yields in the two-parametric mixing time characteristics

$$n\theta = f(\mathrm{Re}) \tag{44}$$

For the three stirrer types treated in this example, the mixing time characteristics are presented in Figure 15.

One should not be mistaken by the course of the $n\theta$ (Re) curves: The mixing time does not increase with higher Re numbers, it simply diminishes more slowly until at Re $\approx 10^6$ the minimum achievable mixing time is reached:

$$n\theta \propto \mathrm{Re} \rightarrow \theta \propto \frac{d^2}{\nu} \ (\mathrm{Re} \geq 10^6) \tag{45}$$

From Eq. (45) we learn that the minimum achievable mixing time corresponds to the square of the stirrer diameter: bigger volumes require longer mixing times.

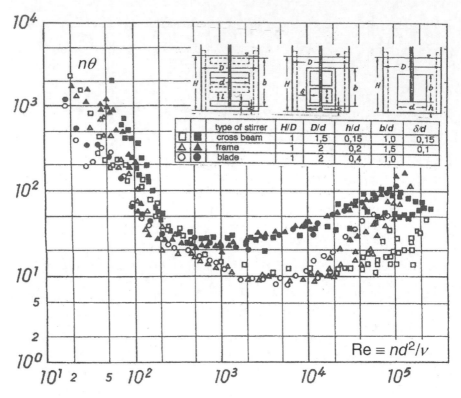

FIGURE 15 Mixing time characteristics of three slowly rotating stirrers (leaf, frame, cross-beam stirrer) in a vessel with and without baffles. To correlate the data in order to emphasize the similarity, $n\theta$ values of the cross-beam stirrer were multiplied by 0.7 and of the leaf stirrer by 1.25. *Source*: From Ref. 10.

Example 7.3: Minimum mixing work ($P\theta$ = min) for homogenization

To gain the information on minimum mixing work ($P\theta$ = min) necessary for a homogenization, the mixing time characteristics as well as the power characteristics have to be combined in a suitable manner. Both of them contain the stirrer speed n and the stirrer diameter d, the knowledge of which would unnecessarily constrict the statement. Therefore, also the ratio D/d, tank diameter/stirrer diameter, which is known for the often-used stirrer types, has to be incorporated.

From the pi frame

$$\{\text{Ne}, n\theta, \text{Re}, D/d\} \tag{46}$$

the following two dimensionless numbers can now be formed:

$$\prod_1 \equiv \text{Ne}\,\text{Re}\,(D/d) = \frac{PD}{\rho\nu^3} = \frac{PD\rho^2}{\mu^3} \tag{47}$$

$$\prod_2 \equiv n\theta\text{Re}^{-1} = \frac{\theta\nu}{D^2} = \frac{\theta\mu}{D^2\rho} \tag{48}$$

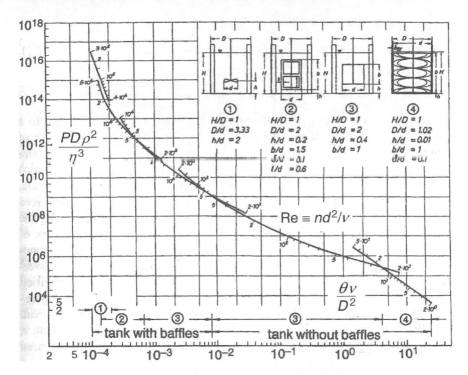

FIGURE 16 Working sheet for the determination of optimum working conditions in the homogenization of liquid mixtures in mixing vessels. *Source*: From Ref. 10.

Figure 16 shows this relationship $\prod_1 = f(\prod_2)$ for those stirrer types that exhibit the lowest $\prod_1$ values within a specific range of $\prod_2$, that is, the stirrers requiring the least power in this range. It represents the working sheet for the determination of optimum working conditions on the homogenization of liquid mixtures in mixing vessels.

This graph is extremely easy to use. The physical properties of the material system, the diameter of the vessel, D, and the desired mixing time, θ, are all known, and this is enough to generate the dimensionless number $\prod_2$.

1. From the numerical value of $\prod_2$, the *stirrer type* and baffling conditions can be read off the abscissa. The diameter of the stirrer and the installation conditions can be determined from data on stirrer geometry in the sketch.
   The curve $\prod_1 = f(\prod_2)$ then provides the following information:
2. The numerical value of $\prod_1$ can be read off at the intersection of the $\prod_2$ value with the curve. The *power consumption P* can then be calculated from this.
3. The numerical value of Re can be read off the Re scale at the same intersection. This, in turn, makes it possible to determine the *rotational speed n* of the stirrer.

Example 8: Scale-up of mixers for mixing of solids

In the final state, the mixing of solids (e.g., powders) can only lead to a stochastically homogeneous mixture. We can therefore use the theory of random

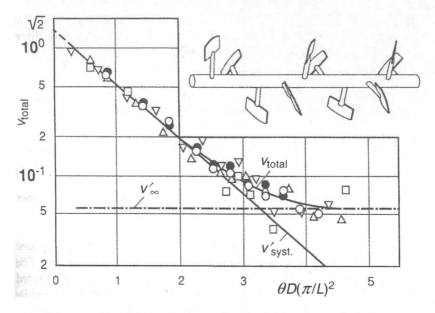

FIGURE 17 Variation coefficient ν as a function of the dimensionless mixing time for different L/D ratios. Copper and nickel particles of $d_p = 300$–400 μm, fill degree of the drum $\varphi = 35\%$, Froude number of the paddle shaft Fr $= 0.019$. *Source*: From Ref. 17.

processes to describe this mixing operation. In the present example (17), we will concentrate on a mixing device in which the position of the particles is adequately given by the x coordinate. Furthermore, we will assume that the mixing operation can be described as a stochastic process without "aftereffects." This means that only the actual condition is important and not its history. The temporal course of this so-called *Markov* process can be described with the second *Kolmogorov* equation. In the case of a mixing process without selective convectional flows (requirement: $\Delta\rho \approx 0$ and $\Delta d_p \approx 0$), the solution of *Fick's* diffusion equation gives a cosine function for the local concentration distribution, the amplitude of which decreases exponentially with the dimensionless time θ $D_{eff}(\pi^2 L^2)$ (Figure 17). (The variation coefficient, v, is defined as the standard deviation σ divided by the arithmetic mean $\bar{x}$: $v \equiv \sqrt{\sigma^2/\bar{x}}$.)

Let us now consider this process using dimensional analysis. At plow mixer, see sketch in Figure 17, we have the following parameters:

Target quantity:	v	variation coefficient as a measure for quality of mixture
Geometric parameters	D	diameter and length of the drum
	d	diameter of the shovels
	d_p	mean particle diameter
	φ	degree of fill of the drum
Material properties	D_{eff}	effective axial dispersion coefficient
	ρ	density of the particles
Process parameters	n	rotational speed of the mixer
	θ	mixing time
	$g\rho$	solid gravity

The relevance list contains 11 parameters

$$\{v; D, L, d, d_p, \phi; D_{eff}, \rho; n, \theta, g\rho\} \tag{49}$$

After the exclusion of the dimensionless quantities v and ϕ and the obvious geometric pi numbers L/D, d/D, and d_p/D, the remaining three pi numbers are obtained via dimensional matrix:

$\theta\, n$	Mixing time number
$D_{eff}/D^2 n \equiv Bo^{-1}$	Bo (Bodenstein number)
$g\rho/(\rho\, Dn^2) \equiv Fr^{-1}$	Fr (Froude number)

The complete pi set contains eight pi numbers and reads:

$$\{v, L/D, d/D, d_p/D, \phi, \theta n, \text{Bo}, \text{Fr}\} \tag{50}$$

To keep the rotational speed of the drum only in the process number Fr, we combine the other two accordingly with Fr and obtain: $\theta\, D_{eff}/D^2$ and gD^3/D_{eff}^2.

The experimental results presented in Figure 17 were obtained in one single model ($D = 0.19$ m) with different lengths ($L/D = 1; 1.5; 2; 2.5$). The geometric and material numbers d/D, d_p/D, ϕ, and gD^3/D_{eff}^2 remained unchanged as did Fr because of the constant rotational speed of the paddle shaft $n = 50/\text{min}$. As a result, the measurements can only be depicted in the pi space

$$\{v, \theta D_{eff}/D^2, L/D\} \tag{51}$$

whereby d/D, d_p/D, ϕ, gD^3/D_{eff}^2, Fr = idem.
The result of these measurements is

$$v = f\left(\frac{\theta D_{eff}}{L^2}\right) \tag{52}$$

In other words, the mixing time (at Fr = const) required to attain a certain mixing quality increases with the square of the drum length L. In order to reduce the mixing time, the component to be mixed would have to be added in the middle of the drum or simultaneously at several positions.

Figure 17 shows experimental results in a single logarithmic graph. They are compared with the theoretical prediction of a stochastic *Markoff*'s process (for details see Ref. 17).

Entrop (18) reported the process characteristics of the *Nauta*® mixer. The *Nauta* mixer utilizes an orbiting action of a helical screw, rotating on its own axis, to carry material upward, while revolving about the centerline of the cone-shaped housing near the wall for top-to-bottom circulation (Fig. 18). *Nauta* mixers of different sizes are not build geometrically similar to each other: the diameter of the helical screw and its pitch are kept equal.

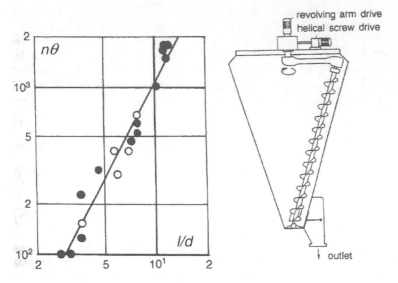

FIGURE 18 Mixing time characteristic of the *Nauta*® mixer and its drawing. *Source*: From Ref. 18.

Mixing time characteristic of the Nauta cone and screw mixer

Relevance list: In case of a pure convective mixing and $\Delta\rho$, $\Delta d_p \approx 0$, the particle size d_p is of no influence.

Target quantity:	θ	mixing time
Geometric parameters	d, l	diameter and length of the helical screw
Material properties	ρ	density of the particles
Process parameters	n, n_b	rotational speed of the helical screw and its beam
	$g\rho$	solid gravity

$$\{\theta; d, l; \rho; n, n_b, g\rho\} \tag{53}$$

$7 - 3 = 4$ numbers will be produced. The pi set reads:

$$\{n\theta, l/d, n_b/n, Fr \equiv n^2 d\rho/g\,\rho \equiv n^2 d/g\} \tag{54}$$

The measurements were executed under the following conditions: Mixer volume $V = 0.05$–10 m^3; diameter of the helical screw $d = 0.15$–0.63 m; rotational speed of the helical screw $n = 30$–120/min; $n_b/n = 20$–70; Fr = 0.24–4. Material systems: sand and fine-grained limestone.

The mixing time characteristic of the *Nauta* mixer is given in Figure 18. It can be shown that the type of material has a negligible influence (proof that the density ρ is irrelevant indeed). Likewise, the number n_b/n has, within the used range, no effect. In contrast, the influence of the parameter l/d is very pronounced. The process equation reads:

$$n\theta = 13\left(\frac{l}{d}\right)^{1.93} \quad \frac{n_b}{n} = 20 - 70 \quad Fr = 0.24 - 4 \tag{55}$$

This means, in practice, that the mixing time is lengthened by the square of the length (compare with Eq. 45).

The power characteristic of the *Nauta* mixer has been found:

$$\text{Ne Fr} \equiv \frac{P}{nd^4g\rho} \propto \left(\frac{l}{d}\right)^{1.62} \tag{56}$$

By multiplication of both process characteristics Eqs. (55) and (56), the expression for the mixing work can be obtained, this being necessary for a given mixing quality.

$$W = P\theta \propto d^{0.45}l^{3.55}\rho g \tag{57}$$

From the energy point of view, it is therefore advantageous to construct mixers of low heights and to provide them with helical screws of large diameters.

Example 9: Scale-up of single-screw extruders for mixing highly viscous media

Single-screw extruders are important mixing devices for highly viscous media. The mixing action is due to the cross-channel flow ("leak flow") in the full flights of the extruder caused by the combined actions of drag and pressure flows. The pressure flow can be greatly enhanced and varied by combining single-screw extruder with a gear-type rotary pump.

The pressure characteristics of such an extruder/pump combination is given by

$$Y \equiv \text{Eu Re} \, d/L \equiv f_1(Q) \tag{58}$$

where Q represents the flow rate number, $Q \equiv q/(nd^3)$; q, volumetric through-put; n, rotational speed; and d, L, diameter and length of the screw housing. In the creeping flow (Re < 100) of Newtonian liquids, this is a linear dependency described by the analytical expression:

$$\frac{1}{y_1}Y + \frac{1}{q_1}Q = 1 \tag{59}$$

where y_1 and q_1 are the respective axis intercepts (Fig. 19).

In this representation, the throughput number Q is standardized by the intercept A_1. It is the numerical value of Q where the screw machine is conveying without pressure formation. With this kinematic flow parameter, $\Lambda \equiv Q/A_1$, the state of flow of a screw machine can be outlined more distinctly.

From the three ranges of the conveying characteristics, only the middle one $0 < \Lambda < 1$ (the so-called "active conveying range" of the screw machine) can be implemented by suitable throttling and/or a change in the rotational speed alone, without an additional conveying device. At $\Lambda = 0$, the screw machine is fully choked and the highest pressure builds up. At $\Lambda = 1$, the highest throughput is achieved without a pressure buildup.

In other two ranges, the gear-type rotary pump has to enter into action. If the pump pushes the liquid in the same direction as the screw, the range $\Lambda > 1$ results. The conveying action of the screw machine is "run over" by the conveying action of the pump. In this operation, an excellent heat transfer between the housing and the liquid can be obtained (19).

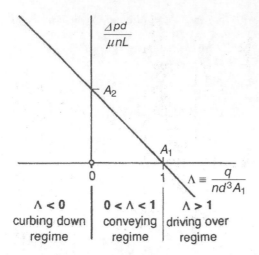

FIGURE 19 Subdivision of the typical working ranges of an extruder/pump combination by the kinematic flow parameter $\Lambda \equiv Q/A_1$.

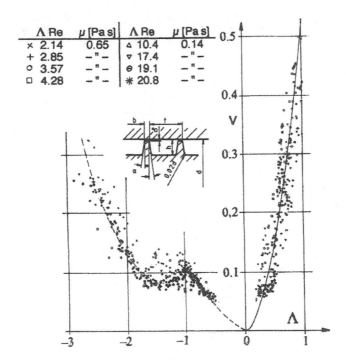

FIGURE 20 Homogenization effect of the extruder/pump combination. Influence of the kinematic flow parameter Λ on the variation coefficient ν at the distribution of iron powder in silicone oil. $d = 60$ mm; $L/d = 5.23$. (For geometry of the profile parameters of the screw machine see Ref. 19, Fig. 1.4.1.)

At $\Lambda < 0$, the pump pushes the liquid against the conveying sense of the screw. In this flow range, the screw machine is an excellent mixing device.

Figure 20 depicts the mixing characteristics in the frame $v(\Lambda)$ of the extruder/pump combination and confirms the above statement. At $\Lambda = 0$, the liquid throughput is zero and the residence time unlimited. Here, the stochastic homogeneity is surely reached and corresponding v value is $v \approx 0$. The fitting line in the range $0 < \Lambda < 1$ corresponds to the analytical expression $v = 0.52\ \Lambda^{1.79}$. Monograph (19) contains a series of suggestions concerning the scale-up of a combination single-screw extruder/gear-type rotary pump for homogenization as well as for heat transfer.

Example 10: Scale-up of liquid atomization (liquid-in-gas-dispersion)

Liquid atomization is an important unit operation, which is employed in a variety of processes. They include fuel atomization, spray drying, metal powder production, coating of surfaces by spraying, and so on.

In all these tasks, the achievable (as narrow as possible) droplet size distribution represents the most important target quantity. It is often described merely by the mean droplet size, the so-called "*Sauter* mean diameter" d_{32} (20), which is defined as the sum of all droplet volumes divided by their surfaces. Mechanisms of droplet formation are as follows:

1. Liquid jet formed by a pressure nozzle is inherently unstable. The breakup of the laminar jet occurs by a symmetrical oscillation, a sinusoidal oscillation, and, finally, atomization.
2. Liquid sheet formation by an appropriate nozzle is followed by rim disintegration, aerodynamic wave disintegration, and turbulent breakup.
3. Liquid atomization by a gas stream.
4. Liquid atomization by centrifugal acceleration.

For all of these operations, dimensionless process equations exist (21); some of them will be represented in the following.

As discharge velocity at the nozzle outlet increases, the following states appear in succession: dripping, laminar jet breakup, wave disintegration, and atomization. These states of flow are described in a pi space {Re, Fr, We$_p$}, whereby $We_p \equiv \rho v^2 d_p / \sigma$ represents the Weber number, formed by the droplet diameter, d_p. To eliminate the flow velocity, v, these numbers are combined to give

$$\text{Bond number } Bd_p \equiv \frac{We}{Fr} \equiv \frac{\rho g d_p}{\sigma} \qquad (60)$$

and

$$\text{Ohnesorge number } Oh_p \equiv \frac{We^{1/2}}{Re} \equiv \frac{\mu}{(\sigma \rho d_p)^{1/2}} \qquad (61)$$

The subscript p indicates that these pi numbers are formed with the droplet diameter.

For a liquid, dripping from a tiny capillary with diameter, d, it follows:

$$\frac{d_p}{d} = 1.6\left(\frac{\rho g d^2}{\sigma}\right)^{-1/3} = 1.6\,Bd^{-1/3} \qquad (62)$$

Broader tubes (Bd > 25) exert no influence of d. Then we obtain

$$\text{Bd}_p \equiv \frac{\rho g d_p^2}{\sigma} = 2.9 - 3.3 \qquad (63)$$

On the jet surface, waves are formed, which, at wave lengths of $\lambda > \pi d_j$ (d_j, jet diameter), grow rapidly. The fastest wave disturbance takes place at the optimum wave length of

$$\frac{\lambda_{opt}}{\pi d_j} = \sqrt{2 + 6\,\text{Oh}} \qquad (64)$$

For a low liquid viscosity $d/d_j \approx 1.9$ applies. If liquid output pulsates, uniformly spaced droplets are obtained; here, $d/d_j \approx 1$.

With higher discharge velocities, laminar jets are produced, which disintegrate to droplets in a certain distance from the capillary. The transition from dripping to liquid jet disintegration occurs at higher Weber numbers:

$$\text{We} \equiv \frac{\rho v^2 d}{\sigma} = 8 - 10 \qquad (65)$$

At We < 8, gravitational acceleration also has to be considered, thereby the Bond number has to be included into the process equation.

The working principle of hollow cone nozzles is that the liquid throughput is subjected to rotation by a tangential inlet and is then further accelerated in the conical housing toward the orifice (Fig. 21). A liquid film with a thickness, δ, is thereby produced, which, at the discharge from the orifice, spreads to a hollow cone sheet and disintegrates to droplets.

At low discharge velocities and low film thicknesses, the sheet disintegration is due to the oscillations caused by air motion. In this case, the film thickness has a large impact on the droplet size. In contrast, it is insignificant whether a pure liquid or a lime-water suspension (mass portion $\varphi = 16-64\%$) is treated (22).

By exceeding a certain discharge velocity, turbulence forces increase to such an extent that film disruption takes place immediately at the orifice. Now, the droplet size is independent of the film thickness. This state of atomization is described by the critical Weber number. Measuring data obtained with hollow

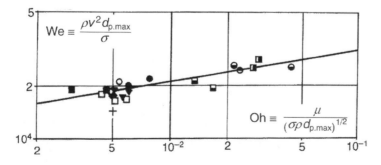

FIGURE 21 Liquid film atomization with hollow cone nozzles by turbulent forces. (For an explanation of signs see the original publication.) *Source*: From Ref. 22.

cone nozzles of different geometry and pure liquids as well as lime-water suspensions are represented in Figure 21. $We_{p,crit}$ and the Ohnesorge number are formed by the largest stable droplet diameter, $d_{p,max}$. The pi equation reads:

$$We_{p,\,crit} = 4.5 \times 10^4 \, Oh_p^{1/6}$$

This equation is useless for scaling up purposes, because the (unknown!) target quantity $d_{p,max}$ appears also in the process number Oh. In the combination

$$We_{p,\,crit}Oh_p^2 \equiv \frac{We}{Re} \equiv \frac{v\mu}{\sigma} \qquad (66)$$

a new pi number is obtained, which does not contain $d_{p,\,max}$:

$$We_{p,\,crit} \equiv \frac{\rho v^2 d_{p,crit}}{\sigma} = 1.97 \times 10^4 \left(\frac{v\mu}{\sigma}\right)^{0.154} \qquad (67)$$

This process equation can now serve for scaling up $d_{p,max}$.

DIMENSIONAL ANALYSIS AND SCALE-UP OF MILLS FOR EMULSIFICATION AND FOR GRINDING

In this paragraph, two unit operations will be discussed that are often encountered in the pharmaceutical industry.

Example 11: Emulsification of nonmiscible liquids

Liquid/liquid emulsions consist of two (or more) nonmiscible liquids. Classical examples for oil-in-water (O/W) emulsions are milk, mayonnaise, lotions, creams, water-soluble paints, photo emulsions, etc. As appliances serve dispersion and colloid mills, as well as high-pressure homogenizers, all of them utilize a high energy input to produce finest droplets of the disperse (mostly oil) phase. The aim of this operation is the narrowest possible droplet size distribution. It is normally characterized by the "Sauter mean diameter" d_{32} (20) or by the median d_{50} of the size distribution. Therefore, d_{32} or d_{50}, respectively, have to be regarded as the target quantity of this operation.

The characteristic length of the dispersion chamber, for example, the slot width between rotor and stator in dispersion mills or the nozzle diameter in high pressure homogenizers (utilizing high-speed fluid shear) will be denoted as "d."

As material parameters, the densities and the viscosities of both phases as well as the interfacial tension σ must be listed. We incorporate the material parameters of the disperse phase ρ_d and μ_d in the relevance list and note separately the material numbers ρ/ρ_d and μ/μ_d. Additional material parameters are the (dimensionless) volume ratio of both phases φ and the mass portion c_i of the emulsifier (surfactant) (e.g., given in ppm).

The process parameters have to be formulated as intensive quantities. In appliances where liquid throughput q and the power input P are separated from each other as two freely adjustable process parameters, the volume-related power input P/V and the period of its duration ($\tau = V/q$) must be considered:

$$\left(\frac{P}{V}\right)\tau = \frac{E}{V}\,[ML^{-1}T^{-2}] \qquad (68)$$

In appliances with only one degree of freedom (e.g., high-pressure homogenizers), the power is being introduced by the liquid throughput. Here, the relevant intensively formulated power P is therefore power per liquid throughput, P/q. Because of the fact that in nozzles $P \propto \Delta pq$, this results in

$$\frac{P}{q} = \frac{(\Delta pq)}{q} = \Delta p [ML^{-1}T^{-2}] \tag{69}$$

Therefore, the volume-related energy input E/V and the throughput-related power input $P/q \triangleq \Delta p$) represent homologous quantities of the same dimension. For the sake of simplicity, Δp will be introduced in the relevance list.

Now, this six-parametric relevance list of the dimensional parameters (the dimensionless parameters ρ/ρ_d, μ/μ_d, φ, c_i are excluded) reads

$$\{d_{32}; d; \rho_d, \mu_d, \sigma, \Delta p\} \tag{70}$$

The corresponding dimensional matrix delivers the remaining three dimensionless numbers:

$$\prod_1 \equiv \frac{\Delta pd}{\sigma} \equiv Eu\,We \equiv La\,(Laplace\;number)$$

$$\prod_2 \equiv \frac{\mu_d}{(\rho_d d\sigma)^{1/2}} \equiv \frac{We^{1/2}}{Re} \equiv Oh\,(Ohnesorge\;number)$$

$$\prod_3 \equiv \frac{d_{32}}{d}$$

The complete pi set is given as

$$\{d_{32}/d,\,La,\,Oh,\,\rho/\rho_d,\,\mu/\mu_d,\,\varphi,\,c_i\} \tag{71}$$

Assuming a quasi-uniform power distribution in the throughput or in the volume, a characteristic length of the dispersion space becomes irrelevant. In the relevance list (Eq. 70) the parameter d must be cancelled. The target number $\prod_3 \equiv d_{32}/d$ has to be dropped and the dimensionless numbers La* and Oh* have to be built by d_{32} instead of d. At given and constant material conditions (ρ/ρ_d, μ/μ_d, φ, c_i = const), the process characteristics will be represented in the following pi space:

$$Oh^{*-2} = f(La^*Oh^{*2}) \rightarrow d_{32}\left(\frac{\rho_d\sigma}{\mu_d^2}\right) = f\left\{\Delta p\left(\frac{\mu_d^2}{\rho_d\sigma^2}\right)\right\} \tag{72}$$

This dependency has been confirmed on two colloid mills in the scale 1:2.2 (23) (Fig. 22). For a material system of vegetable oil/water and $\varphi = 0.5$, the following correlation is found:

$$d_{32} = 4.64 \times 10^5 \Delta p^{-2/3} \quad d_{32}[\mu m]; \; \Delta p[M/(LT^2)] \tag{73}$$

Similar results have been presented for other two-parametric appliances (23).

It should be pointed out that the dimensional representations in the form of Eq. (73) as $d_{32} = f(\Delta p)$ presents a serious disadvantage as compared to the

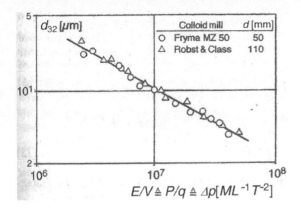

FIGURE 22 The relationship $d_{32} = f(\Delta p)$ for two colloid mills of different size. Material system: vegetable oil/water and $\varphi = 0.5$. *Source*: From Ref. 23.

dimensionless one: Eq. (73) is valid only for the investigated material system and tells nothing about the influence of the physical parameters.

Example 12: Fine grinding of solids in stirred ball mills

The fine grinding of solids in mills of different shape and mode of operation is used to produce finest particles with a narrow particle size distribution. Therefore, as in the previous example, the target quantity is the median value d_{50} of the particle size distribution.

The characteristic length of a given mill type is d.

The physical properties are given by the particle density ρ_p, the specific energy of the fissure area β, and the tensile strength σ_Z of the material. Should there be additional material parameters of relevance, they can be easily converted to material numbers by the above mentioned ones.

As process parameter, the mass-related energy input $E/\rho V$ must be taken into account. The relevance list reads:

$$\{d_{50}; d; \rho_p, \beta, \sigma_Z; E/\rho V\} \tag{74}$$

From this relevance list the following pi set follows

$$\{d_{50}/d, (E/\rho V)\rho d/\beta, \sigma_Z d/b\} \tag{75}$$

Assuming a quasi-uniform energy input in the mill chamber, its characteristic diameter d will be irrelevant. Then the pi set is reduced to

$$\left\{ \left(\frac{E}{\rho V}\right)\frac{\rho d_{50}}{\beta}, \frac{\sigma_Z d_{50}}{\beta} \right\} \rightarrow d_{50}\left(\frac{\sigma_Z}{\beta}\right) = f\left\{ \left(\frac{E}{\rho V}\right)\left(\frac{\rho}{\sigma_Z}\right) \right\} \tag{76}$$

In case of unknown physical properties, σ_Z and β, Eq. (76) is reduced to $d_{50} = f(E/\rho V)$, which is then used for the scale-up of a given type of mill and a given grinding material.

For fine grinding of, for example, limestone for paper and pottery manufacturing, bead mills are widely used. The beads of steel, glass, or ceramic have a diameter of 0.2 to 0.3 mm and occupy up to 90% of the total mill volume ($\phi \leq 0.9$). They are kept in motion by perforated stirrer discs while the liquid/solid suspension is pumped through the mill chamber. Mill types frequently in use are stirred disc mill, centrifugal fluidized bed mill, and ring gap mill.

Karbstein et al. (25) pursued the question of the smallest size of the laboratory bead mill that would still deliver reliable data for scale-up. In different-sized rigs ($V = 0.25$–25 L), a sludge consisting of limestone ($d_{50} = 16$ μm) and 10% aqueous Luviscol solution (mass portion of solids $\varphi = 0.2$) was treated. It was found that the minimum size of the mill chamber should be $V = 1$ L. A further, unexpected but dramatic result was that the validity of the process characteristics

$$d_{50} \propto \left(\frac{E}{\rho V}\right)^{-0.43} \qquad \frac{E}{\rho V} \leq 10^4 \qquad (77)$$

expires at $E/\rho V \approx 10^4$, and the finest particle diameter cannot fall below $d_{50} \approx 1$ μm.

These facts and the scattering of the results made a systematic investigation of the grinding process necessary (26). The grinding process in bead mills is determined by the frequency and the intensity of the collision between beads and grinding medium. According to this assumption, the grinding result will remain constant if both these quantities are kept constant. The intensity of the collision is essentially given by the kinetic energy of the beads:

$$L_{\mathrm{kin}} \propto m_{\mathrm{M}} u^2 \propto V_{\mathrm{M}} \rho_{\mathrm{M}} u^2 \propto d_{\mathrm{M}}^3 \rho_{\mathrm{M}} u^2 \qquad (78)$$

(d_{M}, ρ_{M} are diameter and density of the mill beads and u is the tip velocity of the stirrer). On the other hand, the frequency depends on the size of the mill chamber and therefore on the overall mass-related energy input. To achieve the same grinding result in different-sized bead mills, E_{kin} as well as $E/\rho V$ have to be kept idem. The input of the mechanical energy can be measured from the torque and the rotational speed of the perforated discs and the kinetic energy can be calculated from Eq. (78).

The above assumption was examined with the same material system and the same grinding media (beads). Three different-sized bead mills were used (V [l] = 0.73, 5.54, 12.9). Figure 23 shows the results. To achieve a satisfactory correlation, the size of the mill chamber d will have to be introduced in the relevance list. A further finding is that under the same conditions a smaller mill delivers a coarser product. This has been found already in the previously cited paper (25).

As to the course of the function $d_{50} = f(E_{\mathrm{kin}})$ at $E/\rho V = 10^3$ kJ/kg = const, the following explanation is given in Ref. 26. With E_{kin} increasing, the particle size first diminishes but later increases. This is plausible if the introduced specific energy is viewed as a product of the frequency and the intensity of the collision. At $E/\rho V =$ const and increasing the intensity of the collision, the frequency has to diminish, resulting in a coarser product.

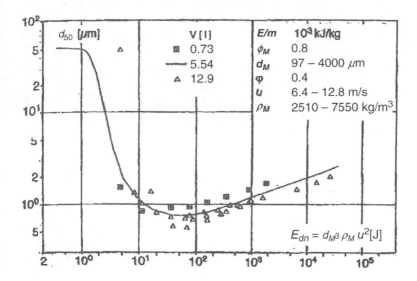

FIGURE 23 The relationship $d_{50} = f(E_{kin})$ for three colloid mills of same type but different size. Identical material system and constant $E/\rho V = 10^3$ kJ/kg. *Source*: From Ref. 26.

DIMENSIONAL ANALYTICAL TREATMENT OF HEAT TRANSFER PROCESSES
Driving Force and the Target Quantity of the Process

At first it is to be pointed out that heat transfer is normally an indirect process. In the case of cooling, for example, the part that receives heat is divided by a wall from the part where heat is produced. We deal with three different heat transfer steps, two of which belong to heat transfer by convection (under obviously different conditions) and the third one is heat conduction through a solid wall.

In the following, we will investigate only that part of the mixing vessel where a reaction takes place and the reaction heat produced has to be removed through the wall. The driving force of the process is the temperature difference ΔT between both spaces separated by the wall because temperature stands for energy levels of the systems that are to be equalized.

The target quantity of this process is heat transfer coefficient at the inner wall, h. It can be regarded as the heat conductivity, k, in the boundary layer, divided by its thickness, δ: $h = k/\delta$. Because of the unknown δ, h is not measurable. It can only be calculated from the general heat transfer equation by using it as the determining equation for h:

$$h \equiv \frac{Q}{A\Delta T}$$

(Q is the heat flow through the heat exchanger area A)

Steady State Heat Transfer in Mixing Vessels

The pi space of the heat transfer characteristics of a mixing vessel is obtained by the following relevance list:

Target quantity: heat transfer coefficient at the inner wall, h
Geometric parameters: vessel and stirrer diameters: D, d
Material parameters: density, ρ; viscosity of liquid bulk, μ; and at the inner wall, μ_w; heat capacity, C_p; heat conductivity, k
Process parameters: stirrer speed, n.

The complete nine-parametric relevance list reads as follows:

$$\{h; D, d; \rho, \mu, \mu_w, C_p, k; n\} \tag{79}$$

Here two characteristic lengths were introduced. D stands for that geometri part of the device where the heat is transferred (in the case of cooling coils, coil diameter D_c had to be introduced instead), whereas d is the stirrer diameter, which, together with n, governs the hydrodynamics in the vessel.

This nine-parametric relevance list leads to $9 - 4 = 5$ dimensionless numbers, the fourth base dimension being the temperature Θ:

$$\{\text{Nu}, \text{Pr}, \text{Re}, \text{Vis}, D/d\} \tag{80}$$

Legend:

Nu $\equiv hD/k$ (Nusselt number, the target number)
Pr $\equiv C_p\mu/k$ (Prandtl number, pure material number)
Re $\equiv nd^2\rho/\mu$ (Reynolds number, the process number)
Vis $\equiv \mu_w/\mu$ (viscosity ratio)
D/d (wall clearance, the geometric number)

Figure 24 shows the dependence (Eq. 80) for an anchor stirrer with two arms and a close wall clearance ($D/d = 1.02$). The figure consists of two parts representing the same measuring results in two different pi spaces: above as Nu $= f$ (Re), below as Nu $= f$ (Re, Pr).

A comparison of both representations verifies that the consideration of the Prandtl number by $\text{Pr}^{1/3}$ only starts gaining weight increasingly from ca. Re > 200; in the range Re < 200 its contemplation is rather negative. (For the heat transfer from tube wall to the fluid flowing under laminar conditions, Levêque (28) found that the heat transfer coefficient h is proportional to the third root of the shear rate at the wall.)

The scattering of the measuring data in the range of Re < 200 is well founded by the measuring technique applied here. The mean bulk temperature in the vessel in the laminar flow region could not be measured with a thermometer because round its wall an insulating border layer was formed. In this range, the average temperature of the bulk liquid had to be calculated from the heat balance. In the range Re > 200, the correspondence between the calculated and measured values was approximately 10% (27).

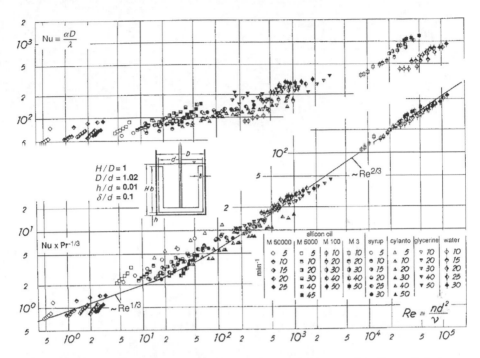

FIGURE 24 Heat transfer characteristics of a mixing vessel with an anchor stirrer with two arms and $D/d = 1.02$. *Source*: From Ref. 27.

The fitting lines in the lower figure verify the following dependences:

$$\text{Re} > 200 : Nu = 0.28 \, \text{Re}^{2/3} \, \text{Pr}^{1/3} \tag{81}$$

$$\text{Re} < 200 : Nu = 0.8 \, \text{Re}^{1/3} \, \text{Pr}^{1/3} = 0.8 \, \text{Pe}^{1/3} \tag{82}$$

This is compulsory. If in the creeping flow range (Re < 200) the influence of the Prandtl number is considered by $\text{Pr}^{1/3}$, then the Reynolds number must also have the same exponent. Only then the result is a number (Peclet number, Pe) that does not contain the liquid viscosity, and the liquid density ρ is combined with the *mass*-related heat capacity C_p to produce the *volume*-related one. In the creeping flow range, liquids behave like solid bodies and then neither viscosity nor density affect heat transfer:

$$\text{Pe} \equiv \text{Re} \, \text{Pr} \equiv nd^2 \rho C_p / k \equiv nd^2 / a$$

$a \equiv k/(\rho C_p)$ means thermal conductivity.

H. Judat (see in Ref. 33, sect. 7.2.2) investigated heat transfer in a mixing vessel with an anchor stirrer with four arms equipped with wipers ($D/d = 1$). With the wipers, the liquid border layer at the wall is completely removed. As a result, the Nu values ($\triangleq a_i$ values in the creeping flow area are increased by a full decade and, in addition, the creeping flow range expands up to Re = 2×10^3 because the stirrer beams dip into the laminar border layer. Here, too, Nu $\propto$ Pe$^{1/3}$ holds.

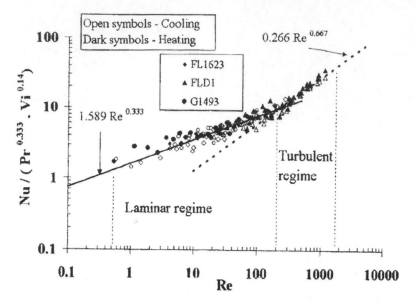

FIGURE 25 Heat transfer characteristics of a mixing vessel equipped with an *Ekato*-Paravisc stirrer (*D/d* = 1.06) and measured with three different Newtonian fluids. *Source*: From Ref. 29.

Delaplace et al. (29) studied heat transfer in a vessel (*D* = 0.346 m) equipped with a *Ekato*-Paravisc stirrer (*d* = 0.32 m, *D/d* = 1.08) and found for Newtonian as well as for non-Newtonian liquids the same heat transfer equations (Fig. 25):

$$\text{Re} > 200 : \text{Nu} = 0.27 \ \text{Re}^{2/3} \ \text{Pr}^{1/3} \ \text{Vis}^{-0.14} \tag{83}$$

$$\text{Re} < 200 : \text{Nu} = 1.59 \ \text{Pe}^{1/3} \ \text{Vis}^{-0.14} \tag{84}$$

The fact that no difference between heat transfer in Newtonian and in non-Newtonian liquids was found (fluids of the pseudoplastic and yield stress type were investigated and their viscosity considered according to the Metzner–Otto concept) verifies that non-Newtonian fluid behavior affects only the turbulent flow region. A comparison of process equations between the Paravisc stirrer and the old fashioned anchor stirrer (at *D/d* ≈ similar) shows that the Paravisc stirrer delivers, by a factor of 2, better heat transfer values only in the creeping flow area (Re < 200). In the turbulent region every stirrer delivers the same results.

In the optimization of stirrers to achieve the optimum heat removal in a cooling process, it should not be forgotten that the removable heat flow, *Q* (kW), increases in the range of Re > 200 (in technical mixing vessels Re < 100 is seldom achieved) according to the heat transfer characteristic with $\text{Re}^{2/3} \propto n^{2/3}$, whereas the thereby associated stirrer power (≙ stirring heat) increases substantially overproportionally according to the power characteristic of the stirrer with *P* (kW) $\propto n^3$. Thus, it follows that there is an optimum stirrer speed at

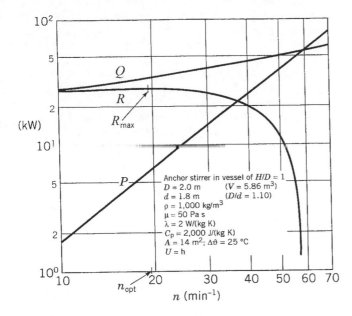

FIGURE 26 Graphical representation of the course of $R \equiv Q - P$ as a function of the stirrer speed n for the example given in the plot. *Source*: From Ref. 30.

which the maximum process heat, for example, chemical reaction heat, R, can be removed:

$$R \equiv Q - P$$

Figure 26 illustrates this situation with a concrete example. It shows that the optimum range with respect to the stirrer speed is very flat, 90% of the maximum value being removed in the range $n_{opt} = 20/\text{min} \pm 60\%$.

To compare an anchor stirrer (at $D/d = 1.02$) with *Ekato*-Paravisc stirrer (at $D/d = 1.08$), their power characteristics have to be taken into account. In the range of Re < 100 they read:

anchor stirrer: $\quad$ NeRe = 420
Ekato-Paravisc stirrer: $\quad$ NeRe = 250

For Re > 100, see Refs. 27 and 29. Obviously, the Paravisc stirrer is more suitable for heat removal than the anchor stirrer. The reason for this advantage lies possibly in the pumping action of the stirrer, with which the liquid is more effectively removed from the wall.

DIMENSIONAL ANALYTICAL TREATMENT OF MASS TRANSFER PROCESSES
Driving Force and Target Quantities of the Process
In mass transfer processes, mass is transferred from one phase to the other through an interface. This can be either solid (dissolution in the systems S/L) or

a fluid one: L/L, G/L (absorption and desorption processes). In the first case the interface is known, in the second case the fluid interface is neither known nor measurable. This distinction has a big impact on dimensional analytical treatment of the process.

In mass transfer, the driving force consists in the removal of an equilibrium disturbance and concerns a thermodynamic quantity, namely the chemical potential, μ.

It is often presumed that the leveling out of concentration differences Δc between two phases is the cause for mass transfer. That is not the case. This fact can easily be demonstrated with a number of examples. It should suffice to remark that a material system consisting of granular cooking salt in saturated aqueous solution is in equilibrium. The chemical potential in both phases is equal, but the concentration of NaCl in granular cooking salt is 100%, whereas in the saturated aqueous solution it is only 26.4% (at 20°C).

The bridge between the chemical potential, which is very difficult to determine, and the concentration difference, which is easily determined, was erected by *Lewis* and *Whiteman* in 1923/1924, who postulated in their "*Two-Film Theory*" (with regard to the system G/L) the following:

1. On both sides of the interface, laminar boundary layers exist which the gas can pass only by *diffusion*.
2. In the interface, the thermodynamic equilibrium *immediately* occurs.

In the material system G/L, the transfer from the gas phase to the interface can be neglected because it is at least by 50 times faster than the transfer from the interface through the laminar liquid boundary layer to the bulk of a liquid. If—as postulated—a thermodynamic equilibrium always exists in the interface, then also the saturation concentration c_s of the gas is always present. Under these conditions the driving force of mass transfer is in fact given by concentration difference:

$$\Delta c = c_s - c \qquad (85)$$

Thus, the general mass transfer equation is given by the following relationship:

$$G = k_L A \Delta c \qquad (86)$$

Legend:

G (kg gas/sec)	mass transfer rate through the interface
A (m²)	interfacial area (e.g., the sum of the surfaces of all gas bubbles)
k_L (m/sec)	liquid-side mass transfer coefficient
Δc (kg/m³)	characteristic concentration difference of the dissolved gas between the interface and the liquid bulk

k_L can physically be comprehended as $k_L \propto D/x_L$, where D is the diffusion coefficient of the gas in the liquid-side laminar boundary layer of thickness x_L. Thus, k_L represents a definition quantity, which is as little measurable as the interfacial area A. Both of them are influenced by the kinematics of the process and by material conditions. In surface aeration, they are combined into only one quantity, which can easily be determined by constituents of the overall mass transfer Eq. (86):

$$k_L A \equiv \frac{G}{\Delta c} \tag{87}$$

$k_L A$ represents the target quantity of mass transfer in *surface aeration*.

In volume (bulk) aeration it is assumed that the process takes place in a liquid, which is turbulently mixed and thus an equal number of gas bubbles of an equal size exists in each volume element. Under these circumstances, it is advisable to formulate the general mass transfer Eq. (86) as a volume-related one:

$$\frac{G}{V} = k_L \left(\frac{A}{V}\right) \Delta c \tag{88}$$

(This contains an additional advantage because Δc, too, is a volume-related quantity per definition.) A/V is abbreviated to $a \equiv A/V$ and—since it is not measurable—combined with k_L to the "overall liquid-side mass transfer coefficient" $k_L a$:

$$k_L a \equiv \frac{G}{V \Delta c} \tag{89}$$

$k_L a$ is easily measured by Eq. (89) and represents the target quantity of mass transfer in *bulk aeration*.

From the viewpoint of dimensional analysis, there is a considerable distinction between the two target quantities $k_L A$ and $k_L a$.

$k_L A$ is an *extensively* defined quantity, which therefore must compulsorily depend on extensive parameters like the stirrer diameter d and the stirrer speed n.

$k_L a$, in contrast, is a volume-related *intensive* quantity, which therefore must compulsorily depend on intensively formulated process parameters like power per liquid volume P/V and gas throughput q per aerated cross-sectional area S, the so-called superficial velocity, $v_G \propto q/S$.

Mass Transfer G/L in Surface Aeration

The supply of atmospheric oxygen to municipal sewage purification plants has been performed for decades by turbine surface aerators installed in the liquid surface of shallow wastewater treatment ponds ($H \leq 4$ m). The stirrers work as water pumps: they suck in wastewater, spray it over the liquid surface, and, in addition, whirl it up. In this way, the mass transfer G/L is effected.

Target quantity: mass transfer coefficient in surface aeration, $k_L A$
Geometric parameter: diameter of the turbine stirrer, d
Material parameters: density and kinematic viscosity of the liquid, ρ, ν
Process parameters: stirrer speed of the turbine, n acceleration due to density, g

The acceleration due to gravity, g, is essential in this process because it influences the parabolic throw of the ejected liquid. Two further possible parameters, the diffusion coefficient D and the surface tension σ, will be renounced, because in wastewater treatment the only liquid of interest is water. Thus, the constricted relevance list reads:

$$\{k_L A; d; \rho, \nu, n, g\} \tag{90}$$

This six-parametric set delivers the following three dimensionless numbers:

$$(k_L A)^* \equiv \frac{G}{d^3 \Delta c} \left(\frac{\nu}{g^2}\right)^{1/3} \qquad \text{sorption number}$$

$$\text{Re} \equiv \frac{nd^2}{\nu} \qquad\qquad \text{Reynolds number}$$

$$\text{Fr} \equiv \frac{n^2 d}{g} \qquad\qquad \text{Froude number}$$

To achieve that the only variable process parameter, n, does not appear in both process numbers (Fr and Re), we first determine which of the two process numbers is essential, and then we free the other one by combining it with the first one from n.

The process takes place in water, and the state of flow will be a turbulent one. Hence, Re cannot play an important role. The process will be governed essentially by the Froude number. We will combine Re with Fr and obtain

$$\text{Ga} \equiv \frac{\text{Re}^2}{\text{Fr}} \equiv \left(\frac{d^3 g}{\nu^2}\right) \qquad \text{(Galilei number)}$$

Thus, the pi space reads:

$$\{(k_L A)^*, \text{Fr}, \text{Ga}\} \tag{91}$$

Because of the circumstance that the second essential parameter, acceleration due to gravity, g, cannot be varied on Earth, measurements must be performed with measuring devices of different scale. (This is the only way to decouple Fr and Re.)

The process equation for a turbine stirrer ("Rushton turbine"), the disk of which was installed in the water surface, reads:

$$(k_L A)^* = 1.41 \times 10^{-4} \text{Fr}^{1.205} \text{Ga}^{0.115}; \quad \text{Fr} = 0.02 - 0.34; \quad \text{Ga} = 1.5 \times 10^9 - 2 \times 10^{11}$$

The investigated range of the scale-up factor was $\mu = 1:5$ (for details, see Ref. 31).

Mass Transfer G/L in Bulk Aeration in Mixing Vessels

There are a number of chemical and biotechnological reactions between gas (G) and liquid (L) that take place in mixing vessels: hydrogenation, oxidation, chlorination, phosgenization, and aerobic bioconversion. The relevance list for this operation reads as follows:

Target quantity:	volume-related mass transfer coefficient, $k_L a$
Geometric parameters:	none
Material parameters:	density and kinetic viscosity of the liquid, ρ, ν
	diffusivity of the gas in the liquid, D
	bubble coalescence behavior of the liquid, S_i
Process parameters:	volume-related mixing power, P/V
	superficial velocity of the gas, v
	gravitational acceleration, g

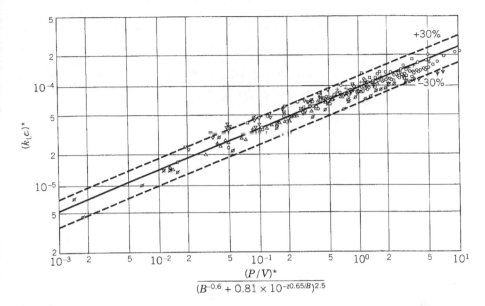

FIGURE 27 Sorption characteristic of a mixing vessel with a turbine stirrer for a coalescing material system (water/air). *Source*: From Ref. 33.

Here, some remarks are to be made. First, despite extensive research, bubble coalescence phenomena have still not been clarified to such an extent as to permit explicit formulation of the coalescence parameters (see Ref. 7, sect. 4.10). In the following, they will be taken into consideration in a lump as S_i. Second, the decision in favor of P/V and v instead of P/V and q/V is based on extensive research results (Fig. 27).

We start from the relevance list:

$$\{k_L a, \rho, \mu, D, S_i, P/V, v, g\} \tag{92}$$

and obtain the pi space

$$\{(k_L a)^*, (P/V)^*, v^*, Sc, S_i^*\} \tag{93}$$

Legend:

$$(k_L a)^* \equiv k_L a \left(\frac{v}{g^2}\right)^{1/3} \quad \text{(sorption number)}$$

$$(P/V)^* \equiv \frac{P/V}{\rho(vg^4)^{1/3}} \quad \text{(dimensionless } P/V \text{ number)}$$

$$v^* \equiv \frac{v}{(vg)^{1/3}} \quad \text{(dimensionless superficial velocity number)}$$

$$Sc \equiv D/\nu \quad \text{(Schmidt number)}$$

$$S_i^* \qquad \text{(unknown numbers describing the bubble } coalescence)$$

Figure 27 shows a correlation of mass transfer measurements in this pi space. The measurements were performed under unsteady state conditions by several authors in a water/air system, which is bubble coalescent, using a turbine stirrer as a mixing device. The measurements cover an extreme experimental scale of $\mu \approx 1$–80. The geometric parameters were broadly varied: $d = 0.05$–3.1 m; $D = 0.15$–12.2 m; $H = 0.15$–6.1 m, $V = 1.5$ L–906 m³. Between B and v^*, the following correlation exists: $B = (\pi/4)v^*$.

The process equation reads:

$$(k_L a)^* = \frac{9.8 \times 10^{-5}(P/V)^{*0.40}}{\left(B^{-0.60} + 0.81 \times 10^{-0.65/B}\right)^{2.5}}$$

Ignoring the additive term in this equation, we find $(k_L a)^* \propto (P/V)^{*0.40} B^{0.60}$.

In contrast, Figure 28 shows the results of mass transfer in the system: aqueous 1 N sodium sulfite solution/air. These measurements were carried out under steady state conditions in vessels with hollow stirrers on the scale $\mu = 1$:5 (35,36). In this material system, the high salt concentration (70 g Na₂SO₃/L) fully suppresses bubble coalescence. In the case of the self-aspirating hollow stirrer, the stirrer power and gas throughput were coupled via the stirrer speed and were therefore dependent on each other.

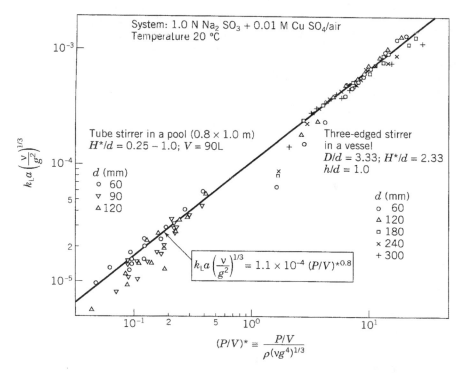

FIGURE 28 Sorption characteristic of a mixing vessel with a self-aspirating hollow stirrer in a material system with fully suppressed coalescence. *Source*: From Refs. 34,35.

Consequently, v^* does not occur explicitly in the representation in Figure 28 because it is a function of $(P/V)^*$.

Here, the process equation reads:

$$(k_L a)^* = 1.1 \times 10^{-4} \left(\frac{P}{V}\right)^{*0.80} \tag{94}$$

TABLE 4　Important, Named Dimensionless Numbers

Name	Symbol	Group	Remarks
		A. Mechanical unit operations	
Reynolds	Re	vl/ν	$\nu \equiv \mu/\rho$
Froude	Fr	$v^2/(lg)$	
	Fr*	$v^2\rho/(lg\Delta\rho)$	$\equiv$ Fr $(\rho/\Delta\rho)$
Galilei	Ga	gl^3/ν^2	$\equiv$ Re^2/Fr
Archimedes	Ar	$g\Delta\rho l^3/\nu^2\rho$	$\equiv$ Ga $(\Delta\rho/\rho)$
Euler	Eu	$\Delta p/(\rho v^2)$	
Newton	Ne	$F/(\rho v^2 l^2)$	Force
		$P/(\rho v^3 l^2)$	Power
Weber	We	$\rho v^2 l/\sigma$	
Ohnesorg	Oh	$\mu/(\rho\sigma l)^{1/2}$	$\equiv$ We$^{1/2}$/Re
Mach	Ma	v/v_s	V_s, velocity of sound
Knudsen	Kn	λ_m/l	λ_m, molecular free path length
		B. Thermal unit operations (heat transfer)	
Nusselt	Nu	hl/λ	
Prandtl	Pr	ν/a	$a \equiv \lambda/(\rho C_p)$
Grashof	Gr	$\beta\Delta Tgl^3/\nu^2$	$\equiv \beta\Delta T$ Ga
Fourier	Fo	at/l^2	
Péclet	Pe	vl/a	$\equiv$ RePr
Rayleigh	Ra	$\beta\Delta Tgl^3/(a\nu)$	$\equiv$ GrPr
Stanton	St	$h/(v\rho C_p)$	$\equiv$ Nu/(RePr)
		C. Thermal unit operations (mass transfer)	
Sherwood	Sh	kl/D	k, mass transfer coefficient
Schmidt	Sc	ν/D	
Bodenstein	Bo	vl/D_{ax}	D_{ax}, axial dispersion coefficient
Lewis	Le	a/D	$\equiv$ Sc/Pr
Stanton	St	k/v	$\equiv$ Sh/(Re Sc)
		D. Chemical reaction engineering	
Arrhenius	Arr	$E/(R\,T)$	E, activation energy
Hatta	Hat$_1$	$(k_1 D)^{1/2}/k_L$	1st order reaction
	Hat$_2$	$(k_2 c_2 D)^{1/2}/k_L$	2nd order reaction
Damköhler	Da	$\dfrac{c\Delta H_R}{\rho C_p T_0}$	genuine, see Ref. 5
	Da$_I$	$k_1\tau$	τ, residence time
	Da$_{II}$	$k_1 l^2/D$	$\equiv$ Da$_I$ Bo
			$\equiv$ Da$_I$ Re Sc
	Da$_{III}$	$k_1\tau\left(\dfrac{c\Delta H_R}{\rho C_p T_0}\right)$	$\equiv$ Da$_I$$\left(\dfrac{c\Delta H_R}{\rho C_p T_0}\right)$
	Da$_{IV}$	$\dfrac{k_1 c\Delta H_R l^2}{\lambda T_0}$	$\equiv$ Da$_I$Re Pr$\left(\dfrac{c\Delta H_R}{\rho C_p T_0}\right)$

These results can be summarized as follows. In the case of a coalescent material system, for example, in pure liquids of low viscosity (e.g., water), the absorption rate depends to an equal extent on P/V and on $v \propto q/D^2$:

$$(k_L a) \propto \left(\frac{P}{V}\right)^{0.4} v^{0.5} \tag{95}$$

In completely coalescence suppressed systems, for example, in many highly concentrated aqueous salt solutions (see Ref. 7, sect. 4.10) in contrast to the above, the following applies:

$$(k_L a) \propto \left(\frac{P}{V}\right)^{0.7} v^{0.2} \tag{96}$$

Only with self-aspirating hollow stirrers, where v^* is not an independent process parameter, the correlation (94) was found.

From the above, the following conclusion can be made. High-power inputs (P/V) are justified only in coalescence inhibited material systems. In other words, the generation of very fine primary gas bubbles in coalescent-prone systems is not economically justified.

Dimensional analysis and scale-up rules for two component nozzles ("injectors") for mass transfer in the G/L system in bubble columns are given in Ref. 36.

REFERENCES

1. West GB. Scale and dimensions—from animals to quarks. Los Alamos Sci 1984; 11: 2–20.
2. Bridgman PW. Dimensional Analysis. New Haven: Yale University Press, 1922, 1931, 1951. Reprint by AMS Press, New York, 1978.
3. Lord Rayleigh. The principle of similitude. Nature 1915; 95(2368): 66–68.
4. Zlokarnik M. Scale-up in Chemical Engineering. 2nd ed. Wiley-VCH Verlag GmbH & Co. KGaA 2006, ISBN 3-527-31421-0.
5. Pawlowski J. Theory of Similarity in Physico-Technological Research (in German). Berlin, New York: Springer, 1971.
6. Zlokarnik M. Mixing power in gassed liquids (in German). Chem Ing Tech 1973; 45:689–692.
7. Zlokarnik M. Stirring—Theory and Practice. Wiley-VCH Verlag GmbH 2001, ISBN 3-527-29996-3.
8. Zlokarnik M. Design and scale-up of mechanical foam breakers. Ger Chem Eng 1986; 9:314–320.
9. Zlokarnik M. Scale-up under conditions of partial similarity. Int Chem Eng 1987; 27:1–9.
10. Zlokarnik M. Suitability of different stirrer types for the homogenisation of liquid mixtures (in German). Chem Ing Tech 1967; 39:539–548.
11. Henzler H-J. Rheological material properties—explanation, measurement, recording and importance (in German). Chem Ing Tech 1988; 60:1–8.
12. Böhme G, Stenger M. Consistent scale-up procedure for power consumption in agitated non-Newtonian fluids. Chem Eng Technol 1988; 11:199–205.
13. Metzner AB, Otto RE. Agitation of non-Newtonian fluids. AIChE J 1957; 1:3–10.
14. Sánchez Pérez JA, Rodríguez Porcel EM, Casas López JL, et al. Shear rate in stirred tank and bubble column bioreactors. Chem Eng J 2006; 124:1–5.
15. Pawlowski J. Process Relationships for non-Newtonian fluids—criticism of the Metzner-Otto concept. Chem Eng Technol 2006; 28:37–41.

16. Henzler H-J. Scale-up of fermenter vessels under consideration of the non-Newtonian properties of the fermenter mixtures (in German). Chem Ing Tech 2007; 79:951–965.
17. Müller W, Rumpf H. Mixing of powders in mixers with axial motion (in German). Chem Ing Tech 1967; 39:365–965.
18. Entrop W. Scaling-up solid-solid mixers. Int Symp Mixing, B–Mons 1978, paper D1.
19. Pawlowski J. Transport Phenomena in Single Screw Extruders (in German). Frankfurt/M: Salle+Sauerländer, 1990. ISBN 3-7935-5528-3 (Salle).
20. Sauter J. Size determination of fuel droplets (in German). Forschungsarbeiten Heft 279 (1926).
21. Walzel P. Spraying and atomizing of liquids. In: Ullmann's Encyclopedia of Industrial Chemistry. Vol. B2, chapter 6. Weinheim, Germany: VCH, 1988.
22. Dahl HD, Muschelknautz E. Atomization of liquids and suspensions with hollow cone nozzles. Chem Eng Technol 1992; 15:224–231.
23. Schneider H, Roth T. Emulsification in Food Industry (in German). Universität Karlsruhe 1996, XIII-1/18:
24. Karbstein H, Schubert H. Parameters influencing the choice of devices for production of fine-disperse O/W emulsions (in German). Chem Ing Tech 1995; 67:616–619.
25. Karbstein H, Müller F, Polke R. Scale-up of centrifugal fluidized be mills (in German). Aufbereitungstechnik 1996; 37:469–479.
26. Kwade A, Stender H-H. Constant comminution results in scale-up of centrifugal bed mills (in German). Aufbereitungstechnik 1998; 39:373–382.
27. Zlokarnik M. Heat transfer at the wall of a mixing vessel at cooling and heating in the range of $10^0 < Re < 10^5$. Chem Ing Tech 1969; 41:1195–1202.
28. Levêque MA. Le lois de la transmission de la chaleur par convection. Ann Mines 1928; 12:201, 305, 381.
29. Delaplace G, Torrez C, Leuliet J-C, et al. Experimental and CFD simulation of heat transfer to highly viscous fluids in an agitated vessel equipped with a non standard hellical ribbon impeller. Trans IChemE 2001; 79A:927–937.
30. Pawlowski J, Zlokarnik M. Optimisation of stirrers for an optimum removal of reaction heat (in German). Chem Ing Tech 1972; 44:982–986.
31. Zlokarnik M. Scale-up of surface aerators for wastewater treatment. Adv Biochem Eng 1979; 11:158–180.
32. Zlokarnik M. Suitability and efficiency of surface aerators for the biological waste water treatment (in German). Korresp Abwasser 1980; 27:14–21.
33. Judat H. Mass transfer gas/liquid in mixing vessels—a critical assessment. Ger Chem Eng 1982; 5:357–363.
34. Zlokarnik M. Scale-up of hollow stirrers. Part II: Determination of achievable mass and heat transfer (in German). Chem Ing Tech 1966; 38:717–723.
35. Zlokarnik M. Sorption characteristics for gas-liquid contacting in mixing vessels. Adv Biochem Eng 1978; 8:133–151.
36. Zlokarnik M. Sorption characteristics of slot injectors and their dependency on the coalescence behaviour of the system. Chem Eng Sci 1979; 34:1265–1271.

2 Engineering approaches for pharmaceutical process scale-up, validation, optimization, and control in the PAT era

Fernando J. Muzzio

INTRODUCTION AND BACKGROUND

The time and expense required to develop new drug products are enormous. A recent public FDA report (1) estimates that the cost of bringing a new drug to market is between $0.8 and $1.7 billion, which represents a 50% increase in just five years (Fig. 1). This cost escalation has very substantial consequences: The number of new drugs and devices submitted to the FDA is dropping rapidly and *today it is less than half than five years ago* (Fig. 2). Because of these rising costs, innovators concentrate their efforts on products with potentially high market return, and the decreasing pool of new products is one of the main drivers for the major recent wave of mergers and acquisitions across the pharmaceutical industry.

The humanitarian cost of the state of affairs is very significant. Many therapies of proven medical efficacy never reach the market because the target disease only affects a "small" population ("orphan drugs"). Therapies for "third-world diseases" receive low priority. Development cost is one of the key factors for the rapidly rising costs in health care, which correlates to the growth of uninsured or underinsured populations. The FDA unambiguously identifies the situation as "an impending crisis in public health" caused largely by inadequate product development practices (Ref. 1, p. 6).

To invoke a cliché, pharmaceutical product development is an "art" form (2) (Fig. 3). Pharmaceutical products and processes are developed primarily by recipe-driven trial-and-error methods. Typically, the first stage (drug synthesis) yields a drug substance in powder form. In the second stage (formulation), the material is turned into a preliminary product using small-scale iterative experiments following one of a few available recipes that are expected to achieve the desired release profile (immediate release, delayed release, sustained release) in a certain environment within the body (stomach, intestine, colon). In the next stage, the process is scaled up to a pilot plant, and later on, to manufacturing scale, simply by attempting to replicate the bench-scale recipe in larger-size equipment.

A paucity of predictive science hinders every step of this lengthy and expensive process. Typically, at stage I, the particle properties needed to formulate the material in the desired manner are unknown. At stage II, it is not known how ingredient choices will affect product performance and manufacturability. Later on, scale-up is done simply by attempting to execute the "recipe" using larger equipment. Engineering principles (predictive simulations, dimensional analysis, scale-up factors) are seldom, if ever, used. Product and process "equivalence" are established a posteriori by examining the product in vivo and in vitro and processing parameters are "tweaked" until the desired

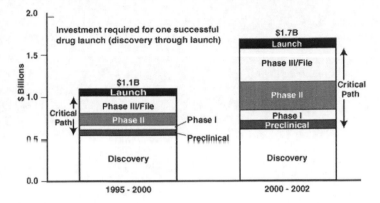

FIGURE 1 Cost of bringing a new drug to market, showing the rapid increase in drug development costs in the last five years. *Source*: From Ref. 1.

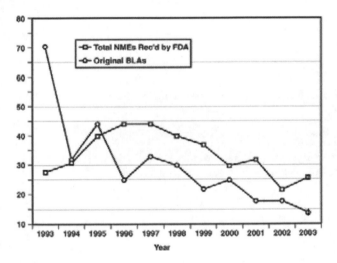

FIGURE 2 New Molecular Entities (NME) and Biological License Applications (BLA) received by FDA in the last 10 years show *the rapid decrease in new products developed*.

performance is achieved. Once this is accomplished, it is very difficult to introduce changes into the manufacturing process because, simply put, neither industry nor governmental agencies can reliably predict the impact of material or process changes on the final product.

Typically, due to a need to develop the product as quickly as possible, information is only transferred in the downstream direction. This practice significantly hinders true product and process optimization, continuous improvement, and incorporation of new technologies. While in the past this approach might have been tolerable, in recent years these methods are becoming rapidly obsolete. This is due, in part, to significant advances in understanding the genetic basis of disease. New drugs are much more potent (and toxic),

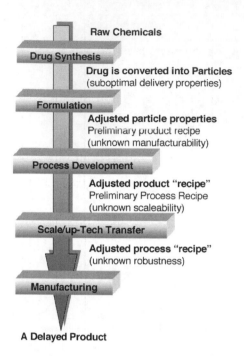

FIGURE 3 The current product development process showing the major stages and their outcomes.

requiring very precise manufacturing. They are also increasingly specific, insoluble, chemically vulnerable, and have poor membrane permeability. Thus, they must be delivered in much smaller doses and much more precisely, making product development and manufacturing significantly more difficult, and regulatory expectations much harder to meet. The net result of this rapid progress in drug discovery and this stagnation in process development is an industry where "developers are forced to use the tools of the last century to evaluate this century's advances" (Ref. 1, p. 4).

In the author's opinion, the situation just described is not an unavoidable consequence of the intrinsic complexity of pharmaceutical products. In fact, other industries with products that are equally complex (e.g., microelectronics) have developed and implemented predictive methods for product and process development, optimization, and control, capable of much higher quality standards (as defined by allowed variability in product functionality) than the pharmaceutical industry. Rather, current practices in the industry largely reflect two factors: the business model, which disproportionately rewarded introduction of new products over optimization of existing ones, and the regulatory framework that, for decades, has discouraged innovation and continuous improvement.

Fortunately, product and process development in the pharmaceutical industry appear to be entering a period of deep transformation, initially driven by recognition at FDA that a higher technological standard was a desirable and achievable goal, and fueled by an intense desire for improvement on the part of many industrial scientists and engineers.

Let us describe the desired future state of pharmaceutical product and process development by comparison to another industry: airplane construction. The design of an airplane begins by selection of its desired performance: We wish to build a device capable of flying at a given speed, carrying a given load, while optimizing cost (e.g., fuel consumption). The laws of aerodynamics are then invoked in developing predictive computer models, which are used to design and optimize the structure of the intended airplane *before a single piece is ever built*. A small-scale model is then constructed and tested under conditions that are predictive of the performance of the full-scale device (e.g., a wind tunnel operated under specifically selected conditions). Once theory is verified by experiment, the final product is built, and it performs as intended (or very close to it).

We would be hard pressed to accept a situation where airplane development was conducted by the methods used in 1903 by the Wright brothers, that is, by building many aircraft, all slightly different, and testing them in the field in order to select for subsequent use those that perform appropriately (i.e., those that did not crash). Yet, in essence, that is how pharmaceutical products are developed. At the present time, a formulation/manufacturing method is proposed, tried in the field, and retained if the product performs as intended; otherwise, it is slightly modified, tried again, and so on. A whole century of model-based product and process design has somehow gone largely unnoticed.

Far from being unique to the aerospace industry, model-based design and optimization is standard practice across a great many industries, including microelectronics, petrochemicals, automobiles, etc. All of these industries share four characteristics:

- Materials used to build products are well understood and their performance is predictable.
- The fundamental laws that govern product and process performance across scales are known, and have been articulated in the form of predictive mathematical models.
- Model-based methods for product and process design, optimization, and control have been developed and tested.
- A human resource skilled in the use of such methods has been developed and incorporated into organizational structures that take full advantage of their capabilities.

In the author's view, these four characteristics summarize the desired (and achievable) state of product and process design and development in the pharmaceutical industry. These views are largely espoused by the FDA (http://www.fda.gov/cder/gmp/gmp2004/GMP_finalreport2004.htm), which in recent regulatory language has defined "process understanding" (now accepted to be the central goal of the Process Analytical Technology Initiative) as *the ability to predict performance* (http://www.fda.gov/AboutFDA/CentersOffices/CDER/ucm088828.htm). Much has been said and written about the evolving regulatory views, and only a brief review is warranted here [for details, the reader is encouraged to visit the FDA website (http://www.fda.gov) and review the documentation posted there].

Process Analytical Technologies (PAT) and Quality by Design (QbD) are intimately linked subjects, and have been intertwined (in a sometimes confusing manner) both in the discussion and in the documentation put forward by regulatory bodies. In its simplest form, PAT is a collection of tools (sensors, analyzers, data analysis software) that enables the monitoring of process variables. These tools can be used to determine the state of the process, or its completion, both in batch and in continuous modes. However, in order to use PAT tools in an effective manner, we usually need to answer three questions:

1. What to measure?
2. What does the measurement mean?
3. What do we do with the results?

The answer to the first two questions requires determining which material attributes and process parameters are critical to product quality and performance. The answer to the last question, pro forma, is to use the results to manage variability and maximize product quality and process performance. This requires development of sufficient understanding about the process to enable formulation of a control policy, so that the process can be operated flexibly and purposefully to minimize the impact of variability sources on product quality. In fact, QbD can be defined as both the process used to answer these three questions and the implemented outcome. In this context, QbD, a model-driven approach to process design, is clearly enabled by PAT tools.

It has taken the pharmaceutical sciences community a bit over half a decade to develop these definitions. The evolution of events and guidance documents underlying PAT and QbD is shown in Figure 4, which displays a chart often used by FDA. While discussions about model-based design of pharmaceutical products and processes go back several decades, attention on the need to upgrade design methods was brought into sharp focus by publication of the Critical Path Initiative strategic plan in 2004, which outlined the need to transcend empirical methods and incorporate model-based design and optimization for both products and processes. This document was shortly followed by the PAT guidance, which provided many stepping stones,

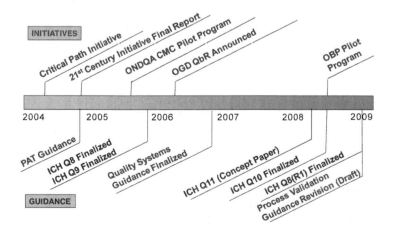

FIGURE 4 A chronological chart of main initiatives and guidance documents related to PAT and QbD. *Source*: From http://www.FDA.gov.

including an articulation of the purpose of such tools (real-time quality assurance) and the framework for their integration into development and manufacturing (predictive product design, leading to closed loop process control).

Events unfolded quickly after the PAT guidance was released. The Office of New Drug Quality Assurance launched a pilot program for application of QbD methods and PAT tools to both new and existing products that attracted nine original and three supplemental New Drug Applications (3), 11 of which were subsequently approved. The same year, the International Conference on Harmonization (ICH) (http://www.ich.org) issued two major guidelines: (*i*) ICH Q8, which focuses on the applications of QbD principles to pharmaceutical development, introduced important concepts such as design space. This guideline was later revised in 2009 to provide examples and more terse definitions. (*ii*) ICH Q9, which emphasizes quality risk management, introduced additional tools, and provided a formal framework for risk identification, evaluation, acceptance, and management. These guidelines were followed by several additional FDA guidance documents and by another ICH guideline, ICH Q10, which was issued in Europe in 2008 and adopted in the United States in 2009 and which emphasizes implementation of quality systems across the life cycle of a pharmaceutical product.

Meanwhile, companies continued to incorporate QbD and PAT methods into submissions. Following the pilot program, over 30 additional applications (original and supplemental NDAs and INDs) had been submitted to FDA incorporating QbD methodologies, many of which had been approved by late 2009. Reflecting a broadening of the initiative, the FDA announced a new QbD pilot program through the Office of Biotechnology Products.

At the time of this writing, most major pharmaceutical companies based in the United States and Europe have implemented efforts to incorporate PAT tools into development and manufacturing, and many of them have launched in-house programs seeking to develop expertise in QbD. Hardly a month goes by without a workshop or a conference on this topic, and major conferences (IFPAC, ISPE, AIChE, AAPS, FIP) now routinely devote large sections of their program to QbD and PAT. In fact, to a very large extent, QbD has become part of the standard lexicon in product development and process design, and the use of these tools and methods is quickly propagating to smaller pharmaceutical companies, generic drug manufacturers, contract manufacturers, and throughout academia.

In the remainder of this chapter, we focus on providing an engineering perspective for achieving the above-mentioned desired state. The chapter is organized as follows: First, to establish a common language, we define some common terms from both a pharmaceutical and an engineering perspective. Subsequently, we review model-based design and optimization as a framework for product and process development and optimization, process scale-up, and continuous improvement activities. The role of PAT methods and principles in this framework is discussed. Finally, the main areas requiring effort are identified.

MODEL-BASED OPTIMIZATION

Certain engineering terms are often used in industrial pharmacy practice with a loose meaning, generating significant confusion. Consider, for example, the term "optimization," which in industrial pharmacy often refers to the practice of examining process performance empirically, for a small set of parameter values often chosen based on experience (such as three different blending times) and then selecting the value that gives the results that are deemed most adequate. The choice is often made without resorting to statistical comparison of results. "Scale-up" refers to a process development stage (Fig. 3) where the process recipe is carried out in larger equipment, and scale equivalence is "established" by demonstrating the ability to manufacture adequate product. A process is said to be "in control" when it is possible to make many batches of product within specification.

To an engineer, these terms have radically different meanings. Optimization is the use of a predictive model to determine the best possible design of a product, or the best possible operating condition for a process. To find "the best," the *design space* (the permissible region of parameters given technical, regulatory, or economic constraints) is identified. A quantitative target function describing the property to be optimized is developed. The target function can be a single performance attribute (quality, technical performance, profit) or a combination of multiple parameters after they are assigned a given weight. Once the design space and the target function are known, the absolute minimum (or maximum) of this function is found (Fig. 5).

Typically, the optimization process is conducted in iterative fashion (Fig. 6), beginning with the development of a model of the process. The model can be statistical (4) or mathematical. In early stages of product or process design, relatively little is known, and only a preliminary version of the model can be developed. A "first-pass" optimization exercise is conducted. Model predictions are compared with actual performance and results are used to improve the model itself. Results are also used to refine knowledge about design space boundaries. The more refined model is used to generate higher quality performance predictions, which are again used to predict an optimum operating regime. Comparison of prediction and practical observations are used to further improve the model, the target function, and the design space. The process continues ad infinitum following a virtuous cycle that leads to ever better predictive power.

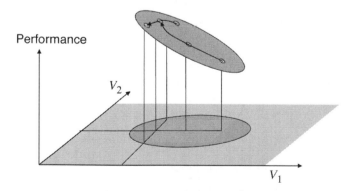

FIGURE 5 Schematic of the model-based optimization process, where performance depends on two variables (V_1 and V_2). Model-based methods would explore the entire oval domain, seeking the "global best." Common OVAT practices only explore a few points along orthogonal trajectories.

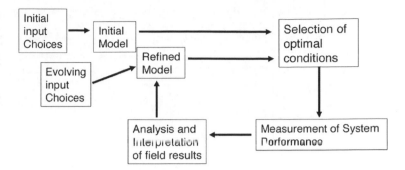

FIGURE 6 The iterative optimization process. An initial model is developed, used to predict process performance, tested by comparison with experiment, refined, and used to improve prediction. The process naturally accommodates changes in economic or regulatory constraints.

Since economic conditions, process capabilities, and regulatory require-ments change over time, both the design space and the target function are dynamic structures, and the optimum product or process design, in fact, a moving target. Model-based optimization is ideally suited to respond to these dynamics. Once a high-quality model is available, the change in conditions can be incorporated into the process, and a new iteration along the virtuous cycle is performed to generate the new selection of optimum processing conditions.

Oil refining is perhaps the best-developed example of a process operated in this "continuous optimization mode." A refinery receives a different mixture of petroleum every day, and the prices of its various products fluctuate continuously. Exquisite knowledge of the process is used to determine the precise conditions (temperatures, pressures, recycle rates, etc.) that would product the optimum product mix for the available raw materials and market conditions. As the factory is operated, model predictions are compared to actual performance, and deviations are used to *optimize model performance.*

True optimization process can be challenging. The design space can be a complex, irregularly shaped region (or set of disconnected regions) in an *n*-dimensional space. The target function can have local minima that can "trap" the trajectory of the solution-seeking algorithm. To avoid such "non-convex" situations, searching algorithms have been developed that incorporate a certain measure of randomization in the sequential selection of process conditions to be examined. Ample literature exists on the topic and is not reviewed here in the interest of brevity, for an introduction, see Refs. 5 and 6.

Current practices in industrial pharmacy can now be put in perspective. Typically, the method of choice is univariate (OVAT, "one variable at a time"). One variable is examined for a few conditions, which, in practice, are selected within a "safe" subset of the permissible design space. A value of this parameter is selected and kept subsequently constant. Another variable is then examined, a value is chosen, and the process continues sequentially. Unless the target function is essentially a plane, if the end result is anywhere near the global optimum, is only by chance. A historical reason for this dated practice is that the regulatory framework greatly discouraged implementation of the virtuous cycle mentioned above, which is the heart of the optimization process. Once a process was approved, the cost of implementing improvements (and the risk of examining process performance outside approved sets of parameters) were simply too high. As a result, while the rest of the industrial world embarked in wave after wave of quality revolutions, pharmaceutical process development practices stayed frozen in decades-old paradigms from a time before computer models.

PROCESS SCALE-UP

Development of PAT approaches for process scale-up is likely to take place at several levels. At the conceptually simplest level, PAT presupposes the development of sensing instruments capable of monitoring process attributes online and in real time. Once the analytical method is validated for accuracy at the laboratory scale, it can be used to obtain extensive information of process performance (blend homogeneity, granulation particle size distribution, moisture content) under various conditions (blender speed, mixing time, drying air temperature, humidity, and volume, etc.). Statistical models can then be used to relate the observable variables to other performance attributes (e.g., tablet hardness, content uniformity, and dissolution) in order to determine ranges of measured values that are predictive of acceptable performance.

Typically, for batch processes such as blending or drying, this entails the determination of process end-point attributes. The PAT method then becomes the centerpiece of the scale-up effort. Process scale-up can be undertaken under the assumption that the relationships between observables and performance are independent of scale, and if this assumption is verified in practice, the manufacturing process in full scale can be monitored (typically, to completion), providing a higher level of assurance that the product is likely to be within compliance.

For continuous or semicontinuous processes (such as tablet compression), the main role of PAT methods is not process end-point determination, rather it is to serve as a component of a feedback or feed-forward control strategy devoted to keeping process (and product) performance within the desired range along the life of the process. This is conceptually more complex and requires a greater level of predictive understanding regarding the dynamic effect of controlled variables on performance attributes (see later in the chapter). However, once the development of suitable controls is achieved, scale-up itself is greatly simplified for continuous (or semicontinuous) processes, typically involving running the process for longer times.

At a more sophisticated level of articulation, PAT will involve the use of analytical methods, coupled with modeling approaches, to develop models capable of predicting quantitatively the relationship between input parameters (raw materials properties, process parameters, environmental inputs) and product performance. In the author's opinion, this is the true definition of "process understanding." On an early stage, models can be statistical (correlation-based), seeking only to determine directional relationships and covariances. Over time, predictive mathematical models can be developed, once mechanistic relationships between inputs and outputs are established.

Predictive models make it possible to perform true process scale-up, which consists of the use of a predictive model to find quantitative criteria for establishing process similarity across scales. The model is also used to determine the changes in both the design space and the target function across scales, and to predict optimum conditions of manufacturing facilities yet to be built.

Even more, a predictive model allows the designer to explore beforehand the effect of uncertainty in raw material properties, market conditions, and regulatory constraints, thus making it possible to design flexible manufacturing systems that have built-in capabilities for accommodating changing conditions. The methodology, known as "design under uncertainty" is currently an active area of research in the systems engineering community.

PROCESS CONTROL

As mentioned above, process controls entails monitoring a process continuously, and whenever necessary, taking corrective action (by acting on controlled variables) in order to keep the system under control. While a large number of control strategies have been developed and studied (7,8), in essence, all control systems involve the same components (Fig. 7): (*i*) instrumentation capable of measuring on-line, in real time, the values of controlled variables, input parameters (e.g., environmental variables, process inputs), and process conditions; (*ii*) a set of specifications for the desired process conditions; (*iii*) a predictive model describing the effect of controlled variables on process conditions; and (*iv*) a control policy prescribing the manner in which controlled variables must be modified in response to measured deviations in either input parameters or process conditions.

Two main control schemes exist: feedback control and feed-forward control (Fig. 7). In feedback control (by far the most common), system performance is monitored, deviations from desired conditions are quantified, and controlled variables are modified to return the system to the desired state. In feed-forward control, process inputs are monitored. As they deviate from desired values, their effect on the system is predicted, and controlled variables are modified to minimize their effect. Feedback control is "safer," since it guarantees performance by controlling it directly, but it is also slower: corrective action is taken

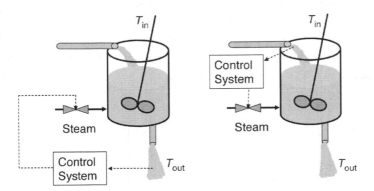

FIGURE 7 Schematic of a control system, using a stirred tank as an example. A stream enters the tank at temperature T_{in}. The system is designed to maintain the exit temperature at T_{out}. In a feedback mode, the exiting temperature is measured, and the steam feed is opened or closed as necessary. T_{out} is known, but the effects of variability are corrected only after they have entered the system. In a feed-forward mode, the incoming temperature is measured and the steam feed is modified to prevent its variability from entering the system. However, T_{out} is unknown.

only after the perturbation has affected process performance. Feed-forward control is faster: it acts on input deviations as soon as they are detected. However, it is riskier: if the detected deviation is a measurement error, the control system will purposefully move the system *away* from the desired set point.

It is apparent that a predictive model is the hearth of a control algorithm. Unless the relationship between process inputs and process performance is known, deviations can be detected, but effective corrective action cannot be taken. However, fast, error-free monitoring is also essential: unless inputs and state variables can be quickly and accurately quantified, the control system is blind and devoid of value.

As with scale-up, two levels of implementation are possible. The first level only entails the ability to sense and a directional characterization of the effect of variables. PAT methods can be extremely effective for this purpose by generating large datasets of process inputs and outputs that can then be correlated to generate statistical or polynomial control models. Provided that (*i*) deviations from desired set points are small, (*ii*) interactions between inputs are weak, and (*iii*) the response surface does not depart too much from linearity, such systems can provide the basis of an initial effort to control a system.

However, for many systems, more sophisticated control systems capable of overcoming these restrictions are likely to be desirable. To develop such systems, we need to expand the predictive models mentioned above to incorporate the "dynamic" effects of input, control, and process variables. The model needs to be able to answer questions such as how quickly do deviations in input conditions propagate through the system, how does the system respond over time under different control policies, what is the effect of lags in sensing and responding. The control system, itself, becomes part of these dynamics: depending on the control policy, the response of the system as a whole will be different. Moreover, the model can be used to optimize the control system by allowing the user to determine what the optimum number and location of the sensing points are, what the ideal control policy for a given system is, etc. Since lags, capacities, and propagation rates are almost always scale-dependent, the control system developed under laboratory conditions needs to be adjusted in the scaled-up version of the system. The outcome, however, is highly desirable: a system where variability sources are known, understood, and managed.

CONCLUSIONS

This brief chapter summarized some of the main roles of PAT for process optimization, scale-up, and control. In the author's view, the development of models capable of predicting the effects of raw material properties and process parameters on process performance is not only desirable but also a highly necessary condition for the development of modern approaches for optimal design and control of manufacturing processes. Given the complexity and diversity of materials and products and the tight quality requirements, the task might appear to be daunting. However, it is an achievable task, as demonstrated by the daily track record of other industries that deal with highly complex products and processes. An important reason is that generic process models usually only need to be developed once: the better the model, the more universal it is.

Arguably, given its immediate and direct impact on public health, the pharmaceutical industry has additional reasons to achieve a higher level of technological execution, where product quality is assured by effective automated systems and where variability sources are understood and minimized. Even removing this motivation, industry should embrace model-based optimization enthusiastically, since it has reduced cost and accelerated product development across many industries.

In the last five years, recognition of the need to achieve the goals described here has motivated an active dialogue between regulatory agencies, pharmaceutical companies, and academia. A recognition is emerging that sustained efforts and substantial resources will be needed in years to come. It is also becoming clear that the path ahead is no longer optional: a consensus has emerged that the state of the art is inadequate, and that positive change is possible.

An important final thought is that substantial efforts need to be given to the development of properly trained human resources both at companies and at regulatory agencies. Application of the methods mentioned in this chapter requires a substantial level of expertise that has not been part of the traditional training of industrial pharmacists and chemists, and engineers have, by and large, not been integrated into product development teams at companies or in regulatory bodies.

REFERENCES

1. FDA. Challenge and Opportunity on the Critical Path to New Medical Products, 2004. http://www.fda.gov/downloads/Drugs/ScienceResearch/ResearchAreas/ucm079290.pdf
2. Muzzio FJ, Shinbrot T, Glasser BJ. Powder technology in the pharmaceutical industry: the need to catch up fast. Powder Technol 2002; 124:1–7.
3. Winkle HN. Quality by Design (QbD) and Process Analytical Technologies (PAT): Current Status and Future Direction. IFPAC Program, 2010.
4. Hicks CR, Turner KV. Fundamental Concepts in the Design of Experiments. New York: Oxford University Press, 1999.
5. Horst R, Pardalos PM, Nguyen Van Thoai. Introduction to Global Optimization. New York: Springer-Verlag, 1995.
6. Floudas CA, Pardalos PM. A Collection of Test Problems for Constrained Global Optimization Algorithms. New York: Springer-Verlag, 1990.
7. Stephanopoulos G. Chemical Process Control. Englewood Cliffs, NJ: Prentice Hall, 1984.
8. Marlin TE. Process Control: Designing Processes and Control Systems for Dynamic Performance. New York: McGraw-Hill, 1995.

3   Understanding scale-up and quality risks on the interface between primary and secondary development

Frans L. Muller, Kathryn A. Gray, and Graham E. Robinson

INTRODUCTION: THE DEVELOPMENT OF MEDICINES

The development of a new drug product based on a new molecule or a "new chemical entity" (NCE) starts with the discovery of the molecule's activity. Once preclinical testing has indicated the drug's safety and toxicity levels, companies can file a Notice of Claimed Investigational Exemption for a New Drug (or IND) with the FDA to start clinical trials. Clinical trials are typically done in three phases[a] (1):

- Phase 1: Aims to ascertain the highest dose level that can be tolerated. This is usually done in tens of healthy volunteers, or volunteers with the target disease if potential side effects are severe.
- Phase 2: Aims to establish the efficacy of the drug and monitor side effects. These trials typically include hundreds of volunteers who have the disease. The patients are split in groups and given licensed drugs, a placebo, or a new drug. These are "blinded" trials in which the patient is not aware which medication is given.
- Phase 3: Aims to demonstrate unequivocally that the new drug successfully treats or improves the treatment of patients. This typically involves thousands of patients (although this does depend on the disease area), and neither the doctor nor the patient will know what treatment is given (a so-called "double-blinded" trial).

Before a clinical phase can start, animal toxicity studies need to be completed to give confidence that the drug is safe for the period of the trial in humans. Long-term carcinogenic effects and effects on reproduction are also studied. In addition, companies also need to demonstrate that the drug product is stable for the duration of the trial. It can take anywhere from four to six years to complete the clinical trials phases. If successful the company will file a New Drug Application (NDA) with the FDA. The total cost of bringing an NCE to market is estimated by DiMasi et al. (2) at about $800M but this is now seen as a low estimate (3).

Medicine development, in the context of this chapter, is defined as the development required to convert an NCE, that is, a molecule, into a drug product that is suitable to treat patients and can be manufactured consistently and economically. The key steps of medicine development are (*i*) the identification of a suitable physical form of the drug substance (DS, also referred to as the "active pharmaceutical ingredient," or API); (*ii*) the design of processes to generate the drug substance; (*iii*) the design of the drug product (DP or "formulation"); and finally (*iv*) the drug product–manufacturing process.

---

[a] There is a phase 4, which starts after the drug enters the market and is based on the monitoring of adverse events.

The development teams also support the submissions of IND and NDAs. They generate the DS and DP quantities required for development and clinical trials and, on a successful submission, they will transfer the processes to manufacturing departments, or external suppliers (4). Suresh and Basu (3) estimate the development of the drug product to be 30% to 35% of the total cost of bringing a drug to market. From their work it may be concluded that more efficient, science-based medicine development will improve the quality of pharmaceuticals manufactured and significantly reduce time to market, the cost of new drug development, and the manufacturing cost.

Clearly, development, clinical trials and toxicological studies have interwoven timelines. Figure 1 shows a typical series of activities for the development of DS and DP and the quantity of drug substance generated is overlaid on the clinical trials and safety studies (see for instance Ref. 4). At the bottom of the figure is the relative number of compounds present at that stage of development to demonstrate the degree of attrition of potential NCEs. Different companies will have different names for the development activities (5), and the time at which the activities are executed may vary depending on the development model of the company (6).

Early in development, DS and DP quantities required are small. Since at the end of phase 1 a significant number of potential NCEs will have failed, minimizing cost and time are important. The focus in development here is often on manufacturing trial quantities that are "fit for purpose." As development proceeds, the focus shifts from manufacture to process and product design. Decisions taken early on in development can have a wide-ranging impact on the final drug product; for example, physical form is important to bioavailability as well as long-term DP physical stability (7,8), and the chemical route selection is important to the nature of the impurities in the DP as well as to the cost and sustainability of the DS.

After these key decisions are made, the focus shifts to understanding, design, scale-up, and optimization of processes that must provide the required quality and stability while being cost efficient and environmentally acceptable. These processes are manufactured at ever-increasing scale to keep up with the demands of clinical trials as well as the development community; formulation scale-up can use up large quantities of drug substance.

In the last stages of development, the focus shifts to *control* of the product quality. Here, the sensitivity of the DS and DP quality to changes in process parameters (e.g., composition, temperature, time, etc.) is established. The aim is to demonstrate in the NDA that the drug product is effective and safe to the patient. This is especially difficult for metastable, or kinetically stabilized, drug products, for which small parameter changes can cause large changes toward a thermodynamically more stable state. The development aspects of the drug substance manufacture are described in more detail in section "DS Development."

From the above, it may be clear that there are important interactions between the development of DS and DP (also known as primary and secondary development). The fact that development of a DP represents 30% to 35% of the total NCE project cost means that problems arising from changes in drug substance processes or raw materials can have a significant impact on a project (3).

We found that the risk assessment of manufacturing processes can be very successful in helping development teams to focus their efforts on key issues. We introduced risk assessment for a variety of reasons. In early development, it was driven by the aim to bring "large-scale thinking" upstream in development, and

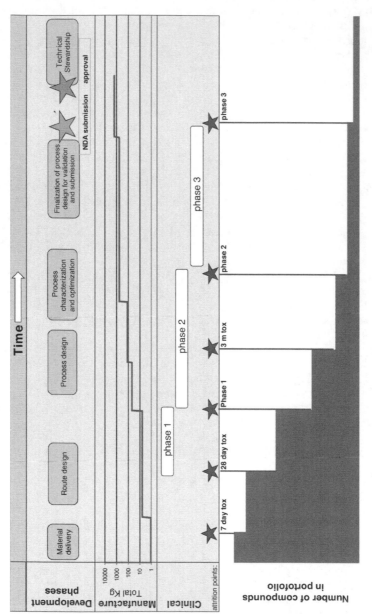

FIGURE 1 Lining up clinical trials, attrition, and process development.

reduce scale-up issues by anticipating them early in development and resolving the issues by closer collaboration between process engineers and process chemists.

Later in development, quality risk assessments (QRAs) are a fundamental aspect of "Quality by Design" (QbD) (9).

This chapter describes the application of risk assessment on manufacturing processes. In section "The Principles of Risk Assessment in Development," the general principles of risk assessment (RA) are discussed. The key risks in medicine development impact on the critical quality attributes (CQAs), the more common drug products CQAs are reviewed in section "The Interface Between Primary and Secondary Development: CQAs." An overview of primary development is given in section "DS Development" to understand which DS development activities impact on DP development and at what stage of development they are likely to do so. This is followed by a discussion on the generation of scenarios and assessing their likelihood. Finally, we give two examples of risk assessment processes that have been applied in AstraZeneca.

THE PRINCIPLES OF RISK ASSESSMENT IN DEVELOPMENT

For all types of organizations, there is a need to understand the risks being taken when seeking to achieve a particular objective. Organizations need to understand the overall level of risk within their processes and activities to develop cost-effective development programs resulting ultimately in successful products and processes. Individuals inherently think in risk terms, however often two people would have a different view of the risks involved in a particular activity. Actively applying risk management techniques allow the development teams to build a collective view of risk that can be communicated.

ICH Q9 (9) describes risk management as a systematic process for the assessment, control, communication, and review of risks (to the quality of the drug product) across the product life cycle. Although this description was specifically developed for pharmaceutical products, it is applicable to all risk management processes. Risk management can typically be considered to involve three steps:

1. Risk assessment—the identification and evaluation of risk
2. Risk control—the prioritization and mitigation of risks followed by the acceptance of residual risk
3. Risk review—review through the life cycle of the product or process to take in to consideration new information/knowledge

Figure 2 gives an overview of risk management used by ICH Q9 and in a range of other literature sources.

The first step in risk management is risk assessment. This is the act of asking three questions: (*i*) What can go wrong? (*ii*) What are the consequences if it goes wrong? and (*iii*) How likely is to go wrong? Over the last century, a wide range of risk assessment techniques have been developed, some examples are given below:

- Failure mode and effect analysis (FMEA) was developed in the 1940s by the U.S. armed forces (10). It seeks to identify cause and effect relationships to help prevent quality problems. This process is often combined with criticality analysis (FMECA) to consider the probability, severity, and detectability of each failure occurring.

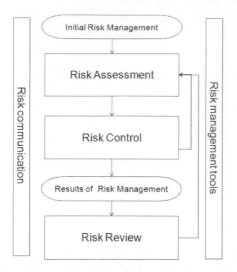

FIGURE 2 High-level description of the important elements of a risk management protocol.

- In chemical industries, hazard and operability (HAZOP) studies were introduced during the 1960s by Imperial Chemical Industries (ICI) as a structured methodology for understanding how a process may deviate from the desired outcome (11) It was designed to improve the safety of increasingly complex and hazardous process plants.
- Potential problem analysis is a technique developed by Kepner and Tregoe (12) and published in their book the new rational manager. It provides a general tool for considering the risks and opportunities facing an organization.

The above processes are similar in that the answer to question (*i*) results in identification of risk scenarios, question (*ii*) leads to evaluation of the scale of the impact, and question (*iii*) gives an idea of the frequency things will go wrong. Typically, the *risk* is considered high if both the impact is severe and the likelihood is high.

The use of risk management in the pharmaceutical industry is not new, but the industry has been slow to adopt some of the formal risk management techniques especially in their application to managing the drug development process and in particular the development of efficient and effective drug substance and drug product–manufacturing processes. With the advent of QbD philosophies and in particular ICHQ9, the use of risk management is becoming an increasingly important aspect of pharmaceutical development.

When to Do Risk Assessment

The development of pharmaceutical processes has a range of drivers: patient safety, manufacturability, and cost. In each of these areas, risk management provides a valuable tool to understand important areas and develop control measures. It allows efficient prioritization of resources and a means to communicate issues outside the project team. The approach and level of rigor should be balanced with the stage of development and level of risk.

In phase 1, prior knowledge and experience can be used to assess risks and opportunities associated with the intrinsic properties of the API, to aid formulation selection or chose the best synthetic route.

During development for phase 2, the level of process understanding will increase. As discussed in section "The Interface between Primary and Secondary Development: CQAs," it is during this phase that the first scale-up to pilot plant manufacture will occur. Risk assessment provides a valuable tool to consider the unexpected events that may occur during the scale-up, which present a risk to achieving the desired yield, quality, or cycle time.

In the later stages of process development (during phase 3), process development resources are focused on preparing the process for transfer from development to the commercial supply organization and finalizing documentation for regulatory submissions. At this stage, risk assessment facilitates knowledge transfer and can support change control in manufacturing.

How to Generate the Risk Assessment Document

All risk assessment techniques require a rigorous application of a systematic process. To be effective, the risk assessment team should have an appropriate breadth and depth of knowledge, skills, and experience. An independent facilitator is required to ensure that the risk assessment process is followed and avoid the temptation to try to resolve or mitigate risks within the assessment meeting. A generic list of team roles are given below:

- Leader/facilitator—provides knowledge of the risk assessment process and has sufficient general technical experience of the subject being studied to chair the meeting
- Recorder—records the risk scenarios and assessment
- Designer—provides detailed knowledge of the process being studied
- User—advises on operational matters
- Expert—independent person with knowledge and experience in the field of study

The first step in the process is to identify risks scenarios. Each scenario is then assessed to consider the likelihood of the risk being realized and severity of its impact. A structured identification process and the use of an agreed set of guide words increase the number of scenarios. A well-designed risk assessment process, with the right people will thus reduce the possibility that an important risk is missed.

As the risks are identified, they should be recorded in a standard format. This can be done using basic tables or by using a more complex knowledge management tool.

Using the Risk Assessment Document in Development

Once the risk scenarios have been generated and assessed mitigation work should be prioritized on the basis of the magnitude of the risk, the project strategy, and the optimized use of project resources.

Early in development, work packages are likely to focus on areas of the process where risk assessment has identified limited knowledge. The aim of this is to improve understanding and remove potential risks. As process knowledge increases, the focus of mitigation work is likely to involve reducing the severity of risks by designing in steps, which act as risk mitigation, for example, additional purification steps.

Where risks cannot be removed or reduced, control strategies must be developed to reduce the residual risk. This may be through introducing tests to ensure desired conditions are met or by improving plant control systems to ensure the process stays within defined boundaries.

At each stage the risk assessment should be updated and the residual risk considered to decide if further risk mitigation is required.

At technology transfer, the risk assessment document should be transferred to the commercial manufacturer along with the other project documentation. It provides a valuable tool when changes to the process are considered and must be updated as further process knowledge is gained.

THE INTERFACE BETWEEN PRIMARY AND SECONDARY DEVELOPMENT: CQAS

The tangible aspect of the interactions between primary and secondary manufacture is clearly the API, now also frequently referred to as the drug substance. Clearly, there are aspects of the physical and chemical properties of the drug substance that impact on the formulation manufacturing processes, or even the safety or effectiveness of the final medicine, or drug product. As a result, the final quality of a medicine is a function of both the primary and secondary processes and manufacturing. In this section, we focus on the aspects of the quality that are commonly impacted by drug substance. The focus is on small-molecule manufacture and excludes biological drug substances.

Definition of "Critical Quality Attribute"

Woodstock (13) defines "pharmaceutical quality" as a drug product that is free of contamination and reproducibly delivers patients the clinical performance as promised on the label. Clearly, a change that poses a risk of a reduction in pharmaceutical quality is a risk to the patient taking the medicine. Lionberger et al. (14) review the QbD concept. They explain how pharmaceutical quality is captured with a target product profile[b] (TPP) that summarizes the patient needs and the contents of the label. As the TPP is a predominately a qualitative document, a target product quality profile[c] (TPQP) is required to describe measurements that provide quantitative information, which can be related to the safety and efficacy of the medicine. Examples of such measurements are chemical analysis, dissolution tests, and stability tests; note that the TPQP is not a "specification" as it also includes efficacy and stability measurements.

With the TPQP is established, development teams can evaluate how changes in the drug product impact on the pharmaceutical quality. Whereas some aspects of the drug product do not need to be controlled, some others may need to be kept within a certain range. Those drug substance or product properties and characteristics that require control or limits are typically described as CQA[d]. Lionberger et al. (14) (Fig. 3) point out that the interpretation of the term CQA does vary rather widely in literature; for example, some authors would define "particle size" as a

---

[b] The ICH guideline Q8(R2) (15) refers to it as the quality target product profile (QTPP).
[c] The International Society for Pharmaceutical Engineers (ISPE) Product Quality Lifecycle Implementation (PQLI) refers to a pharmaceutical target product profile (PTPP, see Ref. 14).
[d] In ICH Q8(R2) (15), a CQA is defined as follows: "A CQA is a physical, chemical, biological, or microbiological property or characteristic that should be within an appropriate limit, range, or distribution to ensure the desired product quality. CQAs are generally associated with the drug substance, excipients, intermediates (in-process materials), and drug product."

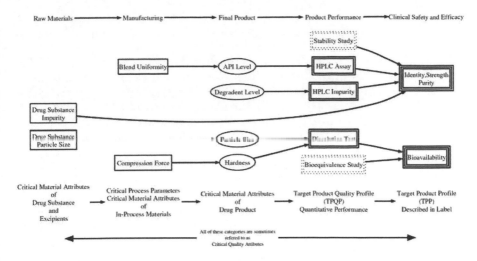

FIGURE 3 An overview of how pharmaceutical quality is linked to materials and manufacturing processes. *Source*: From Ref. 14.

CQA, while others would define the outcome of a "dissolution test" as the relevant CQA. They suggest that critical material attributes (CMAs), that is, directly measurable aspects of drug substance or product, could be used to identify the manufacturing goals. Particle size, hardness, and chemical purity are examples of such CMAs, but a dissolution test would not be considered a CMA.

Although the use of the term CMA is a useful distinction between independent material properties and test evaluations that depend on a range of those properties, here we will continue to use the term CQA in-line with the ICH Q8 (15) definition to describe aspects of the drug substance and product that need to be controlled or limited to ensure pharmaceutical quality.

Common Drug Substance CQAs

Early in development, the understanding of the outcome of measurements in the TPQP cannot yet be correlated to the pharmaceutical quality. As a result, early in development, the CQAs cannot yet be identified with certainty. The ICH guideline Q6A (16) identifies, however, characteristics of the drug substance that universally need to be tested, as well as characteristics that may be relevant to the quality of the drug substance and/or drug product. Ganzer et al. (17) suggests that the characteristics identified in Q6A represent common CQAs for a drug substance. Following his suggestion allows the development team to identify "potential CQAs" (i.e., aspects of the drug substance or product for which lack of control or limits is likely to have an impact on the pharmaceutical quality). These potential CQAs can be groups in three distinct categories:

CQA Related to the Drug Substance's Chemical Composition

- *Identification:* The chemical structure of the drug substance should be confirmed by a method that is specific to the drug substance, for example, infrared spectroscopy. Identification solely by a single chromatographic retention time.

- *Assay:* The content of the new drug substance must be determined.
- *Chiral purity*: Where a new drug substance is predominantly one enantiomer, the opposite enantiomer is excluded from the qualification and identification thresholds given in the ICH guidelines on Impurities in New Drug Substances and Impurities in New Drug Products because of practical difficulties in quantifying it at those levels. However, that impurity in the chiral new drug substance and the resulting new drug product(s) should otherwise be treated according to the principles established in those guidelines.
- *Impurities:* Organic impurities, degradation products, materials extracted from equipment or containers, and residual solvents are included in this category.
- *Inorganic impurities:* The need testing for inorganic impurities (e.g., catalysts, salts) should be evaluated during development and based on knowledge of the manufacturing process.
- *Water content:* This test is important in cases where the new drug substance is known to be hygroscopic or degraded by moisture or when the drug substance is known to be a stoichiometric hydrate.

CQA Related to the Drug Substance's Physical Properties

- *Description*: A qualitative statement about the state (e.g., solid, liquid) and color of the drug substance. If the description of the drug substance changes during storage, action is required.
- *Polymorphic forms:* Some new drug substances exist in different crystalline forms that differ in their physical properties. Polymorphism may also include solvation or hydration products (also known as pseudopolymorphs) and amorphous forms. Differences in these forms could, in some cases, affect the quality or performance of the new drug products (7,8). The appropriate solid state should be specified for cases where differences exist, which have been shown to affect drug product performance, bioavailability, or stability.

  It is generally technically very difficult to measure polymorphic changes in drug products. Polymorph content should only be tested for as a last resort. A surrogate test like dissolution could be used to monitor product performance.
- *Particle size*: Particle size can have a significant effect on dissolution rates, bioavailability, and/or stability.
- *Physicochemical properties:* These are properties such as pH of an aqueous solution, melting point/range, and refractive index.

CQA Related to the Drug Substance's Biological Composition

- *Microbial limits:* There may be a need to specify the total count of aerobic microorganisms, the total count of yeasts and moulds, and the absence of specific objectionable bacteria (e.g., *Staphylococcus aureus, Escherichia coli, Salmonella, Pseudomonas aeruginosa*).

DRUG SUBSTANCE DEVELOPMENT

To understand the impact of development on the DS CQAs, we discuss the development process. First of all, it should be stated that the key outputs of the development process are as follows:

1. An efficient, robust manufacturing process that delivers DS fit for formulation and with no residual risk to the patient.

2. Demonstrated control of CQAs on implementation of a manufacturing process.
3. Manufacture of material for testing and generation of the associated documentation that will support regulatory submission.

For clarity, it is worth defining the terms process and route as used in the context of DS manufacture:

- A process is a sequence of unit operations that are necessary to achieve a chemical transformation and isolate the product (e.g., formation of an amido, hydrolysis of an ester, reduction of a ketone). A process normally comprises several sections: the chemical reaction itself (this involves mixing reactants and reagents, usually in a solvent, and causing them to react), the workup and isolation (this can involve extraction, pH adjustment, precipitation, or distillation), and the purification (this is normally achieved by crystallization or distillation but in exceptional circumstances might require chromatography). It is worth noting that the chemical reaction usually occupies a relatively small proportion of the overall processing time.
- A route (or synthetic route) is a sequence of chemical transformations that will produce the DS. Depending on the complexity of the DS molecule, the number of separate chemical transformations required can vary considerably. The number of synthetic steps in a route depends on the commercial availability of suitable starting materials. It is not uncommon for a synthetic route to contain 10 to 20 chemical transformations. It can be advantageous to avoid some isolations by telescoping two or more sequential chemical transformations into a single process. This strategy saves valuable processing time and can avoid safety health and environment (SHE) issues (exposure of the chemist or operator to toxic intermediates or potent sensitizers) but the approach can be risky if the chemistry is not well understood and yield or quality is not reproducible. For these reasons, in the early stages of development it is generally advisable to isolate the product from every chemical transformation in a synthesis. This allows the quality of each intermediate to be assessed before use in the next stage and ensures components present in a reaction mixture do not interfere with the chemistry in the next stage.

Skills and People Involved
The successful development of manufacturing processes for DS can only be achieved through a multidisciplinary effort involving process chemists (PCs), analytical chemists (ACs), process engineers (PEs), development manufacturing (DM) personnel, and chemical hazard (CH) experts. In early manufacturing campaigns, the approach is likely to be dominated by PC resource because of the rapidly evolving nature of the chemistry, but as the development progresses, other functions play an increasingly important role (18).

Overview
The amount of DS required to support toxicity, formulation, and clinical studies escalates significantly throughout the course of development. Manufacture takes place in a series of campaigns. The size (in kilos) of a particular campaign can vary considerably depending on the development model being followed, the nature of the drug indication, the potency of the drug, and its toxicity profile.

The nature of the DP formulation can also affect the requirement for DS. Typical DS campaign sizes might be as follows:

- Campaign 1: about 100 g for preclinical use only
- Campaign 2: about 5 kg for preclinical and phase 1 clinical studies
- Campaign 3: about 50 kg for toxicity and phase 2 clinical studies
- Campaign 4: about 500 kg for toxicity and phase 3 clinical studies
- Campaign 5: about 500 kg for further phase 3 clinical studies and pivotal stability studies
- Technology transfer campaign: several batches at manufacturing scale to establish the processes in the final manufacturing plant
- Validation campaign: three consecutive batches at manufacturing scale to validate the processes and supply launch stocks of DS

The timescale required to complete these manufacturing campaigns depends on several key factors: the availability of suitable starting materials and reagents, the level of difficulty of the chemistry, the availability of resources (people and equipment). In addition to the time required for procurement of starting materials and operation of the chemical processes, time must also be allowed for particle size reduction and analysis of the DS. Campaigns 1 and 2 are undertaken in glassware (up to 100 L). Because of the undeveloped nature of the processes a significant degree of flexibility in approach, planning, and execution is required to meet the delivery timescale. Typically, the lead time for these campaigns (the time from ordering the starting materials to availability of analytically cleared DS) will be at least 6 months. For campaign 3, manufacture will be carried out in pilot plant equipment and the lead time will be 6 to 12 months. For subsequent campaigns involving larger amounts of DS, the lead time will be more than 1 year. In view of these timescales, it is essential that the estimated amount of DS required from a manufacturing campaign should be as accurate as possible when placing an order for starting materials and making detailed plans for the manufacture. Starting material requirements are calculated from predicted process yields which, in the early stages of development, might be based on relatively little practical experience. A small contingency factor is usually built into the stage planning yields and hence the material requirements. However, if a request to deliver an increased amount of DS is made after the campaign has started it might be impossible to satisfy this demand unless significant improvements to the stage yields are achieved.

Drug syntheses are often complex, involving many and diverse chemical steps. It would be impractical for most pharmaceutical companies to have the resource (plant and people) to undertake all the manufacture and associated process development in-house. In addition, the number of candidate drug projects that are actively being progressed at any time can fluctuate widely. To solve this problem, pharmaceutical companies arrange for supply of key intermediates or even the final drug substance by contract manufacture from an external company. Many such contract manufacturing organizations exist worldwide. In the early stages of development when drug substance supply is on the critical path, key factors in the selection of a contract manufacturer for a particular job are speed of response, quality, and reliability. Sometimes contract manufacturing organizations are chosen because they have expertise in particular types of chemistry or have special plant facilities.

As the candidate drug progresses through development, the quantities of intermediates required increase and other factors (e.g., cost, experience of regulatory submissions) become increasingly important in the selection of a contractor. The company chosen to supply the early quantities of intermediate will generally be unsuitable for later stages of development and commercial production when much larger scale manufacturing plant is needed.

To ensure a successful outcome, it is vital to maintain close contact between technical representatives on the DS project team and their counterparts at the manufacturing organization or contract manufacturing company. The project team will want assurance that manufacture of a key intermediate is proceeding according to plan. If technical problems arise during manufacture, the technical representatives might be able to offer useful advice and in any case will want to know what steps are being taken to solve the problem. In the early stages of manufacture, when the processes are not well understood, there is a significant risk of failure. The need to stop manufacture, investigate the cause of the failure, and implement a modified process will result in a delay to the delivery of DS and probably a shortfall in the quantity. If all the material is being processed in a single batch, failure could involve complete loss of the material if the wrong product is obtained or if purification is impossible. The risk is mitigated by manufacturing two or more batches of each stage, but, of course, this extends the manufacturing time. The project team must balance the risks and benefits involved before deciding which strategy to adopt.

Initial Compound Manufacture

The medicinal chemist prepares novel compounds for characterization and biological screening on a scale of milligrams, frequently with the aid of automated, parallel synthesizers. Compounds of interest will undergo repeat synthesis on a scale-up to a few grams for further evaluation. These syntheses will be carried out using the most expedient route. The first manufacture of a potential candidate drug on a significant scale will typically produce in the order of 100 g, and this will also use the medicinal chemistry route. Because of the desire for speed and the high attrition rate at this point in development, the manufacture is carried out with little or no development. Often the processes are highly inefficient, and there is extensive use of chromatography to purify intermediates and the final product.

The product is used in short-term or sighting toxicity studies (typically up to 7 days) and is not generally made to good manufacturing practice (GMP) standard. Clearance of the DS for use is based on a limited amount of analysis, for example, assay by high pressure liquid chromatography (HPLC) or nuclear magnetic resonance (NMR), organic impurities, chiral purity if relevant. The limits on the potential CQA are therefore not firmly specified. The limits are tightened as development progresses through phase 1 to phase 3 and commercialization and other clauses are introduced to control specific items (e.g., catalyst residues).

Simultaneously with this initial manufacture, plans are made for campaign 2, which is typically 5 kg in size and is made according to GMP. Campaign 2 supplies DS for key one-month toxicity studies and usually the first clinical studies (phase 1). The procedures used in manufacture of campaign 1 might be totally unsuitable for such a large increase in scale but, in view of the time and resource pressures, it is not appropriate to develop a perfectly optimized synthetic route for campaign 2. The focus will be on developing processes that are fit for purpose only. It is unlikely there will be sufficient time to develop an alternative route and prove its viability. However, some of the processes used to make campaign 1 might require considerable modification or improvement before they can be scaled up. It is essential that they can be operated safely and any processes proposed for scale-up must be subjected to appropriate evaluation of the chemical hazards. Availability and cost of key starting materials and reagents are important factors. If the materials are relatively cheap, they can be ordered in advance to give the manufacture a head start. However, there is a risk they will be wasted if the likely candidate drug is not nominated for development.

Batch failures and processing abnormalities are common in early development manufacture. The reasons are diverse but common examples include incomplete removal of the plant cleaning solvent, failure to follow the operating instructions, failure to adhere to the required process conditions because of plant limitations, inadequate understanding of the chemistry, misinterpretation of in-process test information. With a good level of experience, many of the problems that occur could be predicted and possibly prevented.

Route Design

To make large quantities of any drug substance for development or commercialization, it is essential to consider the feasibility of the synthetic route. Sometimes, the medicinal chemistry route is acceptable with minor modifications but often it is not. The reasons for the medicinal chemistry route not being suitable for scale-up are many and varied: very difficult chemistry, extreme processing conditions, hazardous or toxic reagents, low yield, starting materials too expensive or not available in commercial quantities, and IP concerns (19,20).

Sometimes the expected amount of drug substance cannot be delivered in full by the required date (e.g., because the processes are not reliable or insufficient starting material has been supplied). In this case, a split delivery of drug substance might be the only option. This requires agreement within the project team to a revised delivery plan. Splitting the manufacturing campaign is inefficient in terms of process chemistry and production resource although there is the benefit of learning from the first part of the campaign that could lead to improvements being implemented in later parts. With a split campaign, there is a risk that the quality of DS could vary between the different parts.

If the medicinal chemistry synthesis is deemed unacceptable for scale-up, it will be necessary for the process development chemist to generate alternative potential routes for evaluation. This is normally the role of the chemist with appropriate input from other functions. The process of generating ideas for alternative routes varies: the chemist might generate ideas based on personal experience or precedent but, to ensure the ideas are broadly based, group "brainstorming" sessions are often used. The human input can be supplemented by using one of the proprietary computer programs. These are based on databases of known reactions or commercially available materials. Such exercises can generate a large number of ideas, so it is necessary to decide which of the suggested routes are worth investigating or developing. First, it will be necessary to establish that all the stages in the synthesis actually work. Many will be based on good precedent so their feasibility is not in doubt but usually at least one stage in a proposed new route is doubtful. Therefore, it is a priority to demonstrate the feasibility of this potentially difficult step before developing any of the easier stages.

Many factors must be taken into account when selecting a manufacturing route: chemical efficiency, ease of purification, cost, availability of starting materials and reagents, plant requirements, quantity of drug substance required, safety and environmental considerations, intellectual property. Nearly always, the selection is made by carefully balancing these factors against each other.

Butters et al. (21) introduce the acronym "SELECT" to describe the six key business drivers for the pharmaceutical business:

- Safety
- Economy
- Legal
- Ecological
- Control
- Throughput

These drivers concisely summarize the factors that impact on route selection.

To make the selection as objective as possible, a Kepner–Tregoe analysis can be used (12). The participants in the analysis agree a relative weighting for all the factors affecting the route selection, and subsequently the routes under consideration are given an agreed score for each of the factors; in many cases, there is no information on a factor, so the score is based on judgment and experience. The score for each factor is multiplied by its weighting and the resulting numbers for each factor are added together to give a total score for the route. The route obtaining a significantly higher score is preferred.

Ideally, the final (or commercial manufacturing) route should be in place for campaign 3. In other words, the synthetic route should be frozen at campaign 3. This is so that the nature of impurities in the DS does not change. Changing the synthetic route after campaign 3 might lead to different impurities in the DS that are not qualified by toxicity studies for human dosing. If it becomes necessary to change the synthetic route after campaign 3, additional (or bridging) toxicity studies might be required to qualify new impurities. This could for instance happen to compress project timescales. Phase 2 material may then be required before the commercial route is agreed. This needs to be included in the project plan and a delay to the overall program might be incurred.

The selection of a route has a significant impact on the potential CQA, as outlined in Table 1. As soon as the final manufacturing route has been identified, a PGI (potential genotoxic impurity) risk assessment and an environmental assessment should be carried out. It is also appropriate to propose a registered starting material (RSM) strategy at this point. Ideally, there should be at least two synthetic steps between the RSM and the DS. The two synthetic steps must have demanding analytical control points. The final intermediate should be designated as one that is converted into the DS by covalent bond formation. Early regulatory submissions (IND and clinical trial exemption [CTX]) should describe the synthetic route from the RSMs although the requirement to disclose earlier synthetic steps in the synthesis should be anticipated. The implication is that changes to the processes used to make the RSMs do not need to be notified to the regulatory authorities (provided the quality still meets the agreed specification).

During this phase of work, studies are conducted to aid selection of the best form of the DS for development. This work requires a multifunctional

TABLE 1 **Impact of Route Selection on the Potential CQA**

	On route selection	Comment
CQA related to the chemical composition of the drug substance		
Chiral purity	Enantiomeric excess 90 to 95% ee	Isomer separation by chromatography or salt crystallization. Possible change to stereoselective synthesis or use of enzymes
Impurities	Significant change in the nature of impurities (identity and level)	Change of chemistry with different raw materials and reagents
Inorganic impurities	Potential change in nature of residual inorganic material (including heavy metals)	Dependent on reagents and process used in final stage
Water content	Potential change in level of water	Dependent on presence of water during purification process and hygroscopicity of product
Residual solvent	Potential change in nature of solvent	Level dependent on solvent used in purification process and solvate formation
CQA related to the physical properties of the drug substance		
Salt and polymorphic forms	Form selection occurs at a similar time as route selection, polymorphic form change often occurs at this time	
Particle size	Not specified	
Physicochemical properties	Not specified unless deemed critical	

Abbreviation: CQA, critical quality attributes.

approach (PC and AC supported by a crystallization expert). Once the form has been selected, it is appropriate to begin the search for polymorphs.

Process Design

The process design phase involves selecting the most suitable reaction reagent or catalyst and solvent for achieving a chemical transformation and the type of workup to be used. Changes will again impact on the CQAs, and Table 2 gives an overview of typical changes. Parallel laboratory reactors and automated equipment are being used increasingly in the process design phase (e.g., for screening solvents, reagents, and catalysts). Any process selected for scale-up beyond a few liters of reaction volume must be assessed for chemical and operational safety according to a sliding scale. This consists of measuring such parameters as the heat of reaction, the rate of gas evolution (if any), and the thermal stability of all the reactants and the product. If safety concerns arise from this work, they must be addressed by modifying the process (e.g., by changing a reagent, a temperature, or a process step such as an evaporation or mode of addition).

Processes that yield isolated intermediates frequently involve crystallization of a solid product, and this achieves some degree of purification. When the

TABLE 2 Impact of Process Design on the Potential CQA

	On process design	Comment
CQA related to the chemical composition of the drug substance		
Chiral purity	Enantiomeric excess 95 to 98% ee	Depends on efficiency of resolution process or stereoselective synthesis
Impurities	New impurities introduced, actual levels of impurities might reduce	Change of impurity profile in raw materials (different suppliers using different synthetic routes)
Inorganic impurities	Potential change in nature of residual inorganic material (including heavy metals)	Dependent on process and plant configuration used in final stage
Water content	Potential change in level of water	Dependent on presence of water during purification process and hygroscopicity of product. Also affected by drying conditions on scale-up
Residual solvent content	Potential change in type and level of solvent	Level dependent on solvent used in purification process and solvate formation. Also affected by drying conditions on scale-up
CQA related to the physical properties of the drug substance		
Polymorphic forms	The DS form has been agreed, but it is feasible that a more stable polymorphic form may be identified during development work	

Abbreviation: CQA, critical quality attributes.

final chemical transformation in the synthesis is reached, it is possible that the isolation step will furnish material of acceptable quality (i.e., it will pass the provisional specification). If not, it will be necessary to carry out a further purification step. In either case, special procedures must be incorporated to ensure the DS is fit for clinical use (use of filtered solvents and a designated clean area for the isolation step). The crystallization step in the final process invariably becomes a focus of attention for experimental work because of its potential to affect the quality and physical form of the DS. The final crystallization delivers the DS in the selected form, whether it is a neutral molecule, free base (or acid), or a salt thereof. Equipment is available to measure crystal size and growth rate in situ in both laboratory experiments and plant scale manufacture. The objective of this work is a controlled crystallization that reproducibly gives DS with the desired characteristics. In principle, a single solvent–seeded cooling crystallization is preferred because it is most likely to meet the objective of a controlled crystallization. The crystallization step should be seeded to afford maximum control. However, the solubility and stability characteristics of many candidate drugs dictate the use of mixed solvent systems. The detailed investigation of a crystallization process is best undertaken jointly between the PC and the PE with input of a crystallization expert.

During the course of manufacturing campaigns, it is almost inevitable that some batches of DS will fail to meet their specification. Such failures might arise because of insufficient reduction of impurity levels or contamination with extraneous matter. As a consequence, it will be necessary to reprocess the material (reintroduce it to an existing process) or develop a rework process (a new or nonstandard process) to bring the material within specification. A potential danger with this is that the impurity profile might be distorted from that of typical material by reprocessing or reworking. For example, some impurities might be completely removed.

The application of scale-up risk evaluation (SURE) is generally helpful in identifying the most important development areas (22) (see also sect. "Example 1: Scale-Up Risk Evaluation"). This is occasionally referred to as "tactical risk assessment," as it is only executed on stages where the confidence in the process is low.

Process Characterization and Optimization

This phase of development involves a detailed investigation into key process parameters (e.g., reactant and reagent stoichiometry, temperature, volume of solvent used). It is also the time to develop a detailed understanding of the process including the reaction mechanism, competing pathways, consumption and appearance of dispersed phases, mass transfer, and mixing sensitivity. As demonstrated in Table 3, the impact on the CQA is more in terms of understanding and control, rather than changes. It is beneficial to measure reaction profiles and analyze them with process models that include both kinetic and mass transfer, especially for processes where issues have been experienced on scale-up. Automated equipment is invaluable for gathering experimental data over long periods and sampling reaction mixtures for analysis. Factorial experimental design (FED) is an integral part of the work because it ensures a systematic approach to parameter investigation and helps to minimize the number of experiments needed to reach a conclusion. The work requires special skills and is best carried out within a multidisciplinary team (PC, PE, physical organic chemist, AC). Key objectives of this work cover most areas of the SELECT model: quality, efficiency, output, environmental acceptability, and, to a lesser extent, yield.

At this time, a more formal QRA can be used to identify development drivers that will lead to increased process robustness. Process robustness is defined as the ability of the process to tolerate variability of materials and changes of the process and equipment without an adverse impact on quality. The QRA will identify issues associated with scale-up and the quality of the starting materials, the reagents and solvents. After prioritization of the risk, the development team will then work to gain understanding and mitigate the risks.

TABLE 3   Impact of Process Characterization and Optimization on the Potential CQA

	Impact
CQA related to the drug substance's chemical composition	
Chiral purity	Set at a specific limit, process understanding of potential racemization
Impurities	All relevant impurities identified
	Process understanding around their formation and clean-up in relevant process stages
CQA related to the drug substance's physical properties	
Polymorphic forms	DS form specified and controlled.
	Process understanding of form, form transformations and the impact of processing and impurities on control of form
Particle size	Specified, impact of DS processes on size reduction understood

Finalization of Process Design for Validation and Submission

During this phase of development there are two deliverables: (*i*) the technology transfer of the commercial process the commercial supply organization with associated process validation and (*ii*) generation of regulatory submissions including the finalization of data required to support them.

During this phase, the processes ranges are compared with the capability of the proposed manufacturing equipment to confirm suitability of both the processes and the equipment. Final set points are decided and where parameters have been shown to be important, proven acceptable ranges (PARs) are often established through confirmatory FEDs. At this point, critical parameters are established and analytical methods are validated. All this information is transferred to the commercial supply organization, and a process of confirming that they can reproduce the processes and methods supplied by development is undertaken.

Typically, a comparative transfer of methods is undertaken, then a number of batches are manufactured in the equipment. If this is successful, three validation batches are carried out to confirm the process behaves reproducible. As part of ICH Q8, the idea of replacing validation with continuous verification has been proposed, this is defined as *an alternative approach to process validation in which manufacturing process performance is continuously monitored and evaluated*.

In tandem with this transfer to commercial supply, the development team generates the regulatory submission. The level of process knowledge contained in that documentation is likely to be dependent on the approach of the organization. At a minimum, the following should be included in the submission:

- Identification of the CQAs associated with the drug substance
- Definition of material attributes and process parameters that impact the CQAs
- A defined manufacturing process
- A control strategy

If the company applies an enhanced, QbD approach (as defined by ICH Q8 & Q11) greater levels of process and product understanding will be supplied. This data may have been generated at any point during development, but should support a multivariate understanding of system and design space. Such a QbD approach may allow a more flexible regulatory approach to future changes.

Technology Transfer and Validation

Technology transfer covers transfer of the manufacturing processes from the development function to proposed manufacturing plant. This may involve transfer between different functions or sites of the same company or to an entirely different company. In any case, the importance of a comprehensive package of high-quality, clearly written documentation cannot be overemphasized. Transfer of late-stage manufacture to another company or strategic supplier inevitably involves different plant items and configurations and different ways of working. In some cases, distance and language are obstacles. The outsourcing company must be chosen carefully and the information transfer process must be managed well to minimize the risk of issues arising during manufacture through misunderstandings.

Depending on the TT/validation model that is chosen, the TT campaign will supply three batches of DS for pivotal stability studies. When all the experimental work has been completed and the necessary documents have been written, the Readiness to Proceed to Process Validation document can be approved on a stage-by-stage basis. Success criteria are carefully described in the validation program. The size of the validation campaign is determined by several factors but, most importantly, the need for three consecutive batches to meet the predetermined success criteria. If this is achieved, the manufacturing process is deemed to have been validated.

SCENARIO GENERATION: ANTICIPATING PROCESS VARIATIONS

So far we discussed the general principles of risk assessment and some common CQAs and presented an overview of the primary development activities that generate the manufacturing processes, as well as the understanding of those processes. It may be clear that alongside the CQAs presented in section "The Interface Between Primary and Secondary Development: CQAs," which essentially represent the risk to the patient, there are also business risks.

For instance, financial loss will result if material has to be destroyed or reworked because of quality issues. Manufacturing or operability issues may plague scale-up campaigns potentially delaying clinical trials. So even if the risk to the patient is zero (e.g., full detectability of an issue) lack of delivery can be catastrophic to the company.

A HAZOP risk assessment identifies hazard issues by evaluating the interactions of a process with a real plant. Detailed descriptions of the plant, the process, and the materials used are required in such study. Risk assessment of a process under development is different in that it assesses a process's ability to consistently produce quality material in a "typical plant" that is not specified in detail.

The typical plant referred to is for primary manufacture usually understood to be a jacketed dished end batch vessel, with the height of the vessel typically similar to the diameter of the vessel. The vessel is equipped with an agitator that provides "reasonable" mixing. One does however not tend to specify the nature of the agitation system in detail (although it is assumed the agitation is not by anchor agitators). The impact of agitation is typically covered by evaluation of the impact of lower or higher agitation on the vessel.

The above comments on agitation demonstrate the nature of process risk assessments: the process being assessed is well defined (e.g., the order of operations and the nature and quantities of the material charged), the interaction between the plant and the process is captured by evaluation of the risk associated with a change in that interaction (e.g., more or less agitation). This change can be due to scale-up but it is not limited to that. Other causes of change may be relocation to a different unit, variability in raw materials, cleaning of plant, etc.

In risk assessment, a change is captured by generating a scenario that describes it. The FMEA risk phrase "failure mode" is an often-used synonym for QRA scenarios. A scenario is thus essentially a description of the change of a parameter, physical form or plant or equipment performance, etc. The scenario is evaluated and scored for its impact on product quality (e.g. a particular CQA).

Alternatively it could evaluate a risk to the business, for example the delivery of the required quantity of material at a particular time. The impact of a scenario can be either positive (an opportunity) or negative (a threat).

The generation of scenarios and their scoring should be done by the development team, helped with experienced personnel and a facilitator external to the project. This helps to widen the nature of the scenarios, and introduces large-scale thinking into a development team that up to then may only have worked on 1 L scale or less.

Scenario Generation

As the project progresses, the quantities of both drug substance and product required for toxicology, formulation development, and clinical trials increase. So although process development is typically done in 20 mL to 3 L equipment, the scale of manufacturing of DS material increases to 20 to 100 L in a large-scale (or kilogram) laboratory. For phase 2 and phase 3 trials, material is typically manufactured at 500 to 2000 L scale in a pilot-scale facility or 1000 L agile manufacturing unit.

Clearly, to define scenarios one needs to have an understanding of the nature of equipment and operations used at the various scales. Table 4 provides an overview of equipment characteristics at a range of scales used in development. The table lists a number of physical attributes of the equipment, but also the equipment capabilities like isolation methods, containment, heat, and mass transfer, etc.

It is obvious that as the scale increases, so do material quantities, the time it takes to order the materials, as well as the time it takes to process them. Although obvious, one has to consider whether this change should be captured in one or more scenarios. For instance, is the material purchased in large quantities different from the material we bought in small quantities for the laboratory work? In our experience, particle size, polymorphic form, impurity profile, and solvent content can all change. Some of these may be picked up by the specification of the material (e.g., solvent, impurity levels), but polymorph, particle size, and new unknown impurities are often not specified for raw materials.

Mixing time is also inherently worse at a larger scale. The bulk mixing timescales vary with $1/N$, with N the agitator speed. From Table 4, it follows that on scaling the mixing time reduces from seconds on the small scale to minutes or even 10s of minutes at the larger scale. The impact of this depends on the nature of the operations in the vessel. For operations like mass transfer, drop size reduction and avoiding rheological problems in precipitations, it is sufficient to keep either the tip speed or the power per unit volume constant, and this can be achieved over a wide range of processing scales (23,24).

Heat transfer and heat losses are another classic example of an equipment capability that reduces with scale. This has two major consequences: (i) exothermic reactions need to be controlled, which is typically done by slowing addition rates on scale-up and (ii) to prevent thermal run away reactions, larger scale systems, which resemble adiabatic systems more closely, have a significantly lower maximum safe temperature than small vessels. As a result of the reduction in heat transfer with scale-up, process times increase, which could lead to additional impurities through degradation or overreaction. Alternatively, some species may be supersaturated and, given more time at large scale, may nucleate where this had not been seen on a smaller scale.

TABLE 4 An Overview of Equipment Used at a Range of Scales

Scale	Screening equipment	Synthetic laboratory	Development laboratory	Large-scale laboratory (kg)	Pilot-scale plant
Volume description	10 mL Hydrogenation, stem block, well plates; typically all in reactions	20–250 mL Round-bottom flasks; surface addition	100–5000 mL Glass-jacketed vessels with quick fit lids; surface addition	20–100 L Glass-jacketed reactors; surface addition	200–2000 L Glass-lined mild steel-jacketed reactors, surface addition. Occasional reactors may be Hastelloy
Starting materials	<5 g	1–10 g	10–100 g	1–10 kg	20–50 kg
Ordering time	Day	Day	Day	Days to weeks	Weeks to months
Batch/campaign time	Hours	Hours–days	Hours to days	Days to week	Weeks
PAT	Temperature, pressure	Temperature, pressure	Temperature, pressure, in situ IR, UV, viscosity, particle size	Temperature, pressure, in situ particle size	Temperature, pressure, volume
Auxiliaries	Few, manufacturer specific	Quick fit glass overheads heating mantles, dricold	Overhead stirring and heater chiller external baths, vacuum ovens	Fixed vapor uplift, condensers and receivers. Open nutsche filters, tray drier ovens, some batch centrifuges	Fixed vapor uplift, condensers and receivers. Closed pressure filters or batch centrifuges + dryer
Agitation Tip speed and power per unit volume	Flea, shaking, sometimes overhead agitated	Flee, some overhead stirring, minimal baffling	Glass and metal agitators, minimal baffling. Typical retreat curve or pitch blade. Occasional anchor	Glass retreat curve and general metal impellers (RDT, PBT). Occasional finger baffle	Glass retreat curve and general metal impellers (RDT, PBT). Occasional finger baffle
Attrition, grinding	Severe attrition when stirred with flee	Severe attrition when stirred with flee			
Minimum addition time	Seconds	Seconds	10s of seconds	Minutes	10s of minutes
Heat transfer	High, set point reached in minutes	High, set point reached in minutes. Significant heat losses through top half of vessel	Medium, set point reached in 10s of minutes (limited by jacket). Significant heat losses through lid	Low-medium, Eq. set point reached in 30 min. Limited by internal heat transfer. Significant heat losses through lid and vapor up lift	Low Eq. temperature reached in 30–60 min. Limited by internal heat transfer, low heat loses

Mass transfer	Typically low, but OK for some specialized equipment	Low	Low to high	Low-medium, but typical for hydrogenerators	Low-medium, but typical for hydrogenerators
Solid suspension	In homogeneous	In homogeneous	Well distributed providing agitation is sufficient	Well distributed providing agitation is sufficient	Well distributed providing agitation is sufficient
Isolation	Syringe filter	Buchi filter, open to air, dried by passing air through the cake, and vacuum oven	Buchi filter, open to air, dried by passing air through the cake then vacuum oven	Nutsche filter open to air, dried by passing air through the cake then vacuum oven. Sometimes possibility to use an in-line filter to screen out solids	Pressure filter or centrifuge combined with a drier. Dried by applying vacuum or (hot) nitrogen through the cake. Sometimes possible to use in-line filters (GAF bags, micron sized filters)
Absence of O_2	None	By nitrogen or argon if required	By nitrogen or argon if required	By nitrogen if required	By nitrogen
Distillation	None	High refractionation through heat losses in overheads	High refractionation through heat losses through lid and overheads	High refractionation through heat losses through lid and overheads	Low refractionation, minimum heat losses
Containment	Fumehood	Fumehood	Fumehood	Fumehood	Plant
Risk processes	Paper assessment + DSC	Paper assessment + DSC and adiabatic stability test as required	Paper assessment + DSC and adiabatic stability test as required	Full hazard assessment based on calorimetry adiabatic and isothermal stability tests	Full hazard assessment based on calorimetry, adiabatic and isothermal stability tests. Plant compatibility check

Abbreviations: DSC, differential scanning calorimetry; PAT, Process Analytical Technology; PBT, pitched blade turbine; RDT, Rushton disk turbine.

As a consequence of the reduction in heat transfer on scale-up, distillations will take longer; the rate of evaporation is proportional to the heat input. If solvent mixtures are distilled, and a certain composition has to be achieved (e.g., <0.1% water), it can be difficult to set an end point to the distillation. Reflux and refractionation are typically not controlled at any of the scales, and hence the practice of distilling down to a specified volume can give rise to significant variability in the composition. The alternative, distillation to a specified volume that has built up in a receiver, is also dangerous, as solvent losses at a small scale can be quite significant if leakage rates are high when vacuum distilling.

In addition to the scenarios associated with materials and the scale, design, and operation of equipment, there are also some generally unpredictable aspects of processing. Apart from the impact of delays in processing because of the plant breakdown or malfunction, by far the most unpredictable thing in scale-up is nucleation. In systems under development, it is not always clear if one or other species becomes supersaturated at some point during the processes. The impact of unexpected nucleation ranges from no impact to catastrophic process failure. Nucleation results in a sudden drop in the concentration of the crystallizing species which slows down subsequent reactions to unfeasible speeds. Alternatively the system can "set solid," in which case heat and mass transfer become extremely low (24).

In discussing the scenario generation for the chemical processes developed for primary manufacture, some general points around scenario generation arise:

- Requires a general understanding of the principles and operation of plant/equipment at a range of scales
- Requires a general understanding of the interaction between a process and the equipment; what aspect of the equipment is important to the process
- General understanding of all input materials
- Need to assess the whole process start to finish
- Scenarios need to be realistic where knowledge is available. If a scenario touches on an area where there is a lack of understanding, the team should log it and move on
- Risk assessment should be done by the development team in conjunction with some external peers to widen the range of scenarios

These general points translate also to secondary manufacture.

Scenarios: Assessing the Impact

The scenarios generated are derived from typical changes in the process, scale, equipment, or material used. In development projects, it is often the impact of a scenario on quality that is scored as changes in quality can have significant impact on the overall drug development program:

- Polymorphic form or particle size distribution changes may result in either unstable formulations or reduced bioavailability.
- A change in impurity levels may alter the shelf life of product.
- New impurities formed will require additional toxicity studies.

Examples that occur in development and the potential impact on key CQAs are listed in Table 5. It is clear that the CQAs are affected by a wide range of factors and interactions. As development proceeds, more and more of the factors are controlled. For instance, the risk of finding a new polymorphic form will be

TABLE 5 Impact of Scale-Up and Development on a Range of Drug Substance CQAs

Processing factors		Impact on CQA[a]		
Scale-up and development factors	Impact on operation	Polymorphic form	Particle size and shape	Impurities, color, solvent
Inputs				
Materials supplied: psd and polymorph changes	Processing rates change; yield losses			More and new impurities
Materials supplied: assay, impurities				New impurities
Foreign material [oxygen (air), moisture, rust, fouling, cleaning fluids, etc.]	New reactions, deactivation of catalyst, slower reaction	Hydrates, salts	psd changes	Higher, more water, solvent
Equipment				
Geometry and size of processing equipment	Longer processing times, yield losses, inaccurate solvent compositions	Metastable form	psd changes	Can change
Agitator design/speed	Changes in inhomogeneity caused by mixing leading to changes in processing times, yield losses, emulsification	Metastable form	psd and shape change	Can change
Different material of construction incompatibilities	Incompatible material, plant failure			Higher, new impurities
Pressures changes	Different P leads under or overreaction and wrong solvent composition in distillation	Metastable form	psd and shape change	More and new impurities
Mass transfer				
Solid addition rate	Inhomogeneity, changes in solid dissolution rate			Higher
Liquid addition rate	Different rate of mixing leads to changes in crystallization and/or reaction selectivity	Metastable form, solvate	psd and shape change	More solvent
Gas disengagement	Different inertion protocols and surface movement can lead to buildup of gasses formed in the liquid (especially CO, CO_2 and SO_2)			More and new impurities

(continued)

Table 5   Impact of Scale-Up and Development on a Range of Drug Substance CQAs (*Continued*)

	Processing factors	Impact on CQA[a]		
Scale-up and development factors	Impact on operation	Polymorphic form	Particle size and shape	Impurities, color, solvent
Gas dispersion and absorption	Different equipment systems will have different mass transfer capabilities resulting in different reaction times			More and new impurities
Heat transfer and temperature control				
Temperature fluctuations larger	Unwanted nucleation	Metastable form	psd and shape change	More solvent and associated impurities
Heat losses smaller	Duration of tasks longer resulting in more degradation, over reaction. Crystallization process may be slower	Different form	psd increases	New, more impurities
Physical process mishaps				
Randomness of nucleation	Sudden appearance of a new phase or form, can change both reaction rates and crystallization processes	Different form, solvate	psd and shape change	Higher and new impurities, more solvent
Small compositional changes (volatile losses, pH shifts)	Subtle changes in physical properties (e.g., density, partition coefficient, etc.) resulting in additional phases, changes in wash efficiency, emulsification, reactivity			Higher, new impurities, more solvent and salts
Plant failure	Unexpected extension of processing times, solvent loss, ingress of water/solvents	Solvates		More and new impurities

[a]Assay is related to the impurities CQA; Because of historic specification writing, this tends to be included as a CQA. *Abbreviation:* psd, particle size distribution.
Source: From Ref. 16.

reduced by polymorph screens; the molecule has been evaluated in a wider range of experiments and with wider range of purities. Small, and even pilot-scale experiments may not however reveal that a system is metastable during the processing. It is possible that only after many production runs the system suddenly nucleates. Once it has nucleated, residual seed will remain in the equipment and subsequent batches are very likely to also nucleate (8).

Risk assessment does not need to be limited to QRAs. It can support process development in many different areas: for example, route selection, formulation selection, scale-up, quality, manufacturability. Although the principles will be the same, the key difference between these different applications of risk assessments is the nature of the impact being assessed.

Butters et al. introduce the acronym SELECT to describe the six key business drivers for the pharmaceutical business (Table 6). They applied the SELECT criteria to choose between alternative chemical routes. Manipura et al. (2009) (25) took this a step further and expanded each of the six SELECT business drivers with a larger number of subareas (Fig. 4). The final aim of development is to device a process that will successfully meet all the SELECT criteria. Butters and Aruna both indicate that application and evaluation of the SELECT criteria early in development can have a big beneficial impact on the final process design: Early in design process, issues can be designed out by changing the process, in later-stage development one has to control the issue, which is generally more difficult.

Risk assessment can be applied to evaluate the risk of process, equipment, and scale changes on each of the SELECT drivers separately (i.e., a sustainability risk assessment, a QRA), or it can be applied to a several of the criteria at the same time: for example, a scale-up risk evaluation like described in section

TABLE 6   Description of the SELECT Model

Criteria	Subcriteria	Example of potential issue
Safety	Process safety Exposure to harmful substances	Threat to workers or plant from explosions or exotherms Threat to workers or plant from carcinogens or sensitizers
Environmental	Volume of wasted natural resources Substances harmful to the environment	Quantity and nature of solvents Aquatic toxins and ozone depleting chemicals
Legal	Infringement of intellectual property rights Regulations that control use of reagents and intermediates	Key intermediate patented by competitor Notification of new substances (NONS; EU legislation)
Economics	Cost of good target for market Investment costs to support development	Long synthesis route using expensive materials High cost of process cannot be changed in short term
Control	Control of CQA Control of chemistry and physical parameters	Meeting specification and GMP requirements Nonselective reagents, unstable intermediates
Throughput	Timescale of manufacture in available plant Availability of raw materials	Long route with dilute stages Rare natural products

Source: From Ref. 21.

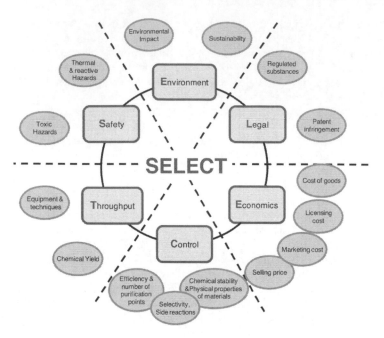

FIGURE 4   Extended SELECT model. *Source*: From Ref. 25.

"Example 1: Scale-Up Risk Evaluation" assesses both the throughput and quality control. Route selection, the original reason for the SELECT model, will compare routes on the basis of an evaluation of all six aspects.

Scoring of Scenarios
When doing the risk assessment, the impact of scenarios and the likelihood they are realized needs to be scored. For briefness, we refer to the combination of likelihood and impact as the "score" of a scenario. The score essentially represents the risk perception of the assessment team. The most subjective element of the score is the likelihood that a particular scenario will occur. The extent of the impact can often be derived from a series of logic steps and extrapolation, but the likelihood score is solely based on the people involved in the risk assessment and their experience.

In order for risk assessments to be relevant and comparable, consistency of scoring across team and projects is much more important than the actual numeric values of a score. This is another reason why risk assessments are usually facilitated: the facilitator has a good understanding of the agreed scoring and applies this across development teams and processes.

The easiest way to achieve a consistent common view is by defining a set of risk phrases that are accepted companywide: each score value has a phrase associated that describes the impact as well as the likelihood. Examples of such scoring definitions are provided in the examples of implemented process risk assessment (see for instance sect. "Example 2: Quality Risk Assessment").

The scoring definitions can be illustrated for the SELECT criteria (excluding Legal, see Table 7). In general, high scores refer to a high impact or

TABLE 7 Generic Scoring for Likelihood and the SELECT Criteria (Excluding Legal) for Scenarios

	Likelihood	Safety on people	Safety and environment	Economics	Control	Throughput
Threat						
High value	Very probable, known to happen in the past	People severely affected: long-term illness or deaths	Catastrophic impact on environmental or assets	Significant negative impact on balance sheet	Wide variability	Significant reduction in output
	...	...	...	...	...	...
Low value	Improbable	Not affected	Not affected	Not affected	Not affected	Not affected
	...	...	...	...	...	...
Opportunity high value	High chance of success in a short time	Better for people	Reduces impact	Beneficial impact on balance sheet	Improved consistency	Increased output

likelihood, while a low score indicates the scenario is unlikely to occur, or there is no effect on a particular element. The highest score tends to relate to extreme events, in this way teams are forced to consider the widest possible range of impacts.

Of course, it is also possible that a scenario might actually improve things. In that case, it is important that the opportunity is logged. Note that scoring opportunities can lead to confusion. This is mainly because for a threat, likelihood is related to the chance something happens. For an opportunity, teams tend to score the likelihood of success. The latter score tends to include not only whether something is possible (as for the threats) but also an evaluation of the amount of effort required to get there, and the companies' willingness to spend that effort.

The numerical values assigned to scenarios are actually not very important, as long as there is a range of values. Early on in development, it is often enough to score "high, medium, or low" as the knowledge of the process is relatively low, and so the likelihood and the impact are not easily defined. Later in development, process knowledge increases and the scoring can be more refined. Typically, the numbers range from, for instance, 1 to 5 or 1 to 10.

To priorities risks, the score for a scenario can be multiplied (likelihood × impact) so as to get a single number that represents the degree of risk: the "risk priority number" (RPN). It is for this reason that the lowest score does not tend to be zero. In such cases, the risk of scenarios with a very high impact will become invisible, as their likelihoods are frequently low. For evaluation purposes and sanity checks, it is preferred to show these as having a low risk, rather than no risk. An alternative to the RPN is to plot the scores in a risk matrix; the scenarios are positioned in a figure with *likelihood* on the y-axis, and *impact* on the x-axis. Thus, high-risk scenarios are in the top right-hand corner, and low risks are in the bottom left-hand corner. These figures are easily generated in a macroenabled spreadsheet. See for instance the risk matrix in section "Example 1: Scale-Up Risk Evaluation" in the example of an implemented process risk assessment (Fig. 5).

EXAMPLES OF IMPLEMENTATION OF RISK ASSESSMENT IN DEVELOPMENT
Example 1: Scale-Up Risk Evaluation

Conventional scale-up aims to design new equipment or unit operations to match the process requirements for commercial manufacture (see for instance Ref. 26). In pharmaceutical development, the major equipment items are generally fixed, and scale-up refers to the smooth operation of a process on a larger scale. Basu et al. (27) identify the importance of a long-term view of the process under development. They propose to model the complete process, which would require data that is typically only available in the later stages of development when process changes can introduce unacceptable delays to the project.

The scale-up risk evaluation (SURE) was designed by Muller and Latimer (22) to facilitate multidisciplinary teams to anticipate scale- and equipment-dependent manufacturing risks and opportunities early on in the development of a new compound. In doing this, it identifies gaps in knowledge of how the process works and focuses work on those gaps that also present the highest risk to successful operation of the process (from a quality or manufacturability

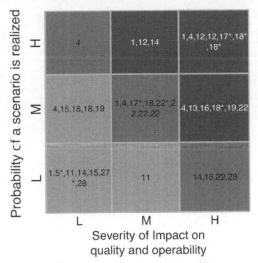

Probability of a scenario is realized

H	4	1,12,14	1,4,12,12,17*,18* ,18*
M	4,15,18,18,19	1,4,17*,18,22*,2 2,22,22	4,13,16,18*,19,22
L	1,5*,11,14,15,27 *,28	11	14,16,22,28

L   M   H

Severity of Impact on
quality and operability

- Numbers represent operations, operations
  with multiple scenarios will appear multiple times
- Starred numbers represent opportunities

FIGURE 5 Example of a risk matrix for a stage with 28 operations (each identified by a number in the risk matrix).

standpoint). The principle of SURE is based on that of a HAZOP study, but is not intended to identify SHE risks.

The process is as follows: a multidisciplinary team evaluates the process; for each operation in a process recipe various scenarios are identified (a scenario is defined as an unplanned change in conditions or equipment). The potential impact of a scenario on the process is then assessed as a "threat" or an "opportunity" and subsequently the scenarios are scored on

1. the *probability* of the scenario will occur in the planned manufacture and
2. the *severity* of the effect on product quality or process operability.

The output of a SURE study is a risk matrix and a summary table of the threats and opportunities. The output is used by the development team to prioritize further development work, which will mitigate the risks.

When to Do a SURE Study

The study can be performed at anytime in the development of a "process" but is best done once both reaction and workup have basic definition. Typically, a SURE study is appropriate when

- the chemistry works with satisfactory yields, reagents and solvents have been selected, and workup has early definition;
- externally developed chemistry is taken up by the team;
- the process is considered "complex," for example,
  - solids being dissolved and formed during the reaction
  - L-L and G-L reactions

- exothermic reactions, sensitive reagents, strong dependency on stoichiometry
- complex intermediates/unknown chemical pathways
- workups with washes, distillations, extractions (e.g., difficult workup).

Studies should not be conducted if the process is very straightforward and well understood and hence is deemed low risk.

Facilitation and Participants
The minimum team requirements are a chemist, an engineer, and a study facilitator. If appropriate, analysts and plant personnel could also attend the meeting.

The facilitator (typically an experienced PE) brings a number of skills to the SURE study: a consistent approach, knowledge of the tool, an independent eye, and experience of other projects.

The inclusion of too many team members or observers can detract from or slow down the study.

Preparation for the Meeting
The process owner is responsible for providing a process description, as well as information that aids the understanding of the process (typically a reaction scheme and some mechanistic information).

The PE is responsible for arranging the meeting and populating the minutes template with the relevant information from the process description. The engineer is also responsible for ensuring the mitigation table is actioned and updated as development proceeds.

Study Description
The study is performed by (i) capture of current knowledge followed by (ii) generation and evaluation of meaningful scenarios. An excel-based tool is used to capture the process and SURE information.

Typically, this process is completed on sections of the process description (typically 10 operations at the time).

Capturing Understanding
The sequence of operations in the process description is described and recorded in order. The operation to add a reactive reagent, for example, would be described by documenting: (i) reagent name, concentration, amount (actual or by reference to other key material), and timescale (rate); (ii) the complexity of the reaction mass, for example, rheology, the number of phases (present, formed, or destroyed); (iii) the intended change or mechanism (A > B reaction); (iv) physical properties (boiling/melting point); and (v) experimental data (heat data/reaction profile). A more simple operation, for example, to heat or cool, would require much less description.

Risk Evaluation
For each step, possible "scenarios" are generated using classic (HAZOP type) guide words; for example, longer time, higher temperature. Any scenario that generates a meaningful outcome is documented, noting the mechanism involved and the nature of its effect on the process (e.g., yield, quality, operability).

Risk Rating

The scenarios are then weighted on two scales: (*i*) the *probability* of a scenario is realized in the manufacture and (*ii*) the *severity of the* potential impact on operability of the process and/or the quality of the product. The probability and effect are scored as "low," "medium," or "high." The impact score is a subjective one, which represents the view of the team. If the assessment of the risk is difficult because information is lacking, it scores automatically as high to drive the development team to generate of understanding in this area.

Output Generation

The Excel template automatically populates a pictorial "risk matrix" (like figure 5) and a "mitigation summary table." The number and magnitude of risks identified can vary significantly. Typically, early in development the risks are spread evenly over the risk matrix. For more mature processes few high risks remain, and these are typically well known to the project team.

Risk Mitigation

The SURE study output is to be reviewed by the development team and should be used to prioritize development work within the technical team. Risks are considered high if the probability/severity combinations are H/M, H/H, or M/H. It is expected that work will be focused on low-risk opportunities and high-risk threats. The outcome of mitigation work should be recorded in the mitigation table.

For instance, for an eight-hour hold during which a reaction progressed to completion, "less agitation" was identified as a high-risk scenario. The development team conducted a lab scale experiment with an agitation rate scaled down from the proposed plant agitation rate and discovered a significant reduced reaction time. As a result they could lower the reaction temperature, which resulted in a reduction in impurities.

Medium risk is represented if either the impact or the probability was deemed low (i.e., LM, MM, ML). An example is product degradation during distillation. A scenario "longer" distillation was identified as medium risk: It was deemed likely for the distillation to take longer on plant. Subsequent lab experiments demonstrated that the product was stable for 24 hours under distillation conditions.

Finally, scenarios pose a low risk for the combinations LL, ML, and LM. Scenarios in this area can be important if they relate to an opportunity rather than a threat: For instance, in a series of washes, we identified a low-risk scenario "omit" (a wash). The operation was later removed from the process description reducing complexity, waste, and processing time.

SURE Review

The mitigation table should be reviewed after the first campaign following the review. It is generally a good idea to transfer high risks into the first QRA.

Participant's Feedback

Clearly, a rigorous approach like SURE requires a significant investment of time from the development team. To ensure the SURE process develops and made best use of people's time, feedback on the methodology is always discussed at the end of a SURE study. Typically, both chemists and engineers are enthused by the process. Chemists are key contributors to the discussions, providing most of the information. They generally find the methodology useful as it gives them additional areas to focus on and increases the development team's confidence in the process. For many engineers, it was the first time they discussed all aspects of a process in detail, which gave them a much better insight in what development was planned, why it is required. This then enables them to collaborate more closely with the chemists and empowers them to contribute more fully to process development.

Example 2: Quality Risk Assessment

QRA is used to provide an effective means of identifying important threats and uncertainties to the *pharmaceutical quality* of drug product. QRA executed on primary manufacturing processes of intermediates and drug substance will provide direction and technical focus for design space definition and control strategies (see ICH Q9). QRA is therefore a strategic tool that influences the long-term process development, and demonstrates that in an NDA the final manufacturing processes will robustly produce medicine with the appropriate pharmaceutical quality.

The principle of FMECA is that a multidisciplinary team identifies the potential ways in which a product may fail (*failure modes* or *scenarios*) and the effect of these failures (*failure effects, impact*). The impact of the failure (*severity*), the likelihood of its occurring (*probability* or *sensitivity of the process*), and the ability to detect the failure (*detectability*) are then assigned numerical scores based on predefined criteria. These individual scores are multiplied to provide an overall risk priority number (RPN) that is used to rank risks and prioritize mitigation activity.

The assessment can be made using the manufacturing process flow as a guide, with each sequential unit operation being assessed in turn for potential failure modes (known as a process parameter or "bottom-up" process). Alternatively the product quality attributes can be used as the starting point for assessment of the relevant manufacturing operations (known as a quality attribute or "top-down" process). In this case, the tool might better be described as failure effect–mode analysis since the failure modes are identified with reference to the effects that they have on the quality attributes—there may be several failure modes identified for each failure effect and the scoring process for each failure mode is the same for both methodologies. Both approaches are considered valid and are available to the project.

The bottom-up approach is preferred when the understanding of the process is poor and the intention is to carry out a rigorous identification of potential failure scenarios. The top-down approach may require less time, and results in a summary of the team's understanding of the current risks that can be part of the regulatory submission as it provides a clear link from CQA to risk mitigation/operational control. Both approaches will highlight gaps in process understanding that need to be addressed.

QRA Team

A multidisciplinary team of experts with the most knowledge of the process and technologies that may be used for risk mitigation should be assembled. The team will typically include the PC, AC, PE, and quality advisor. A facilitator who is independent of the project but who has experience of the technique being applied will normally lead it. When performing a QRA for the pure stage, representation from PAR&D (PD and or AD) is necessary to ensure the drug substance quality attributes are correctly assigned. This is especially important at the first QRA where the physical requirements of the drug substance may not have been fully determined and more scientific judgment is required.

Preparation for the QRA Meeting
Some preparation is required before the QRA meeting to ensure its effectiveness, this includes the following:

- Definition of the scope of the QRA—what process is being assessed
- Agreement on the drug substance quality attributes. In earlier stages of development, those attributes that are believed to be likely CQAs should be used where the definition is incomplete
- Generation of a process map
- Identification of long-term in-process controls that provide risk mitigation

The information should be gathered by the relevant technical personnel and made available in summary form to the QRA team prior to the meeting.

Identification of Drug Substance Quality Attributes
Design space definition should "work back" from the CQAs of the drug substance to ensure that these are adequately controlled by the processes, and the impact of potential process changes on these attributes are understood. The term "critical" describes a process step, condition, test requirement, or other relevant parameter or process item that *must* be controlled within predetermined criteria to ensure the API meets its specification (ICH Q7a), these will not be confirmed until the end of the development process and so the use of the term critical should be avoided until then.

To perform a meaningful QRA the quality attributes pertaining to the process being assessed need to be identified and agreed beforehand. There must also be some understanding of the process already to hand.

The drug substance quality attributes are likely to be similar to the specification clauses and any physical form characteristics thought to have an impact on the formulation or action of the drug (safety and efficacy). This activity should be performed in close cooperation with PAR&D and should review all the quality attributes of the drug substance. The results of a risk analysis should be used to highlight areas where process understanding is lacking and should thereby enable work to be focused on these most important stages.

The risk analysis should be reviewed and updated periodically through development.

Risk Assessment Methodology
All risk assessment methods have three stages: risk identification, risk assessment, and risk mitigation.

For the purposes of quality risks assessment, a failure mode may be defined as a set of circumstances during processing that will lead to the failure of drug substance to meet a CQA. These sets of conditions may be identified using a top-down or bottom-up approach; the only difference between them is in the way in which these failure modes are identified, and in both cases there is a reliance on a good knowledge of the process behaviors. Thereafter, the methods of risk assessment (scoring) and mitigation are the same.

TABLE 8   Examples of Guide Words That Can Be Used to Help Identify Failure Mode Identification

Guide word	Parameters
No (not or none)	Temperature
More of	Time
Less of	Stoichiometry
As well as	Pressure
Sooner/later than	Supersaturation
Part of	pH
Other than	Rate
Reverse	Concentration

The QRA process uses a form of failure mode and effect and criticality analysis (FMECA) to review the process, which is a mechanism for identifying and assessing potential product and process problems.

Process Parameter Failure Mode Identification
In the bottom-up approach, a failure mode is a way in which a step in the process can fail. The team carries out a structured brainstorm using the guide words in Table 8 to identify ways in which a step in the process could fail to complete its intended function.

When identifying the various modes of failure, it should be assumed that routine GMP controls are in place and are effective, it is the specific process that is being assessed, not general manufacturing capability.

The team must now consider, if the failure occurs, what the consequences/effects are. If this failure occurs what will happen? For some failure modes there may be only one effect, for others there may be several effects. Failure effects will normally fall into one of the following categories:

- Material quality issues (input and intermediate)
- Process issues

The failure effects should be documented in the FMECA matrix.

This approach will identify many effects that, although important from a manufacturing standpoint, for example, ability to filter, are not necessarily relevant to the quality of API.

Failure Effects
In a bottom-up approach to risk identification those effects that are identified as irrelevant to the meeting of a CQA may be ignored for the purposes of a QRA. The top-down approach automatically concentrates on those circumstances that will affect the CQAs and will not necessarily identify risks to operational efficiency.

Quality Risk Rating (Risk Assessment)
An FMECA technique is used as a tool for identifying possible risks in the process and assigning values of probability, severity, and detectability. It is important that the three factors are considered separately for example the

probability and severity of a failure occurring should be considered irrespective of how detectable the event is:

1. Probability (P) = probability of a certain failure to occur

    Probability in these assessments is considered to be the sensitivity of the process to operating conditions. For example, if good quality product has been produced over a wide range of temperatures, given that other conditions are met, then the probability of temperature causing a CQA failure is low. If either the demonstrated range is low or there is little knowledge the probability must be rated proportionally higher. The probability is rated on a 1 to 5 scale with 1 indicating the process is insensitive to processing conditions (i.e., has wide ranges) and 5 indicating extreme sensitivity.

    It is useful, but not sufficient, to evaluate historical data from batch records if it already exists. In assessing likelihood, consideration must obviously be given to interactions between the process step under consideration and others, so, for example, if the step under consideration is "heat batch to reaction temperature," the effect of temperature on the reaction must be considered in relation to other factors such as reagent addition time, charges, etc. For the purposes of QbD, it is not sufficient merely to consider the small variations that may normally be expected during processing but a wider view must be taken that encompasses the scope of process knowledge buildup during development.

2. Severity (S) = severity of such a failure

    The team must evaluate the severity of each effect, not failure, to occur. That is the potential effect on drug substance quality attributes and hence potential harm to a patient. A scale of 1 to 5 is used with 1 indicating no effect and 5 indicating a batch that needs to be destroyed.

3. Detectability (D) = detectability of the failure if it occurs

    The team assesses the likelihood of detecting the failure before its impact on a patient is realized. A scale of 1 to 5 is used with 1 indicating that a failure is immediately detectable before the unit operation and 5 indicating that there is no method to detect a failure before the product reaches the customer. Generally, it is the effect of the failure that is detected and not the mode.

Risk Priority Number

The RPN is calculated for all items by multiplying:

(probability of failure) × (severity) × (likelihood of detection)

or

$(P) \times (S) \times (D)$

The worst case (highest risk) is $5 \times 5 \times 5 = 125$; the best case $1 \times 1 \times 1 = 1$ (lowest risk).

This approach is used as a tool for continuous improvements. If, for example, a new measuring technology is introduced the result may be increased detectability of a failure mode and thus a lowered RPN. Changes in procedures may lead to a decreased risk of an error to occur and will lower its RPN. It is also possible that new failure modes are identified, which need to be included in the analysis.

TABLE 9   Summary of the Rating Scheme for Performing a QRA

Severity (S)	Probability (P)	Detectability (D)	Score
Will not affect quality of stage product	Very low/free	Before error made	1
Different material quality, but will process on with no impact to API quality	Low/wide	IPC/during processing	2
Adjustment to downstream processing required to maintain API quality	Medium/limited	Intermediate specification testing	3
Batch requiring rework	High/tight	API testing/drug product processing	4
Destroyed batch/product recall or UNKNOWN	Very high/ very tight	Detected by customer	5

Abbreviations: API, active pharmaceutical ingredient; QRA, quality risk assessment.

Dependent on the scope of the QRA the team may wish to set a threshold values for RPN that require different levels of mitigation, or allow categorization of high medium or low risk rather than using the absolute RPN values. Typical value are <25 for low, 25 to 75 for medium, and >75 for high.

Table 9 summarizes the rating scheme for performing the QRA to make consistent judgments of probabilities, severity, and detectability.

The risk ratings and RPN scores are filled in on the FMECA matrix and any comments are noted.

The completed matrix and minutes of the meeting should be circulated to the QRA team for review and final confirmation of the accuracy of the assessment.

Facilitation

QRAs are much more effective with appropriate facilitation. The facilitator need not be connected to the project technical team; indeed it is recommended that the facilitator be from outside of the project so that he/she can concentrate on running the process and not get drawn into technical discussions. The role involves the following:

- Correctly applying the FMECA process
  - Are all failure modes mentioned and listed?
  - Are effects of the failure modes correct? (no confusion between causes and effects)
- Supporting the QRA leader with the preparation of the meeting and during the FMECA session
- Ensuring P, S, and D scores are assigned for each failure mode/effect
- Keeping the assessment flowing, do not lose time with long discussions about P, S, and D scores. In case of doubt, take the "worst case"
- Ensuring the FMECA worksheet is completely filled in (actions, responsible person, date)

Risk Mitigation Proposal

The risk mitigation proposal is usually generated following completion and final agreement of the QRA. The risk mitigation review meeting will consist of the core team of technical experts with process knowledge. The meeting should evaluate the scope of the mitigation exercise.

The team should review the FMECA matrix and generate mitigation proposals. These should be documented as a series of actions and assigned to responsible individuals. This proposal should form the basis of the project scope document and direct the development of the process.

Reporting
A version-controlled document that has full details of each step of the process should be generated to document the QRA. New versions will be created as the process is reviewed throughout development, establishment, and commercial manufacture.

CONCLUDING REMARKS
The medicine development process takes place over several years. Starting from making fit-for-purpose material for early clinical trials by inefficient processes and administering drugs in undeveloped formulations, development teams explore many avenues to generate economical, safe, robust manufacturing processes that reliably generate drug substance, and drug product that is free of contamination, and reproducible delivers patients the therapeutic benefit promised on the label: drug product with the required *pharmaceutical quality*.

Risk assessment can be applied at the end of development to demonstrate that variability in the operation of manufacturing processes poses an insignificant risk to the pharmaceutical quality. It is used in this way to support Quality by Design submissions.

It is however during development that risk assessment of manufacturing processes truly drives the QbD. By periodically risk assessing the manufacturing processes, development teams collate a good overview of risks associated with the whole manufacturing process. In addition, the risk assessment also provides an opportunity to incorporate the experience from peers and experts that would not otherwise have been involved unless specific problems are encountered.

The output of risk assessments allows the teams to focus on areas where the risk to either the pharmaceutical quality or business objectives is high, as well as areas where understanding is still lacking.

Risk assessment does however require an investment of time and resource. A companywide system will eventually be required, with trained facilitators and agreed protocols. Development teams will have to spend some days per year in risk assessments. However, in analogy with the statement "A week in the lab will save you an afternoon in the library," we would argue that months in the lab and a late-stage quality failure will save days in risk assessment.

REFERENCES
1. DiMasi JA, Hansen RW, Grabowski HJ, et al. Cost of innovation in the pharmaceutical industry. J Health Econ 1991; 10:107–142.
2. DiMasi JA, Hansen RW, Grabowski HJ. The price of innovation: new estimates of drug development costs. J Health Econ 2003; 22:151–185.
3. Suresh P, Basu PK. Improving pharmaceutical product development and manufacturing: impact on cost of drug development and cost of goods sold of pharmaceuticals. J Pharm Innov 2008; 3:175–187.
4. O'Brien MK, Kolb M, Sutherland K, et al. Early process development: the Wyeth approach. Chimia 2006; 60:518–522.

5. Adler C, Brunner J, Fichter C, et al. Process development for active pharmaceutical ingredient following a development cascade. Chimia 2006; 60:523–529.
6. Shultis K. The dilemma of process development. Drug Discov Today 2002; 7(16):850–853.
7. Chemburkar SR, Bauer J, Deming K, et al. Dealing with the impact of Ritonavir Polymorphs on the late stages of bulk drug process development. Org Proc Res Dev 2000; 4:413–417.
8. Bauer J, Spanton S, Henry R, et al. Ritonavir: an extraordinary example of conformational polymorphism. Pharm Res 2001; 18:859–866.
9. ICH Expert working group. ICH Harmonised tripartite guidelines: Quality Risk Management, Q9, 2005. Available at: http://www.ich.org/cache/compo/276-254-1.html. Accessed March 2010.
10. MIL-P-1629 (1949) November 9 and MIL-P-1629A (1980). November 24 Procedure for performing a failure mode effect and criticality analysis, United States Military Procedure.
11. Dunjo J, Fthenakis V, Vilchez J, et al. Hazard and operability (HAZOP) analysis: a literature review. J Hazard Mater 2010; 173:19–32.
12. Kepner CH, Tregoe BB. The New Rational Manager. Princeton, NJ: Princeton Research Press, 1981.
13. Woodstock J. The concept of pharmaceutical quality. Am Pharm Rev 2004; 7(6): 1–3.
14. Lionberger RA, Lee SL, Lee L, et al. Quality by design: concepts for ANDAs. AAPS J 2008; 10(2):268–276.
15. ICH Expert Working Group. ICH Harmonised Tripartite Guidelines Q8(R2): Pharmaceutical Development, 2009. Available at: http://www.ich.org/cache/compo/276-254-1.html. Accessed March 2010.
16. ICH Expert Working Group. ICH Harmonised Tripartite Guideline Q6A: Specifications: Test Procedures and Acceptance Criteria for New Drug Substances and New Drug Products: Chemical Substances, 1999. Available at: http://www.ich.org/cache/compo/276-254-1.html. Accessed March 2010.
17. Ganzer WP, Materna JA, Mitchell MB, et al. Current thoughts on critical process parameters and API synthesis. Pharm Technol 2005; 29(7):46–66.
18. Walker D. Organization. In: The Management of Chemical Process Development in the Pharmaceutical Industry. Hoboken, NJ: John Wiley & Sons, 2007.
19. Andersen NG. Practical Process Research and Development. New York: Academic Press, 2000.
20. Rao S. The Chemistry of Process Development in the Fine Chemical and Pharmaceutical Industry. 2nd ed. New Delhi: Asian Books Pvt Ltd, 2007.
21. Butters M, Catterick D, Craig A, et al. Critical assessment of pharmaceutical processes: a rationale for changing the synthetic route. Chem Rev 2006; 106:3002–3027.
22. Muller FL, Latimer J. Anticipation of scale up issues in pharmaceutical development. Comput Chem Eng 2009; 33:1051–1055.
23. Patterson GK, Paul EL, Kresta SM, Etchells AW. Mixing and chemical reactions. In: Paul EL, Atiemo-Obeng VA, Kresta SM, eds. Handbook of Industrial Mixing. Hoboken, NJ: John Wiley & Sons, 2004.
24. Muller FL. On the rheological behaviour of batch crystallisations. Chem Eng Res Des 2009; 87:627–632.
25. Manipura A, Sharratt PN, Roberts EPL, et al. Decision support system for route selection in pharmaceutical process development. AIChE's 2009 Annual Meeting, Nashville, TN, USA, November 8–13, 2009.
26. Bisio A, Kabel RL. Scaleup of Chemical Processes. New York: John Wiley & Sons, 1985.
27. Basu PK, Mack RA, Vinson JM. Consider a new approach to pharmaceutical process development. Chem Eng Prog 1999; 95(8):82–90.

4 Scale-up and process validation

Steven Ostrove

INTRODUCTION

Validation is providing documented evidence that a process will work as expected with a high degree of assurance. What does this really mean? First of all, the statement implies that the process must be repeatable. Second, it needs to produce the same quality; and third, one needs to be secure in its operation. How does this come about? Above all, the process needs to be clearly defined. It is important to understand the steps, their controls, and thus the results. In addition, the equipment needs to be fully operational. This means that the process should be tested (validated) and the equipment qualified. All parts of the process are included in this procedure. The equipment needs to be qualified before it can be used, and the process needs to be validated to demonstrate robustness and reproducibility.

We often refer to "validation" without thinking of these two major aspects of the term—process *and* equipment. A pharmaceutical company (and I include medical devices and biotechnology companies) needs to operate in a "validated" state, otherwise known as "GMP compliant." These two major pieces are often further subdivided, and are often performed separately and by separate groups within a company. Because of this, it is necessary for every company to assure that both functions are complete and well documented.

This chapter will concentrate on the process validation (PV) portion; however, to do that it is necessary to begin with the equipment qualification (EQ). One cannot perform or even minimally validate a process without a sufficient and complete EQ. So, before delving into the PV aspect of scaling up, the EQ component needs to be briefly discussed.

EQUIPMENT QUALIFICATION

EQ is considered to have three components (which are sometimes combined). These are the installation qualification (IQ), the operational qualification (OQ), and the performance qualification (PQ). As stated, the IQ and OQ are often performed together as an EQ. Also, there is sometimes overlap between the PQ for the equipment and the process qualification. The process qualification is a part of the PV, which will be discussed later in this chapter. If the PQ is not combined with the process qualification, the process qualification will require additional steps (discussed later) (1).

The EQ (here it is comprised of the IQ and OQ) needs to include items that describe the unit that will be performing a task in the process. This includes items such as tanks, blenders, drying units (fluid bed, dry heat ovens), chromatography columns (2) (and associated equipment), filters, granulators, filling machines, etc. That is, any piece of equipment that affects the outcome of the manufacturing process needs to be qualified (3). One function of the EQ that is often overlooked, or at least often not considered, is that it provides the company with a starting point in case of emergency replacement or as a means of helping to define the process parameters. In the later case, existing equipment is often used when a process is scaled up so the process parameters would be dictated by the equipment that is on site.

- The EQ (IQ and OQ combined) is used to establish written proof that the equipment is what you ordered, or need, for the process and that it will work as it is expected or designed to work. The PQ part is used to demonstrate that the unit will operate at the required process set point(s) for the time needed for the process to take place. In addition, the PQ also tests the limits or boundaries of the equipment and shows that while the IQ and OQ (or EQ) test the individual units, the PQ tests the process chain.

To have a complete EQ, the following items should be included:

- Materials of construction [for all parts that come in contact with the product or one of its components (e.g., water, active ingredient, excipients)].
- Physical description of the unit (e.g., size, volume, jacketed)
  - Major components (e.g., motors, compressors, impellers).
- Operating parameters (not necessarily the range to be used in the process).
  - Whenever possible, the full operating range should be tested.
    - Examples.
      - Speed control.
      - Temperature control.
- All functions that pertain to the process (functions that are not used do not necessarily need to be included in the qualification; however, it may be necessary to demonstrate that they do not interfere with the functions used in the process).
- Environmental constraints [maximum or minimum temperature(s) and/or humidity].
- Lubricants used (it is often recommended to use food-grade lubricants especially when there is potential product contact if a leak was to occur).
- Spare parts—only those that are critical to the continued successful operation of the unit.
- Other physical or operational parameters that may influence the operation or performance of the equipment that directly, or indirectly, has impact on the product.
- Are all utilities required for the operation of the equipment connected, commissioned, or qualified (e.g., compress air, electricity)?
- Calibration and preventive maintenance are complete.
- Another point to consider in EQ is the actual increase in size. A 10× increase in size is generally accepted to have the same thermodynamic parameters as the smaller unit. That is, heat, mass distribution, etc., are considered to be the same within the 10× increase.

After reviewing the above information, the question can be asked, How is process scale-up affected by this? In simple terms, the process is developed using "small" equipment. In some cases the equipment may be scaled up to larger sizes or volumes (i.e., pilot scale), in other cases another piece or type of equipment may need to be used. Development work usually does not include validation or qualification. Pilot plant or commercial production certainly does require qualification and validation. The Food and Drug Administration (FDA) has a guideline that deals with some of these issues (SUPAC) (4). If this guidance is employed care must be taken to comply with all aspects of the guidance as there are many requirements that must be met to fully comply.

As the volume produced is increased, the equipment size must also increase. Some things that need to be considered are as follows:

- Height to width ratios (e.g., bioreactors)
- Volume to surface area ratios
- Fill volume ratio
- The effective charging or discharging of the materials
- Cleaning
- Effect/affect of gases (e.g., air, oxygen) sparging
- Geometric vessel design
- Mixing times—proportion of each material in the blender
- Mixing speeds (may vary because of volumes, geometry)
- Heating affects of mixing or chemical reactions (i.e., the thermodynamics of the chemical reactions)

Once the equipment has been shown to be operational it needs to be shown to be appropriate for its intended purpose. The PQ is used to document or otherwise demonstrate that the equipment will perform consistently within the range or set parameters needed by the process. In the IQ and OQ it has been shown to work independently over its full operation range (as specified by the manufacturer). Now some of the questions that need to be asked (and answered) are as follows:

- Can it maintain the needed operation settings for the time required by the process?
- Is the equipment capable of running at the required speed, consistently within a set range, over the time required for the process?
- Do the various pieces of equipment work together as a "train" or are they totally independent?

All equipment used in the production of clinical or commercial products need to be qualified. Each step of the scale-up, development lab through full commercial batch sizes, need to have qualified equipment so that the PV can be completed without questions about the equipment functioning as intended. This means that a process cannot be validated if the equipment is not qualified. And, the equipment cannot be qualified if the utilities that make them work are not commissioned or qualified. SUPAC is not to be relied on to provide the necessary qualification documents. If the equipment is not qualified and the calibrations complete prior to starting the PV, there is always a question as to whether the process is really in control and, thus, compliant.

PROCESS VALIDATION: GENERAL

As stated earlier, process needs to be validated. To do this, one needs to provide documentation that the process will produce the product with definable and measurable characteristics every time with a "high degree of assurance." To accomplish this validation the following needs to be considered:

- Define and determine the "critical process parameters" (CPPs).
- Define and determine the "critical quality attributes" (CQA).

Critical Process Parameters

CPPs are those process parameters that must be met or maintained so that the product will maintain its purity, quality, identity, strength and safety. In selecting or determining a CPP, it needs to be a measurable parameter. A CPP usually determines the critical process or quality attributes (CPA or CQA). CPPs include physical items such as mixing time and temperatures. A range should be validated since it nearly impossible to have an absolute temperature or time achieved. The range should not be too large or too tight so as to keep adequate control on the process.

When scaling up, the CPP(s) identified should be carried over as the process size is increased. However, it must be kept in mind that additional CPPs may be added to the process on the basis of the new size or containers used. Some CPPs are

- temperatures,
- mixing time,
- hold times (holding in a tank during preparation or waiting for the next process step to begin), and
- velocity of flows (between containers, drying—fluid bed dryers).

Critical Process Attributes

CPAs are those process attributes that must be met to release the product. These are directly affected by the CPPs. The CPA is also measurable, that is, you can see or measure the effect of the CPP.

Examples of some CPAs are as follows:

- Solid oral dose
  - Hardness
  - Friability
  - Size (thickness)
  - Weight
  - Dissolution
- Liquids, creams, and ointments
  - Viscosity
  - Clarity
  - Color
  - Volume
  - pH, osmolarity, conductivity
- Parenterals
  - Sterility
  - Concentration
  - Viscosity
  - pH, osmolarity, conductivity
- Medical devices
  - Radio frequency compliance, radio frequency interference (RFI), and electromagnetic interference (EMI)
  - Materials of construction
- Biologics
  - Virus removal
  - Contaminants (impurity)

Throughout the scale-up process, the product needs to maintain its efficacy. This means that parameters contained in the U.S. Pharmacopeia (USP) (5) or other countries' pharmacopeias need to be addressed as part of the validation process. These include items such as: content uniformity and dissolution.

The latest industry approach to the PV as promulgated in the draft guideline on PV from the FDA (6) in late 2008. This document now outlines three (3) stages of the process. Each stage of the process has its own set of expectations. The first two—stage 1, process design, and stage 2, process qualification—are the two that relate to scale-up activities. The third stage, continued process verification, pertains to established processes to assure an ongoing state of control.

Stage 1: Process design emphasizes the need to use good scientific methods for development. As stated, "The goal of this stage is to design a process suitable for routine commercial manufacturing that can consistently deliver a product that meets its critical quality attributes" (6). The use of design of experiment (DOE) protocols can help in the understanding and control of the process. This allows the study of the interactions of all components of the process [active pharmaceutical ingredient (API), excipients, containers, etc.]. The FDA recognizes that changes made during development are not necessarily validated. However, the FDA expects that the information obtained here will be used as the basis for the PV.

Stage 2: Process qualification is concerned with assuring that the facility and equipment are correct for the process. During the scale-up process, since the original development may not have been done on qualified equipment (if as part of R&D), the equipment needs to be qualified. One must make sure that during scale-up, the equipment will fit its intended purpose. The equipment PQ needs to be completed so as to document that the system functions as expected and that the process will operate under the conditions needed for the product.

As mentioned earlier, the PQ can be combined with the process qualification. When this is done the process is tested at several levels of operation (usually high, middle, and low). The equipment PQ tests the operation over the range to be used during production, while the process qualification tests the production over the same range. If the two are not combined, then the process needs to be tested over its expected operating range resulting in additional testing and increased time due to the extra tests needed. The purpose of this is to document that the equipment is able to sustain the conditions necessary to make the product successfully and is robust enough to assure the safety and efficacy of each unit of the drug.

As an example, if a tablet press is to produce 300 tablets (300 rpm)/min, the machine would need to be tested during the equipment PQ over a range of 250 to 350 rpm. And the process qualification needs to test the tablet production over 250 to 350 tablets/min. Thus, an equipment test at 250, 300, and 350 rpm for an extended time period is needed. In addition, tablets need to be made at the 250, 300, and 350 rpm (or tablets/min). By combining the two (PQ and process qualification) at least three tests are eliminated. In addition, a matrix approach may be used in performing these tests if multiple strengths or sizes of the product are to be produced. This would also reduce the number of tests needed to qualify the equipment.

In addition, additional samples are expected to be taken during this phase of the validation to demonstrate the robustness of the process. The PV needs to have a history, or rational as to why and how a step is to be performed and what its function is in the process. Scale-up and development provide this rational.

PROCESS VALIDATION: SPECIFICS

Some examples of specific issues that need to be addressed during the PV (after all of the equipment has been fully qualified) include the following:

- Containers
  - Closure—leak test (7)
  - Configuration
  - Material of construction
- Content uniformity (oral solid dose)
  - Tablet hardness, size/weight
- Cleaning
  - Hold times (clean and dirty)
  - Compatibility with cleaning agents
- Thermodynamic properties
  - Exothermic versus endothermic reactions (volumes, dissipation, etc.)
  - Filtration
  - Chromatography

All of the above (and others specific to each process) need to be tested during the scale-up process if the product is to be used for either clinical or commercial use. As in all PVs, each step needs to be shown to be reproducible and consistent within the product specifications.

Factors such as gas distribution (fermentation), heat (granulation and mixing), and other thermodynamic parameters need to be considered during the scale-up process. In general, a rule of thumb that is useful is a scale-up factor of $10\times$ (8) is about the maximum one can go and maintain the same relative thermodynamic properties. Some specialized processes, such as chromatography, require more careful consideration. Maintaining the height to width ratio here and in bioreactors is very important. Scaling up using different height to width ratios, very often, will not yield the intended product.

Cleaning issues and environmental impact are just as important to the PV as the process itself. Cleaning times (including clean and dirty hold times), and compatibility of all components with the cleaning agents are parameters that are often considered too late in the process. As the process is scaled up, cleaning parameters change. Larger vessels usually require more time to reach temperature (an important factor in depyrogenation as well as general cleaning) or to have the cleaning agent work effectively because of the increased surface area. Port sizes increase in scale-up. This means more possibilities of product or ingredients getting into the atmosphere (room). Protective clothing may be required or certainly extra environmental monitoring will probably be needed.

Another point that should be considered during the validation of scaling up is the increased number of samples that will require analysis. This includes the utility samples (e.g., water) as well as extra process (in process samples). Also, as mentioned in the draft FDA Process Validation guideline, a statistician should be consulted during the PV to assure that the correct interactions have been captured and that these interactions will yield the expected results.

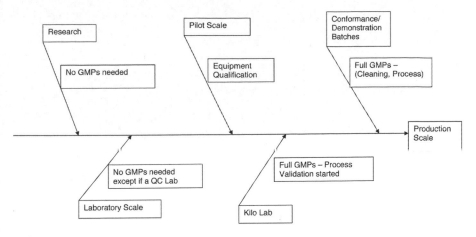

FIGURE 1   Basic flow of GMP requirements—R & D to Production.

SUMMARY

Figure 1 shows a simplified flow from research to Process levels.

It shows that PV during scale-up is not really different than the PV of a commercial product. However, each step in the scale-up needs to use qualified equipment and eventually validated. As the equipment size increases, so does the complexity of the process (e.g., more or larger moving parts, more particle generation, etc.). The equipment used in scaling up needs to be qualified as does the analytical methods used. All factors, such as mix times, hold times, temperatures, flow rates, etc., change as the size increases. SUPAC does not cover all situations and is not intended to be used when going from development to commercial size, although it may apply in some cases.

A carefully thought out validation process is required since there are often several steps needed to bring a laboratory scale process to commercial size. Scaling up validation now requires a complete understanding of the process and how it can and needs to be controlled. Process analytical technology (PAT) (9) can be implemented during the scale-up and, thus, needs to have its own validation included in the process.

As always, know the process, plan the qualification and validation, and document it all.

REFERENCES

1. Agalloco J, Carlton F. Validation of Pharmaceutical Processes. 3rd ed. New York, NY: Informa Health Care, 2007.
2. Ostrove S. Considerations for scaling up to process promatography, LC-GC, Vol. 7, #7.
3. Code of Federal Regulations, 21 CFR 211.
4. Guidance for Industry nonsterile semisolid dosage forms scale-up and postapproval changes: chemistry, manufacturing, and controls; in vitro release testing and in vivo bioequivalence documentation.
5. U.S. Pharmacopeia.

6. Guidance for Industry process validation: general principles and practices—draft guidance.
7. FDA. Guidance for Industry: container closure systems for packaging human drugs and biologics, 1999.
8. Ostrove S. Personal communication.
9. Guidance for Industry PAT—a framework for innovative pharmaceutical development, manufacturing, and quality assurance.

5 Parenteral drug scale-up

Igor Gorsky

INTRODUCTION

The term "parenteral" is applied to preparations administered by injection through one or more layers of skin tissue. The word is derived from the Greek words, *para* and *etheron*, meaning outside of intestine, and is used for those dosage forms administered by routes other than the oral route. Because administration of injectables, by definition, requires circumventing the highly protective barriers of human body, the skin and the mucous membranes, the purity of the dosage form must achieve the exceptional quality. This is generally accomplished by close utilization of Good Manufacturing Practices.

The basic principles employed in the preparation of the parenteral products do not vary from those widely used in other sterile and nonsterile liquid preparations. However, it is imperative, that all calculations are made in an accurate and most precise manner. Therefore, an issue of a parenteral solution scale up essentially becomes a liquid scale-up task, which requires a high degree of accuracy. A practical yet scientifically sound means of performing this scale-up analysis of liquid parenteral systems is presented below. The approach is based on the scale-of-agitation method. For single-phase liquid systems, the primary scale-up criterion is equal liquid motion when comparing pilot-size batches to larger production-size batches.

One of the most important processes involved in the scale-up of liquid parenteral preparations is mixing (1). For liquids, mixing can be defined as a transport process that occurs simultaneously in three different scales during which one substance (solute) achieves a uniform concentration in another substance (solvent). On a large, visible scale, mixing occurs by bulk diffusion in which the elements are blended by the pumping action of the mixer's impeller. On the microscopic scale, elements that are in proximity are blended by the eddy currents, and they form drag where local velocity and shear-stress differences act on the fluid. On the smallest scale, final blending occurs via molecular diffusion whose rate is unaffected by the mechanical mixing action. Therefore, large-scale mixing primarily depends on flow within the vessel whereas small-scale mixing is mostly dependent on shear. This approach focuses on large-scale mixing using three viable approaches, specifically concentrating on the scale-of-agitation method.

GEOMETRIC SIMILARITY

There are several methods to achieve appropriate scale-up of mixing. The first method involves geometric similarity. This technique employs proportional scale-up of geometric parameters of the vessel. The scaled-up parameters may include such geometric ratios as D/T ratio, where D is diameter of the impeller and T is diameter of the tank, and Z/T ratio, where Z is the height of the liquid in the vessel. Similar ratios are compared for both the small-scale equipment (D_1T_1) and the larger-size equipment (D_2T_2). For example,

$$R = D_1T_1 = D_2T_2 \qquad (1)$$

where R is the geometric scaling factor.

After R has been determined, other required parameters such as the rotational speed of the larger equipment can then be calculated by power law relationships. In the above example, the required rotational speed, N, can be calculated as

$$N_2 = N_1 \left(\frac{1}{R}\right)^n \qquad (2)$$

Rotational speeds may be expressed either in terms of rpm or in terms of sec^{-1}. The power law exponent, n, has a definite physical significance. The value of n and the corresponding significance are determined either empirically or through theoretical means. Table 1 lists most common values assigned to n.

The scale-up can be completed by using predicted values of N_2 to determine the horsepower requirements of the large-size system. In most designs, D/T will be in the following range:

$$0.15 \leq \frac{D}{T} \leq 0.6 \qquad (3)$$

and Z/T will be in the range:

$$0.3 \leq \frac{Z}{T} \leq 1.5 \qquad (4)$$

TABLE 1 Most Common Values Assigned to the Power Law Exponent, n, When Comparing Large- to Small-Scale Equipment

N	Physical interpretation
0	Equal blend time.
	This exponent is rarely used due to excessively large equipment requirement to hold speed constant.
1/2	Equal surface motion.
	Equal surface motion is related most often to vortex formation. The depth of the vortex is related by geometric similarity and equal Froude number: $$N_{FR} = \frac{DN^2}{g}$$
2/3	Equal mass transfer rates.
	Scale-up based on the mass transfer rate between phases is directly related to liquid turbulence and motion at the interface. Scale-up of solids dissolution rate or mass transfer between liquid phases is adequately handled utilizing 2/3as an exponent.
3/4	Equal solids suspension.
	Agitation for a desired level of solids suspension is based on an overall appearance of the solid-liquid system. Results of the empirical correlations have been summarized for most types of solids suspension scale-up cases.
1	Equal liquid motion (equal average fluid velocity).
	Analyzing the significance of the scale-up exponent for liquid motion shows that similar results are obtained when equal tip speed (fluid velocity) of torque per volume is applied to geometrically similar agitation system.

These values, in conjunction with N and the horsepower requirements, may completely define the major parameters of the systems. However, in most of the cases, scaled-up bench batches yield atypical agitator speeds and significantly larger power requirements. The number of American National Standards Institute/American Gear Manufacturers Association agitator speeds and standard motor horsepowers available off the shelf is quite sufficient to closely approximate most levels of agitation. It is very seldom that the level of agitation of scaled liquid system requires a nonstandard agitator. Upon identification of the rpm and horsepower requirements, the scale-up procedure follows to engineering and economic evaluation phase. For illustration purposes, equal power per volume with geometric similarity is shown to be equivalent to a scale-up exponent of $n = 2/3$. Turbulent power requirement or a constant power number is proportional to the product of agitator speed cubed and diameter of the impeller diameter to the fifth power:

$$P \propto N^3 D^5 \tag{5}$$

Because of the geometric similarity conventions that hold all length ratios constant, tank dimensions are a fixed multiple of impeller diameter. Therefore, the tank volume is proportional to impeller diameter cubed:

$$V \propto D^3 \tag{6}$$

Subsequently, if power per volume is held constant in two different size systems, the agitator speed must change in relation to the impeller diameter:

$$\frac{P}{V} \propto N^3 D^2 \tag{7}$$

$$N_1^3 D_1^2 = N_2^3 D_2^2 \tag{8}$$

Rearranging Eq. (8) into Eq. (2) demonstrates that this relationship is equivalent to a scale-up exponent of two thirds:

$$N_2 = N_1 \left(\frac{D_1}{D_2}\right)^{2/3} = N_1 \left(\frac{1}{R}\right)^{2/3} \tag{9}$$

It is important to note that the small-scale agitator operations may be described in terms of impeller diameter and agitator speed, manufacturing process equipment is more conveniently specified by horsepower and fluid velocity. For most standard turbine configurations, power number correlations are available to convert impeller diameter and agitator speed into a horsepower value for given fluid properties. Most laboratory bench equipment is designed to provide a torque measurement that can be readily converted to horsepower directly from the conditions of the pilot batches.

DIMENSIONLESS NUMBERS METHOD

The second method uses dimensionless numbers to predict scale-up parameters. The use of dimensionless numbers simplifies design calculations by reducing the number of variables to consider. The dimensionless number approach has been used with good success in heat transfer calculations and to some extent in gas dispersion (mass transfer) for mixer scale-up. Usually, the primary independent variable in a dimensionless number correlation is Reynolds number:

$$N_{RE} = \frac{D^2 \rho N}{\mu} \qquad (10)$$

where

N = shaft speed (sec^{-1})
D = propeller blade diameter (cm)
ρ = the density of the solution dispersion (g/cm^3)
μ = the viscosity of the solution dispersion (g/cm-sec).

Other dimensionless numbers are used widely for various scale-up applications. One example is Froude number:

$$N_{FR} = \frac{DN^2}{g} \qquad (11)$$

where g is acceleration due to gravity in cm-sec^{-2}. The Froude number compares inertial forces to gravitational forces inside the system.

Another example is the power number, which is a function of the Reynolds number and the Froude number:

$$N_P = \frac{Pg_c}{\rho N^3 D^5} \qquad (12)$$

where P is power and g_c is a gravitational conversion factor. This number relates density, viscosity, rotational speed, and the diameter of the impeller. The power number correlation has been used successfully for impeller geometric scale-up. Approximately half a dozen other dimensionless numbers are involved in the various aspects of mixing, heat, and mass transfer, etc.

Both of the above methods belong to a traditional fluid mechanical approach known as dimensional analysis (2). Unfortunately, these methods cannot always achieve results in various manufacturing environments. Therefore, the third method is introduced below, which can be applied easily to the various research and production situations. This method actually is a combination of the first two methods.

SCALE-OF-AGITATION APPROACH

The basis of the scale-of-agitation approach is a geometric scale-up with the power law exponent, $n = 1$ (Table 1). This provides for equal fluid velocities in both large- and small-scale equipment. Furthermore, several dimensionless groups are used to relate the fluid properties to the physical properties of the equipment being considered. In particular, bulk fluid velocity comparisons are made around the largest blade in the system. This method is best suited for turbulent flow agitation in which tanks are assumed to be vertical cylinders.

Although good success may be achieved in applying this technique to marine-type propeller systems, the original development was based on low-rpm, axial, or radial impeller arrangements. Because the most intensive mixing occurs in the volume immediately around the impeller, this discussion focuses

TABLE 2   Nomenclature

Q	Effective pumping capacity or volumetric pumping flow in cm³/sec
N	Shaft speed in sec⁻¹
N_{RE}	Impeller Reynolds number, dimensionless
N_Q	Pumping number, dimensionless
D	Diameter of the largest mixer blade in cm
ρ	Density of the fluid in g/cm³
μ	Viscosity of the fluid in g/cm-sec
v_b	Bulk fluid velocity in cm
T	Diameter of the tank in cm
A	Cross-sectional area of the tank in cm²

on this particular region of mixing. Table 2 describes the nomenclature used to develop the theory behind the approach.

The analysis proceeds as follows. First, determine the D/T ratio of the tank, based on the largest impeller, in which the original (usually Research and Development, R&D) batches had been compounded. It is also necessary to know the rotational speed and the horsepower of the mixer used.

The only two product physical properties needed are density and viscosity. Generally, parenterals, as the most solution-type products, will follow Newtonian fluid behavior and may also be considered incompressible. Therefore, point densities and viscosities can be used satisfactorily.

The next step in the analysis is to calculate the impeller Reynolds number achieved during this original compounding using Eq. (10). The impeller Reynolds number must be >2000 to proceed with analysis (3).

Mixing achieved in the initial R&D processing must be in turbulent range. If the impeller Reynolds number is <2000, then mixing in the pilot tank was either inadequate or represented some other special case such as moderately viscous fluids. In these situations, another D/T ratio curve must be used.

Proceeding further, let us obtain the value of the terminal pumping number in the R&D pilot process by using the following formula:

$$N_Q = 1.1283 - \left[1.07118 \left(\frac{D}{T} \right) \right] \tag{13}$$

Equation (13) is empirical relationship obtained by the linear regression between D/T and terminal pumping numbers (4). It is important to note that a family of curves exists for each D/T ratio when N_Q (pumping number) is plotted versus the impeller Reynolds number (5). In the turbulent range ($N_{RE} > 2000$), the N_Q curves flatten out and thus are independent of the Reynolds number.

The terminal pumping number, $N_{Q/RE>2000}$, plotted against the D/T ratio results in Eq. (13). The cross-sectional area of the pilot-size tank is determined by using Eq. (14).

$$A = \frac{\pi T^2}{4} \, \text{cm}^2 \tag{14}$$

Then, the value of effective pumping capacity for the pilot-size mixer is calculated using Eq. (15).

$$Q = N_Q N D^3 \, \text{cm}^3/\text{sec} \tag{15}$$

TABLE 3 Process Requirements Set Degree of Agitation for Blending and Motion

Scale of agitation	Bulk fluid velocity (cm/sec)	Description of mixing
1	3	Agitation levels 1 and 2 are characteristic of applications requiring minimum fluid velocities to achieve the product result.
2	6	Agitators capable of level 2 will
		a. blend miscible fluids to uniformity if specific gravity differences are less than 0.1 and if the viscosity of the most viscous is less than 100 times of the other;
		b. establish complete fluid-batch control;
		c. produce a flat but moving fluid-batch surface.
3	9	Agitation levels 3 to 6 are characteristic of fluid velocities in most chemical (including pharmaceutical) industries agitated batches.
4	12	Same as 3
5	15	Same as 3 and 4
6	18	Agitators capable of level 6 will
		a. blend miscible fluids to uniformity if specific gravity differences are less than 0.6 and if the viscosity of the most viscous is less than 10,000 times of the other;
		b. suspend trace solids (<2%) with settling rates of 2 to 4 ft/min;
		c. produce surface rippling at lower viscosities.
7	21	Agitation levels 7 to 10 are characteristic of applications requiring high fluid velocities for process result, such as mixing of the high-viscosity suspension preparations.
8	24	Same as 7
9	27	Same as 7 and 8
10	30	Agitators capable of level 10 will
		a. blend miscible fluids to uniformity if specific gravity differences are less than 1.0 and if the viscosity of the most viscous is less than 100,000 times of the other;
		b. suspend trace solids (<2%) with settling rates of 4 to 6 ft/min;
		c. provide surging surface at low viscosities.

Finally, by inserting the values derived in Eqs. (14) and (15) into Eq. (16), the value for bulk fluid velocity around the largest impeller of the system is obtained.

$$v_b = \frac{Q}{A} \, \text{cm/sec} \tag{16}$$

The bulk fluid velocity can be inserted into Table 3 to determine the level of agitation achieved in the original R&D pilot batch. The larger-size production tank and mixer are then designed so that the scale of agitation produced in the larger vessel matches that required for the pilot-size batches. The scale-of-agitation approach was first developed in the mid-1970s by engineers at Chemineer, Inc. (6).

Table 3 summarizes the scale-of-agitation parameters and gives a qualitative description of the type of mixing associated with the various levels. According to this approach, mixing is a similar process if the calculated bulk fluid velocities for the production-size vessels lie within ±1 unit level of the scale of agitation required from an analysis of the R&D pilot batches. It is quite easy to match the required scale of agitation by simply adjusting the rpm when working with a variable-speed equipment. Thus, a given tank equipped with a variable-speed mixer will generally be capable of several agitation levels.

SCALE-OF-AGITATION APPROACH EXAMPLE

To illustrate the actual application of the scale-of-agitation approach to scale-up, the above method was applied to the scale-up of typical injectables solution from 378-L pilot batch to a 3780-L production-size batch. The example product is a Newtonian fluid with density of 1.018 g/cm^3 and a viscosity of 0.0588 g/cm-sec (5.88 cps). The tank used in the manufacturing of the pilot batch had the following parameters:

T = diameter of the tank = 74.6 cm
A = cross-sectional area = 4371 cm^2

The agitation was accomplished with the turbine-type mixer, and the largest axial impeller was 40.64 cm. The pilot batch was mixed at 90 rpm (1.5/sec). From the initial known data, the D/T ratio was determined.

$$\frac{D_{378L}}{T_{378L}} = \frac{40.64 \text{ cm}}{74.60 \text{ cm}} = 0.54 \tag{17}$$

Then the value of the impeller Reynolds number was obtained by plugging known values into Eq. (10).

$$N_{RE(3785 L)} = \frac{D_{378L}^2 \rho N_{378L}}{\mu} = \frac{(40.64 \text{ cm})^2 (1.018 \text{ g/cm}^3)(1.5/\text{sec})}{0.0588 \text{ g/cm/sec}} = 44449 \tag{18}$$

Because the value of the Reynolds number is >2000, Eq. (13) is used to obtain the pumping number. The pumping number is inserted into Eq. (15) to obtain the effective pumping capacity.

$$Q_{378L} = (N_{Q(378L)})(N_{378L})(D_{378L}^3) = (0.55)(1.5/\text{sec})(40.64 \text{ cm})^3$$
$$= 55375 \text{ cm}^3/\text{sec} \tag{19}$$

Knowing the effective pumping capacity of agitation and cross-sectional area of the pilot-batch tank, bulk fluid velocity is obtained by using Eq. (16).

$$v_{b(378L)} = \frac{Q_{378L}}{A_{378L}} = \frac{55375 \text{ cm}^3/\text{sec}}{4371 \text{ cm}^2} = 12.6 \text{ cm/sec} \tag{20}$$

Inserting this bulk fluid velocity into Table 3, one can calculate the level of agitation used in the pilot batch of indictable solution as 4, which is described as characteristic of fluid velocities in most chemical process industries' agitated batches.

Now the appropriate shaft speed for scaled-up production equipment can be calculated. The tank used for production batches has a capacity of 3780 L. It is equipped with a turbine-type agitator, which has a shaft speed range of 20 to 58 rpm. The diameter of this tank is 167 cm. The diameter of the largest axial impeller is 87 cm. Given the diameter of the production tank, the cross-sectional area can be determined as

$$A_{3780\,L} = \frac{\pi T_{3780\,L}^2}{4} = \frac{\pi(167\ \text{cm})^2}{4} = 21904\ \text{cm}^2 \tag{21}$$

The next step is solving Eq. (16) for effective pumping capacity in the larger vessel.

$$Q_{3780\,L} = (v_{b(378\,L)})(A_{3780\,L}) = (12.6\ \text{cm}/\sec)(21904\ \text{cm}^2) = 275990\ \text{cm}^3/\sec \tag{22}$$

Earlier, the analysis established that the mixing of this product occurs in the turbulent flow regime because the Reynolds number obtained far exceeds the minimally required 2000. Therefore, the pumping number can be calculated for 3780-L tank by using Eq. (13) to obtain

$$N_{Q(3780\,L)} = 1.1283 - \left[(1.07118)\left(\frac{87\text{cm}}{167\text{cm}}\right)\right] = 0.57 \tag{23}$$

Finally, Eq. (15) is rearranged to solve for appropriate shaft speed to be used in a 3780-L batch.

$$N_{3780\,L} = \frac{Q_{3780\,L}}{N_{Q(3780\,L)}D_{3780\,L}^3} = \frac{275990\ \text{cm}^3/\sec}{(0.57)(87\text{cm})^3} = 0.73/\sec = 44\ \text{rpm} \tag{24}$$

The shaft speed value obtained is well within the rpm range of the 3780-L tank agitator. To determine the rpm range for production batches, start with level-3 agitation at the low rpm end and level-5 agitation at the high rpm end. Table 3 provides bulk velocities for levels 3 and 5. In turn, these are used to calculate the respective pumping capacities, defined via Eq. (16). The low and high speeds are then calculated, as described above, by rearranging Eq. (15).

This method can be used easily to show the logic behind the scale-up from original R&D batches to production-scale batches. Although scale-of agitation analysis has its limitations, especially in mixing of suspension, non-Newtonian fluids, and gas dispersions, similar analysis could be applied to these systems, provided that pertinent system variables were used. These variables may include superficial gas velocity, dimensionless aeration numbers for gas systems, and terminal settling velocity for suspensions.

LATEST REVISIONS OF THE APPROACH

As was discussed earlier, the scale-of-agitation approach has been successfully used in scale-up of various liquid systems, including parenteral drugs. However, in the late 1990s, it was slightly revised to assure even more accurate results (7). We have already determined that the mixing in the agitated tank must be in the turbulent state in order for Eq. (13) to work properly. Therefore, an assumption is made that, the full turbulence is achieved at $N_{RE} > 2000$. However, one should be aware that this assumption may result in an error of up to 12% in N_Q calculation. One may come to the conclusion that some inadequacies may be encountered in the areas of mixing close to $N_{RE} = 2000$. This later revision of the approach thrived on the fact that because this scale-up process was based on the use of existing equipment, it may not be possible to build in as much safety factor as possible, when engineering a new facility.

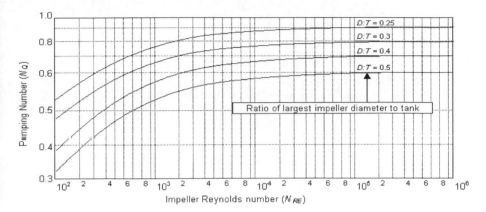

FIGURE 1 Pumping number versus impeller Reynolds number for turbine- and marine-type propeller agitators.

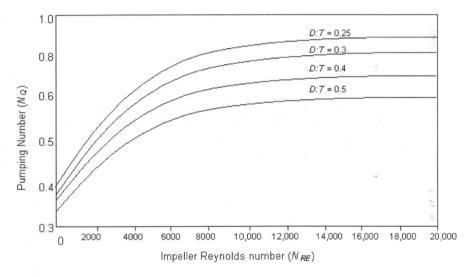

FIGURE 2 Pumping number versus impeller Reynolds number for turbine- and marine-type propeller agitators on linear coordinates.

Therefore, it would be important to determine N_Q very accurately. To achieve this goal plotting of D/T curves onto the N_{RE} versus N_Q grid was reexamined. Upon replotting Figure 1 using linear coordinates, the following trend was observed (Fig. 2). The curves rise sharply at first, which somewhat resemble dissolution profile for a solid dosage form.

The Lagenbucher's equation for a dissolution profile curve is:

$$Y = 1 - \exp\left[\frac{-(X)^a}{b}\right] \tag{25}$$

Similarly, an equation for curves in Figure 2 may be expressed as follows:

$$N_Q = 1 - \exp\left[\frac{-(N_{RE})^a}{b}\right] \tag{26}$$

where a and b are constants.

Further, the equation for constant a was determined by

$$a = -0.272\left(\frac{D}{T}\right) + 0.39 \tag{27}$$

The constant b was found to be independent of the D/T ratio and had a value of 7.7.

However, Eq. (26) only covered applications where N_{RE} was below 1000. Another equation (8) to determine N_Q in the systems, where N_{RE} is higher than 1000 is

$$N_Q = \frac{AN_{RE}}{N_{RE} + B} \tag{28}$$

where both A and B are functions of the D/T ratio and were determined to be

$$A = -1.08\left(\frac{D}{T}\right) + 1.12 \tag{29}$$

and

$$B = 578 - 1912\left(\frac{D}{T}\right) + 1980\left(\frac{D}{T}\right)^2 \tag{30}$$

These equations yield an approximate 5% maximum error as compared to an approximate 10% error in Eq. (13).

However, it is also necessary to mention that the strength of the analysis is in its ability to mathematically transfer mixing environment from the bench scale to the maximum compounding vessel as close to the original pilot batch as possible. In our experience, the maximum rpm ranges empirically achieved during compounding equal 6 to 20 rpm, which are well within maximum 10% error that one may encounter by usage of Eq. (13) in the marginal cases, where N_{RE} is close to 2000. Therefore, it is safe to conclude that the method outlined in Eqs. (13) through (16) is the most efficient to find mixing parameters of the scaled-up system. Yet, Eqs. (26) and (28) show the way of closer N_Q determination, which may be more useful for the systems with higher viscosities, thus lower N_{RE}.

SCALE-OF-AGITATION APPROACH FOR SUSPENSIONS

In order to reduce the problem of adequately dispersing the insoluble drug during formulation of sterile aqueous suspensions, the micronized material, that is, material with a particle size of 10 to 30 μm is used. Uniform distribution of the drug is required to ensure an adequate dose at the concentration per unit volume indicated on the label. Improper formulation or scale-up can result in caking of the insoluble material at the bottom of the container, making it difficult to disperse, to take up in a syringe, and thus to administer. To avoid caking, various flocculating agents are added to the product. Proper scale-up, however, is essential for adequate mixing conditions, which effect caking process. During scale-up of a suspension product, along with already discussed above

TABLE 4 Suspension Products' Percent Solids Vs. Correction Factor f_w

Solids (%)	Factor (f_w)
2	0.8
5	0.84
10	0.91
15	1.0
20	1.10
25	1.20
30	1.30
35	1.42
40	1.55
45	1.70
50	1.85

parameters, the settling rate should be considered. The presence of a two-phase, solid-liquid system classifies an agitation problem as a solid-suspension one. In such problems, the suspension of solid particles having a settling velocity >0.5 ft/min (0.25 cm/sec) within a continuous liquid phase is the purpose of the proper agitation and scale-up. The estimated terminal settling velocity, u_t, of spherical particles of 10 to 30 μm size in low viscosity 1 to 300 cps suspensions is empirically determined as 1. For an ease of analysis, the particle shape is assumed as a sphere, since most of the studies for settling velocities are conducted on the spherical beads. The different particle geometry (cylinders, disks, crushed solids, many crystalline forms) would not compromise the integrity of the analysis due to the usage of micronized materials. First, one must determine design settling velocity u_d, which is a product of terminal settling velocity u_t and a correction factor f_w, from Table 4:

$$u_d = u_t f_w \tag{31}$$

Upon determination of design settling velocity, one must choose the scale of agitation required, using Table 5 (9). It should be noted that Table 5 uses similar concepts as we outlined earlier in Table 3, applying them for suspension products.

The chosen scale of agitation is then plugged into Figure 3 chart to find the value of constant ϕ.

Rearranging Eq. (32) for constant ϕ,

$$\phi = \frac{N^{3.75} D^{2.81}}{u_d} \tag{32}$$

into Eq. (33) for mixer speed we easily find agitation rpm:

$$N = \sqrt[3.75]{\frac{\phi u_d}{D^{2.81}}} \tag{33}$$

HEAT TRANSFER SCALE-UP CONSIDERATIONS

It is important to add heat transfer scale-up considerations to scale up approach for the liquid parenteral solutions as heat transfer applications may play a considerable role in preparation of these products. For the heat transfer applications, constant horsepower per unit volume is used to achieve approximately similar heat transfer coefficient for the same type of impeller. This

TABLE 5   Process Requirements Set Degree of Agitation for Solids Suspension

Scale of agitation	Description of mixing
1–2	Agitation levels 1 and 2 are characteristic of applications requiring minimal solids suspension levels to achieve the process result. Agitators capable of scale levels of 1 will a. produce motion of all of the solids of the design settling velocity in the vessel; b. permit moving fillets of solids on the tank bottom, which are periodically suspended.
3–5	Agitation levels 3 and 5 are characterize most chemical process industries solids suspension applications and are typically used for dissolving solids. Agitators capable of scale levels of 3 will a. suspend all the solids of design settling velocity completely off the vessel bottom; b. provide slurry uniformity to at least one-third of fluid batch height; c. be suitable for slurry draw-off at low-exit nozzle elevations.
6–8	Agitation levels 6 and 8 characterize applications, where the solids suspension levels approach uniformity. Agitators capable of scale levels of 6 will a. provide concentration uniformity of solids to 95% of the fluid batch height; b. be suitable for slurry draw-off up to 80% of fluid batch height.
9–10	Agitation levels 9 and 2 characterize applications, where the solid-suspension uniformity is the maximum practical. Agitators capable of scale levels of 9 will a. provide slurry uniformity of solids to 98% of the fluid batch height; b. be suitable for slurry draw-off by means of overflow.

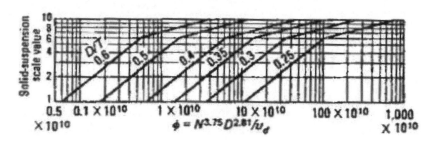

FIGURE 3   Solid suspension scale value versus ϕ.

approach is close approximation since the effect of horsepower (hp) on the heat transfer coefficient (h_0) is relatively small:

$$h_0 = hp^{0.22} \tag{34}$$

Therefore, even a moderate error in the mixer scale-up will have only a small effect on the agitator-side heat transfer coefficient. Other factors that include heat transfer area per unit volume are considerably more significant. For instance, in the jacketed tank, the heat transfer area per unit volume decreases upon scale-up. In order to assure the same proportionate heat removal or addition per unit batch size, additional heat transfer area (e.g., coils) may be required. Additionally, other variables, such as temperature driving force may have to be adjusted to compensate for decreased heat transfer area. As an aid in preliminary approximation of agitator-side heat transfer coefficients, Figure 4 may be utilized.

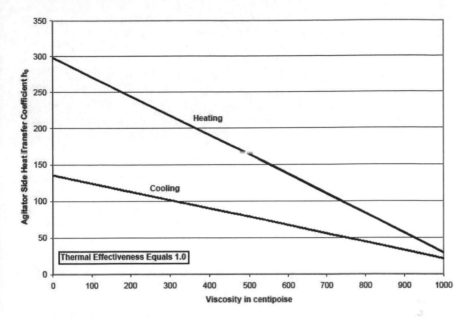

FIGURE 4 Typical agitator-side heat transfer coefficient of organic fluids.

Figure 4 shows typical agitator-side film coefficient for cooling or heating of organic fluids that serves to provide an "order-of-magnitude" estimate of the agitator-side heat transfer coefficient to embark on preliminary scale-up design work. The heat transfer coefficient will change depending on the specific physical characteristics of the system and the exact agitator selection. The numbers have been generated for the case of the vertical cylinder tubes or a single bank of helical coils. For properly baffled jacketed tanks, approximately 65% decrease of the values shown in Figure 4 may be expected. For the inorganic aqueous solutions, the values of heat transfer coefficient shown in Figure 4 may be expected to increase three or four times.

CONCLUSIONS
Above scale-up approach for the liquid parenteral solutions provides a precise transfer of the compounding mixing equipment environment to the production scale. Because of the unsurpassed importance of proper agitation during preparation of injectables, lion's share of this chapter is devoted to scale-up of agitating equipment. Other pieces of equipment used during manufacturing of parenteral drugs, such as sterilization equipment, filtration systems, various pumps, and packaging equipment are geometrically scaleable and are easily selected from the wide variety available on the market vendors.

One must also stress the importance of quality considerations during compounding and full adherence to current Good Manufacturing Practices, while producing parenteral products. Personnel responsible for the process design and scale-up of the equipment must assure proper documentation of the scale-up with tractability of all the preparatory work from the pilot batch(es) to the manufacturing of the marketed products. One can recommend usage of the spreadsheet programs for documenting of equipment parameters and subsequent calculations required for proper scale-up.

In a light of SUPAC (Scale-Up and Post-Approval Changes) guidance to the Industry, possible ramifications of the scale-up approach described in this chapter must be considered, as possibilities of interchanging from lower-energy to higher-energy agitation and vice versa are evident. SUPAC guidance should be followed for appropriate body of evidence to be gathered including sufficient stability studies and appropriate submissions to the agency to be prepared.

The last decade have shown that utilization of such tools as the scale-of-agitation approach for parenteral liquids scale-up have proven to be practical as well as time saving. They allow for precise transfer of technological design space parameters attained during drug development stage into production, thus following ICH Q8 (10) guidance. They also provide robust mathematical model of mixing procedure that in turn reduces risk of failure during technology transfer from research and development scale onto production floor thus adhering to principals of ICH Q9 (11) guidance.

REFERENCES

1. Cartensen JT, Ashol M. Scale-up factors in the manufacturing of solution dosage forms. Pharm Technol 1982; 6(11):64–77.
2. Von Essen JA. Liquid Mixing: Scale-Up Procedures. Presented at: Inter-American Congress and VII Chilean Congress of Chemical Engineering, Santiago, Chile, November 6–11, 1983.
3. Hollman PR. Consistent Mixing: The Key to Uniform Quality. Conference College of Engineering, Department of Engineering Professional Development, University of Wisconsin-Madison, May 1991.
4. Gorsky I, Nielsen RK. Scale-up methods used in liquid pharmaceutical manufacturing. Pharm Technol 1992; 16(9):112–120.
5. Oldshue JY. Fluid Mixing Technology. New York: McGraw-Hill, 1983.
6. Morton JR, Hicks RW, Fenic JG. How to design agitators for desired process response. Chem Eng 1976; 102–110.
7. Klein GF. A new approach to the scale-up of liquid pharmaceuticals. Pharm Technol 1999; 23(3):136–144.
8. Tao BY. Optimization via the simplex method. Chem Eng 1988; 95(2):85.
9. Gates LE, Morton JR, Fondy PL. Selecting agitator system to suspend solids in liquid. Chem Eng 1976; 144–150.
10. ICH Harmonized Tripartite Guidance, Guidance for Industry Q8(R2) Pharmaceutical Development, June, 2009.
11. ICH Harmonized Tripartite Guidance, Quality Risk Management, November 9, 2005.

6 Nonparenteral liquids and semisolids

Lawrence H. Block

INTRODUCTION

A manufacturer's decision to scale-up (or scale-down) a process is ultimately rooted in the economics of the production process, that is, in the cost of material, personnel, and equipment associated with the process and its control. While process scale-up often reduces the unit cost of production and is therefore economically advantageous per se, there are additional economic advantages conferred on the manufacturer by scaling up a process. Thus, process scale-up may allow for faster entry of a manufacturer into the marketplace or improved product distribution or response to market demands and correspondingly greater market-share retention[a]. Given the potential advantages of process scale-up in the pharmaceutical industry, one would expect the scale-up task to be the focus of major efforts on the part of pharmaceutical manufacturers. However, the paucity of published studies or data on scale-up—particularly for nonparenteral liquids and semisolids—suggests otherwise. On the other hand, one could argue that the paucity of published studies or data is nothing more than a reflection of the need to maintain a competitive advantage through secrecy.

One could also argue that this deficiency in the literature attests to the complexity of the unit operations involved in pharmaceutical processing. If pharmaceutical technologists view scale-up as little more than a ratio problem, whereby

$$\text{Scale-up ratio} = \frac{\text{large-scale production rate}}{\text{small-scale production rate}}, \tag{1}$$

then the successful resolution of a scale-up problem will remain an empirical, trial-and-error task—rather than a scientific one. In 1998, in a monograph on the scale-up of disperse systems, Block (3) noted that due to the complexity of the manufacturing process that involves more than one type of unit operation[b] (e.g., mixing, transferring, etc.), process scale-up from the bench or pilot plant level to commercial production is not a simple extrapolation:

---

[a] On the other hand, the manufacturer may determine that the advantages of process scale-up are compromised by the increased cost of production on a larger scale and/or the potential loss of interest or investment income. Griskey (1) addresses the economics of scale-up in some detail in his chapter on engineering economics and process design, but his examples are taken from the chemical industry. For a more extensive discussion of process economics, see Holland and Wilkinson (2).

[b] The term *unit operations*, coined by Arthur D. Little in 1915, is generally used to refer to distinct *physical* changes or unit actions (e.g., pulverizing, mixing, and drying), while unit operations involving *chemical* changes are sometimes referred to as *unit processes*. The physical changes comprising unit operations primarily involve contact, transfer of a physical property, and separation between phases or streams.

The successful linkage of one unit operation to another defines the function-ality of the overall manufacturing process. Each unit operation *per se* may be scalable, in accordance with a specific ratio, but the composite manufacturing process may not be, as the effective scale-up ratios may be different from one unit operation to another. Unexpected problems in scale-up are often a reflection of the dichotomy between *unit operation* scale-up and *process* scale-up. Furthermore, commercial production introduces problems that are not a major issue on a small scale: e.g., storage and materials handling may become problematic only when large quantities are involved; heat generated in the course of pilot plant or production scale processing may overwhelm the system's capacity for dissipation to an extent not anticipated based on prior laboratory-scale experience. (3)

Furthermore, unit operations may function in a rate-limiting manner as the scale of operation increases. When Astarita (4) decried the fact, in the mid-1980s, that "there is no scale-up algorithm which permits us to rigorously predict the behavior of a large-scale process based upon the behavior of a small scale process," it was presumably as a consequence of all of these problematic aspects of scale-up.

A clue to the resolution of the scale-up problem for liquids and semisolids resides in the recognition that their processing invariably involves the unit operation of mixing. Closer examination of this core unit operation reveals that flow conditions and viscosities during processing can vary by several orders of magnitude depending on the scale of scrutiny employed, that is, whether on a *micro*scopic (e.g., µm to cm) or *macro*scopic (e.g., cm to m) scale. The key to effective processing scale-up is the appreciation and understanding of micro-scale and macroscale transport phenomena, that is, diffusion and bulk flow, respectively. Transport by diffusion involves the flow of a property (e.g., mass, heat, momentum, electromagnetic energy) from a region of high concentration to a region of low concentration as a result of the microscopic motion of electrons, atoms, molecules, etc. Bulk flow, whether convection or advection, however, involves the flow of a property as a result of macroscopic or bulk motion induced artificially (e.g., by mechanical agitation) or naturally (e.g., by density variations) (5).

TRANSPORT PHENOMENA IN LIQUIDS AND SEMISOLIDS AND THEIR RELATIONSHIP TO UNIT OPERATIONS AND SCALE-UP

Over the last four decades or so, transport phenomena research has benefited from the substantial efforts made to replace empiricism by fundamental knowl-edge based on computer simulations and theoretical modeling of transport phenomena. These efforts were spurred on by the publication in 1960 by Bird et al. (6) of the first edition of their quintessential monograph on the interrela-tionships among the three fundamental types of transport phenomena: mass transport, energy transport, and momentum transport[c]. All transport phenom-ena follow the same pattern in accordance with the generalized diffusion equation (GDE). The unidimensional *flux*, or overall transport rate per unit

---

[c] The second edition of *Transport Phenomena* was published in 2002, 42 years later, an indication of the utility of the first edition and its continuing acceptance by the engineering discipline.

area in one direction, is expressed as a system property multiplied by a gradient (5):

$$\frac{\partial \Gamma}{\partial t}\bigg|_x = \delta\left(\frac{\partial^2 \Gamma}{\partial x^2}\right) = \delta\left(\frac{(\partial \Gamma / \partial x)}{\partial x}\right) = \delta\left(\frac{\partial E}{\partial x}\right), \tag{2}$$

Γ represents the concentration of a property Q (e.g., mass, heat, electrical energy, etc.) per unit volume, that is, $\Gamma = Q/V$, t is time, x is the distance measured in the direction of transport, δ is the generalized diffusion coefficient, and E is the gradient or driving force for transport.

Mass and heat transfer can be described in terms of their respective concentrations Q/V. While the concentration of mass, m, can be specified directly, the concentration of heat is given by

$$\frac{mC_pT}{V} = \rho C_p T, \tag{3}$$

where Cp is the specific heat capacity and T is temperature. Thus, the specification of $\rho C_p T$ in any form of the generalized diffusion equation will result in the elimination of ρC_p, assuming it to be a constant, thereby allowing the use of temperature as a measure of heat concentration (5). In an analogous manner, momentum transfer can be specified in terms of the concentration of momentum $\mathbf{u}$, when its substantial derivative is used instead of its partial derivative with respect to time:

$$\frac{D\mathbf{u}}{Dt} = v\nabla^2\mathbf{u}, \tag{4}$$

where v is the kinematic viscosity. If pressure and gravitational effects are introduced, one arrives at the Navier–Stokes relationships that govern Newtonian fluid dynamics.

When the flux of Γ is evaluated three dimensionally, it can be represented by Eq. (5):

$$\frac{d\Gamma}{dt} = \frac{\partial \Gamma}{\partial t} + \frac{\partial \Gamma}{\partial x}\frac{dx}{dt} + \frac{\partial \Gamma}{\partial y}\frac{dy}{dt} + \frac{\partial \Gamma}{\partial z}\frac{dz}{dt} \tag{5}$$

Equations (2) and (5) are represented schematically in Figure 1. At the simplest level, as Griskey (1) notes, Fick's law of diffusion for mass transfer and Fourier's law of heat conduction characterize mass and heat transfer, respectively, as vectors, that is, they have magnitude and direction in the three coordinates, x, y, and z. Momentum or flow, however, is a tensor that is defined by nine components rather than three. Hence, its more complex characterization at the simplest level is, in accordance with Newton's law,

$$\tau_{yx} = -\eta\left(\frac{dv_x}{dy}\right) \tag{6}$$

where τ_{yx} is the shear stress in the x-direction, (dv_x/dy) is the rate of shear, and η is the coefficient of Newtonian viscosity. The solution of Eq. (2), the generalized diffusion equation,

$$\Gamma = f(t, x, y, z), \tag{7}$$

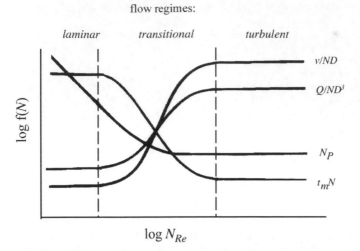

FIGURE 1 Various dimensionless parameters (dimensionless velocity, $v^* = v/ND$; pumping number, $N_Q = Q/ND^3$; power number, $N_p = Pg_c/\rho N^3 D^5$; and dimensionless mixing time, $t^* = t_m N$) as a function of the Reynolds number for the analysis of turbine-agitator systems. *Source:* Adapted from Dickey and Fenic (20).

will take the form of a parabolic partial differential equation (Eq. 5). However, the more complex the phenomenon—for example, with convective transport a part of the model—the more difficult it is to achieve an analytic solution to the GDE. Numerical solutions, however, where the differential equation is transformed to an algebraic one, may be somewhat more readily achieved.

Transport Phenomena and Their Relationship to Mixing as a Unit Operation[d]

As noted earlier, virtually all liquid and semisolid products involve the unit of operation of mixing[e]. In fact, in many instances, it is the primary unit operation. Even its indirect effects, for example, on heat transfer, may be the basis for its inclusion in a process. Yet, mechanistic and quantitative descriptions of the mixing process remain incomplete (7–9). Nonetheless, enough fundamental and empirical data are available to allow some reasonable predictions to be made.

---

[d] Reprinted in part, with revisions and updates, by courtesy of Marcel Dekker, Inc. from Ref. 3.
[e] *Mixing*, or *blending*, refers to the random distribution of two or more initially separate phases into and through one another, while *agitation* refers only to the induced motion of a material in some sort of container. Agitation does not necessarily result in an intermingling of two or more separate components of a system to form a more or less uniform product. Some authors reserve the term *blending* for the intermingling of miscible phases while *mixing* is employed for materials that may or may not be miscible.

The diversity of dynamic mixing devices is unsettling: the blades of their dynamic, or moving, components may be impellers in the form of propellers, turbines, paddles, helical ribbons, Z-blades, or screws. In addition, one can vary the number of impellers, the number of blades per impeller, the pitch of the impeller blades, and the location of the impeller, and thereby affect mixer performance to an appreciable extent. Furthermore, while dispersators or rotor/stator configurations may be used rather than impellers to effect mixing, mixing may also be accomplished by jet mixing or static mixing devices. The bewildering array of mixing equipment choices alone would appear to make the likelihood of effective scale-up an impossibility. However, as diverse as mixing equipment may be, evaluations of the rate and extent of mixing and of flow regimes[f] make it possible to find a common basis for comparison.

In low-viscosity systems, miscible liquid blending is achieved through the transport of unmixed material, via flow currents (i.e., bulk or convective flow), to a mixing zone (i.e., a region of high shear or intensive mixing). In other words, mass transport during mixing depends on *streamline* or *laminar* flow, involving well-defined paths, and *turbulent* flow, involving innumerable, variously sized, eddies or swirling motions. Most of the highly turbulent mixing takes place in the region of the impeller, fluid motion elsewhere serving primarily to bring fresh fluid into this region. Thus, the characterization of mixing processes is often based on the flow regimes encountered in mixing equipment. Reynolds' classic research on flow in pipes demonstrated that flow changes from laminar to irregular, or turbulent, once a critical value of a dimensionless ratio of variables has been exceeded (10,11). This ratio, universally referred to as the Reynolds number, N_{Re}, is defined by Eqs. (8a) and (8b) as

$$N_{Re} = \frac{Lv\rho}{\eta} \qquad \text{(a)}$$

$$N_{Re} = \frac{D^2N\rho}{\eta} \qquad \text{(b)}$$

(8)

where ρ is the density, v is the velocity, L is a characteristic length, and η is the Newtonian viscosity; Eq. (8b) is referred to as the *impeller* Reynolds number, as D is the impeller diameter and N is the rotational speed of the impeller. N_{Re} represents the ratio of the inertia forces to the viscous forces in a flow. High values of N_{Re} correspond to flow dominated by motion while low values of N_{Re} correspond to flow dominated by viscosity. Thus, the transition from laminar to turbulent flow is governed by the density and viscosity of the fluid, its average velocity, and the dimensions of the region in which flow occurs (e.g., the diameter of the pipe or conduit and the diameter of a settling particle). For a straight circular pipe, laminar flow occurs when $N_{Re} < 2100$; turbulent flow is evident when $N_{Re} > 4000$. For $2100 \leq N_{Re} \leq 4000$, flow is in transition from a laminar to a turbulent regime. Other factors such as surface roughness, shape, and cross-sectional area of the affected region have a substantial effect on the critical value of N_{Re}. Thus, for particle sedimentation, the critical value of N_{Re} is 1; for some mechanical mixing processes, N_{Re} is 10 to 20 (12). The erratic, relatively unpredictable nature of turbulent eddy flow is further

---

[f] The term flow regime is used to characterize the hydraulic conditions (i.e., volume, velocity, and direction of flow) within a vessel.

influenced, in part, by the size distribution of the eddies, which are dependent on the size of the apparatus and the amount of energy introduced into the system (10). These factors are indirectly addressed by N_{Re}. Further insight into the nature of N_{Re} can be gained by viewing it as inversely proportional to eddy advection time, that is, the time required for eddies or vortices to form.

In turbulent flow, eddies move rapidly with an appreciable component of their velocity in the direction perpendicular to a reference point, for example, a surface, past which the fluid is flowing (13). Because of the rapid eddy motion, mass transfer in the turbulent region is much more rapid than that resulting from molecular diffusion in the laminar region, with the result that the concentration gradients existing in the turbulent region will be smaller than those in the laminar region (13). Thus, mixing is much more efficient under turbulent flow conditions. Nonetheless, the technologist should bear in mind potentially compromising aspects of turbulent flow: for example, increased vortex formation (14) and a concomitant incorporation of air, increased shear and a corresponding shift in the particle size distribution of the disperse phase.

Although continuous-flow mixing operations are employed to a limited extent in the pharmaceutical industry, the processing of liquids and semisolids most often involves batch processing in some kind of tank or vessel. Thus, in the general treatment of mixing that follows, the focus will be on batch operations[8] in which mixing is accomplished primarily by the use of dynamic mechanical mixers with impellers, although jet mixing (16,17) and static mixing devices (18)—long used in the chemical process industries—are being used to an increasingly greater extent now in the pharmaceutical and cosmetic industries.

Mixers share a common functionality with pumps. The power imparted by the mixer, via the impeller, to the system is akin to a pumping effect and is characterized in terms of the shear and flow produced:

$$\left.\begin{array}{c} P \propto Q\rho H \\ or \\ H \propto \dfrac{P}{Q\rho} \end{array}\right\} \tag{9}$$

where P is the power imparted by the impeller, Q is the flow rate (or pumping capacity) of material through the mixing device, ρ is the density of the material, and H is the velocity head or shear. Thus, for a given P, there is an inverse relationship between shear and volume throughput.

The power input in mechanical agitation is calculated using the *power number*, N_P,

$$N_P = \frac{P g_c}{\rho N^3 D^5}, \tag{10}$$

where g_c is the force conversion factor ($g_c = \text{kg} \cdot \text{m/sec}^2/\text{Newton} = \text{g} \cdot \text{cm}/\text{sec}^2/\text{dyne}$), N is the impeller rotational speed (sec^{-1}), and D is the diameter of the impeller. For a given impeller/mixing tank configuration, one can define a

---

[8] The reader interested in continuous-flow mixing operations is directed to references that deal specifically with that aspect of mixing such as the monographs by Oldshue (15) and Tatterson (16).

specific relationship between the Reynolds number (Eq. 8^h) and the power number (Eq. 10) in which three zones (corresponding to the laminar, transitional, and turbulent regimes) are generally discernible. Tatterson (16) notes that for mechanical agitation in laminar flow, most *laminar* power correlations reduce to $N_P N_{Re} = B$, where B is a complex function of the geometry of the system[i], and that this is equivalent to $P \propto \eta$. $\eta N^2 D^3$; "if power correlations do not reduce to this form for laminar mixing, then they are wrong and should not be used." Turbulent correlations are much simpler: for systems employing baffles[j], $N_P = B$; this is equivalent to $P \propto \rho \cdot N^3 D^5$. On the basis of this function, slight changes in D can result in substantial changes in power.

Impeller size relative to the size of the tank is critical as well. If the ratio of impeller diameter D to tank diameter T is too large (D/T is $> \sim 0.7$), mixing efficiency will decrease as the space between the impeller and the tank wall will be too small to allow a strong axial flow due to obstruction of the recirculation path (19). More intense mixing at this point would require an increase in impeller speed but this may be compromised by limitations imposed by impeller blade thickness and angle. If D/T is too small, the impeller will not be able to generate an adequate flow rate in the tank.

Valuable insights into the mixing operation can be gained from a consideration of system behavior as a function of the Reynolds number, N_{Re} (20). This is shown schematically in Figure 1 in which various dimensionless parameters (dimensionless velocity, v/ND; pumping number, Q/ND^3; power number, $N_P = Pg_c/\rho N^3 D^5$; and dimensionless mixing time, $t_m N$) are represented as a log-log function of N_{Re}. Although density, viscosity, mixing vessel diameter, and impeller rotational speed are often viewed by formulators as independent variables, their interdependency, when incorporated in the dimensionless Reynolds number, is quite evident. Thus, the schematic relationships embodied in Figure 1 are not surprising[k].

Mixing time is the time required to produce a mixture of predetermined quality; the rate of mixing is the rate at which mixing proceeds toward the final state. For a given formulation and equipment configuration, mixing time, t_m, will depend on material properties and operation variables. For geometrically similar systems, if the geometrical dimensions of the system are transformed to ratios, mixing time can be expressed in terms of a dimensionless number, that is, the dimensionless mixing time, θ_m or $t_m N$:

$$t_m N = \theta_m = f(N_{Re}, N_{Fr}) \Rightarrow f(N_{Re}). \tag{11}$$

The Froude number, $N_{Fr} = v/\sqrt{Lg}$, is similar to N_{Re}: it is a measure of the inertial stress to the gravitational force per unit area acting on a fluid. Its inclusion in Eq. (11) is justified when density differences are encountered; in the

---

[h] Here, the Reynolds number for mixing is defined in SI derived units as $N_{Re} = (1.667 \times 10^{-5} ND^2\rho)/\eta$, where D is the impeller diameter, in mm; η is the viscosity, in Pa sec; N is the impeller speed, in rpm; and ρ is the density.

[i] An average value of B is 300, but B can vary between 20 and 4000 (16).

[j] Baffles are obstructions placed in mixing tanks to redirect flow and minimize vortex formation. Standard baffles—comprising rectangular plates spaced uniformly around the inside wall of a tank—convert rotational flow into top to bottom circulation.

[k] The interrelationships are embodied in variations of the Navier–Stokes equations, which describe mass and momentum balances in fluid systems (6).

absence of substantive differences in density, for example, for emulsions more so than for suspensions, the Froude term can be neglected. Dimensionless mixing time is independent of the Reynolds number for both laminar and turbulent flow regimes as indicated by the plateaus in Figure 1. Nonetheless, as there are conflicting data in the literature regarding the sensitivity of θ_m to the rheological properties of the formulation and to equipment geometry, Eq. (11) must be regarded as an oversimplification of the mixing operation. Considerable care must be exercised in applying the general relationship to specific situations.

Empirical correlations for *turbulent* mechanical mixing have been reported in terms of the following dimensionless mixing time relationship (16):

$$\theta_m = t_m N = K\left(\frac{T}{D}\right)^a,$$ (12)

where K and a are constants, T is the tank diameter, N the is impeller rotational speed, and D is the impeller diameter. Under *laminar* flow conditions, Eq. (12) reduces to

$$\theta_m = H_0$$ (13)

where H_0 is referred to as the mixing number or homogenization number. In the *transitional* flow regime,

$$H_0 = C(N_{Re})^a,$$ (14)

where C and a are constants, with a varying between 0 and -1.

Flow patterns in agitated vessels may be characterized as radial, axial, or tangential relative to the impeller but are more correctly defined by the direction and magnitude of the velocity vectors throughout the system, particularly in a transitional flow regime: while the dimensionless velocity, v^*, or v/ND, is essentially constant in the laminar and turbulent flow zones, it is highly dependent on N_{Re} in the transitional flow zone (Fig. 1). Initiation of tangential or circular flow patterns, with minimal radial or axial movement, is associated with vortex formation, minimal mixing, and, in some multiphase systems, particulate separation and classification. Vortices can be minimized or eliminated altogether by redirecting flow in the system through the use of baffles[1] or by positioning the impeller so that its entry into the mixing tank is off-center. For a given formulation, large tanks are more apt to exhibit vortex formation than small tanks. Thus, full-scale production tanks are more likely to require baffles even when smaller (laboratory or pilot plant scale) tanks are unbaffled.

Mixing processes involved in the manufacture of disperse systems, whether suspensions or emulsions, are far more problematic than those employed in the blending of low-viscosity miscible liquids due to the multiphasic character of the systems and deviations from Newtonian flow behavior. It is not uncommon for both laminar and turbulent flow to occur simultaneously in different regions of the system. In some regions the flow regime may be in transition, that is, neither laminar nor turbulent but somewhere in between. The

---

[1] The usefulness of baffles in mixing operations is offset by increased clean-up problems (due to particulate entrapment by the baffles or congealing of product adjacent to the baffles). Furthermore, "overbaffling"—excessive use of baffles—reduces mass flow and localizes mixing, which may be counterproductive.

implications of these flow regime variations for scale-up are considerable. Nonetheless, it should be noted that the mixing process is only completed when Brownian motion occurs to a sufficient extent that uniformity is achieved on a molecular scale.

Viscous and Non-Newtonian Materials

Mixing in high-viscosity materials ($\eta > \sim 10^4$ m Pa·sec) is relatively slow and inefficient. Conventional mixing tanks and conventional impellers (e.g., turbine or propeller impellers) are generally inadequate. In general, due to the high viscosity, N_{Re} may well be below 100. Thus, laminar flow is apt to occur rather than turbulent flow. As a result, the inertial forces imparted to a system during the mixing process tend to dissipate quickly. Eddy formation and diffusion are virtually absent. Thus, efficient mixing necessitates substantial convective flow that is usually achieved by high-velocity gradients in the mixing zone. Fluid elements in the mixing zone, subjected to both shear and elongation, undergo deformation and stretching, ultimately resulting in the size reduction of the fluid elements and an increase in their overall interfacial area. The repetitive cutting and folding of fluid elements also result in decreasing inhomogeneity and increased mixing. The role of molecular diffusion in reducing inhomogeneities in high-viscosity systems is relatively unimportant until these fluid elements have become small and their interfacial areas have become relatively large (21). In highly viscous systems, rotary motion is more than compensated for by viscous shear so that baffles are generally less necessary (15).

Mixing equipment for highly viscous materials often involves specialized impellers and configurations that minimize high-shear zones and heat dissipation. Accordingly, propeller-type impellers are not generally effective in viscous systems. Instead, turbines, paddles, anchors, helical ribbons, screws, and kneading mixers are resorted to, successively, as system viscosity increases. Multiple impellers or specialized impellers (e.g., sigma blades, Z-blades) are often necessary along with the maintenance of narrow clearances, or gaps, between impeller blades and between impeller blades and tank (mixing chamber) walls in order to attain optimal mixing efficiency (15,21). However, narrow clearances pose their own problems. Studies of the power input to anchor impellers used to agitate Newtonian and shear-thinning fluids showed that the clearance between the impeller blades and the vessel wall was the most important geometrical factor: N_P at constant N_{Re} was proportional to the fourth power of the clearance divided by tank diameter (22). Furthermore, although mixing is promoted by these specialized impellers in the vicinity of the walls of the mixing vessel, stagnation is often encountered in regions adjacent to the impeller shaft. Finally, complications (wall effects) may arise from the formation of a thin, particulate-free, fluid layer adjacent to the wall of the tank or vessel that has a lower viscosity than the bulk material and allows slippage (i.e., nonzero velocity) to occur, unless the mixing tank is further modified to provide for wall-scraping.

Rheologically, the flow of many non-Newtonian materials can be characterized by a time-independent power law function (sometimes referred to as the Ostwald–deWaele equation):

$$\tau = K\dot{\gamma}^a$$

or   (15)

$$\log \tau = K' + a(\log \dot{\gamma}),$$

where τ is the shear stress, $\dot{\gamma}$ is the rate of shear, K' is the logarithmically transformed proportionality constant K with dimensions dependent on a, the so-called flow behavior index. For pseudoplastic or shear-thinning materials, $a < 1$; for dilatant or shear-thickening materials, $a > 1$; for Newtonian fluids, $a = 1$. For a power law fluid, the average apparent viscosity, η_{avg}, can be related to the average shear rate by the following equation:

$$\eta_{avg} = K' \left(\frac{dv}{dy}\right)_{avg}^{n'-1}, \tag{16}$$

On the basis of this relationship, a Reynolds number can be derived and estimated for non-Newtonian fluids from

$$\left[N_{Re} = \frac{Lv\rho}{\eta}\right] \Rightarrow \left[N_{Re,\, nonN} = \frac{ND_i^2\rho}{K'(dv/dy)_{avg}^{n'-1}}\right]. \tag{17}$$

Dispersions that behave, rheologically, as Bingham plastics, require a minimum shear stress (the yield value) in order for flow to occur. Shear stress variations in a system can result in local differences wherein the yield stress point is not exceeded. As a result, flow may be impeded or absent in some regions compared to others, resulting in channeling or cavity formation and a loss of mixing efficiency. Only if the yield value is exceeded *throughout* the system, will flow and mixing be relatively unimpeded. Helical ribbon and screw impellers would be preferable for the mixing of Bingham fluids, in contrast to conventional propeller or turbine impellers, given their more even distribution of power input (16). From a practical vantage point, monitoring power input to mixing units could facilitate process control and help to identify problematic behavior. Etchells et al. (23) analyzed the performance of industrial mixer configurations for Bingham plastics. Their studies indicate that the logical scale-up path from laboratory to pilot plant to production, for geometrically similar equipment, involves the maintenance of constant impeller tip speed that is proportional to $N{\cdot}D$, the product of rotational speed of the impeller (N) and the diameter of the impeller (D).

Oldshue (15) provides a detailed procedure for selecting mixing times and optimizing mixer and impeller configurations for viscous and shear-thinning materials that can be adapted for other rheologically challenging systems.

Gate and anchor impellers, long used advantageously for the mixing of viscous and non-Newtonian fluids, induce complex flow patterns in mixing tanks: both primary and secondary flows may be evident. *Primary* flow or circulation results from the direct rotational movement of the impeller blade in the fluid; *secondary* flow is normal to the horizontal planes about the impeller axis (i.e., parallel to the impeller axis) and is responsible for the interchange of material between different levels of the tank (24). In this context, rotating viscoelastic systems, with their normal forces, establish stable secondary flow patterns more readily than Newtonian systems. In fact, the presence of normal stresses in viscoelastic fluids subjected to high rates of shear ($\sim 10^4$/sec) may be substantially greater than shearing stresses, as demonstrated by Metzner et al. (24). These observations, among others, moved Fredrickson (25) to note "... neglect of normal stress effects is likely to lead to large errors in theoretical calculations for flow in complex geometries." However, the effect of these secondary flows on the efficiency of mixing, particularly in viscoelastic systems, is equivocal. On the one hand, vertical velocity near the impeller blade in a Newtonian system might be 2% to 5% of the horizontal velocity, whereas, in a non-Newtonian system, vertical velocity can be 20% to 40% of the horizontal. Thus, the overall circulation can improve considerably. On the other hand, the relatively small, stable toroidal vortices that tend to form in viscoelastic systems may result in substantially incomplete mixing. Smith (26) advocates the asymmetric placement of small deflector blades on a standard anchor arm as a means of achieving a dramatic improvement in mixing efficiency of viscoelastic fluids without resorting to expensive alternatives such as pitched blade anchors or helical ribbons.

In highly shear-thinning fluids, as well as in Bingham plastic or viscoplastic fluids, impeller agitation may lead to the formation of an agitated volume—referred to as a cavern—around the impeller surrounded by a stagnant region wherein the local shear stress is less than the fluid's apparent yield stress (27). When caverns form, it may be difficult to ensure homogeneity. This is particularly problematic when opaque, multiphase fluids (e.g., emulsions, suspensions) are involved, as visualization of this phenomenon is difficult at best. Electrical resistance tomography and positron emission projection imaging have been used to facilitate the characterization of cavern size (28), but less sophisticated techniques have been used as well. One such procedure employs the injection of glitter into the mixing tank followed by the freezing of the mixing tank contents and the subsequent dissection of the frozen solid to reveal cavern boundaries (27).

Side wall clearance, that is, the gap between the vessel wall and the rotating impeller, was shown by Cheng et al. (29) to be a significant factor in the mixing performance of helical ribbon mixers not only for viscous and viscoelastic fluids but also for Newtonian systems. Bottom clearance, that is, the space between the base of the impeller and the bottom of the tank, however, had a negligible, relatively insignificant effect on power consumption and on the effective shear rate in inelastic fluids. Thus, mixing efficiency in nonviscoelastic fluids would not be affected by variations in bottom clearance. For viscoelastic fluids, on the other hand, bottom clearance effects were negligible only at lower rotational speeds ($\leq$60 rpm); substantial power consumption increases were evident at higher rotational speeds.

The scale-up implications of *mixing*-related issues such as impeller design and placement, mixing tank characteristics, new equipment design, and the mixing of particulate solids are beyond the scope of this chapter. However, extensive monographs are available in the chemical engineering literature (many of which have been cited herein[m]) and will prove to be invaluable to the formulator and technologist.

---

[m] The reader is directed to previously referenced monographs by Oldshue and by Tatterson as well as to standard textbooks in chemical engineering, including the multivolume series authored by McCabe et al., and the encyclopedia *Perry's Chemical Engineers' Handbook*. An excellent resource is the *Handbook of Industrial Mixing: Science and Practice*, edited by Paul EL, Atiemo-Obeng VA, and Kresta SM, and published in 2004.

Particle Size Reduction

Disperse systems often necessitate particle size reduction, whether it is an integral part of product processing, as in the process of liquid-liquid emulsification, or an additional requirement insofar as solid particle suspensions are concerned. (It should be noted that solid particles suspended in liquids often tend to agglomerate. Although milling of such suspensions tends to disrupt such agglomerates and produce a more homogeneous suspension, it generally does not affect the size of the unit particles comprising the agglomerates.) For emulsions, the dispersion of one liquid as droplets in another can be expressed in terms of the dimensionless Weber number, N_{We}:

$$N_{We} = \frac{\rho v^2 d_0}{\sigma}, \qquad (18)$$

where ρ is the density of a droplet, v is the relative velocity of the moving droplet, d_0 is the diameter of the droplet, and σ is the interfacial tension. The Weber number represents the ratio of the driving force causing partial disruption to the resistance due to interfacial tension (30). Increased Weber numbers are associated with a greater tendency for droplet deformation (and consequent splitting into still smaller droplets) to occur at higher shear, that is, with more intense mixing. This can be represented by

$$N_{We} = \frac{D_i^3 N^2 \rho_{cont}}{\sigma}, \qquad (19)$$

where D_i is the diameter of the impeller, N is the rotational speed of the impeller, and ρ_{cont} is the density of the continuous phase. For a given system, droplet size reduction begins above a specific critical Weber number (31); above the critical N_{We}, average droplet size varies with $N^{-1.2} D_i^{-0.8}$, or, as an approximation, with the reciprocal of the impeller tip speed. In addition, a better dispersion is achieved, for the same power input, with a smaller impeller rotating at high speed (31).

As the particle size of the disperse phase decreases, there is a corresponding increase in the number of particles and a concomitant increase in interparticulate and interfacial interactions. Thus, in general, the viscosity of a dispersion is greater than that of the dispersion medium. This is often characterized in accordance with the classical Einstein equation for the viscosity of a dispersion,

$$\eta = \eta_0 (1 + 2.5\phi), \qquad (20)$$

where η is the viscosity of the dispersion, η_0 is the viscosity of the continuous phase, and ϕ is the volume fraction of the particulate phase. The rheological behavior of concentrated dispersions may be demonstrably non-Newtonian (pseudoplastic, plastic, or viscoelastic), and its dependence on ϕ more marked due to disperse phase deformation and/or interparticulate interaction.

A further complication ensues with the realization that the fluid dynamics in an impeller-agitated mixing vessel containing immiscible fluids comprise a near-blade region and a circulation region. Turbulent energy is dissipated far more efficiently (about two orders of magnitude) near the impeller than in the circulation region. Kichatov et al. (32) explored the effect of impeller blade geometry on emulsion drop size and concluded that maximum drop size, d_{max}, depended primarily on the viscosity of the dispersed phase and on the rotational speed of the impeller. The effect of impeller geometry weakens with increasing fluid viscosity (33). At low rotational speeds, $d_{max} : N^{-1.5}$, while at high rotational speeds, $d_{max} : N^{-0.5 \Rightarrow -0.75}$.

Maa and Hsu (34) investigated the influence of operation parameters for rotor/stator homogenization on emulsion droplet size and temporal stability in order to optimize operating conditions for small- and large-scale rotor/stator homogenization. Rotor/stator homogenization effects emulsion formation under much more intense turbulence and shear than that encountered in an agitated vessel or a static mixer. Rapid circulation, high shear forces, and a narrow rotor/stator gap (<0.5 mm) contribute to the intensity of dispersal and commingling of the immiscible phases since turbulent eddies are essential for the breakup of the dispersed phase into droplets. Maa and Hsu's estimates of the circulation rates in small and large scale rotor/stator systems—based on the total area of the rotor/stator openings, the radial velocity at the openings (resulting from the pressure difference within the vortex that forms in the rotor/stator unit) and the centrifugal force caused by the radial deflection of fluid by the rotor—appear to be predictive for the scale-up of rotor/stator homogenization (34).

Dobetti and Pantaleo (35) investigated the influence of hydrodynamic parameters per se on the efficiency of a coacervation process for microcapsule formation. They based their work on that of Armenante and Kirwan (36) who described the size of the smallest eddies or vortices generated in a turbulent regime on a microscopic scale in the vicinity of the agitation source, that is, microeddies[n], as

$$d_e = \left(\frac{v^3}{P_s}\right)^{1/4} \tag{21}$$

where d_e is the diameter of the smallest microeddy, v is the kinematic viscosity of the fluid (i.e., η/ρ, or viscosity/density), and P_S is the specific power, that is, power input per unit mass. Hypothetically, if mass transfer of the coacervate and particle encapsulation occurred only within the microeddies, then the diameter of the hardened microcapsules would depend on the size of the microeddies produced by the agitation in the system. They dispersed a water-insoluble drug in a cellulose acetate phthalate (CAP) solution to which a coacervation-inducing agent was gradually added to facilitate microencapsulation by the CAP coacervate phase. The stirring rate and the tank and impeller configuration were varied to produce an array of microeddy sizes. However, the actual size of the hardened microcapsules was less than that calculated for the corresponding microeddies (Fig. 2). The authors attributed the inequality in sizes, in part, to relatively low agitation energies. Their conclusion is supported by their calculated N_{Re} values, ranging from 1184 to 2883, which are indicative of a flow regime ranging from laminar to transitional, rather than turbulent.

Comminution, or particle size reduction of solids, is considerably different from that of the breakup of one liquid by dispersal as small droplets in another. Particle size reduction is generally achieved by one of four mechanisms:

---

[n] Deduced in 1941 by A. N. Kolmogorov, it is generally referred to the Kolmogorov length or dissipation scale (9).

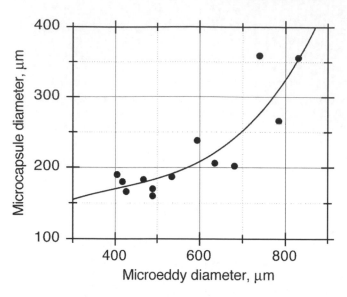

FIGURE 2 Microcapsule size as a function of microeddy size. *Source*: Adapted from Dobetti and Pantaleo (35).

(*i*) compression, (*ii*) impact, (*iii*) attrition, or (*iv*) cutting or shear. Equipment for particle size reduction or milling includes *crushers* (which operate by compression, e.g., crushing rolls), *grinders* (which operate principally by impact and attrition, although some compression may be involved, e.g., hammer mills, ball mills), *ultrafine grinders* (which operate principally by attrition, e.g., fluid-energy mills), and *knife cutters*. Accordingly, a thorough understanding of milling operations requires an understanding of fracture mechanics, agglomerative forces (dry and wet) involved in the adhesion and cohesion of particulates, and flow of particles and bulk powders. These topics are dealt with at length in the monographs by Fayed and Otten (37) and Carstensen (38,39).

As Austin (40) notes, the formulation of a general theory of the unit operation of size reduction is virtually impossible given the multiplicity of mill types and mechanisms for particulate reduction. The predictability of any comminution process is further impaired given the variations among solids in surface characteristics and reactivity, molecular interactions, crystallinity, etc. Nonetheless, some commonalities can be discerned. First, the particle size reduction rate is dependent on particle strength and particle size. Second, the residence time of particles in the mill is a critical determinant of mill efficiency. Thus, whether a given mill operates in a single-pass or a multiple-pass (retention) mode can be a limiting factor insofar as characterization of the efficacy of comminution is concerned. Third, the energy required to achieve a given degree of comminution is an inverse function of initial particle size. This is due to (*i*) the increasing inefficiency of stress or shear application to each particle of an array of particles as particle size decreases and (*ii*) the decreasing incidence of particle flaws that permit fracture at low stress (40).

If monosized particles are subjected to one pass through a milling device, the particle size distribution of the resultant fragments can be represented in a cumulative form. Subsequent passes of the comminuted material through the milling device often result in a superimposable frequency distribution when the particle sizes are normalized, for example, in terms of the weight fraction less than size y resulting from the milling of particles of larger size x. The mean residence time, τ, of material processed by a mill is given by

$$\tau = \frac{M}{F},\qquad(22)$$

where M is the mass of powder in the mill and F is the mass flow rate through the mill. Process outcomes for retention mills can be described in terms of residence time distributions defined by the weight fraction of the initial charge at time $t = 0$, which leaves between $(t + dt)$. If the milling operation is scalable, the particle size distributions produced by a large and a small mill of the same type would be comparable and would differ only in the time scale of operation, that is, the operation can be characterized as $f(t/\tau)$. The prospect for scalability may be further enhanced when the weight fraction remaining in an upper range is a log-linear (first-order) function of total elapsed milling time[o] (39). Corroboration of the likelihood of scalability of milling operations is Mori's finding that most residence time distributions for milling conform to a log-normal model (41).

One estimate of the efficacy of a crushing or grinding operation is the crushing efficiency, E_c, described as the ratio of the surface energy created by crushing or grinding to the energy absorbed by the solid (33):

$$E_c = \frac{\sigma_s(A_{wp} - A_{wf})}{W_n},\qquad(23)$$

where σ_s is the specific surface or surface per unit area, A_{wp} and A_{wf} are the areas per unit mass of product particulates and feed particulates, that is, after and before milling, respectively, and W_n is the energy absorbed by the solid per unit mass. The energy absorbed by the solid, per unit mass, is less than the energy W supplied to the mill per unit mass, that is, $W_n < W$. While a substantial part of the total energy input W is needed to overcome friction in the machine, the rest is available for crushing or grinding. However, of the total energy stored within a solid, only a small fraction is converted into surface energy at the time of fracture. As most of the energy is converted into heat, crushing efficiency values tend to be low, that is, $0.0006 \leq E_c \leq 0.01$, principally due to the inexactness of estimates of σ_s (33).

A number of quasi-theoretical relationships have been proposed to characterize the grinding process: Rittinger's "law" (1867),

$$\frac{P}{\dot{m}} = K_R \left(\frac{1}{\bar{D}_p} - \frac{1}{\bar{D}_f} \right),\qquad(24)$$

which states that the work required in crushing a solid is proportional to the new surface created, and Kick's "law" (1885),

$$\frac{P}{\dot{m}} = K_K \ln \frac{\bar{D}_f}{\bar{D}_p},\qquad(25)$$

---

[o] Total elapsed milling time encompasses the time during which solids are subjected to a milling operation, whether the particulates undergo single or multiple passes through the mill.

which states that the work required to crush or grind a given mass of material is constant for the same particle size reduction ratio. In Eqs. (24) and (25), $\bar{D}_p$ and $\bar{D}_f$ represent the final and initial average particle sizes[P], P is the power (in kilowatts), and $\dot{m}$ is the rate at which solids are fed to the mill (in tons/hr). K_R and K_K are constants for the Rittinger equation and the Kick equation, respectively.

Bond's "law" of particle size reduction provides an ostensibly more reasonable estimate of the power required for crushing or grinding of a solid (42):

$$\frac{P}{\dot{m}} = \frac{K_B}{\sqrt{D_p}},\tag{26}$$

where K_B is a constant that is *mill*-dependent and *solids*-dependent, and D_p is the particle size (in mm) produced by the mill. This empirical equation is based on Bond's hypothesis that the work required to reduce very large particulate solids to a smaller size is proportional to the square root of the surface to volume ratio of the resultant particulate product. Bond's work index, W_i, is an estimate of the gross energy required, in kilowatt hours per ton of feed, to reduce very large particles [80% of which pass a mesh size of Df (mm)] to such a size that 80% pass through a mesh of size D_p (mm):

$$W_i = \frac{K_B}{\sqrt{D_p}},\tag{27}$$

Combining Bond's work index (Eq. 27) with Bond's law (Eq. 26) yields

$$\frac{P}{\dot{m}} = W_i \cdot \sqrt{D_p}\left(\frac{1}{\sqrt{D_p}} - \frac{1}{\sqrt{D_f}}\right),\tag{28}$$

which allows one to estimate energy requirements for a milling operation in which solids are reduced from size D_f to D_p. [N.B. W_i for wet grinding is generally smaller than that for dry grinding: $W_{i,wet}$ is equivalent to $(W_{i,dry})^{3/4}$ (33).]

These relationships are embodied in the general differential equation

$$dE = -\frac{CdX}{X^n},\tag{29}$$

where E is the work done and C and n are constants. When $n = 1$, the solution of the equation is Kick's law; when $n = 2$, the solution is Rittinger's law; and, when $n = 1.5$, the solution is Bond's law (41).

Although these relationships (Eq. 24–29) are of some limited use in scaling up milling operations, their predictiveness is limited by the inherent complexity of particle size reduction operations. Virtually all retentive or multiple-pass milling operations become increasing less efficient as milling proceeds since the specific comminution rate is smaller for small particles than for large particles. Computer simulations of milling for batch, multiple pass, and continuous modes have been outlined by Snow et al. (44). They describe a differential

---

[P] In this section, particle size refers to the nominal particle size, that is, the particle size based on sieving studies or on the diameter of a sphere of equivalent volume.

equation for batch grinding for which analytical and matrix solutions have been available for some time:

$$\frac{dw_k}{dt} = \sum_{u=1}^{k} [w_u S_u(t) \Delta B_{k,u}] - S_k(t) w_k \tag{30}$$

Equation (30) includes a term S_u, a grinding-rate function that corresponds to

$$S_u = -\frac{dw_u/dt}{w_u}, \tag{31}$$

that is, the rate at which particles of upper size u are selected for breakage per unit time relative to the amount, w_u, of size u present, and a term $\Delta B_{k,u}$, a breakage function that characterizes the size distribution of particle breakdown from size u into all smaller sizes k. Equation (30) thus defines the rate of accumulation of particles of size k as the difference between the rate of production of particles of size k, from all larger particles, and the rate of breakage of particles of size k into smaller particles. Adaptation of Eq. (30) to continuous milling operations necessitates the inclusion of the distribution of residence time, $\tau = M/F$ as discussed above.

Additional complications in milling arise as fines build up in the powder bed (40): (*i*) the fracture rate of *all* particle sizes decreases, the result, apparently, of a cushioning effect by the fines, which minimizes stress and fracture; (*ii*) fracture kinetics become nonlinear. Other factors, such as coating of equipment surfaces by fines, also affect the efficiency of the milling operation.

Nonetheless, mathematical analyses of milling operations, particularly for ball mills, roller mills, and fluid-energy mills, have been moderately successful. There continues to be a pronounced need for a more complete understanding of micromeritic characteristics, the intrinsic nature of the milling operation itself, the influence of fines on the milling operation, and phenomena including flaw structure of solids, particle fracture, particulate flow, and interactions at both macroscopic and microscopic scales.

Mass Transfer

Movement of liquids and semisolids through conduits or pipes from one location to another is accomplished by inducing flow with the aid of pumps. The induction of flow usually occurs as a result of one or more of the following energy transfer mechanisms: gravity, centrifugal force, displacement, electromagnetic force, mechanical impulse, or momentum transfer. The work expended in pumping is the product of pump capacity, Q, that is, the rate of fluid flow through the pump (in m³/hr), and the dynamic head, H:

$$P = \frac{HQ\rho}{3.670 \times 10^5}, \tag{32}$$

where P is the pump's power output, expressed in kW, H is the total dynamic head, in N·m/kg, and ρ is the fluid density, in kg/m. Because of frictional heating losses, power input for a pump is greater than its power output. As pump efficiency is characterized by the ratio of power output to power input, the pumping of viscous fluids would tend to result in decreased pump efficiency due to the increase in power required to achieve a specific output.

Another variable, ε, the surface roughness of the pipe, has an effect on pump efficiency as well and must also be considered. The Fanning friction factor f is a dimensionless factor that is used in conjunction with the Reynolds number to estimate the pressure drop in a fluid flowing in a pipe or conduit. The relative roughness, ε/D, of a pipe—where D is the pipe diameter—has an effect on the friction factor f. When *laminar* flow conditions prevail, f may be estimated by

$$f = \frac{16}{N_{Re}},\tag{33}$$

when *turbulent* flow in smooth pipes is involved,

$$f = \frac{0.079}{N_{Re}^{0.25}}.\tag{34}$$

A useful discussion of incompressible fluid flow in pipes and the influence of surface roughness and friction factors on pumping is found in *Perry's Chemical Engineer's Handbook* (45).

The transfer of material from mixing tanks or holding tanks to processing equipment or to a filling line, whether by pumping or by gravity feed, is potentially problematic. Instability (chemical or physical) or further processing (e.g., mixing; changes in the particle size distribution) may occur during the transfer of material (by pouring or pumping) from one container or vessel to another due to changes in the rate of transfer or in shear rate or shear stress. While scale-up related changes in the velocity profiles of time-*independent* Newtonian and non-Newtonian fluids due to changes in flow rate or in equipment dimensions or geometry can be accounted for, time-dependency must first be recognized in order to be accommodated.

Changes in mass transfer *time* as a consequence of scale-up are often overlooked. As Carstensen and Mehta (46) note, mixing of formulation components in the laboratory may be achieved almost instantaneously with rapid pouring and stirring. They cite the example of pouring 20 mL of liquid A, while stirring, into 80 mL of liquid B. On a production scale, however, mixing is unlikely to be as rapid. A scaled-up batch of 2000 L would require the admixture of 400 L of A and 1600 L of B. If A were pumped into B at the rate of 40 L/min, then the transfer process would take at least 10 minutes, while additional time would also be required for the blending of the two liquids. If, for example, liquids A and B were of different pH (or ionic strength, or polarity, etc.), the time required to transfer all of A into B and to mix A and B intimately would allow some intermediate pH (or ionic strength, or polarity, etc.) to develop and persist, long enough for some adverse effect to occur such as precipitation, adsorption, and change in viscosity. Thus, transfer times on a production scale need to be determined so that the temporal impact of scale-up can be accounted for in laboratory or pilot plant studies.

Dissolution

When dissolution is a necessary part of a manufacturing process, the ultimate objective—the formation of a homogeneous solution—can only be achieved through mixing of solute and solvent. Dissolution or mass transfer from the solute phase to a well-mixed solution phase may be characterized by a mass transfer coefficient, k, that relates the interfacial flux, j_i, or the amount of mass transferred per unit time per unit area, to the concentration difference between the bulk solution and the solution in the interfacial phase, that is, immediately adjacent to the solute/solvent interface. That is, $k = (j_i)/\Delta C$. Most dissolution processes involve a turbulent flow regime in order to enhance the rate of mass transfer per unit area. For relatively large particles, the rate of increase in k is exponentially related to the increase in agitation intensity, that is, $k \propto N^p$, where N is the impeller speed (rpm) and the exponent p may range from 0.1 to 0.8, depending on the solid and liquid characteristics and the type and dimensions of the mixing tank and the impeller (47). As solute particles undergo dissolution, particle size decreases and fluid flow in the vicinity of the particles becomes laminar. As a result, k becomes independent of agitation intensity and diffusivity becomes the principal determinant of dissolution.

Maximal dissolution occurs when the contact between the dissolving solute and the dissolution medium is maximal. Thus, as dissolution is hampered when solute particles settle to the bottom of the tank, off-bottom suspension or fluidization of solute particles facilitates dissolution. Solid suspension in the fluid is the result of the drag and lift forces of the fluid on the solid particles and the turbulent eddies that result from the agitation imparted to the system. When complete off-bottom suspension is achieved, all particles remain suspended in the fluid or do not remain on the bottom of the tank for more than one or two seconds (47). Further increases in agitation intensity beyond this "just-suspended" state do not result in a corresponding increase in k as the accompanying increases in interfacial contact between solute and solvent are relatively small. Dead zones in the mixing tank (where particles tend to accumulate) at the conjunction of the tank wall and tank base are more apt to occur in a flat-bottomed mixing tank than in a dish-bottomed mixing tank.

Heat Transfer

On a laboratory scale, heat transfer occurs relatively rapidly as the volume to surface area ratio is relatively small; cooling or heating may or may not involve jacketed vessels. However, on a pilot plant or production scale, the volume to surface area ratio is relatively large. Consequently, heating or cooling of formulation components or product takes a finite time during which system temperature, T (°C), may vary considerably. Temperature-induced instability may be a substantial problem if a formulation is maintained at suboptimal temperatures for a prolonged period of time. Thus, jacketed vessels or immersion heaters or cooling units with rapid circulation times are an absolute necessity. Carstensen and Mehta (46) give an example of a jacketed kettle with a heated surface of A cm^2, with inlet steam or hot water in the jacket maintained at a temperature T_0°C. The heat transfer rate (dQ/dt) in this system is proportional to the heated surface area of the kettle and the temperature gradient, $T_0 - T$ (i.e., the difference between the temperature of the kettle contents, T, and the temperature of the jacket, T_0) at time t:

$$\frac{dQ}{dt} = C_p\left(\frac{dT}{dt}\right) = kA(T_0 - T) \tag{35}$$

where C_p is the heat capacity of the jacketed vessel and its contents and k is the heat transfer coefficient. If the initial temperature of the vessel is $T_1°C$, Eq. (35) becomes

$$T_0 - T = (T_0 - T_1)e^{-at}, \tag{36}$$

where $a = kA/C_p$. The time t required to reach a specific temperature T_2 can be calculated from Eq. (36), if a is known, or estimated from time-temperature curves for similar products processed under the same conditions. Scale-up studies should consider the effect of longer processing times at suboptimal temperatures on the physicochemical or chemical stability of the formulation components and the product. A further concern for disperse system scale-up is the increased opportunity in a multiphase system for nonuniformity in material transport (e.g., flow rates and velocity profiles) stemming from nonuniform temperatures within processing equipment.

HOW TO ACHIEVE SCALE-UP[q]

Full-scale tests using production equipment, involving no scale-up studies whatsoever, are sometimes resorted to when single-phase low-viscosity systems are involved and processing is considered to be predictable and directly scalable. By and large, these are unrealistic assumptions when viscous liquids, dispersions, or semisolids are involved. Furthermore, the expense associated with full-scale testing is substantial: commercial-scale equipment is relatively inflexible and costly to operate. Errors in full-scale processing involve large amounts of material. Insofar as most liquids or semisolids are concerned, full-scale tests are *not* an option.

On the other hand, scale-up studies involving relatively low scale-up ratios and few changes in process variables are not necessarily a reasonable alternative to full-scale testing. For that matter, experimental designs employing minor, incremental changes in processing equipment and conditions are unacceptable as well. *These* alternative test modes are inherently unacceptable as they consume time, an irreplaceable resource (48) that must be utilized to its maximum advantage. *Appropriate* process development, by reducing costs and accelerating lead times, plays an important role in product development performance. In *The Development Factory: Unlocking the Potential of Process Innovation*, author Gary Pisano (49) argues that while pharmaceuticals compete largely on the basis of product innovation, there is a hidden leverage in process development and manufacturing competence that provides more degrees of freedom, in developing products to more adroit organizations than to their less adept competitors. Although Pisano focuses on drug synthesis and biotechnology process scale-up, his conclusions translate effectively to the manufacturing processes for drug dosage forms and delivery systems. In effect, scale-up issues need to be addressed jointly by pharmaceutical engineers and formulators as soon as a dosage form or delivery system appears to be commercially viable. Scale-up studies should not be relegated to the final stages of product development, whether initiated at the behest of FDA (to meet regulatory requirements) or marketing and sales divisions (to meet marketing directives or sales quotas).

---

[q] Reprinted in part, with revisions and updates, by courtesy of Marcel Dekker, Inc. from Ref. 3.

The worst scenario would entail the delay of scale-up studies until after commercial distribution (to accommodate unexpected market demands).

Modular scale-up involves the scale-up of individual components or unit
operations of a manufacturing process. The interactions among these individual
operations comprise the potential scale-up problem, that is, the inability to
achieve sameness when the process is conducted on a different scale. When the
physical or physicochemical properties of system components are known, the
scalability of some unit operations may be predictable.

Known scale-up correlations thus may allow scale-up even when laboratory
or pilot plant experience is minimal. The *fundamental approach* to process scaling
involves mathematical modeling of the manufacturing process and experimental validation of the model at different scale-up ratios. In a paper on fluid
dynamics in bubble column reactors, Lübbert et al. (50) noted:

> Until very recently fluid dynamical models of multiphase reactors were
> considered intractable. This situation is rapidly changing with the develop-
> ment of high-performance computers. Today's workstations allow new
> approaches to ... modeling.

Insofar as the scale-up of pharmaceutical liquids (especially disperse
systems) and semisolids is concerned, virtually no guidelines or models for
scale-up have generally been available that have stood the test of time. Uhl and
Von Essen (51), referring to the variety of rules of thumb, calculation methods,
and extrapolation procedures in the literature, state "Unfortunately, the
prodigious literature and attributions to the subject [of scale-up] seemed to
have served more to confound. Some allusions are specious, most rules are
extremely limited in application, examples give too little data and limited
analysis ...." Not surprisingly, then, the *trial-and-error* method is the one most
often employed by formulators. As a result, serendipity and practical experience
continue to play large roles in the successful pursuit of the scalable process.

Principles of Similarity

Irrespective of the approach taken to scale-up, the scaling of unit operations and
manufacturing processes requires a thorough appreciation of the principles of
similarity."*Process* similarity is achieved between two processes when they
accomplish the same process objectives by the same mechanisms and produce
the same product to the required specifications." Johnstone and Thring (52) stress
the importance of four types of similarity in effective process translation: (*i*)
geometric similarity, (*ii*) mechanical (static, kinematic, and dynamic) similarity,
(*iii*) thermal similarity, and (*iv*) chemical similarity. Each of these similarities
presupposes the attainment of the other similarities. In actuality, approximations
of similarity are often necessary due to departures from ideality (e.g., differences
in surface roughness, variations in temperature gradients, and changes in
mechanism). When such departures from ideality are not negligible, a correction
of some kind has to be applied when scaling up or down: these scale effects must
be determined before scaling of a unit operation or a manufacturing process can
be pursued. It should be recognized that scale-up of multiphase systems,
based on similarity, is often unsuccessful since only one variable can
be controlled at a time, that is, at each scale-up level. Nonetheless, valuable

mechanistic insights into unit operations can be achieved through similarity analyses.

Geometric Similarity

Point-to-point geometric similarity of two bodies (e.g., two mixing tanks) requires three-dimensional correspondence. Every point in the first body is defined by specific x, y, and z coordinate values. The corresponding point in the second body is defined by specific x', y', and z' coordinate values. The correspondence is defined by the following equation

$$\frac{x'}{x} = \frac{y'}{y} = \frac{z'}{z} = L \tag{37}$$

where the linear scale ratio L is constant. In contrasting the volume of a laboratory scale mixing tank (V_1) with that of a geometrically similar production scale unit (V_2), the ratio of volumes (V_1/V_2) is dimensionless. However, the contrast between the two mixing tanks needs to be considered on a linear scale: for example, a 1000-fold difference in volume corresponds to a 10-fold difference, on a linear scale, in mixing tank diameter, impeller diameter, etc.

If the scale ratio is not the same along each axis, the relationship among the two bodies is of a *distorted geometric similarity* and the axial relationships are given by

$$\frac{x'}{x} = X, \quad \frac{y'}{y} = Y, \quad \frac{z'}{z} = Z \tag{38}$$

Thus, equipment specifications can be described in terms of the scale ratio L or, in the case of a distorted body, two or more scale ratios (X, Y, Z). Scale ratios facilitate the comparison and evaluation of different sizes of functionally comparable equipment in process scale-up.

Mechanical Similarity

The application of force to a stationary or moving system can be described in static, kinematic, or dynamic terms, which define the mechanical similarity of processing equipment and the solids or liquids within their confines. *Static* similarity relates the deformation under constant stress of one body or structure to that of another; it exists when geometric similarity is maintained even as elastic or plastic deformation of stressed structural components occurs (51). In contrast, *kinematic* similarity encompasses the additional dimension of time while *dynamic* similarity involves the forces (e.g., pressure, gravitational, centrifugal) that accelerate or retard moving masses in dynamic systems. The inclusion of time as another dimension necessitates the consideration of *corresponding times*, t' and t, for which the time scale ratio t, defined as $t = t'/t$, is a constant.

Corresponding particles in disperse systems are geometrically similar particles that are centered on corresponding points at corresponding times. If two geometrically similar fluid systems are kinematically similar, their corresponding particles will trace out geometrically similar paths in corresponding intervals of time. Thus, their flow patterns will be geometrically similar and heat or mass transfer rates in the two systems will be related to one another (51).

Pharmaceutical engineers may prefer to characterize disperse systems' *corresponding velocities*, which are the velocities of corresponding particles at corresponding times:

$$\frac{v'}{v} = v = \frac{L}{t} \tag{39}$$

Kinematic and geometric similarity in fluids ensures geometrically similar streamline boundary films and eddy systems. If forces of the same kind act upon corresponding particles at corresponding times, they are termed *corresponding forces*, and conditions for dynamic similarity are met. While the scale up of power consumption by a unit operation or manufacturing process is a direct consequence of dynamic similarity, mass and heat transfer—direct functions of kinematic similarity—are only indirect functions of dynamic similarity.

Thermal Similarity
Heat flow, whether by radiation, conduction, convection, or the bulk transfer of matter, introduces temperature as another variable. Thus, for systems in motion, thermal similarity requires kinematic similarity. Thermal similarity is described by

$$\frac{H'_r}{H_r} = \frac{H'_c}{H_c} = \frac{H'_v}{H_v} = \frac{H'_f}{H_f} = \mathbf{H} \tag{40}$$

where H_r, H_c, H_v, and H_f are the heat fluxes or quantities of heat transferred per second by radiation, convection, conduction, and bulk transport, respectively, and $\mathbf{H}$, the thermal ratio, is a constant. Geometric similarity is a necessary requirement as well and, insofar as thermal similarity is concerned, extends even to the thickness of tank walls, impeller shafts, and blades, etc.

Chemical Similarity
This similarity state is concerned with the variation in chemical composition from point to point as a function of time. Chemical similarity, that is, the existence of comparable concentration gradients, is dependent on both thermal and kinematic similarity.

Interrelationships Among Surface Area and Volume upon Scale-Up
Similarity states aside, the dispersion technologist must be aware of whether a given process is volume dependent or area dependent. As the scale of processing increases, volume effects become increasingly more important while area effects become increasingly *less* important. This is exemplified by the dependence of mixing tank volumes and surface areas on scale-up ratios (based on mixing tank diameters) in Table 1 [adapted from Tatterson (16)]. The surface area to volume ratio is much greater on the small scale than on the large scale: surface area effects are thus much more important on a small scale than on a large one. Conversely, the volume to surface area ratio is much greater on the large scale than on the small scale: volumetric effects are thus much more important on a large scale than on a small scale. Thus, volume-dependent processes are more difficult to scale-up than surface area–dependent processes. For example, exothermic processes may generate more heat than can be

TABLE 1 Area- and Volume-Dependence on Scale-Up Ratios

Scale	Tank diameter (m)	Area (m²)	Volume (m³)	Area/volume	Volume/area
1	0.1	0.0393	0.000785	50	0.02
10	1	3.93	0.785	5	0.2
20	2	15.7	6.28	2.5	0.4
50	5	98.2	98.2	1	1

Assumptions: tank is a right circular cylinder; batch *height* = tank *diameter*; area calculations are the sum of the area of the convex surface and the area of the bottom of the cylinder.

tolerated by a formulation, leading to undesirable phase changes or product degradation unless cooling coils, or other means of intensifying heat transfer, are added. A further example is provided by a scale-up problem involving a 10-fold increase in tank volume, from 400 to 4000 L, and an increase in surface area from 2 to 10 m². The surface area to volume ratio is 1/200 and 1/400, respectively. In spite of the 10-fold increase in tank volume, the increase in surface area is only 5-fold, necessitating the provision of additional heating or cooling capacity to allow for an additional 10 m² of surface for heat exchange.

As Tatterson (16) notes, "there is much more volume on scale-up than is typically recognized. This is one feature of scale-up that causes more difficulty than anything else." For disperse systems, a further mechanistic implication of the changing volume and surface area ratios is that particle size reduction (or droplet breakup) is more likely to be the dominant process on a small scale while aggregation (or coalescence) is more likely to be the dominant process on a large scale (16).

Interrelationships Among System Properties upon Scale-Up

When a process is dominated by a mixing operation, another gambit for the effective scale-up of geometrically similar systems involves the interrelationships that have been established for impeller-based systems. Tatterson (16) describes a number of elementary scale-up procedures for agitated tank systems that depend on operational similarity. Thus, when scaling up from level 1 to level 2,

$$\frac{(P/V)_1}{(P/V)_2} = \begin{cases} \left(\dfrac{N_1}{N_2}\right)^3 \left(\dfrac{D_1}{D_2}\right)^2 & \text{for turbulent flow} \\ \left(\dfrac{N_1}{N_2}\right) & \text{for laminar flow} \end{cases} \tag{41}$$

power per unit volume is dependent principally on the ratio N_1/N_2 since impeller diameters are constrained by geometric similarity.

A change in size on scale-up is not the sole determinant of the scalability of a unit operation or process. Scalability depends on the unit operation mechanism(s) or system properties involved. Some mechanisms or system properties relevant to dispersions are listed in Table 2 (53). In a number of instances, size has little or no influence on processing or on system behavior. Thus, scale-up will not affect chemical kinetics or thermodynamics although the thermal effects of a reaction could perturb a system, for example, by affecting convection (53).

TABLE 2   Influence of Size on System Behavior or Important Unit Operation Mechanisms

System behavior or unit Operation mechanisms	Important variables[a]	Influence of size
Chemical kinetics	C,P,T	None
Thermodynamic properties	C,P,T	None
Heat transfer	Local velocities, C,P,T	Important
Mass transfer within a phase	N_{Re}, C, T	Important
Mass transfer between phases	Relative phase velocities, C,P,T	Important
Forced convection	Flow rates, geometry	Important
Free convection	Geometry, C,P,T	Crucial

[a]C, P, and T are concentration, pressure, and temperature, respectively.
Source: Adapted from Ref. 51.

Heat or mass transfer within or between phases is indirectly affected by changes in size while convection is directly affected. Thus, since transport of energy, mass, and momentum are often crucial to the manufacture of disperse systems, scale-up can have a substantial effect on the resultant product.

Dimensions, Dimensional Analysis, and the Principles of Similarity

Just as process translation or scaling-up is facilitated by defining similarity in terms of dimensionless ratios of measurements, forces, or velocities, the technique of dimensional analysis per se permits the definition of appropriate composite dimensionless numbers whose numeric values are process specific. Dimensionless quantities can be pure numbers, ratios, or multiplicative combinations of variables with no net units.

Dimensional analysis is concerned with the nature of the relationship among the various quantities involved in a physical problem. An approach intermediate between formal mathematics and empiricism, it offers the pharmaceutical engineer an opportunity to generalize from experience and apply knowledge to a new situation (33,54). This is a particularly important avenue as many engineering problems—scale-up among them—cannot be solved completely by theoretical or mathematical means. Dimensional analysis is based on the fact that if a theoretical equation exists among the variables affecting a physical process, that equation must be dimensionally homogeneous. Thus, many factors can be grouped, in an equation, into a smaller number of dimensionless groups of variables (33).

Dimensional analysis is an algebraic treatment of the variables affecting a process; it does not result in a numerical equation. Rather, it allows experimental data to be fitted to an empirical process equation that results in scale-up being achieved more readily. The experimental data determine the exponents and coefficients of the empirical equation. The requirements of dimensional analysis are that (*i*) only one relationship exists among a certain number of physical quantities and (*ii*) no pertinent quantities have been excluded nor extraneous quantities included.

Fundamental (primary) quantities, which cannot be expressed in simpler terms, include mass (M), length (L), and time (T). Physical quantities may be expressed in terms of the fundamental quantities: for example, density is ML^{-3}; velocity is LT^{-1}. In some instances, mass units are covertly expressed in terms of force (F) in order to simplify dimensional expressions or render them more identifiable. The MLT and FLT systems of dimensions are related by the equations

$$\left. \begin{array}{l} F = Ma = \dfrac{ML}{T^2} \\[3mm] M = \dfrac{FT^2}{L} \end{array} \right\}$$

According to Bisio (55), scale-up can be achieved by maintaining the dimensionless groups characterizing the phenomena of interest constant from small scale to large scale. However, for complex phenomena this may not be possible. Alternatively, dimensionless numbers can be weighted so that the untoward influence of unwieldy variables can be minimized. On the other hand, this camouflaging of variables could lead to an inadequate characterization of a process and a false interpretation of laboratory or pilot plant data.

Pertinent examples of the value of dimensional analysis have been reported recently in a series of papers by Maa and Hsu (18,34,56). In their first report, they successfully established the scale-up requirements for microspheres produced by an emulsification process in continuously stirred tank reactors (CSTRs) (56). Their initial assumption was that the diameter of the microspheres, d_{ms}, is a function of phase *quantities, physical properties* of the dispersion and dispersed phases, and *processing equipment parameters*:

$$d_{ms} = f(D\omega, D/T, H, B, n_{imp}, g_c, g, c, \eta_o, \eta_a, \rho_o, \rho_a, v_o, v_a, \sigma) \qquad (42)$$

Gravitational acceleration, g, is included to relate mass to inertial force. The conversion factor, g_c, was included to convert one unit system to another. The subscripts o and a refer to the organic and aqueous phases, respectively. The remaining notations are as follows:

D	impeller diameter (cm)
ω	rotational speed (angular velocity) of the impeller(s) (sec^{-1})
T	tank diameter (cm)
H	height of filled volume in the tank (cm)
B	total baffle area (cm^2)
n	number of baffles
n_{imp}	number of impellers
v_o, v_a	phase volumes (mL)
c	polymer concentration (g/mL)
η_o and η_a	phase viscosities (g/cm·sec)
ρ_o and ρ_a	phase densities (g/mL)
σ	interfacial tension between organic and aqueous phases (dyne/cm)

The initial emulsification studies employed a 1-L "reactor" vessel with baffles originally designed for fermentation processes. Subsequent studies were successively scaled up from 1 to 3, 10, and 100 L. Variations due to differences in reactor configuration were minimized by utilizing geometrically similar reactors with approximately the same D/T ratio (i.e., 0.36–0.40). Maa and Hsu contended that separate experiments on the effect of the baffle area (B) on the resultant microsphere diameter did not significantly affect d_{ms}. However, the number and location of the impellers had a significant impact on d_{ms}. As a result, to simplify the system, Maa and Hsu always used double impellers ($n_{imp} = 2$) with the lower one placed close to the bottom of the tank and the other located in the center of the total emulsion volume. Finally, Maa and Hsu determined that the volumes of the organic and aqueous phases, in the range they were concerned with, played only a minor role in affecting d_{ms}. Thus, by the omission of D/T, B, and v_o, and va, Eq. (42) was simplified considerably to yield

$$d_{ms} = f(D\omega, g_c, g, c, \eta_o, \eta_a, \rho_o, \rho_a, \sigma) \tag{43}$$

Equation (43) contains 10 variables and 4 fundamental dimensions (L, M, T, and F). Maa and Hsu were able to subsequently define microsphere size, d_{ms}, in terms of the processing parameters and physical properties of the phases:

$$\frac{g(\rho_o - \rho_a)d_{ms}^2}{\sigma} = \prod_2^{-0.280} \prod_3^{-0.108} \prod_4^{0.056} \left(0.0255 \prod_5^e + 0.0071\right), \tag{44}$$

where $\prod_i$ are dimensionless multiplicative groups of variables. (The transformation of Eq. (43) into (44) is described by Maa and Hsu (56) in an appendix to their paper.) Subsequently, linear regression analysis of the microsphere size parameter, $g(\rho_o - \rho_a)d_{ms}^2/\sigma$, as a function of the right-hand side of Eq. (43), that is, $\left[\prod_2^{0.280} \prod_3^{-0.108} \prod_4^{0.056}(0.0255 \prod_5^e + 0.0071)\right]$, resulted in $r \approx 0.973$ for 1, 3, 10, and 100 L reactors, at two different polymer concentrations. These composite data are depicted graphically in Figure 3.

Subsequently, Maa and Hsu (18) applied dimensional analysis to the scale-up of a liquid-liquid emulsification process for microsphere production, utilizing one or another of three different static mixers that varied in diameter, number of mixing elements, and mixing element length. Mixing element design differences among the static mixers were accommodated by the following equation:

$$d_{ms} = 0.483 d^{1.202} V^{0.556} \sigma^{0.556} \eta_a^{-0.560} \eta_o^{0.004} \eta^h c^{0.663}, \tag{45}$$

where d_{ms} is the diameter of the microspheres (μm) produced by the emulsification process, d is the diameter of the static mixer (cm), V is the flow rate of the continuous phase (mL/sec), σ is the interfacial tension between the organic and aqueous phases (dyne/cm), η_a and η_o are the viscosities (g/cm·sec) of the aqueous and organic phases, respectively, n is the number of mixing elements, h is an exponent the magnitude of which is a function of static mixer design, and c is the polymer concentration (g/mL) in the organic phase. The relative efficiency of the three static mixers was readily determined in terms of emulsification efficiency, ε, defined as equivalent to $1/d_{ms}$: better mixing results in smaller microspheres. In this way, Maa and Hsu were able to compare and contrast CSTRs with static mixers.

Houcine et al. (57) used a nonintrusive laser-induced fluorescence method to study the mechanisms of mixing in a 20 dm^3 CSTR with removable baffles, a conical bottom, a mechanical stirrer, and two incoming liquid jet streams. Under certain conditions, they observed an interaction between the flow induced by the

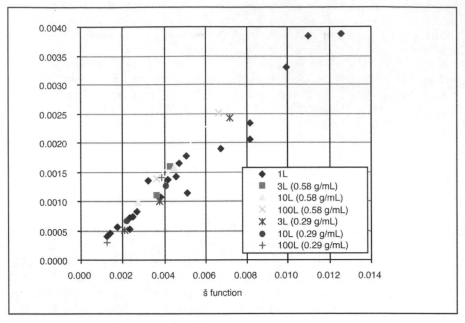

Π function value

FIGURE 3 Microsphere diameter parameter, d_{ms}, as a function of processing parameters and physical properties of the phases [$\prod$ functions of the right-hand side of Eq. (31)]. *Source*: From Maa and Hsu (56).

stirrer and the incoming jets, which led to oscillations of the jet stream with a period of several seconds and corresponding switching of the recirculation flow between several metastable macroscopic patterns. These jet feed-stream oscillations or intermittencies could strongly influence the kinetics of fast reactions such as precipitation. The authors used dimensional analysis to demonstrate that the intermittence phenomenon would be less problematic in larger CSTRs.

Additional insights into the application of dimensional analysis to scale-up can be found in the chapter in this volume by Zlokarnik (58) and in his earlier monograph on scale-up in chemical engineering (59).

Mathematical Modeling and Computer Simulation

Basic and applied research methodologies in science and engineering are undergoing major transformations. Mathematical models of "real-world" phenomena are more elaborate than in the past, with forms governed by sets of partial differential equations that represent continuum approximations to microscopic models (60). Appropriate mathematical relationships would reflect the fundamental laws of physics regarding the conservation of mass, momentum, and energy. Euzen et al. (53) list such balance equations for mass, momentum, and energy (e.g., heat) for a single-phase Newtonian system (with constant density, ρ, viscosity, η, and molar heat capacity at constant pressure, C_p) in which a process takes place in an element of volume, ΔV (defined as the product of dx, dy, and dz):

$$\frac{\partial C_i}{\partial t} = -\left\{ v_x \frac{\partial C_i}{\partial x} + v_y \frac{\partial C_i}{\partial y} + v_z \frac{\partial C_i}{\partial z} \right\} + \left\{ D_{ix} \frac{\partial^2 C_i}{\partial x^2} + D_{iy} \frac{\partial^2 C_i}{\partial y^2} + D_{iz} \frac{\partial^2 C_i}{\partial z^2} \right\} + R_i$$

Mass balance

$$\rho\left\{ \frac{\partial v_x}{\partial t} + v_x \frac{\partial v_x}{\partial x} + v_y \frac{\partial v_x}{\partial y} + v_z \frac{\partial v_x}{\partial z} \right\} = -\frac{\partial P}{\partial x} + \eta\left\{ \frac{\partial^2 v_x}{\partial x^2} + \frac{\partial^2 v_x}{\partial y^2} + \frac{\partial^2 v_x}{\partial z^2} \right\} + \rho g_x \qquad (46)$$

Momentum balance (e.g., in direction)

$$\rho C_p\left\{ \frac{\partial T}{\partial t} + v_x \frac{\partial T}{\partial x} + v_y \frac{\partial T}{\partial y} + v_z \frac{\partial T}{\partial z} \right\} = \left\{ k_x \frac{\partial^2 T}{\partial x^2} + k_y \frac{\partial^2 T}{\partial y^2} + k_z \frac{\partial^2 T}{\partial z^2} \right\} + S_R$$

Energy balance

wherein P is pressure, T is temperature, t is time, v is fluid flow velocity, k is thermal conductivity, and R_i, g_x, and S_R are kinetic, gravitational, and energetic parameters, respectively. Equation (46) is presented as an example of the complex relationships that are becoming increasingly more amenable to resolution by computers rather than for its express utilization in a scale-up problem. Pordal et al. (61) reviewed the potential role of computational fluid dynamics (CFD) in the pharmaceutical industry. Kukura et al. (62) and McCarthy et al. (63,64) have used CFD software to simulate the hydrodynamic conditions of the USP dissolution apparatus. Their results demonstrate the value of CFD in analyzing hydrodynamic conditions in mixing processes. A more extensive review of CFD can be found in the publication by Marshall and Bakker (65).

However, most CFD software programs available to date for simulation of transport phenomena require the user to define the model equations and parameters and specify the initial and boundary conditions in accordance with the program's language and code, often highly specialized. A practical interim solution to the computational problem presented by Eq. (46) and its non-Newtonian counterparts is available in the form of software developed by Visimix Ltd. (66)—VisiMix Laminar, VisiMix Turbulent, and VisiMix DI[r]—for personal computers. These interactive programs utilize a combination of classical transport equations in conjunction with algorithms for computation of mixing processes and actual laboratory, pilot plant, and production data to simulate macro- and microscale transport phenomena. VisiMix's user friendly, menu-driven software is based on physical and mathematical models of mixing phenomena based on fundamental transport equations and on extensive theoretical and experimental research (67–69). Graphical menus allow the user to select and define process equipment from a wide range of options including vessel shape, agitator type, jacketing, and baffle type. VisiMix not only addresses most unit operations with a mixing component (e.g., blending, suspension of solids, emulsification, dissolution, gas dispersion) but also

---

[r] VisiMix Laminar simulates mixing in Newtonian and non-Newtonian media in laminar and transitional flow regimes, while VisiMix Turbulent addresses the turbulent flow regime. VisiMix DI complements VisiMix Turbulent by enabling hydrodynamic modeling and calculations for mixing equipment with different impellers on the same shaft.

TABLE 3 Shear Rates at Different Processing Scales

Scale	Agitator speed (rpm)	Tip velocity (m/sec)	Average shear rate = (tip speed/ distance from tip to baffle) (1/sec)	VisiMix simulation: shear rate in bulk volume (1/sec)	VisiMix simulation: shear rate near the impeller blade (1/sec)	VisiMix simulation: shear rate near baffle (1/sec)
Laboratory reactor	700	3.11	37	902	12,941	902
Pilot plant reactor	250	5.98	118	2,470	12,883	4,146
Production plant reactor	77	8.60	15	1,517	11,116	1,678

Source: Adapted from Ref. 67.

evaluates heat transfer/exchange (e.g., for jacketed tanks). Tangential velocity distributions, axial circulation, macro- and microscale turbulence, mixing time, equilibrium droplet size distribution, and droplet breakup and coalescence are just some of the calculations or simulations that VisiMix can provide.

Liu and Neeld (70) used VisiMix software to calculate shear rates in laboratory, pilot plant, and production-scale vessels. Their results (Table 3) showed marked differences, by as much as two orders of magnitude, in the shear rates calculated in the conventional manner (from tip speed and the distance from impeller tip to baffle, that is, $\dot{\gamma} = ND/(T - D)$ and the shear rates computed by VisiMix. The latter's markedly higher shear rates resulted from VisiMix's definition of the shear rate in terms of Kolmogorov's model of turbulence and the distribution of flow velocities. Note that VisiMix's estimates of the respective shear rates, in the vicinity of the impeller blade, are comparable at all scales while the shear rates in the bulk volume or near the baffle are not, except on the laboratory scale. If the efficacy of the mixing process were dependent on the shear achieved adjacent to the impeller, the VisiMix scaling simulations would predict comparable outcomes for the equipment parameters employed. However, if the shear rate in the vicinity of the impeller were not the controlling factor in achieving similitude, then scale-up relying on adjustments in agitator speed or tip velocity would be unsuccessful.

Experimental Aspects

Tools and techniques for obtaining qualitative and quantitative measurements of mixing processes have been described and critiqued in detail by Brown et al. (71). Scale-up experimentation involving mixing in stirred tanks generally entails vessels between ~0.2 and 2 m in diameter. At the low end, geometric similarity may be difficult to achieve and probes may not be small enough to avoid altering flow patterns or fluid velocities, especially on a microscopic scale. Bubble, droplet, or particle sizes may also be of the same order of magnitude as the probes or equipment components (baffles, impellers, etc.), thereby decreasing the applicability of the experimental data to larger-scale systems.

SCALE-UP PROBLEMS

As Baekeland (72) said, "Commit your blunders on a small scale and make your profits on a large scale." Effective scale-up mandates an awareness of the relative importance of various process parameters at different scales of scrutiny. Heat transfer, molecular diffusion, and microscopic viscosity operate on a so-called microscopic scale. On a macroscopic scale, these parameters may not appear to have a noticeable effect, yet they cannot be ignored: were there no energy, mass, or momentum transport at the microscopic scale, larger-scale processes would not function properly (16). On the other hand, a system's flow regimes operate at both microscopic and macroscopic levels. Turbulent flow, characterized by random swirling motions superimposed on simpler flow patterns, involves the rapid tumbling and retumbling of relatively large portions of fluid or eddies. While turbulence, encountered to some degree in virtually all fluid systems, tends to be isotropic on a small scale, it is anisotropic on a large scale.

Ignoring or misinterpreting unit operations or process fundamentals. Among some of the more common scale-up errors are the following:

- Scaling based on wrong unit operation mechanism(s)
- Incompletely characterized equipment (e.g., multishaft mixers/homogenizers)
- Insufficient knowledge of process; lack of important process information
- Utilization of different types of equipment at different levels of scale-up
- Unrealistic expectations (e.g., heat dissipation)
- Changes in product or process (e.g., altered formulation, phase changes, and changes in order of addition) during scale-up

These last issues, in particular, are exemplified by the recent report of Williams et al. (73) on problems associated with the scale-up of an o/w cream containing 40% diethylene glycol monoethyl ether and various solid, waxy excipients (e.g., cetyl alcohol; polyoxyethylene-2-stearyl ether). Preparation of 300 g batches in the laboratory in small stainless steel beakers proceeded without incident while 7 kg batches made with a Brogli-10 homogenizer were subject to precipitation in or congealing of the external phase in the region between the sweep agitation blade and the discharge port. Low levels of congealed or precipitated excipient that went undetected on the laboratory scale, marked differences in the rate and extent of heat exchange at the two levels of manufacturing, and the presence of cold spots or nonjacketed areas in the Brogli-10 homogenizer contributed to the problem.

Unfortunately, the publication by Williams et al. is one of the only reports of a scale-up problem involving liquids or semisolids in the pharmaceutical literature. A number of papers that purport to deal with scale-up issues and even go so far as to compare the properties of small versus large batches fail to apply techniques such as dimensional analysis or CFD that could have provided the basis for a far more substantial assessment or analysis of the scale-up problem for their system. Worse yet, there is no indication of how scale-up was achieved or what scale-up algorithm(s), if any, were used. Consequently, their usefulness, from a pedagogical point of view, is minimal. In the end, effective scale-up requires the complete characterization of the materials and processes involved and a critical evaluation of all laboratory and production data that may have some bearing on the scalability of the process.

CONCLUSIONS

Process scale-up of liquids and semisolids not only is an absolutely essential part of pharmaceutical manufacturing but also is a crucial part of the regulatory process. The dearth of research publications to date must reflect either the avoidance of scale-up issues by pharmaceutical formulators and technologists due to their inherent complexity or a concern that scale-up experimentation and data constitute trade secrets that must not be disclosed lest competitive advantages be lost. The emergence of pharmaceutical engineering as an area of specialization and the advent of specialized software capable of facilitating scale-up should ultimately change these attitudes.

REFERENCES

1. Griskey RG. Chemical Engineering for Chemists. Washington, D.C.: American Chemical Society, 1997:283–303.
2. Holland EA, Wilkinson JK. Process economics. In: Perry RH, Green DW, Maloney JO, eds. Perry's Chemical Engineers' Handbook. 7th ed. New York: McGraw-Hill, 1997:9-1-9-79.
3. Block LH. Scale-up of disperse systems: theoretical and practical aspects. In: Lieberman HA, Rieger MM, Banker GS, eds. Pharmaceutical Dosage Forms: Disperse Systems. 2nd ed., Vol 3. New York: Marcel Dekker, 1998:363, 366–378, 378–388.
4. Astarita G. Scaleup: overview, closing remarks, and cautions. In: Bisio A, Kabel RL, eds. Scale-up of Chemical Processes: Conversion from Laboratory Scale Tests to Successful Commercial Size Design. New York: Wiley, 1985:678.
5. Gekas V. Transport Phenomena of Foods and Biological Materials. Boca Raton, FL: CRC Press, 1992:5–62.
6. Bird RB, Stewart WE, Lightfoot EN. Transport Phenomena. New York: John Wiley & Sons, 1960:71–122.
7. Dickey DS, Hemrajani RR. Recipes for fluid mixing. Chem Eng 1992; 99(3):82–89.
8. Ottino JM. The mixing of fluids. Sci Am 1989; 260(1):56–57, 60–67.
9. Frisch U. Turbulence: The Legacy of A. N. Kolmogorov. Cambridge: Cambridge University Press, 1995.
10. Bershader D. Fluid physics. In: Lerner RG, Trigg GL, eds. Encyclopedia of Physics. 2nd ed. New York: VCH Publisher, 1991:402–410.
11. Stokes RJ, Evans DF. Fundamentals of Interfacial Engineering. New York: Wiley-VCH, 1997:88–89.
12. Sterbacek Z, Tausk P. Mixing in the Chemical Industry. Oxford: Pergamon Press, 1965:8.
13. Treybal RE. Mass-Transfer Operations. 3rd ed. New York: McGraw-Hill, 1980:45.
14. Lugt HJ. Vortices and vorticity in fluid dynamics. Am Sci 1985; 73:162–167.
15. Oldshue JY. Fluid Mixing Technology. New York: McGraw-Hill, 1983:338–358, 72–93, 295–337.
16. Tatterson GB. Scale-up and Design of Industrial Mixing Processes. New York: McGraw-Hill, 1994:125–131, 15–18, 67–74, 117–125, 97–101, 112–113, 243–262.
17. Gladki H. Power dissipation, thrust force and average shear stress in the mixing tank with a free jet agitator. In: Tatterson GB, Calabrese RV, Penny WR, eds. Industrial Mixing Fundamentals with Applications. New York: American Institute of Chemical Engineering, 1995:146–149.
18. Maa Y-F, Hsu C. Liquid-liquid emulsification by static mixers for use in micro-encapsulation. J Microencapsul 1996; 13:419–433.
19. Dickey DS, Fasano JB. Mechanical design of mixing equipment. In: Paul EL, Atiemo-Obeng VA, Kresta SM, eds. Handbook of Industrial Mixing: Science and Practice. Hoboken, NJ: Wiley, 2004:1308.
20. Dickey DS, Fenic JG. Dimensional analysis for fluid agitation systems. Chem Eng 1976; 83(1):139–145.

21. Coulson JM, Richardson JF, Backhurst JR, et al. Chemical Engineering: Fluid Flow, Heat Transfer and Mass Transfer. 4th ed., Vol 1. Oxford: Pergamon Press, 1990: 227–230.

22. Beckner JL, Smith JM. Trans Inst Chem Eng 1966; 44: T224; through Fowler HW. Progress report in pharmaceutical engineering. Manuf Chem Aerosol News 1966; 37(11):60.

23. Etchells AW, Ford WN, Short DGR. Mixing of Bingham plastics on an industrial scale. In: Fluid Mixing III, Symposium Series 108, Institution of Chemical Engineers. Rugby, U.K.: Hemisphere Publisher Corporation, 1985:271–285.

24. Metzner AB, Houghton WT, Sailor RA, et al. A method for measurement of normal stresses in simple shearing flow. Trans Soc Rheol 1961; 5:133–147.

25. Fredrickson AG. Viscoelastic phenomena in thick liquids: phenomenological analysis. In: Acrivos A, ed. Modern Chemical Engineering. Vol. I: Physical Operations. New York: Reinhold Publisher, 1963:197–265.

26. Smith JM. The mixing of Newtonian and non-Newtonian fluids. J Soc Cosmet Chem 1970; 21:541–552.

27. Wilkens RJ, Miller JD, Plummer JR, et al. New techniques for measuring and modeling cavern dimensions in a Bingham plastic fluid. Chem Eng Sci 2005; 60:5269–5275.

28. Simmons MJH, Edwards I, Hall JF, et al. Techniques for visualization of cavern boundaries in opaque industrial mixing systems. Am Inst Chem Eng 2009; 55: 2765–2772.

29. Cheng J, Carreau PJ, Chabra RP. On the effect of wall and bottom clearance on mixing of viscoelastic fluids. In: Tatterson GB, Calabrese RV, Penny WR, eds. Industrial Mixing Fundamentals with Applications. New York: American Institute of Chemical Engineers 1995:115–122.

30. Skidmore JA. Some aspects of the mixing of liquids. Am Perf Cosmet 1969; 84(1): 31–35.

31. Hinze J. Fundamentals of the hydrodynamic mechanism of splitting in dispersion processes. Am Inst Chem Eng J 1955; 1:289–295; through Sterbacek Z, Tausk P. Mixing in the Chemical Industry. Oxford: Oxford: Pergamon Press, 1965:47–48.

32. Kitchatov BV, Korshunov AM, Boiko IV, et al. Effect of impeller blade geometry on drop size in stirring of immiscible liquids. Theor Found Chem Eng 2003; 37(1):19–24.

33. McCabe WL, Smith JC, Harriott P. Unit Operations of Chemical Engineering. 5th ed. New York: Mc-Graw Hill, 1993:276, 960–993, 16–18.

34. Maa Y-F, Hsu C. Liquid-liquid emulsification by rotor/stator homogenization. J Control Release 1996; 38:219–228.

35. Dobetti L, Pantaleo V. Hydrodynamics in microencapsulation by coacervation. American Association of Pharmaceutical Scientists, Annual Meeting and Exposition, Indianapolis, IN, October 29–November 2, 2000.

36. Armenante PM, Kirwan DJ. Mass transfer to microparticles in agitated systems. Chem Eng Sci 1989; 44(12):2781–2796.

37. Fayed ME, Otten L, eds. Handbook of Powder Science and Technology. New York: Van Nostrand Reinhold, 1984.

38. Carstensen J. Solid Pharmaceutics: Mechanical Properties and Rate Phenomena. New York: Academic Press, 1980.

39. Carstensen J. Advanced Pharmaceutical Solids. New York: Marcel Dekker, 2000.

40. Austin LG. Size reduction of solids: crushing and grinding equipment. In: Fayed ME, Otten L, eds. Handbook of Powder Science and Technology. New York: Van Nostrand Reinhold, 1984:562–606.

41. Mori S. Chem Eng (Japan) 1964; 2(2):173; through Perry RH, Green DW, Maloney JO, eds. Perry's Chemical Engineers' Handbook. 7th ed. New York: McGraw-Hill, 1997:20–19.

42. Bond FC. Crushing and grinding calculations. Br Chem Eng 1965; 6:378.

43. Walker WH, Lewis WK, McAdams WH, et al. Principles of Chemical Engineering. 3rd ed. New York: McGraw-Hill, 1937.

44. Snow RH, Allen T, Ennis BJ, et al. Size reduction and size enlargement. In: Perry RH, Green DW, Maloney JO, eds. Perry's Chemical Engineers' Handbook. 7th ed. New York: McGraw-Hill, 1997:20-13–20-22.

45. Boyce MP. Transport and storage of fluids. In: Perry RH, Green DW, Maloney JO, eds. Perry's Chemical Engineers' Handbook. 7th ed. New York: McGraw-Hill, 1997:10-20–10-23.

46. Carstensen JT, Mehta A. Scale-up factors in the manufacture of solution dosage forms. Pharm Technol 1982; 6(11):64, 66, 68, 71, 72, 77.

47. Nagata S. Mixing: Principles and Applications. Tokyo: Kodansha Ltd, 1975:268–269.

48. Dale WJ. The scale-up process: optimize the use of your pilot plant. Abstract 108c, Session 108 on Experimental Strategies for Pilot Plants, 1996 Spring Meeting, American Institute of Chemical Engineers, New York.

49. Pisano GP. The Development Factory: Unlocking the Potential of Process Innovation. Boston: Harvard Business School Press, 1997.

50. Lübbert A, Paaschen T, Lapin A. Fluid dynamics in bubble column bioreactors: experiments and numerical simulations. Biotechnol Bioeng 1996; 52:248–258.

51. Uhl VW, Von Essen JA. Scale-up of equipment for agitating liquids. In: Uhl VW, Gray JB, eds. Mixing Theory and Practice. Vol 3. New York: Academic Press, 1986:200.

52. Johnstone RE, Thring MW. Pilot Plants, Models, and Scale-up Methods in Chemical Engineering. New York: McGraw-Hill, 1957:12–26.

53. Euzen JP, Trambouze P, Wauquier JP. Scale-Up Methodology for Chemical Processes. Paris: Editions Technip, 1993:13–15.

54. Taylor ES. Dimensional Analysis for Engineers. Oxford, UK: Clarendon Press, 1974:1.

55. Bisio A. Introduction to scaleup. In: Bisio A, Kabel RL, eds. Scaleup of Chemical Processes: Laboratory Scale Tests to Successful Commercial Size Design. New York: Wiley, 1985:15–16.

56. Maa Y-F, Hsu C. Microencapsulation reactor scale-up by dimensional analysis. J Microencaps 1996; 13(1):53–66.

57. Houcine I, Plasari E, David R, et al. Feedstream jet intermittency phenomenon in a continuous stirred tank reactor. Chem Eng J 1999; 72:19–29.

58. Zlokarnik M. Dimensional analysis and scale-up in theory and industrial application. In: Levin M, ed. Process Scale-Up in the Pharmaceutical Industry. New York: Marcel Dekker, 2001.

59. Zlokarnik M. Dimensional Analysis and Scale-Up in Chemical Engineering. Berlin: Springer, 1991.

60. Karniadakis GE. Simulation science? Brown Faculty Bull 1996; 8(3). Available at: http://www.cfm.brown.edu/crunch/article.html.

61. Pordal HS, Matice CJ, Fry TJ. The role of computational fluid dynamics in the pharmaceutical industry. Pharm Technol 2002; 26(2):72, 74, 76, 78, 79.

62. Kukura J, Arratia PE, Szalai ES, et al. Engineering tools for understanding the hydrodynamics of dissolution tests. Drug Dev Ind Pharm 2003; 29(2):231–239.

63. McCarthy LG, Kosiol C, Healy AM, et al. Simulating the hydrodynamic conditions in the United States Pharmacopeia paddle dissolution apparatus. AAPS PharmSciTech 2003; 4(2):Article 22.

64. McCarthy LG, Bradley G, Sexton JC, et al. Computational fluid dynamics modeling of the paddle dissolution apparatus: agitation rate, mixing patterns, and fluid velocities. AAPS PharmSciTech 2004; 5(2):Article 31.

65. Marshall EM, Bakker A. Computational fluid mixing. In: Paul EL, Atiemo-Obeng VA, Kresta SM, eds. Handbook of Industrial Mixing: Science and Practice. Hoboken, NJ: Wiley, 2004:257–343.

66. VisiMix Ltd., P.O. Box 45170, Jerusalem, Israel. Available at: http://www.visimix.com.

67. Braginsky LN, Begachev VI, Barabash VM. Mixing in Liquid Media: Physical Foundations and Methods of Technical Calculations. Jerusalem: VisiMix, 1996; excerpts from the Russian edition published by Khimya, Leningrad, 1984.

68. A Review of Main Mathematical Models Used in the VisiMix Software. Jerusalem: VisiMix, 1998.
69. Selected Verification and Validation Examples: The Comparison between Published Experimental Data and VisiMix Calculations. Jerusalem: VisiMix, 1999.
70. Liu K, Neeld K. Simulation of mixing and heat transfer in stirred tanks with VisiMix®. Conference on Process Development from Research to Manufacturing: Industrial Mixing and Scale-Up, Annual Meeting, American Institute of Chemical Engineers, 1999.
71. Brown DAR, Jones PN, Middleton JC, et al. Experimental methods. In: Paul EL, Atiemo-Obeng VA, Kresta SM, eds. Handbook of Industrial Mixing: Science and Practice. Hoboken, NJ: Wiley, 2004:145–256.
72. Baekeland LH. Practical life as a complement to university education—medal address. J Ind Eng Chem 1916; 8:184–190.
73. Williams SO, Long S, Allen J, et al. Scale-up of an oil/water cream containing 40% diethylene glycol monoethyl ether. Drug Dev Ind Pharm 2000; 26:71–77.

7 Scale-up considerations for biotechnology-derived products

Marco Cacciuttolo, John Chon[†], and Greg Zarbis-Papastoitsis

INTRODUCTION

This revised chapter covers the general principles involved in the scale-up of biotechnology-derived products obtained from cell culture. The section "Fundamentals: Typical Unit Operations" focuses on technologies currently used in the manufacture of commercial products. The rest of the sections include a practical guide to process design and scale-up strategies typically used to translate process development into large-scale production of biologics.

Advantages of Biologics as Therapeutic Agents

The main advantage of biologics over traditional small molecule drugs is that biologics are usually proteins that can be normally found in the body. If the biology of these proteins is well understood, the regulatory approval is facilitated as toxicology and immunogenicity could be demonstrated at a much faster pace than in traditional small drug product approval cycles. In addition, biologics offer the advantage of multiple sites of interaction between the drug and the target, which is not usually possible to achieve with the use of small molecule drugs.

The introduction of biologics as credible therapies is evidenced by the large growth of the biologics market (Table 1). Additionally, "Big Pharma" (non-biotech companies with annual revenues >\$10 billion), which have historically focused on small molecules, have been focusing more and more on biologics as of late. Indeed, the forecasted 2010 compound annual growth rate (CAGR) of revenue among the Big Pharma for biologics is 13.0%, compared to a mere 0.9% predicted for small molecules (1).

With increasing market demand for biotechnology-derived products, the global manufacturing capacity for cell culture at one point was estimated not to be able to meet the projected needs. However, within a few years, significant technology advancements have been made in the areas of expression vectors, host cell lines, and media development. For example, typical expression levels for antibodies have gone up from less than 500 mg/L in the late 1990s to over 2 g/L in cell culture by around 2003 or 2004. More recently, reports of 5 g/L have become common with sporadic reports of over 10 g/L making appearances (2). This improvement has made it possible not only to meet the demand with existing capacity but also to make biopharmaceutical production much more cost-effective.

However, in the case of protein separation technologies, further scale-up or multiple cycles will be needed until the challenges of increased throughput from cell culture are successfully met with; for instance, the use of improved resins having much higher binding capacities combined with good resolution.

[†]While this chapter was being prepared for publication, our coauthor Dr. John Chon sadly passed away. We would like to dedicate this work to his wife Kristin and son Aidyn, as well as to his parents and sisters, in loving memory of our dear colleague, partner, and friend.

TABLE 1   Classes of Biologics Products and Their Sales for 2007 and 2008[a]

Class of products	2008 sales (US$ billion)	2007 sales (US$ billion)	Selected branded products
Anti-TNF antibodies	16.36	12.98	Enbrel, Remicade, Humira, Cimzia
Major cancer antibodies	15.59	15.74	Rituxan/MabThera, Herceptin, Avastin, Erbitux, Vectibix
Insulin and insulin analogs	10.9	11.19	Humalog, Humulin, Lantus, Levemir, Novorapid, Actrapid, Novolin
Erythropoietins	10.05	11.82	Aranesp, Procrit, Eprex, Epogen, NeoRecormon, ESPO, Dynepo, Binocrit
Interferon-β	5.35	5.35	Avonex, Rebif, Betaferon/Betaseron
G-CSF	5.18	4.82	Neulasta, Neupogen, Neutrogin, GRAN
Rec. coagulation factors	4.94	5.39	Novoseven, Kogenate, Helixate, Refacto, Advate, Recombinate, Benefix
Enzyme replacement	2.8	2.29	Cerezyme, Fabrazyme, Aldurazyme, Myozyme, Replagal, Naglazyme, Elaprase
Human growth hormone	2.68	2.77	Genotropin, Norditropin, Humatrope, Nutropin, Saizen, Serostim, Omnitrope
Interferon-α	2.56	2.74	Pegasys, Peg-Intron, Intron A
Ophthalmic antibody	1.76	1.36	Lucentis
Antiviral antibody	1.23	>1.13	Synagis
Follicle-stimulating hormone	1.16	~1.28	Gonal-F, Puregon/Follistim

[a]Adapted from La Merie Business Intelligence R&D Pipeline News—Top 20 Biologics 2008—March 9, 2009.
Abbreviations: G-CSF, granulocyte colony-stimulating factor; TNF, tumor necrosis factor.

General Considerations in the Development and Scale-Up of Cell Culture Processes

One obvious reason for scale-up in biologics is to meet market demand. Usually, small lots of product are produced during early evaluation of the drug as the cost of manufacturing can be quite onerous. As the product candidate advances in clinical trials, more material is required and an increase in production scale or process yield, or both, is usually implemented. Another powerful reason to scale-up is to decrease the unit cost of manufacturing. The scale of manufacturing and process improvements both have profound effects on the direct cost of manufacturing (Fig. 1).

If the product candidate is considered to be promising, then the next phase of planning is perhaps the most challenging one: when to scale-up and to what scale? Figure 2 can be used to make an estimation of production scale for a batch-based process depending on estimated product demand and process yield. This decision to scale-up is usually made two to three years before the projected regulatory filing date for the approval of the product, which in turn means about three to four years before the launch of the product. Consequently, the decision to scale-up is in direct opposition to the process development timeline, and special care has to be taken when developing a process for biologics in order for manufacturing not to be the limiting step in product approval.

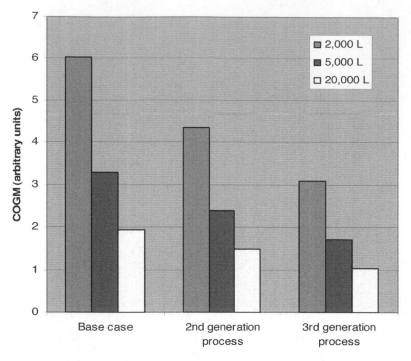

FIGURE 1 The impact of process scale and yield on direct cost of manufacturing.

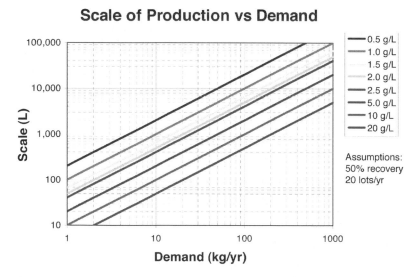

FIGURE 2 Scale of manufacturing as a function of product demand and cell culture yield.

In addition to basic engineering design principles, the scale-up of bio-technology products requires a thorough understanding of process operations and limitations. Additionally, the design and operation of the facility, including appropriate segregation of products, personnel, and equipment at each stage of manufacturing, must comply with current regulatory guidelines. Ultimately, the true measure of successful tech transfer and scale-up is the successful validation of the process at manufacturing scale and ultimate approval of the biopharma-ceutical product.

Because of the complexity of biologic systems and the physical and biochemical characteristics of the protein products, the design and scale-up of biologic processes can be challenging. Batch sizes for the production of bio-technology-derived products can reach 10,000 (3), 12,500 (4,5), and even up to 20,000 L (6). Although these scales of operation are often smaller than conven-tional bacterial or yeast fermentation, the high value of individual production lots requires careful planning and process control. For this reason, laboratory and pilot-scale data together with actual experience are essential for the effective selection of scale-up strategies, equipment, and process parameters (7).

The efficient and timely completion of scale-up to commercial manufac-ture is critical to biotechnology companies. In some cases, novel unit operations or techniques are required to achieve adequate expression, recovery, quality, or integrity of the product. However, this may cause costly delays in product approval because the implementation of new technologies is usually associated with a greater degree of uncertainty as the scale of the operation increases. In addition, the ease of process validation may be an important factor influencing the selection between novel or conventional process techniques (4,8). For exam-ple, cell culture processes can be conducted either as a batch or as a continuous process. However, the time required to validate a continuous process may be longer than that for a batch process. As a consequence, this may impact the time required for preparation and submission of documents to regulatory agencies as well as the time needed for review and approval. For many companies, the duration of clinical development and the strategy for efficacy studies may determine the difference between success and failure of the company.

The timelines needed to complete technology transfer may vary with the complexity of the process. A team composed of manufacturing and develop-ment personnel is responsible for facility design or integration of a process into an existing facility. The team is also responsible for equipment specifications and defining the physical relationship of process operations in order to comply with regulatory standards. The team must be aware of the relevant scale-up criteria to be used because their misapplication can lead to significant perfor-mance differences between bench-top and manufacturing plant scales (9). For this reason, stepwise scale-up is recommended. In addition, successful scale-up requires that manufacturing personnel be properly trained on process requirements and Good Manufacturing Practices (GMPs) to provide an efficient and seamless transition into commercial production within the shortest time possible.

Recent advances in safety, selectivity, quality, and integrity of molecules obtained from recombinant microorganisms and immortalized cell lines have provided a wide range of products used as therapeutic agents. Marketed biotechnology products can be classified into five categories (3): coagulation factors, enzymes, hormones and growth factors, molecular inhibitors/antagonists, and vaccines. Examples of marketed biotechnology products are presented in Table 2. This table illustrates the diversity of cell lines (bacteria, yeast, and mammalian cells) used to produce licensed products. In addition to the expression systems listed below, other expression systems such as insect cells, plant cells, and transgenic animals and plants are currently being evaluated at preclinical and clinical stages.

As seen in Table 2, most of the cell lines used to manufacture biologics employ recombinant cells, in particular Chinese hamster ovary (CHO) cells and myeloma cell lines, which can be optimized to express complex proteins at high yields and are amenable to scale-up. Current trends in the industry show that in addition to these cell lines, human cell lines such as HEK293 and PER.C6® (10), yeasts (11), and molds (12) could also be alternatives to express recombinant proteins. The incentive to use a human cell line is to mimic human proteins and to express recombinant proteins that otherwise could not be expressed in other cell lines. The use of yeast and fungi is intended to primarily decrease the cost of manufacturing. In addition, significant advances have been made recently in yeast and fungi to express glycosylated proteins (11). It is expected that more data will be generated using these expression systems in the near future.

TABLE 2 Examples of Biotechnology-Derived Products

Protein	Clinical application	Production process
Coagulation factors		
Recombinate (F VIII)	Hemophilia	rCHO, bleed-feed
Kogenate (F VIII)	Hemophilia	rBHK-21, bleed-feed
NovoSeven (F VIIa)	Hemophilia A	rBHK
Bene Fix (FIX)	Hemophilia B	rCHO
Atryn (Antithrombin III)	AT III hereditary deficiency	Transgenic goat
Enzymes		
Pulmozyme (DNase I)	Cystic fibrosis	rCHO, suspension
Cerezyme	Gaucher's disease	rCHO, microcarriers
Activase (tPA)	Thrombolytic agent	rCHO, suspension
Abbokinase (Urokinase)	Pulmonary embolism	Human kidney cells
Aldurazyme (Laronidase)	Mucopolysaccharidosis I (MPS I)	
CathfloActivase (Alteplase)	Restoration of function to central venous access devices	
Fabrazyme (Agalsidase-β)	Fabry disease	rCHO, microcarriers
Welferon (IFN alfa)	Hep C treatment	Namalva
Roferon (IFN alfa-b)	Hep C treatment	r*E. coli*
Infergen (IFN alfa)	Hep C treatment	r*E. coli*
Intron A (IFN alfa)	Hairy cell lymphoma	r*E. coli*
Epogen (Epo)	Stimulation of erithropoiesis	rCHO, Roller bottles
Avonex (IFN-β)	Multiple sclerosis	rCHO
Betaseron (IFN-β)	Multiple sclerosis	r*E. coli*
Proleukin (IL)	Metastatic renal carcinoma	r*E. coli*
Gonal F (FSH)	Induction of ovulation	rCHO
Saizen (hGH)	Growth hormone deficiency	rC127, Roller bottles
PEGASYS (peginterferon alfa-2a)	Hepatitis C	
PEG-Intron (peginterferon alfa-2b)	Chronic hepatitis C	

Table 2 *(Continued)*

Protein	Clinical application	Production process
Antibodies		
Rituxan (Mab)	B-cell non-Hodgkin's lymphoma	rCHO
Synagis (Mab)	Prevention of RSV disease	rNS/0, suspension
Herceptin (Mab)	Breast cancer	rCHO, suspension
OKT3 (Mab)	Rescue of acute renal rejection/GVHD	Mouse ascites
Zenapax (Mab)	Prevention of acute renal rejection	rNS/0, suspension
Reopro (Mab)	Prevention of cardiac ischemic complications	rSP2/0
Leukine (GMCSF)	Induction chemotherapy for acute leukemia	rYeast
Neupogen (GCSF)	Treatment of neutropenia	*rE. coli*
Remicade (Mab)	Rheumatoid arthritis	rSP2/0
Simponi (Mab)	Rheumatoid arthritis, psoriasis, arthritis, ankylosing spondylitis	rSP2/0
Stelara (Mab)	Psoriasis	rSP2/0
Ilaris	Cryopirin-associated periodic syndromes	rSP2/0
Arzerra	Chronic lymphocytic leukemia	
Enbrel	Rheumatoid arthritis	rCHO
Avastin (Mab)	Metastatic colorectal cancer	rCHO
Bexxar (Mab radioconjugate)	Non-Hodgkin's lymphoma	B cell
Zevalin (Mab radioconjugate)	Non-Hodgkin's lymphoma	B cell
Botox (Toxin)	Muscle relaxation activity, cervical dystonia	*Botulinum* spp.
Campath (Mab)	B-cell chronic lymphocytic leukemia	rCHO
Erbitux (Mab)	Metastatic colorectal cancer	SP2/0
Humira (Mab)	Rheumatoid arthritis	rCHO
Kinerect (Anakinra)	Rheumatoid arthritis	*rE. coli*
MYOBLOC (botulinum toxin type B)	Cervical dystonia	Botulinum sps.
Ontek (denileukin diftox)	Cutaneous T-cell lymphoma	*rE. coli*
Xolair(Mab)	Metastatic colorectal cancer	rCHO
Vaccines		
Vaqta	Hep A vaccine	MRC5 cells
Recombivax (HbsAg)	Hep B vaccine	rYeast
Engerix-B (HbsAg)	Hep B vaccine	rYeast
GenHevac B (HbsAg)	Hep B vaccine	rCHO, microcarriers
HB Gamma (HbsAg)	Hep B vaccine	rCHO
Comvax (HbsAg)	Combination of PedvaxHIB and Recombivax HB	Microbial fermentation
Infanrix	Tetanus toxoids, diphtheria, acellular Pertussis vaccine	Bacterial fermentation
Certiva	Tetanus toxoids, diphtheria, acellular Pertussis vaccine	Bacterial fermentation
LYMErix (OspA)	Lyme disease vaccine	*rE. coli*
RotaShield	Rotavirus vaccine	FRhk2
Varivax	Varicella vaccine	MRC5 cells
FluMist	Influenza virus vaccine	Eggs

Abbreviations: FCH, follicle-stimulating hormone; GMCSF, granulocyte macrophage colony-stimulating factor; GVHD, graft versus host disease; hGH, human growth hormone; rCHO, recombinant CHO; RSV, respiratory syncytial virus.

FUNDAMENTALS: TYPICAL UNIT OPERATIONS

Comprehensive descriptions of the basic unit operations commonly used in the production of biotechnology products are available in the literature (13). This section focuses on the typical unit operations currently used for the production of biologic molecules in cell culture and the technologies used for the purification of pharmaceutical proteins.

Bioreactor Operation

Commercial manufacturing operations in biotechnology usually employ bioreactors or fermentors for product expression. In this discussion, the term fermentor will refer to bacterial or fungal processes and the term bioreactor to animal cell cultures. While extensive description of the operation of fermentors and bioreactors is available elsewhere (9,13), this chapter will focus on bioreactors used in the manufacture of complex proteins.

There are a variety of types of bioreactors described in the literature. Among them, the stirred tank bioreactor is the most commonly employed due to performance record and ease of operation. Cells growing in bioreactors take up nutrients from the culture medium and release products, by-products, and waste metabolites. Mass transport phenomena required for adequate supply of nutrients and removal of waste metabolites are greatly influenced by mixing and aeration rates. Agitation is used to maintain cells in suspension, to provide a homogeneous mix of nutrients, and to prevent the accumulation of toxic gases (14).

Aeration is also an essential requirement for aerobic cell lines. The design of aeration devices includes single-orifice tubes, sparger rings, and diffuser membranes. Bubble sizes may vary with each device and optimization is required to achieve the maximum ratio of surface area to gas volume transfer rate, which generates a minimal of foaming to prevent damaging effects on cell viability (15,16). The effect of aeration on cell productivity is complex and depends on cell line, medium components (including cell proteins), and characteristics of foam formation and collapse. Thus, the optimal aeration rate is determined empirically at each scale.

In the case of air-lift bioreactors, air flowing upward in a column-shaped bioreactor vessel is used to generate enough mixing of gases and cells simultaneously, thereby replacing the need for conventional impellers of stirred tank bioreactors (17). High volume of airflow can result in foaming in this type of bioreactors, which could be suppressed with the addition of appropriate antifoam agents. The existing production scales in air-lift bioreactors are 2000 and 5000 L.

Bioreactor technology also involves the application of single-use or "disposable" bioreactors such as hollow fiber bioreactors. More recently, the concept of disposable stirred tank bioreactors up to 2000 L scale has been introduced (18). This type of single-use or disposable technologies could make current stainless steel bioreactor equipment and facility design obsolete and may facilitate introduction of clinical stage manufacturing in a far more flexible format and faster than conventional hard-piped designs. This is an important innovation for minimizing capital expenditure, turnaround time from product campaigns, time to commissioning, and for facilitating concurrent product manufacturing.

Filtration Operations

Filtration technologies are used extensively throughout the biotechnology industry (19,20). Membranes and filters can be used for medium exchange during cell growth, cell harvest, product concentration, resin protection, diafiltration, formulation, removal of viruses, and control of bioburden. For example, microfiltration is used to replace spent medium with fresh medium (21) or to recover secreted proteins (5,21). Ultrafiltration membranes with submicron pore sizes are used for product concentration and buffer exchange by diafiltration. This is of particular value because, unlike in affinity capture step with Protein A (where binding is very specific and relatively insensitive to the feed pH and conductivity), ion-exchange capture steps are most effective when the load is more uniform. Preconditioning of the cell culture harvest by diafiltration into defined buffer composition can dramatically improve the consistency of this step.

Nanometer ultrafiltration using filters with tightly controlled pore sizes can be used for virus removal (22). Filtration with 0.2 μm dead-end filters is used for removal of microorganisms (23). Such sterilizing-grade filters are validated with a product-specific bubble point, which is correlated with microbial retention.

Depth filtration with disposable filter modules has been extensively used to clarify mammalian cell culture or to polish the clarified supernatants due to ease of operation, high flow rates, good product recoveries, and reduced validation requirements. Currently, charged depth filters that have the added advantage of viral removal are entering into biopharmaceutical processing, especially in the case of purification processes with limited viral clearance capability (24). Depth filters may also contribute to the removal of process contaminants, such as DNA and endotoxin, and could be integrated into the process at various stages of the protein purification scheme. Various studies have demonstrated that charged depth filters are a powerful tool in host cell protein reduction (25,26) and are expected to play an increasing role in downstream processing. Because of the cost of these filters, it is preferred to use them wherever process volumes are low. In addition, concerns over leachables from the materials of construction and product loss continue to be a source of concern for process engineers.

The key process parameters for filtration scale-up are transmembrane pressure, filtration area, shear rate, operating time, temperature, flux rate, protein concentration, and solution viscosity (5).

Centrifugation

Centrifugation is frequently used in blood serum fractionation. However, fermentation processes also make use of this technology, primarily as a first step in removing solids from the crude harvest fluid. Scale-up of operations for separation of product-containing cells from supernatant fluid or secreted products from host cells is well established (27). Although batch centrifugation is often used at the laboratory scale, continuous centrifugation is preferred at production scale. When centrifugation is used for biotechnology applications, it is preferable to use high-throughput, low-shear centrifuges due to the shear sensitivity of animal cells. The centrifugation step is typically followed by depth filtration to remove suspended solids not completely removed by centrifugal forces and minimize their impact on downstream purification.

Filtration may be the preferable unit operation for separating secreted products from host cells because of its relatively mild operating conditions. Another advantage of filtration is that the cleaning validation is relatively simple compared to the elaborated cleaning validation required for continuous centrifuges. However, as the process volume increases, the economic benefits of using filters decreases and the space required to accommodate large filtration units become a concern. The complexity and the high costs associated with operating large filter units at high flow rates while maintaining low shear makes this technology unsuitable for very large-scale operations.

Because of the above considerations, it is preferred to use filtration as a clarification step for small scales (<2000 L of culture harvest), whereas centrifugation might be the choice for larger scales of operation. Regardless of the harvest method used, high cell density mammalian cultures create a serious challenge for recovering secreted product and argue for innovative harvest/ clarification technologies.

Chromatography

Chromatography is a commonly used unit operation for the purification of proteins in biotechnology applications. It is capable of combining relatively high throughputs with high selectivity. The selection of the appropriate gel is very much dependent on an understanding of the physical and chemical characteristics of the target protein product and the impurities. Chromatography steps can be designed to either capture the product or to remove contaminants.

For ion-exchange gels, contaminant removal is achieved by optimizing the pH and conductivity of the equilibration, wash, and elution buffers. This technique exploits differences in the charge of the target molecule (product) and the charges of product-related and host cell impurities.

Affinity chromatography is often used as an initial capture step to provide high specificity and volume reduction. However, affinity chromatography gels such as Protein A or Protein G are costly, especially in early process steps with crude product streams. The use of crude material on affinity matrices may require extensive cleaning, which contributes to the cost and can reduce the effective lifetime of the gel. Recent advances in Protein A resins have resulted in media with higher capacity (40–50 g/L) and resistance to harsher cleaning protocols such as 0.5 N sodium hydroxide (MabSelect SuRe, GE Healthcare, Piscataway, New Jersey, U.S.). The cost of these resins still remains a significant factor in cost of goods considerations.

Hydrophobic interaction chromatography (HIC), which takes advantage of the different hydrophobicities of proteins and contaminants, is also commonly employed. Because proteins bind effectively to HIC gels at high conductivity, HIC can be integrated effectively with both ion exchange and affinity chromatography. Exposure of the product and equipment to denaturing and corrosive salts remains a significant drawback to HIC chromatography.

Mixed mode resins such as ceramic hydroxyapatite, which has both ion- and cation-exchange modes of separation, are commonly used as polishing steps. Another example is hydrophobic charge induction chromatography (HCIC). This resin is less expensive than Protein A but still selective for antibodies (28). The lower binding capacity (~20–30 mg/L) when compared to Protein A represents a significant limitation of this media. Nevertheless, it can be used in place of costlier Protein A resins to capture antibodies from process feed streams at high conductivity such as fermentation or cell culture supernatants.

Key parameters for chromatography scale-up are gel capacity, linear velocity, residence time, buffer volume, bed height, temperature, cleaning regiment, and gel lifetime.

Dimensional Analysis

Dimensional analysis is a useful tool for examining complex engineering problems by grouping process variables into sets that can be analyzed separately. If appropriate parameters are identified, the number of experiments needed for process design can be reduced and the results can be described in simple mathematical expressions. In addition, the application of dimensional analysis may facilitate the scale-up for selected biotechnology unit operations. A detailed description of dimensional analysis is reviewed by Zlokarnik (29).

These analysis techniques provide a macroscopic description of the process and offer the possibility of qualitative assessment although detailed mechanistic information is not captured. Because of the complexity of living systems, it may be impractical to provide a detailed description of the reaction parameters or to determine the specific dimensionless parameters for modeling cell growth and protein production. Models for mixing and aeration are well described in the literature. Similarly, for chromatography steps, it is often difficult to describe the purification of a single protein from a complex mixture of contaminants that range in concentration. However, parameters such as column volumes of solution (liter solution per liter of gel volume) or residence time (contact time of product with chromatography media) may be used to maintain similarity between scales.

The scale-up of fermentors and bioreactors has been based on chemical industry methods for design and operation of reactors. Most of the correlations typically used in the scale-up of fermentors and bioreactors pertain to mixing and aeration. Although the effect of mechanical agitation on cell culture has been examined extensively (30,31), it should be noted that models describing mass transfer in agitated vessels are of limited value when scaling-up biologic processes (11). Because they have such strong effect on cell culture performance, traditional engineering correlations and "rule-of-thumb" strategies for determining agitation rates at various scales are typically used as a starting point only. To achieve optimal performance, the agitation rates must be fine-tuned empirically at each production scale. Additionally, while the experience available from fermentation technology has been adapted for scale-up of suspension cultures of animal cells, the scale-up of anchorage-dependent cell lines is more complicated (32) and will not be addressed here.

In a 1991 study by van Reis et al. (33), a filtration operation as applied to harvest of animal cells was optimized by the use of dimensional analysis. The fluid dynamic variables used in the scale-up work were the length of the fibers (L, per stage), the fiber diameter (D), the number of fibers per cartridge (n), the density of the culture (ρ), and the viscosity of the culture (μ). From these variables, scale-up parameters such as wall shear rate (γ_w) and their effects on performance such as flux (L/m^2/hr) were derived. On the basis of these calculations, an optimum wall shear rate for membrane utilization, operating time, and flux was found. However, because there is no single mathematical expression relating all of these parameters simultaneously, the optimal solution required additional experimental research.

SCALE-UP OF UPSTREAM OPERATIONS

Unit operations for biologic products obtained from fermentation or cell culture can largely be subdivided into four parts: medium preparation, inoculum expansion, bioreactor, and harvest operations.

Medium Preparation

In development or small clinical production runs, complete liquid medium may be most convenient. Economic issues may dictate that at large scale, powdered or liquid concentrate medium be used. Shipment and storage of large volumes of complete liquid medium is less practical at scales greater than 1000 L.

Culture medium is typically prepared by addition of the base powder or liquid concentrate mixtures to appropriate grade water. These base media mixtures usually contain carbon sources, amino acids, vitamins, salts, trace elements, cell membrane precursors, and antioxidants to mention some major categories. Additional components such as growth factors or lipids may need to be added separately since they are usually not compatible in powder blends.

At present, powdered medium is the formulation of choice for large-scale operations. Powdered medium is easy to ship and store, and has a longer shelf life compared to liquid formulations. Medium components are reduced in particle size by ball milling or micronization, mixed, and charged into appropriate-sized containers. Regardless of which process is used to prepare the powder, homogeneity of the powder blend has always been a concern. Because each component will have a different particle size distribution, it may be difficult to be certain that each container of powder will have the exact same composition. Ray (34) reported on a study examining blend uniformity in powder medium production. A model powder was used to demonstrate homogeneity of medium components that are present at high (glucose) and low (phenol red) concentrations. Large drums of powdered medium were sampled from several locations within the drum to demonstrate homogeneity of amino acids. One issue that has not been adequately addressed yet is whether powder medium components settle and segregate during the course of shipping and storage.

Liquid concentrate medium has emerged recently as an alternative to powdered medium (35,36). For liquid concentrate preparation, medium components are grouped according to solubility criteria. Liquid medium concentrates allow for the preparation of medium in-line, by automated dilution of the concentrates with water of the appropriate quality (37). This would be particularly useful in continuous or perfused processes that require constant preparation of medium. Medium cost and component stability make it a secondary option for batch or fed-batch processes.

Cell Culture Inoculum Expansion

The objective of inoculum expansion is to increase the number of cells to an appropriate amount for inoculation of the production bioreactor. Cells are cultured in successively larger flasks by adding fresh medium during exponential growth phase. Cells should be maintained in a rapidly growing state to ensure a vigorous culture for the production stage. If the cells in the culture are allowed to reach the plateau phase, growth of the culture may lag or cease depending on the cell line and growth medium used. Each step of expansion is determined in laboratory experiments where culture growth curves are measured. There is a minimum seed cell density necessary to minimize the lag phase, as well as a maximum cell density to avoid losing the culture due to starvation or accumulation of toxic metabolites. In the case of fermentation of bacteria and fungi, the usual culture expansion ratio is 1 volume of inoculum to 10 to 100 or higher volumes of fresh medium. In the case of animal cells, this ratio may be as low as one volume of inoculum to four volumes of fresh medium.

For the cultivation of animal cells, inoculum expansions have traditionally been conducted in T-flasks, shake flasks, spinner flasks, or roller bottles. Typically, T-flasks and shake flasks are used for smaller volumes at the beginning of inoculum expansion, roller bottles, or spinner flasks for the larger volumes. However, one drawback of roller bottle inoculum expansion is that an increase in process scale requires an increase in the number of bottles rather than an increase in the volume of the roller bottles in order to keep the optimum surface to volume ratio. This approach, however, can quickly become cumbersome and labor-intensive. Unlike roller bottles, spinner flasks offer the convenience of using larger size of flasks as the amount of inoculum increases. Thus, the number of inoculum vessels can be kept to a minimum reducing the number of manipulations conducted under sterile conditions. However, it should be noted that in many cases the expansion of inoculum in these types of vessels may have significant oxygen transfer limitations. If larger flasks are to be used in the preparation of an inoculum train, an aeration strategy should be considered. Spinner flasks can be aerated either through the headspace or by sparging through a dip-tube. The inoculum can be expanded to 10 to 20 L using these types of flask systems. Beyond that volume, bioreactors of successively large volume will be used for expansion of the cells until the working volume of the production bioreactor is reached. An alternative method for inoculum expansion is to grow cells in a disposable plastic bag on a rocking platform (38). The bag can be configured with sterile hydrophobic filters to allow for aeration of the culture. Systems are currently available for culture volumes up to 100 L. Ultimately, the decision of choosing among the alternative methods will depend on cost, reliability, and confidence in the technique used to expand the inoculum.

One consideration to bear in mind during the design of inoculum expansion is to demonstrate the genetic stability of the cell line beyond the expected number of generations required to operate at large scale. This is usually accomplished by conducting measurements of product expression and genetic markers in cells from an extended cell bank (ECB).

Bioreactor Operation

Several different bioreactor configurations have been described for use in cell culture and fermentation applications. These include stirred tanks, air-lift, and hollow fiber systems. The majority of bioreactor systems in use today for cell culture applications are still of the stirred tank type.

Stirred Tank Bioreactor

It would not be possible to adequately cover the field of stirred tank scale-up in the space available here. Instead, this section will touch briefly on the important issues in bioreactor scale-up. For more detailed methodologies on stirred tank bioreactor scale-up, the reader is referred to several review papers on the topic (31,39,40).

As a stirred tank bioreactor is scaled-up, the majority of operating parameters would stay the same as found at bench-scale. The optimal range for parameters such as temperature, dissolved oxygen, and pH are scale-independent. Among the scale-dependent parameters are the mixing efficiency given by the impeller rate and aeration rate, and hydrostatic pressure. Agitation and aeration rates determine the quality of mixing, the gas-liquid mass transfer rates, and the hydrodynamic stress that the cells experience. Poor mixing can result in heterogeneities in pH, nutrient concentration, and metabolic by-product concentrations. In addition to the oxygen gas–liquid transfer rate, the carbon dioxide gas–liquid transfer rate should be taken into account. In the case of animal cells, carbon dioxide is a metabolic by-product that can accumulate to inhibitory levels unless adequate ventilation is provided (14,41). Strategies to minimize gas sparging (to reduce sparging induced cell damage) can inadvertently result in accumulation of carbon dioxide (42,43).

The basic problem in scaling up a stirred tank bioreactor used in animal cell cultivation is that at larger scales, quality of mixing, gas-liquid mass transfer rates, and hydrodynamic stress to the cells cannot all be kept identical to conditions at bench-scale. An impeller rate and sparge rate must be chosen that provides adequate mixing and gas-liquid mass transfer rates but minimizes cell damage due to shear stress. Animal cells are especially sensitive to mechanical stress as they lack the protective cell wall of bacteria and fungi. Although many correlations have been described for quality of mixing, gas-liquid mass transfer rates, and hydrodynamic stress, they should be used as guidelines rather than a predictor of bioreactor performance at large scale. They will rarely predict accurately the properties of a bioreactor system under real operating conditions. For example, measurements of glucose and lactate in a murine hybridoma culture showed a shift toward anabolic metabolism at the 200 L scale, which was not observed at the 3 L scale. This observation indicated that oxygen limitation was present at the larger scale, even by using constant impeller tip speed as a scale-up criteria. This problem could be obviated by, for instance, increasing the agitation rate at production scale or the set point for dissolved oxygen tension (21).

Quality of mixing is usually described in terms of a mixing (or circulation) time. Mixing times are generally determined by injecting a tracer into a bioreactor and monitoring the signal until it decays to a predetermined level (e.g., 99% of the final value). The simplest tracer is either acid or base with pH probes to monitor pH fluctuations. As bioreactor volumes increase, mixing times for equivalent impeller tip speeds inevitably increase. For instance, calculations of the theoretical mixing time in a 10-L bioreactor and a 10,000-L bioreactor, under typical operating conditions, show that this parameter can increase by an order of magnitude (44).

Aeration of stirred tank bioreactors can be accomplished by several methods including direct sparging of gas through the culture, surface aeration, and silicon tubing aeration. Of these possibilities, direct sparging is the simplest method for supplying a production bioreactor with oxygen. The most commonly used parameter to quantify the gas transfer efficiency is the mass transfer coefficient expressed in terms of the total transfer area, or k_La. Correlations for oxygen mass transfer rates based on tank and impeller geometry can be found in many sources (9,41). However it may not always be possible to find a correlation for a specific reactor configuration, that is, geometry, impeller types, number of impellers, etc. Therefore, these correlations should be used as a rough estimation of the power input required to reach a certain gas transfer efficiency. Gas sparging has also been implicated in damaging animal cells (16). The high velocity gradients that develop around bursting bubbles can generate enough mechanical stress to damage animal cells. Addition of surfactants to the culture medium such as Pluronic F-68^{TM} may prevent the attachment of cell to rising bubbles, reducing their exposure to shear stress (15).

The impact of hydrodynamic stress on animal cells has been reviewed extensively (30,45). Most of the work reported in the literature on cell damage in agitated bioreactors has been done at bench-scale. Kunas and Papoutsakis (46) reported that in 1- to 2-L bioreactors equipped with a 7-cm diameter pitched-blade impeller, cell damage was not observed until the impeller rate was raised to above 700 rpm (tip speed: 513 cm/sec) as long as air entrapment did not occur. However, it is not clear how these bench-scale observations translate into damaging impeller rates at manufacturing scale.

Air-lift Bioreactors

Fundamentally, air-lift bioreactors are a modification of the bubble columns that generate air flow for medium circulation unidirectionally by having at least two columns, a raiser column and a downer column. They are either a draft tube or an external loop bioreactor. The bubbles sparged into a draft tube generate upward flow and medium pours into the annular space between the draft tube and bioreactor vessel and flows downward. Essential design feature to consider is the bioreactor ratio of the height (H) to the diameter (D). Values of H/D of 5 or more are needed for sufficient mixing (17). Efficiency of medium circulation depends on the rate of aeration and on the ratio of the cross-sectional area of the draft tube to the total cross-sectional area of the bioreactor vessel. Air-lift bioreactors are superior for product yield and biomass production when applied to cells that are susceptible to shear under turbulence. Cell breakage caused by mechanical stirring could be minimized by the gentler mixing that air-lift bioreactors offer. Bacteria, yeast, plant and animal cell culture have been cultivated in these systems. Not only the simplicity of construction and main-tenance but also approximately 50% of reduction in the power requirements makes them more attractive due to operating cost reductions. However, due to geometry considerations, the scalability of this system is questionable, and it has never caught on as a routine cell culturing system.

Mode of Operation of Bioreactors

The mode of operation of bioreactors described can be largely classified as batch or continuous. The advantages or disadvantages of using either method are still the subject of controversy as proponents and detractors for each method are always well prepared to defend their positions.

Batch cultivation is perhaps the simplest way to operate a fermentor or bioreactor. It is easy to scale-up, easy to operate, and offers a quick turnaround and reliable performance. Batch sizes of 15,000 L have been reported for animal cell cultivation (4), and vessels of over 100,000 L for fermentation are also available. Continuous processes offer the advantage of minimizing the "down-time" of the production units, and homogeneity of product quality throughout the production cycle as cells are kept in a physiological steady state. Continuous processes can be classified into cell retention and noncell retention. The devices typically used for cell retention are spin filters, hollow fibers, and decanters. Large-scale operation of continuous processes can reach up to 2000 L of bioreactor working volume. Typically, the process is operated at one to two bioreactor volumes exchanged per day. Perfusion is one variation of a continuous process in which cells are retained within the bioreactor to achieve the highest level of product expression possible (47). Usually, high productivity in cell culture is achieved by a high specific productivity and/or high cell density. The major limitation of a batch is the accumulation of toxic metabolites and the depletion of nutrients. This is resolved in continuous systems such as perfusion where spent medium is continuously removed from the culture vessel and is replaced by fresh medium. It is claimed to sustain high productivity for months of continuous operation (48).

The main disadvantage of a continuous system is the long time required for validation and timely submission of product application to the appropriate regulatory agency. This timeline is drastically reduced with the use of a batch system of equivalent volumetric productivity.

Harvest Operation

Biotechnology products expressed by living cells are either contained within the cells (intracellular) or are secreted by the cells into the liquid broth (extracellular). A clarification step is employed to remove the product from cells (lysed or intact) and debris before the purification process is initiated. Typical unit operations available for performing the clarification step include tangential-flow filtration (5,21,49), dead-end or depth filtration (50), and centrifugation (51). Tangential-flow filtration is the most extensively used method because it minimizes cell damage and maximizes effective membrane surface use, flux, and membrane lifetime. It is readily scalable and can provide high processing rates with good efficiency without adversely affecting the cell viability. Critical operating parameters for optimizing the filtration condition are transmembrane pressure, retentate flowrate, and permeate flux. High-shear conditions should be avoided to minimize cell rupture that leads to increased levels of contaminating cellular proteins and nucleic acids. Otherwise, the resulting increase in cell debris will reduce the capacity of downstream sterile filters.

Dead-end membrane filters are designed for sterile filtration of relatively clean fluids. While this system was useful when the typical cell concentrations in harvest were low (1–2 million cells/mL), with current cultures typically reaching well above 20 million cells/mL, this system is no longer practical for use as a primary clarification step. A viable alternative is the use of depth filters that typically have graded pore structure allowing substantially higher processing capacities. A subsequent in-line sterile filtration step is then used to eliminate the remaining debris and control bioburden. Another advantage of the depth filtration system is the development of completely disposable modules (Cuno, Millipore, Pall, Sartorius) requiring no cleaning validation.

Both batch and continuous centrifugation offer scalability and high processing rates. Its disadvantages include higher equipment and maintenance costs. Typically, the clarification efficiency of centrifugation is lower than that of the filtration operations because of the lower resolution of particle densities compared to size differences. This leads to an increased burden for downstream sterile filtration and additional efforts to remove remaining process contaminants such as DNA.

Recent advances in cell culture conditions with the PER.C6 cell line have resulted cell densities of >40 million cells/mL in fed-batch cultures and >150 million cells/mL in the XD® (52) process. These high cell densities are posing an enormous pressure on established clarification techniques such as depth filtration and centrifugation and require new innovations. Enhanced cell settling (ECS™) was recently developed (26) to address this challenge. ECS enables the harvest of high cell density bioreactors by settling the cells and recovering the product in the supernatant. Maximum recovery of the product can be achieved by successive washes of the settled cells.

DOWNSTREAM OPERATIONS
Design of Purification Processes

From the many options available for purification, process design should be based on ease of use, product purity, and overall yield while minimizing the cost of operation. In general, a simple stepwise purification design utilizing orthogonal methods of purification with maximum compatibility between steps is preferred. The use of orthogonal purification techniques is important for the removal of process contaminants to trace levels and for robust viral clearance. The number of product manipulations as well as the quantities and number of buffers can be minimized by maximizing the compatibility of process steps. This consideration should be exercised early in the development of the process as it may have a huge impact later on buffer handling operations at large scale. Initial steps using highly selective capture chromatography facilitate volume reduction and effective removal of the most problematic process contaminants. Effective intermediate and final polishing steps are necessary for the removal of process contaminants to trace levels and virus inactivation and/or removal. The formulation step is designed to produce the final bulk dosage form of the product at an appropriate concentration and long-term product stability. Careful optimization for all process steps is essential for successful scale-up to manufacturing.

For purification, scale-up considerations are important even in the earliest phases of development. It is important to avoid the use of purification techniques of limited scalability potential even for early clinical production because thorough justification of process changes and demonstration of biochemical comparability are necessary prior to product licensure. For successful scale-up, it is important to understand the critical parameters affecting the performance of each purification step at different scales. Conversely, it is important to verify that the scaled-down process is an accurate representation of the scaled-up process so that process validation studies such as viral clearance and column lifetime studies can be performed at the laboratory scale.

TABLE 3 Antibody Purification Process Scale-up and Performance for Different Column Scales

Scale	Target load (g/L)	Yield (%)	Purity (%)	Aggregates (%)	HCP reduction (%)
Small scale	90–95	97	99.4	0.6	95.5
IS Run 1	90–95	98	98.8	1.2	92.6
IS Run 2	90–95	98.5	98.8	1.2	92.5
IS Run 3	90–95	100	98.7	1.3	92.2

Small-scale chromatography was done with a 2.6 × 14.5 cm column while intermediate scale (IS) chromatography was done with a 5 × 14.3 cm column. The same residency time was maintained for the two different scales.
Source: From Ref. 53.

Table 3 describes an antibody purification scale-up from laboratory scale (77 mL) to intermediate scale (281 mL) (53). Product quality and contaminant levels were maintained throughout the scale-up. Thorough analysis of the performance of each column is essential in order to sustain the process robustness at different scales of operation.

Chromatography

The majority of the processes currently used to manufacture biotechnology products employ chromatography columns as the main tool for effective product recovery and purification. The scale-up (54) and validation (55) of this vastly popular unit operation is key for successful implementation of the overall production strategy at large scale and eventual product approval for commercialization.

If an ion-exchange step will be used as an initial capture chromatography step, pH or conductivity adjustment of the conditioned medium might be necessary. At large scale, conductivity adjustment can be accomplished by in-line dilution without increasing the number or volume of the vessels required. Some manufacturers carry out a concentration and/or diafiltration for buffer exchange and volume reduction prior to the capture chromatography step. In this case, whatever time and effort saved in loading the initial capture chromatography must be weighed against the time for the concentration/diafiltration, the time for cleaning and preparation of ultrafiltration cartridges, and the additional buffer preparation time. Finally, attention should be paid to the stability of the clarified media upon pH and conductivity manipulation. Precipitation phenomena are often observed upon lowering of pH and conductivity of clarified harvest prior to loading onto the capture step. This undesirable situation can be usually mitigated by in-line filtration.

Many manufacturers prefer to use an initial capture affinity chromatography step. The affinity gels are highly selective and generally require little or no manipulation of the feedstream. Some possible disadvantages of using an initial affinity column step are the expense of the affinity matrix and the fact that repetitive exposure of the matrix to conditioned medium may require stringent cleaning procedures that may reduce the effective lifetime of the gel. The cost issue can be obviated somewhat by using smaller columns and multiple cycles. However, this will extend processing time and increase labor cost. Unpublished data from an economic analysis using a proprietary cost model demonstrated

COG Comparison of Protein A vs. Non Protein A (NPA) Mab Process at 7 g/L Bioreactor Volumetric Productivity

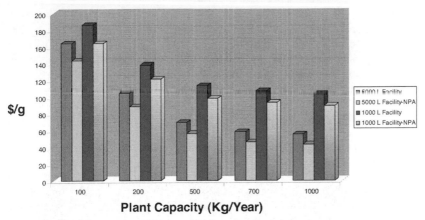

FIGURE 3 Cost comparison of affinity versus nonaffinity downstream process for MAbs. Cost analysis data were generated using a DSM proprietary model generated by BioPlan Associates and members of the DSM and PERCIVIA LLC teams.

that substituting Protein A chromatography for a high-capacity cation-exchange step reduces cost of goods by at least 10% to 15% in a monoclonal antibody process (Fig. 3). In HIC, the product is often eluted at low salt concentrations, which are compatible with the low conductivity necessary for binding to ion-exchange gels. Conversely, an ion-exchange product is often eluted at high salt conditions, which may provide conditions compatible with HIC chromatography. When HIC chromatography is placed at the end of a purification process, it can be a highly effective tool for removing aggregates generated during the previous steps. The use of ion-exchange chromatography during intermediate purification as a flow through step, where the product flows through but impurities bind, provides an excellent unit of operation in terms of cost and ease of operation. The column size is generally much smaller since lower capacity is required and the operational complexity and the volumes of buffers used are greatly reduced.

Finally, it is worth mentioning that manufacturers of biologics are increasingly replacing traditional column chromatography with membrane chromatography in polishing steps. Mustang Q, Sartobind Q, and ChromaSorb are some of the ion exchangers available in membrane form that are used for the reduction of DNA, endotoxin, host cell proteins, and viruses.

Viral Clearance

Viral inactivation and/or removal steps are a critical part of the process design for biotechnology products derived from mammalian cell culture systems. Regulatory agencies are concerned with the presence of endogenous and adventitious agents in the cell lines and/or raw materials employed to manufacture pharmaceutical proteins from cell culture (56). The best approach to ensure adequate viral clearance is to have multiple orthogonal virus removal steps and at least one viral inactivation step. Virus removal, demonstrated with spiking studies using model viruses, should be carried out with a scaled-down version of the purification process that accurately represents the process used in manufacturing. In addition, it is recommended that studies include the use of typical critical operating parameters for each step as well as conditions that represent a worst case for virus removal. For instance, for process validation of chromatography steps extremes of linear velocity, protein concentration, reduced bed height or contact time, and total protein loading should be tested. Although it is often difficult to adequately quantify viruses in some column fractions, it is important whenever possible to quantify the amount of virus in not only the load and product fractions but also in the flowthrough, wash, and strip fractions. Viral inactivation steps using chemical or physical conditions such as low pH, heat, irradiation, or chemical agents should be characterized by performing kinetic inactivation studies. For these studies, typical and worst case conditions should be evaluated. For example, if a product is eluted with a low pH buffer, a manufacturer might consider holding the product at the low pH as the viral inactivation step. However, because the product has some inherent buffering capacity, the final pH value of the eluted product may change based on the protein concentration. Also as the process is scaled-up, the eluted product pH may shift slightly due to subtle modifications in the collection of the product peak. The low pH tested in viral inactivation studies must be based on the maximum eluted product pH, which may not be known prior to scale-up. For these reasons, it may be preferable to define a separate inactivation step in a single vessel with subsurface addition and mixing of the inactivating agent to provide precise control of the hold time, temperature, and pH.

PROCESS CONTROLS
Adequate monitoring of the process can ensure proper and successful operation of the process at any scale. The design and logical integration of process-associated analytical testing has gained importance in the monitoring and controlling of processes. This technique has culminated in the introduction of the PAT (Process Analytical Technology) initiative for biologics by regulatory agencies as previously applied in pharmaceutical processing. As a result, adequate testing of process performance and product quality at relevant process steps can be implemented to ensure process robustness, ultimately leading to lot-to-lot consistency. Identification of relevant analytical technique(s) and critical process steps should be done at the process development stage. The analytical methods could later be integrated into the manufacturing process and be used in process characterization and validation stages. The ultimate goal is to rely on process monitoring to reduce lot-to-lot testing, expedite lot release, and even to eliminate the need for process validation.

SCALE-DOWN MODELS
The development of scale-down models for various process steps plays a significant role in predicting the outcome of the process at the manufacturing scale. An example of a well accepted use of scale-down models in the manufacturing of biologics is the viral removal and inactivation studies as part of the protein purification scheme. Similarly, a well-designed scale-down model can serve as a basis for setting the ranges for critical process parameters that are

essential for the consistent ability of the process to yield the desired product, with acceptable quality attributes. At the same time, these models can also predict the conditions that could lead to failure of the process, and can also set the stage for process validation at manufacturing scale.

The recent introduction of small-volume mini-bioreactor setups (57) makes it possible to conduct experiments by statistical design using multiple and cell culture conditions simultaneously. Feed composition development can be facilitated by using these multiunit devices. This type of arrangements tied to high-throughput data acquisition and analysis software, is becoming a more widely used tool to minimize the cell culture development time and costs In downstream processing, resins were tested in batch mode using 96 well plates. Their performance compared favorably to the performance of column chromatography steps for the cGMP purification process (58).

FACILITY DESIGN

Facility design is also an important consideration in process design and scale-up. An important observation to be made up front is that the market size for biologics does not necessarily translate directly to the size or volume of production (Table 4). Therefore, the market size for biologics does not necessarily result in a decision to build a new facility or to design large-scale equipment. The decisions are largely dependent on the product's intrinsic nature, potency, and demand (i.e., amount of product needed).

Unlike the manufacture of small molecule pharmaceuticals where unit operations, layout, and equipment could be used for multiple products, biologics manufacturing facilities are usually designed for a specific product in mind, with little room for flexibility to match the process developed for other products in the pipeline. This makes the decision to design and build a manufacturing facility for biologics even more difficult. The case of monoclonal antibodies provides one of the few examples where manufacturing facilities can accommodate different products within this category with relative ease.

Retrofitting an existing facility for commercial manufacture can be costly. Sometimes the design of a process has to consider the constraints imposed by an

TABLE 4 Market Size for Selected Biologics

Product	2008 Sales ($billions)	2008 Demand (kg)[a]
Enbrel	6.50	860.79
Remicade	5.30	779.41
Rituxan	5.10	858.82
EPOGEN	5.10	1.77
Herceptin	4.40	661.00
Humira	4.50	238.37
Avastin	4.50	654.55
Erbitux	1.47	183.75
Avonex	2.20	0.16
Rebif	1.70	0.23
Betaseron	1.40	3.32
Neupogen (G-CSF)	1.34	1.69
NovoSeven (F VII)	1.10	0.70

[a]Estimated by the authors based on total sales and average wholesale price.

existing plant. In this case, it is helpful to create a spreadsheet template for scale-up calculations to test and evaluate the operation of the process in an existing environment with minimal changes in existing equipment. Examples of such calculations are found for buffer preparation, bioreactor and harvest operations, filtration operations, product and buffer tanks, chromatography controllers, hard piping, and flow patterns. For example, if existing product tanks are too small, chromatography column sizes can be reduced and multiple cycles need to be performed. However, the long-term costs associated with smaller chromatography columns and extended processing times must be weighed against the initial costs of purchasing and installing larger vessels or columns. The operational segregation of pre- and postviral clearance steps may also require redesign of a facility and should be considered in the early stages of process development.

The advent of new technologies using self-contained unit operations and disposable systems (18) may actually change the current philosophy of facility layout in the near future. For example, with the advances in disposable systems, fully functional and GMP-ready bioreactors of up to 2000 L working volume may be implemented for manufacturing. These units require much smaller footprint and very little by the way of support structures, including utilities such as clean and plant steams, cleaning in place systems and solutions, and cooling waters. Combined with disposable buffer and media prep systems and transportation, it is possible to design a plant in which multiple 2000-L disposable bioreactors are laid out in an open manufacturing floor, with each dedicated to a product or multiple bioreactors combined for a single campaign. Similarly, disposable purification trains could be dedicated to each bioreactor system for maximum flexibility.

With the advances in productivity, these 2000 L disposable bioreactors may be sufficient to meet market demand. For example, productions at 10,000 L scale with 1 g/L productivity could be replaced with 2000 L bioreactors if the productivity is increased to 5 g/L. Indeed, the paradigm of the future for scale-up may be in increasing the process productivity rather than the brute-force method of increasing process size. With productivities of over 20 g/L reported with the XD process, the days of three-story-tall 12,000-L stainless steel bioreactors may be limited. Also, the next generation of high-capacity chromatography resins and high-throughput chromatography and filtration membranes enables downstream processing of high-titer harvests (53,59). These scenarios point to facilities of reduced footprint and complexity (60).

EXAMPLES OF PROCESS SCALE-UP

Once process design is complete and each of the process steps is characterized, the process is ready for scale-up to pilot or manufacturing scale. A spreadsheet template for scale-up calculations is important and provides a mass balance of buffer volumes, column volumes, priming volumes, product volumes, and waste volumes as well as the tank, pump, and column sizes. Product volumes can be expressed relative to column volume or can be calculated from a constant concentration depending on the process step. In addition, starting volumes and titers of conditioned medium as well as step yields and gel or membrane capacity are necessary to calculate bed volumes and membrane surface areas for the purification steps. A worst case approach assuming maximum step yields, product volume, and starting titer is recommended except for cases where underloading a column or a membrane step is problematic.

Some general observations were made during the scale-up of a process using microfiltration to harvest the bioreactor (24). One was that when using tangential-flow filtration, the ratio between retentate flow and permeate flow has to be at least 5:1 in order to avoid the effect know as "dead-end filtration." This finding clearly indicated the need for an additional control on the permeate flow that was not necessary in the small-scale experiments. Another observation was that the ratio of filtration area (FA) to process volume (PV), usually employed as a rule for scale-up, may actually decrease as the scale of operation increases. This is due to a more efficient utilization of the membrane surface with the consequent savings in filtration equipment.

It is also important to recognize the interaction between the scaling parameters. Simply multiplying an existing process by the next scale-up factor may lead to errors. For example, if a single 10-in. filter is used at 66% capacity in the pilot scale, a fourfold increase in scale does not require four 10-in. filters. Rather, three 10-in. filters or a single 30-in. filter can be used at 88% capacity.

Another example demonstrating the interaction between scaling factors comes from chromatography operation. As the process scale increases, the available column volume must increase, either by packing larger columns or by running multiple cycles. Columns are generally available with 30-, 45-, 60-, and 100-cm diameters. It is necessary to select a column diameter when doing calculations and then determine the resulting bed height based on the required volume. Using a narrower diameter column will result in increased processing time if the linear velocity is held constant instead of residence time during scale-up. The alternative is to use a shorter, wider column but there is a minimum bed height that can be used at large scales, generally ≥ 10 cm. The use of a larger diameter column will increase flow rate and decrease operating time. However, the use of a wider column may necessitate packing a column of larger volume than necessary based on the resin capacity. The larger volume column means that greater volumes of buffer are needed and that the product volumes will likely increase. It is important to determine if tanks are available for the additional volumes of product and buffers. In this example (Table 5), as the effective gel loading decreases, the processing time decreases and the buffer volumes increase.

For buffer exchange or formulation steps using ultrafiltration, membrane loading and processing time are closely linked. In contrast with the previous example focusing on chromatography loading, as membrane loading decreases there is no dramatic increase in buffer usage. In general, decreasing the membrane capacity reduces processing time because the gel layer is thinner and has less impact on permeate flux. However, as the membrane surface area is increased, a larger-size ultrafiltration system is required and larger pumps are required to maintain the recirculation flux. For a highly concentrated product, a large system holdup volume increases the potential for product loss. Scale-up of concentration/diafiltration operations may require reoptimization of process parameters, especially if membrane loadings are changed. However, every effort should be made to keep recirculation flux constant with similar feed and retentate pressures.

TABLE 5 Sample Scale-Up Calculation for a Chromatography Step

Assumptions:		Units
Titer	0.5	g/L
Harvest volume	2000	L
Total product	1000	g
Maximum gel capacity	20.0	g/L gel
Minimum gel volume	50	L
Minimum bed height	10.0	cm
Linear velocity	300	cm/hr

	Case 1	Case 2
Column diameter (cm)	60	100
Calculated bed height (cm)	17.7	6.4
Actual bed height (cm)	17.7	10.0
Actual column volume (L)	50	79
Actual capacity used (g/L gel)	20.0	12.7
Flowrate (L/min)	14.1	39.3

	Case 1			Case 2		
Operation	Solution usage (L/L)	Solution volume (L)	Duration (min)	Solution usage (L/L)	Solution volume (L)	Duration (min)
Equilibration	5	250	17.7	5	393	10.0
Load		2000	141.5		2000	50.9
Postload equilibration	3	150	10.6	3	236	6.0
Wash	5	250	17.7	5	393	10.0
Elution	6	300	21.2	6	471	12.0
Sanitization	3	150	10.6	3	236	6.0
Storage	3	150	10.6	3	236	6.0
Grand totals		3250	229.9		3964	100.9

IMPACT OF SCALE-UP ON PROCESS PERFORMANCE AND PRODUCT QUALITY

One of the chief concerns when scaling up biologic process is the effect of minor variations in the microenvironment at different scales that may affect process yields and product quality. Because of the complex nature of biologic molecules, extensive biochemical characterization of physicochemical parameters is needed to demonstrate product comparability upon scale-up. If any differences are detected, it may be necessary to perform animal and/or human studies to further demonstrate product comparability between scales.

There is so much concern about this issue that in some instances in the past it has been preferred to increase the number of units instead of the scale of each unit of operation to avoid potential differences in product quality. In some other instances a suboptimal process is not replaced with a more advanced one because of concerns over potential changes to the product quality that is not possible to detect except with another clinical trial. The market value of biologics and their complexity justifies this ultraconservative approach. Recently, however, the analytical tools and the regulatory experience available have made it possible to propose reasonable upgrades of production methods to either preapproved or already-approved products.

An example of a typical panel of tests performed on IgGs to demonstrate comparability is shown in Table 6. Glycosylation of proteins has taken the lion's share of the attention among different posttranslational modifications because it is essential for maintaining the efficacy and pharmacokinetics of several therapeutic proteins. Changes in carbohydrate profiles are frequently observed during development and scale-up. Monitoring this parameter throughout process development, starting with clone selection through the various stages of process development (including selection of basal and feed media) and during scale-up, will help avoid surprises.

Different innovative technologies to achieve desirable glycosylation of proteins have been employed. To circumvent the differences that arise from variations in glycosylation, expression hosts such as yeast can be genetically engineered to perform glycosylation reactions similar to those found in human cells (11). Another approach is to engineer CHO cell lines, which are deficient in a specific sugar moiety addition. An example of this approach is the

TABLE 6 Typical Assays Used in the Comparability Testing of Monoclonal Antibodies

Protein chemistry	Carbohydrate chemistry
1. Size exclusion HPLC	1. *N*-glycan profile
2. SDS-PAGE (reduced and nonreduced)	2. *N*-glycan mapping
3. Western blots	3. Monosaccharide composition
4. Isoelectric focusing (IEF)	4. Sialic acid content
5. Capillary IEF (c-IEF)	5. *N*-glycan structure and population
6. C-terminal lysine variants	6. *N*-glycosylation site
7. C-terminal sequence of heavy chain	
8. N-terminal sequence of heavy and light chains	
9. Molecular weight of heavy and light chains	
10. Peptide mapping	
11. Amino acid analysis	
12. Intrinsic fluorescence spectroscopy	
13. Thermal denaturation monitored by fluorescence	
14. Fourier transform infrared spectroscopy	

Abbreviation: HPLC, High-performance liquid chromatography.

development of mutant CHO cells incapable of adding fucose to recombinant antibodies. Fucose-deficient antibodies have shown to have increased antibody-dependent cellular cytotoxicity activity in vitro, which in turn may lead to decrease the required dose of antibodies requiring effector functions in vivo (61,62). Recently, an alternative human cell line known as PER.C6, a transformed human retinoblast cell line, has been proposed as a high-yield production system for recombinant proteins requiring human glycosylation. This cell line can be grown up in standard bioreactors, using standard cell culture techniques, to over 40 million cells/mL with yields of nearly 14 g/L for a monoclonal antibody, and up to 200×10^6 cells/mL in perfusion-like cultures called XD (63).

SUMMARY
Once the scale-up factors have been established, the scale-up of the process from pilot to manufacturing scale should be relatively straightforward. There are, of course, important considerations for working in a commercial manufacturing environment that have not been addressed in this chapter. These include, but are not limited to, cGMP and regulatory issues, segregation of pre- and postviral clearance steps, flow of material and personnel, waste handling, and environmental monitoring (39,64). In order to scale-up and transfer a process successfully from laboratory scale to pilot scale and multiple commercial manufacturing sites and scales, a thorough understanding of the integration of scaling factors, facility design, equipment design, and process performance is necessary. A scale-up template spreadsheet can be a useful tool to provide the critical integration of multiple factors.

FINAL REMARKS AND TECHNOLOGY OUTLOOK
The entire field of biotechnology includes not only cell culture–derived biologics but also transgenic systems (animals, plants, insects), and more recently, the revival of traditional fermentation using yeasts and fungi. The combined efforts in these areas over the last five years are resulting in an astounding improvement of manufacturing yields. For example, IgG titers as high as 14 g/L in fed-batch and approximately 27 g/L in XD cell culture of PER.C6 cells for IgGs have been reported[63] (Fig. 4). These impressive yields have been achieved mostly by maximizing the cell biomass, in some cases reaching over 200 million cells/mL, or over 35% solids, in the final harvest of PER.C6 cells. Higher final product titers will heavily depend on the progress of molecular biology to increase productivity on a per cell basis.

The immediate effect of these improvements in product yield is a dramatic decrease in the cost of manufacturing for the bioreactor step. However, it also means that in order to match this performance, recovery and purification operations need to improve in order to take full advantage of these gains. In the recovery field, major improvements have been made recently. Noteworthy is the development of the ECS approach to clarify high cell concentration harvests in situ. This avoids the use of centrifugation, and it is also possible to perform this step in single-use bioreactors, allowing the disposal of the bioreactor container and the biomass in a single step (26). Further development of chromatography resins with capacities of over 100 mg/mL is needed to absorb this increased product mass from upstream, as are the systems necessary to operate chromatography columns at high flow rates. The development of filter-based

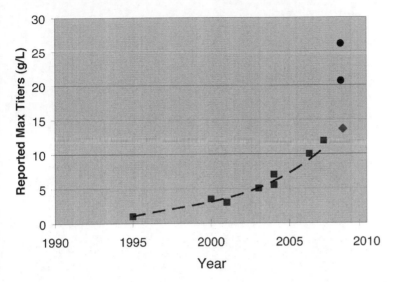

FIGURE 4 Trend of antibody concentrations obtained from cell culture over the past 15 years. Squares are data reported from CHO and NS0 cells, Diamonds are from PER.C6 cells in fed-batch, and circles are from PER.C6 cells in XD process.

separations of proteins using charged membranes offer an alternative to resin-based processes for very high throughput conditions. Also, formulation know-how should be adapted to purification operations for storing in-process and final product solutions at high concentrations in order to reduce the size of storage vessels, which will reduce capital investment. Further modifications in the structure and composition of protein therapeutics could conceivably yield more potent proteins (65), thereby decreasing dose size and thus the scale of manufacturing.

The use of PAT to fully characterize and control the manufacturing process may enable the biotechnology industry in the near future to produce these complex molecules as cheaply and efficiently as traditional small molecule drugs.

REFERENCES

1. 'Big Pharma' Turns to Biologics for Growth to 2010: Financial and Strategic Segmentation of the 'Big Pharma' Sector by Drug Technology. DataMonitor, 2006.
2. Kelley B. Industrialization of mAb production technology: the bioprocessing industry at a crossroads. mAbs 2009; 1:443–452.
3. Resilience: The Americas BioTech Report. New York: Ernst & Young, 2003.
4. Lubiniecki AS, Lupker JH. Purified protein products of rDNA technology expressed in animal cell culture. Biologicals 1994; 22:161–169.
5. Werner RG, Walz F, Noe W, et al. Safety and economic aspects of continuous mammalian cell culture. J Biotechnol 1992; 22:51–68.
6. Palomares L, Ramirez OT. Bioreactor scale-up. In: Spier R, ed. Encyclopedia of Cell Technology. New York: Wiley, 2000.
7. Peters M, Timmerhaus K. Plant Design and Economics for Chemical Engineers. 4th ed. New York: McGraw-Hill, 1991.

8. Griffiths JB. Animal cell culture processes—batch or continuous? J Biotechnol 1992; 22:21–30.
9. Bailey J, Ollis D. Biochemical Engineering Fundamentals. New York: McGraw-Hill, 1986.
10. Jones D, Kroos N, Anema R, et al. High-level expression of recombinant IgG in the human cell line PER.C6. Biotechnol Prog 2003; 19:163–168.
11. Hamilton SR, Bobrowicz P, Bobrowicz B, et al. Production of complex human glycoproteins in yeast. Science 2003; 301:1244–1246.
12. Stuart W. Filamentous fungi as an alternative production host for monoclonal antibodies. In: SRI Antibody Manufacturing and Production. Long Branch, NJ, 2002.
13. Moo-Young M. Comprehensive Biotecnology: The Principles, Applications and Regulations of Biotechnology in Industry, Agriculture, and Medicine. New York: Pergamon Press, 1985.
14. Kimura R, Miller WM. Effects of elevated pCO(2) and/or osmolality on the growth and recombinant tPA production of CHO cells. Biotechnol Bioeng 1996; 52:152–160.
15. Bavarian F, Fan LS, Chalmers JJ. Microscopic visualization of insect cell-bubble interactions. I: Rising bubbles, air-medium interface, and the foam layer. Biotechnol Prog 1991; 7:140–150.
16. Papoutsakis ET. Fluid-mechanical damage of animal cells in bioreactors. Trends Biotechnol 1991; 9:427–437.
17. Takayama S. Bioreactors, airlift. In: Spier R, ed. Encyclopedia of Cell Technology. New York: Wiley, 2000.
18. Sinclair A, Monge M. Biomanufacturing for the 21st century: designing a concept facility based on single-use systems. Bio Process Int 2004; 2(9):26–31.
19. Clooney C. Upstream and downstream processing. In: Moo-Young M, ed. Comprehensive Biotechnology: The Principles, Applications and Regulations of Biotechnology in Industry, Agriculture and Medicine. New York: Pergamon Press, 1985:347–438.
20. Michaels A, Matson S. Membranes in biotechnology: state of the art. Desalination 1985; 53:231–258.
21. Cacciuttolo M, Patchan M, Harrig K, et al. Development of a high yeild process for the production of an IgM by a murine hybridoma. Biopharm 1998; 44:20–27.
22. O'Grady J, Losikoff A, Poiley J, et al. Virus removal studies using nanofiltration membranes. Dev Biol Stand 1996; 88:319–326.
23. FDA Guidelines on Sterile Drug Products Produced by Aseptic Processing. CDER, Food and Drug Administration: Rockville, MD, 1987. Available at: http://www.fda.gov/downloads/Drugs/GuidanceComplianceRegulatoryInformation/Guidances/UCM070342.pdf.
24. Tipton B, Bose J, Larson W, et al. Retrovirus and parvovirus clearance from an affinity column product using adsorptive depth filtration. Biopharm 2002:43–50.
25. Yigzaw Y, Piper R, Tran M, et al. Exploitation of the adsorptive properties of depth filters for host cell protein removal during monoclonal antibody purification. Biotechnol Prog 2006; 22:288–296.
26. Schirmer E, Kuczewski M, Golden K, et al. Primary clarification of very high-density cell culture harvests by enhanced cell settling. BioProcess Int 2010; 8:32–39.
27. Axelsson H. Centrifugation. In: Moo-Young M, ed. Comprehensive Biotechnology: The Principles, Applications and Regulations of Biotechnology in Industry, Agriculture, and Medicine. New York: Pergamon Press, 1985.
28. Egisto B, David J, Warren S, et al. Hydrophobic charge induction chromatography. Genet Eng Biotechnol News 2000; 20:1–4.
29. Zlokarnik M. Dimensional analysis, scale-up. In: Flickinger M, Drew S, eds. Encyclopedia of Bioprocess Technology: Fermentation, bioCatalysis, and Bioseparation. New York: John Wiley and Sons, Inc, 1999:840–861.
30. Hua J, Erickson LE, Yiin TY, et al. A review of the effects of shear and interfacial phenomena on cell viability. Crit Rev Biotechnol 1993; 13:305–328.
31. Tramper J, de Gooijer KD, Vlak JM. Scale-up considerations and bioreactor development for animal cell cultivation. Bioprocess Technol 1993; 17:139–177.

32. Griffiths B, Looby D. Scale-up of suspension and anchorage-dependent animal cells. Methods Mol Biol 1997; 75:59–75.
33. van Reis R, Leonard LC, Hsu CC, et al. Industrial scale harvest of proteins from mammalian cell culture by tangential flow filtration. Biotechnol Bioeng 1991; 38: 413–422.
34. Ray K. Validation of a novel process for large-scale production of powdered media: evaluation of blend uniformity. In: Raw Materials and Contract Services Conference. St. Louis, MO: Williamsburg Bioprocessing Foundation, 1999.
35. Jayme D, Disorbo D, Kubiak J, et al. Use of medium concentrates to improve bioreactor productivity. In: Murakami H, Shirahata S, Tachibana H, eds. Animal Cell Technology: Basic & Applied Aspects. Dordrecht: Kluwer Academic Publishers, 1992:143–148.
36. Jayme D, Fike R, Kubiak J, et al. Use of liquid medium concentrates to enhance biological productivity. In: Kaminogawa S, Ametani A, Hachimura S, eds. Animal Cell Technology: Basic and Applied Aspects. Dordrecht, Netherlands: Kluwer Academic Publishers, 1993.
37. Jayme DW, Kubiak JM, Price PJ. Continuous, automated reconstitution of liquid media concentrates. In: Kobayashi T, Okumura Y, eds. Animal Cell Technology: Basic and Applied Aspects. Vol 6. Dordrecht, Netherlands: Kluwer Academic Publishers, 1994:383–388.
38. Singh V. Disposable bioreactor for cell culture using wave-induced agitation. Cytotechnology 1999; 30:149–158.
39. Reisman HB. Problems in scale-up of biotechnology production processes. Crit Rev Biotechnol 1993; 13:195–253.
40. Leng D. Succeed at scale-up. Chem Eng Prog 1991; 8:23–31.
41. Aunins J, Henzler H. Aeration in cell culture bioreactors. In: Rehm HJ, Reed G, eds. Biotechnology. New York: VCH, 1993.
42. Aunins J, Glazomitsky K, Buckland B. Aeration in Pilot-scale Vessels for Animal Cell Culture. Presented at: AIChE Annual Meeting. Los Angeles, CA, 1991.
43. Taticek R, Peterson S, Konstantinov K, et al. Effect of Dissolved Carbon Dioxide and Bicarbonate on Mammalian Cell Metabolism and Recombinant Protein Productivity in High Density Perfusion Culture. San Diego, CA: Cell Culture Engineering VI, 1998, February 7–12.
44. Tramper J. Oxygen gradients in animal cell bioreactors. In: Beuvery EC, Griffiths JB, Zeijlemaker WP, eds. Animal Cell Technology: Developments Towards the 21st Century. Dordrecht, The Netherlands: Kluwer Academic Publishers, 1195:883–891.
45. Papoutsakis ET. Fluid-mechanical damage of animal cells in bioreactors. Trends Biotechnol 1990; 9:427–437.
46. Kunas KT, Papoutsakis ET. Damage mechanisms of suspended animal cells in agitated bioreactors with and without bubble entrainment. Biotechnol Bioeng 1990; 36:476–483.
47. Deo YM, Mahadevan MD, Fuchs R. Practical considerations in operation and scale-up of spin-filter based bioreactors for monoclonal antibody production. Biotechnol Prog 1996; 12:57–64.
48. Hess P. Using continuous perfusion cell-culture. Presented at: bioLogic, Boston, MA, 2004, Oct. 18–20.
49. Maiorella B, Dorin G, Carion A, et al. Crossflow microfiltration of animal cells. Biotechnol Bioeng 1991; 37:121–126.
50. Brose DJ, Cates S, Hutchison FA. Studies on the scale-up of microfiltration membrane devices. PDA J Pharm Sci Technol 1994; 48:184–188.
51. Dream RF. Centrifugation and its application in the biotechnology industry. Pharm Eng 1992; 12:44–52.
52. Morrow JK. Methods for maximizing antibody yields. Genet Eng Biotechnol News 2008. Available at: http://www.genengnews.com/gen-articles/methods-for-maximizing-antibody-yields/2514.
53. Lain B, Cacciuttolo M, Zarbis-Papastoitsis G. Development of high-capacity MAb capture step based on cation-exchange chromatography. BioProcess Int 2009; 7:26–34.

54. Lode FG, Rosenfeld A, Yuan QS, et al. Refining the scale-up of chromatographic separations. J Chromatogr A 1998; 796:3–14.
55. Levine H, Tarnoski S. Industry perspective on the validation of column-based separation processes for the purification of proteins. PDA J Pharm Sci Technol 1992; 46:87–97.
56. Walter JK, Werz W, Berthold W. Process scale considerations in evaluation studies and scale-up. Dev Biol Stand 1996; 88:99–108.
57. Seewoester T. Development of processes in the fast lane—today's practice and tomorrow's vision. BioProcess International Conference and Exhibition Cell culture and Upstream processing, Boston, MA, 2004.
58. Coffman J, Kramarczyk J, Kelley B. High-throughput screening of chromatographic separations: 1. Method development and column modeling. Biotechnol Bioeng 2008; 100:605–618.
59. Kuczewski M, Fraud N, Faber R, et al. Development of a polishing step using a hydrophobic interaction membrane adsorber with a PER.C6-derived recombinant antibody. Biotechnol Bioeng 2010; 105:296–305.
60. Guldager N. Next-generation facilities for monoclonal antibody production. Pharm Technol 2009; 33:68–73.
61. Yamane-Ohnuki N, Kinoshita S, Inoue-Urakubo M, et al. Establishment of FUT8 knockout Chinese hamster ovary cells: an ideal host cell line for producing completely defucosylated antibodies with enhanced antibody-dependent cellular cytotoxicity. Biotechnol Bioeng 2004; 87:614–622.
62. Shinkawa T, Nakamura K, Yamane N, et al. The absence of fucose but not the presence of galactose or bisecting N-acetylglucosamine of human IgG1 complex-type oligosaccharides shows the critical role of enhancing antibody-dependent cellular cytotoxicity. J Biol Chem 2003; 278:3466–3473.
63. DePalma A. Enhancement of cell culture techniques. Genetic Engineering Biotechnology News 2009: 29(18). Available at: http://www.genengnews.com/gen-articles/enhancement-of-cell-culture-techniques/3073/.
64. Pepper C, Patel M, Hartounian H. CGMP pharmaceutical scale-up: part 4, installation, commissioning, development. BioPharm 2000:28–34.
65. Wooden S. Improving Protein Therapeutics-from Production to Patients. BioProcess International Conference and Exhibition, Cell culture and Upstream processing, Boston, MA, 2004.

8 Powder handling

James K. Prescott

INTRODUCTION

Most pharmaceutical solid dosage forms, suspensions, and powder inhalers involve powder handling at some stage of the production process. Proper handling is critical to achieving quality requirements such as uniform weights, fills, and hardness, as well as content uniformity. Proper handling is also critical to maintaining process efficiencies in terms of maintaining consistent feed rates at maximum production rates, minimizing operator intervention, and maintaining high yields. Understanding the flow behavior in bins and hoppers is a vital necessity for understanding segregation tendencies. Further consideration must be given to maintaining a reliable flow of powder, since no flow or erratic flow can slow production or stop a process altogether.

This chapter focuses on achieving reliable flow, as well as achieving the content uniformity requirements for the product, given that a well-mixed blend of powder has been achieved in the blender. Typical transfer and handling steps are reviewed. The major concerns with powder flow through these steps are illustrated, along with methods to determine the flow behavior in these steps. The mechanisms of segregation and methods to identify problems are presented. Finally, after an understanding of these steps, scaling issues are discussed.

REVIEW OF TYPICAL POWDER TRANSFER PROCESSES

Powder that has been blended in a blender must be discharged for further processing. Often, discharge is driven by gravity alone (such as out of a V-blender), although powder may also be forced out of the blender by way of mechanical agitation (e.g., a ribbon blender). The powder is often discharged into one or more portable containers, such as bins or drums, although some form of conveying system, such as vacuum transfer, may also be used. If drums are used, powder may be hand-scooped from the drums into downstream equipment, or a hopper may be placed on the drum, followed by inversion of the drum for gravity discharge. Powder in bins is usually discharged by gravity alone, although mechanical assistance can also be used. Powder then feeds into one or more press hoppers, either directly or through a single or bifurcated chute, depending on the press configuration. With many modern presses, powder is fed by way of a feed frame or powder feeder from the press hopper into the die cavities.

Each of these transfer and handling steps is deceptively simple. Each of these steps can have a dramatic effect on the product quality, even if no effect is desired. Powder transfer should not be taken for granted and instead should be considered a critical unit operation for which bins, chutes, and press hoppers are major design-critical pieces of equipment.

CONCERNS WITH POWDER-BLEND HANDLING PROCESSES

There are two primary concerns with powder handling that cannot be over-looked when scaling processes: achieving reliable flow and maintaining blend uniformity. To address these issues when scaling processes, knowledge of how powders flow and segregate is required.

How Do Powders Flow?

A number of problems can develop as powder flows through equipment such as bins, chutes, and press hoppers. If the powder has cohesive strength, an arch or rathole may form. An arch is a stable obstruction that usually forms within the hopper section (i.e., converging portion of the bin) near the bin outlet. Such an arch supports the rest of the bin's contents, preventing discharge of the remaining powder. A rathole is a stable pipe or vertical cavity that empties out above the bin outlet. Powder remains in stagnant zones until an external force is applied to dislodge it. Erratic flow is the result of the powder alternating between arching and ratholing or as a result of two-phase (air/solid) flow behavior, while flooding or uncontrolled flow may occur if a rathole sponta-neously collapses. On the other hand, a deaerated bed of fine powder may experience flow rate limitations or no-flow conditions.

One of the most important factors in determining whether powder will discharge reliably from bins or hoppers is establishing the flow pattern that will develop as powder is discharged. The flow pattern is also critical in under-standing segregation behavior.

Flow Patterns

One of two flow patterns can develop in a bin or hopper: funnel flow or mass flow. In funnel flow (Fig. 1), an active flow channel forms above the outlet, which is surrounded by stagnant material. This is a first-in, last-out flow

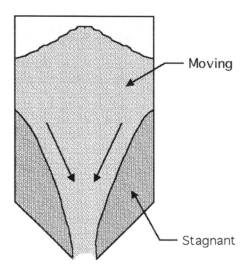

FIGURE 1   Funnel flow behavior in a bin.

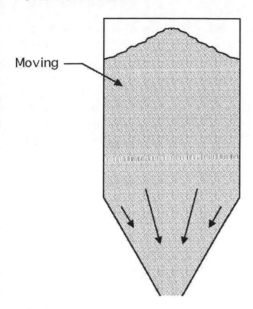

Moving —

FIGURE 2   Mass flow behavior in a bin; all material is moving during discharge.

sequence. As the level of powder decreases, stagnant powder may slough into the flow channel if the material is sufficiently free-flowing. If the powder is cohesive, a stable rathole may remain.

In mass flow (Fig. 2), all of the powder is in motion whenever any is withdrawn. Powder flow occurs throughout the bin, including at the walls.

Mass flow provides a first-in, first-out flow sequence, eliminates stagnant powder, provides a steady discharge with a consistent bulk density, and provides a flow that is uniform and well controlled.

Requirements for achieving mass flow include sizing the outlet large enough to prevent arch formation and ensuring the hopper walls are steep and smooth enough to allow flow along them. Several flow properties are relevant to making such predictions. These properties are based on a continuum theory of powder behavior—namely, that powder behavior can be described as a gross phenomenon without describing the interaction of individual particles. The application of this theory using these properties has been proven over the last 40 years in thousands of installations handling the full spectrum of powders used in industry (1).

Flow Properties
In order to select, design, retrofit, or scale-up powder handling equipment, knowledge of the range of flow properties for all of the powders to be handled is critical. Formulators can also use these properties during product development to predict flow behavior in existing equipment. Although there are many tests that measure "flowability," it is important to measure flow properties relevant to the flow within equipment used in the actual process (2). The flow properties of interest to those involved with scale-up of processes include cohesive strength,

wall friction, and compressibility; permeability is another property of interest that is not covered in this chapter.

Cohesive Strength

The consolidation of powder may result in arching and ratholing within transfer equipment. These behaviors are related to the cohesive strength of the powder, which is a function of the applied consolidation pressure. Cohesive strength of a powder can be measured accurately by a direct shear method. The widely accepted method is described in ASTM International Standard D 6128 (3), although other ASTM standards exist that cover other shear cells.

By measuring the force required to shear a bed of powder that is under various vertical loads, a relationship describing the cohesive strength of the powder as a function of the consolidating pressure can be developed (4). This relationship, known as a flow function, FF, can be analyzed to determine the minimum outlet diameters for bins to prevent arching and ratholing.

Wall Friction

Used in a continuum model, wall friction (friction of powder sliding along a surface) is expressed as the wall friction angle Φ' or coefficient of sliding friction μ (where $\mu = \text{tangent } (\Phi')$]. This flow property is a function of the powder handled and the wall surface in contact with it. The wall friction angle can be measured by sliding a sample of powder in a test cell across a stationary wall surface using a shear tester (Fig. 3) (4). Wall friction can be used to determine the hopper angles required to achieve mass flow. As the wall friction angle increases, steeper hopper walls are needed for powder to flow along them.

Bulk Density

The bulk density of a given powder is not a single or even a dual value but varies as a function of the consolidating pressure applied to it. The degree to which a powder compacts can be measured as a function of the applied pressure (4). For many materials, in a plot of the log of the bulk density, γ, versus log of the consolidating pressure, σ, a straight-line fit is obtained. The resulting data can be used to accurately determine capacities for storage and transfer equipment of any scale, as well as to provide information to evaluate requirements for bin outlet size, hopper wall angle, and feeder operation.

If a flow problem is encountered in solids handling equipment, at any scale, the most likely reason is that the equipment was not based on the flow

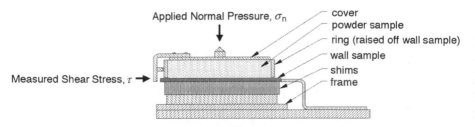

FIGURE 3 Setup of test apparatus for a wall friction test.

properties of the material handled. Often, when flow problems are encountered, the group responsible for selecting handling equipment had little or no knowledge of flow patterns or flow properties.

With an understanding of powder flow behavior and flow properties, segregation can be considered. Ultimately, as material is handled, stored, and transferred, the flow pattern that occurs will dictate how segregated the material will be when fed to downstream equipment.

How Do Powders Segregate?

The goal in any blending operation is to have a properly blended powder mixture at the point in the process where it is needed, for example, during filling of the tablet die. This is not at all the same as requiring that all constituent powders in a blender be properly blended, since subsequent handling of a well-blended powder can result in significant deblending due to segregation. Segregation is often as much a threat to product uniformity as poor or incomplete blending. An ability to control particle segregation during powder handling and transfer is critical to producing a uniform product.

Segregation is the unwanted separation of differing components of a powder blend. This separation action is often referred to as a segregation mechanism. A second action is required for segregation to manifest itself, specifically, the flow from the blender to the creation of the dose. As the powder blend flows, the segregated zones may be reclaimed in such a way as to be effectively reblended; or these zones may be reclaimed one at a time, exacerbating segregation.

Segregation Mechanisms

Segregation can take place whenever forces are applied to the powder, for example, by way of gravity, vibration, or air flow. These forces act differently on particles with different physical characteristics, such as particle size, shape, and density. Most commonly, particles separate as a result of particle size differences. The result of segregation is that particles with different characteristics end up in different zones within the processing equipment (e.g., bin).

Typical pharmaceutical blends separate from each other by three common mechanisms: sifting/percolation, air entrapment (fluidization), and particle entrapment (dusting).

Sifting/Percolation

Under appropriate conditions, fine particles tend to sift or percolate through the gaps between coarse particles. For segregation to occur by this mechanism, there must be a range of particle sizes (a ratio of 2:1 is often more than sufficient). In addition, the mean particle size of the blend must be sufficiently large (greater than about 100 µm), the blend must be relatively free-flowing, and there must be relative motion between particles. This last requirement is very important, since without it even blends of ingredients that meet the first three criteria will not segregate.

Relative motion can be induced, for example, as a pile is being formed, as particles tumble and slide down a chute. The result of sifting/percolation segregation is usually a side-to-side variation of particles. In the case of a bin,

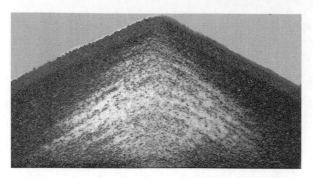

FIGURE 4 Photo of sifting segregation after pile formation; light-colored fines remain in the center, while darker, coarse particles concentrate at the perimeter.

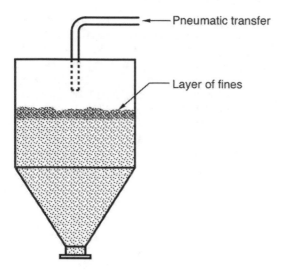

FIGURE 5 Fluidization segregation can take place when a bed of aerated material settles, driving fines to the top of the bin.

the smaller particles will generally be concentrated under the fill point, with the coarse particles concentrated at the periphery of the pile (Fig. 4).

Air Entrainment (Fluidization)

Handling of fine, aerated powders with variations in particle size or particle density often results in a vertical striation pattern, with the finer/lighter particles concentrated above larger/denser ones. This can occur, for example, during the filling of a bin. Whether or not the powder is pneumatically conveyed into the container or simply free-falls through an air stream, it may remain fluidized for an extended period after filling. In this fluidized state, larger and/or denser particles tend to settle at the bottom (Fig. 5). Air counter-flow that occurs while filling an enclosed container can also cause these problems.

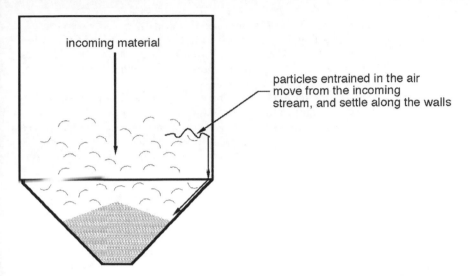

incoming material

particles entrained in the air
move from the incoming
stream, and settle along the walls

FIGURE 6   Dusting segregation can take place when airborne dust settles along the walls of a bin.

Particle Entrainment (Dusting)
Similar to the air entrainment mechanism, particle entrainment, or dusting segregation, occurs primarily with fine powders that vary in particle size or density. Because of these variations, the finer/lighter particles remain suspended in air longer than larger/denser ones. For example, when powder drops into a container, the larger/denser particles will tend to remain concentrated in an area near the incoming stream, whereas smaller/lighter particles will be transported into slower-moving or even stagnant air (Fig. 6). This problem is particularly acute with pyramidal bins, as airborne fines that settle toward the walls eventually slide to the valleys (corners) of the bins. The powder in the corners of the bin discharges last because of the funnel flow pattern that usually develops in pyramidal bins. The resulting trend across one bin usually involves a steady climb in the concentration of the finer components toward the end of the run.

Identifying Segregation Problems
At the Bench Scale
Two basic bench-scale evaluations serve as relative indicators of potential segregation problems. Neither approach provides a quantitative result that correlates to what could be expected at a pilot or production scale; however, they can be used as an indicator of the potential problems that may lie ahead. One approach is to sieve that blend and then assay individual screen cuts. If there is a wide variation of the potency across particle sizes, this serves as a warning that content uniformity problems may occur. The concern with this approach is that the sieving process may separate particles in a more vigorous manner than would be experienced in the actual process.

A second type of bench-scale evaluation is generically called a segregation test. In this type of test, the blend is subjected to forces expected to be induced in a manufacturing setting. If the material is prone to segregation, these forces would segregate the material into different zones of the test apparatus. Samples are then collected and analyzed. Assay or particle size differences across different zones of the tester serve as a warning that segregation problems may occur. The quality of the information gleaned from these segregation tests is highly dependent on the test method (how well the tester reproduces the forces induced in the process), as well as on avoiding sampling error (how samples from the segregation tester are collected, handled, and analyzed). Two examples of segregation test methods are given in ASTM International Standards D6940 and D6941 (5,6).

At a Pilot or Production Scale

The effects of segregation are usually recognized by comparing the standard deviation of samples of the final product (dosage form) to those collected either within a blender or upon blender discharge. The best way to diagnose problems is to take stratified, nested samples of powder from within the blender of dosage forms through the production run (7). Segregation usually results in distinct trends across the run. To diagnose the problem, these trends must be correlated with the flow sequence (from the blender to the dosage formation) and the likely segregation mechanisms.

SCALE EFFECTS

At the smaller scale (such as trials during initial development), powder may be discharged from the blender into one or more containers and then hand-scooped from these containers into a small press hopper. Seldom as part of development trials is a batch left in storage for a significant time after blending prior to compression. At this scale, the forces induced on the particles during bulk transport and handling are lower than full scale; further, distances across which the particles can separate are smaller, thereby reducing the tendency for segregation to occur. Hand-scooping obviates concerns about reliable discharge of powder from a bin. So, if this process works well at the small scale, what must be considered when larger batch sizes are needed?

Analysis of Flow

In situations where a complete description of the physical behavior of a system is unknown, scale-up approaches often involve the use of dimensionless groups, as described in chapter 1. Unlike flow behavior in a blender, the flow behavior of powder through bins and hoppers can be reasonably well predicted by a complete mathematical relationship. In light of this, analysis of powder flow in a bin or hopper by dimensional relationships would be superfluous and, as will be illustrated, irrelevant, since nondimensional groups that connect directly to equipment design parameters cannot be derived.

Bin or Hopper Outlet Size

If gravity discharge is used, the minimum outlet size required to prevent arching is dependent on the flow pattern that occurs. Regardless of the flow

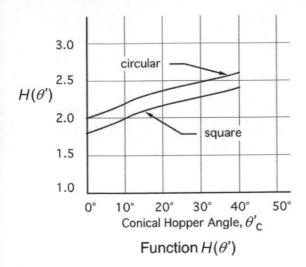

Function $H(\theta')$

FIGURE 7 Plot showing derived function $H(\theta')$ used in calculating arching potential in mass flow bins.

pattern, though, the outlet size is determined with the powder's flow function, which is measured by way of the cohesive strength tests described earlier.

The outlet size required to overcome no-flow conditions depends highly on the flow pattern that develops. If mass flow develops, the minimum outlet diameter, B_c, to overcome arching is (4):

$$B_c = \frac{H(\theta')f_{crit}}{\gamma} \tag{1}$$

$H(\theta')$ is a dimensionless function derived from first principles and is given by Figure 7 [for the complete derivation of $H(\theta')$, which is beyond the scope of this chapter, see Ref. 4]; f_{crit}, with units of force/area, is the unconfined yield strength at the intersection of the hopper flow factor (ff, a derived function based on powder flow properties and the hopper angle) and the powder flow function (FF) (Fig. 8). Bulk density, γ, with units of weight/volume, is determined by compressibility tests described earlier. This calculation yields a dimensional value of B_c in units of length, which is scale independent. The opening size required is not a function of the diameter or the height of the bin or the height-to-diameter ratio.

Putting the above analysis into practice, as a formulation is developed, one can run the shear tests described earlier to determine the cohesive strength (flow function). This material-dependent flow function, in conjunction with Eq. (1), will yield a minimum opening (outlet) size in order to avoid arching in a mass flow bin. For example, this opening size may be calculated to be 8 in. This 8-in. diameter will be needed whether the bin holds 10 kg or 1000 kg, regardless of the hopper or cylinder height or diameter, and is scale independent. In this example, since an 8-in.-diameter opening is required, feeding this material through a press hopper or similarly small openings would pose real problems

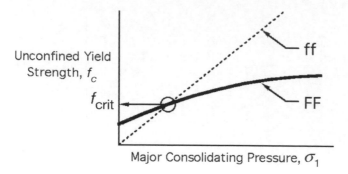

FIGURE 8   Sample flow function (FF) and flow factor (ff), showing f_{crit} at their intersection.

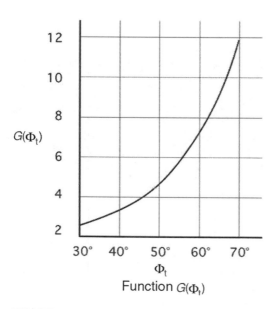

Function $G(\Phi_t)$

FIGURE 9   Plot showing derived function $G(\Phi_t)$ used in calculating ratholing potential in funnel flow bins. Φ_t is the internal friction angle determined via shear tests.

without specially designed equipment; it would be advisable to consider reformulating the product to improve flowability.

If funnel flow develops instead of mass flow, the minimum outlet diameter is given by the tendency for a stable rathole to occur, because this diameter is usually larger than that required to overcome arching. In this case, the minimum outlet diameter is

$$D_f = \frac{G(\Phi_t)f_c(\sigma_1)}{\gamma} \tag{2}$$

$G(\Phi_t)$ is also a derived function and is given in Figure 9; $f_c(\sigma_1)$, the unconfined yield strength of the material, is determined by the flow function (FF) at the actual consolidating pressure, σ_1. The consolidation pressure σ_1 is a function of the head or height of powder above the outlet of the bin, as given by Janssen's equation:

$$\sigma_1 = \frac{\gamma R}{\mu k}(1 - e^{-\mu k h/R}) \tag{3}$$

where R is the hydraulic radius (area/perimeter), μ is the coefficient of friction (tangent Φ', described in the next section), k is the ratio of horizontal to vertical pressures (often, 0.4 is used), and h is the depth of the bed of powder within the bin.

The relationship in Eq. (2) cannot be reduced further, for the function $f_c(\sigma_1)$ is highly material dependent.

Hopper Angle

Design charts describe which flow pattern would be expected to occur, dependent on the hopper shape and hopper angle (e.g., θ_c, as measured from vertical), wall friction angle (Φ'), and effective angle of internal friction (δ) of the material being handled. An example of such a design chart for a conical hopper and a material with $\delta = 40°$ is shown in Figure 10. For any combination of Φ' and θ_c that lies in the mass flow region, mass flow is expected to occur; if the combination lies in the funnel flow region, funnel flow is expected. The uncertain region is an area where mass flow is expected to occur but represents a 4° margin of safety on the design to account for inevitable (minor) variations in test results and surface finish.

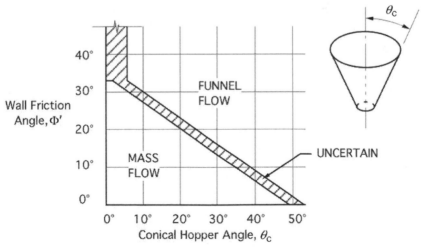

Design chart for conical hopper, $\delta = 40°$

FIGURE 10 Mass flow/funnel flow design chart for a conical hopper handling a bulk material with a 40° effective angle of internal friction.

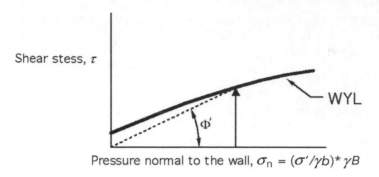

Shear stess, τ

Φ'

Pressure normal to the wall, $\sigma_n = (\sigma'/\gamma b)* \gamma B$

FIGURE 11 Sample wall yield locus generated from wall friction test data. *Abbreviation:* WYL, wall yield locus.

The wall friction angle Φ' is determined by wall friction tests, as described earlier. The resulting wall yield locus (Fig. 11) is a function of the normal pressure against the surface. For many combinations of wall surfaces and powders, the wall friction angle changes depending on the normal pressure. When mass flow develops, the solids pressure normal to the wall surface is given by the following relationship:

$$\sigma_n = \left(\frac{\sigma'}{\gamma b}\right)\gamma B \qquad (4)$$

Ref. (4) provides charts giving $(\sigma'/\gamma b)$. Assuming $(\sigma'/\gamma b)$ and the bulk density γ are constant for a given powder and hopper (a reasonable assumption for a first approximation), the pressure normal to the wall is simply a linear function of the span of the hopper, B, at any given point. Therefore, the critical point is at the outlet of the hopper; this is the smallest span B, with the correspondingly lowest normal pressure to the wall, σ_n. Generally, with decreasing normal pressure, σ_n, the wall friction angle Φ' increases. Hence, the outlet (smallest span) usually has the highest value of wall friction for a given design so long as the hopper interior surface finish and angle remain constant above the outlet. Therefore, the outlet is the critical point for the selection of the hopper angle.

When considering scale effects, the implication of the foregoing analysis is that the hopper angle required for mass flow is principally dependent on the outlet size selected for the hopper under consideration, and not the size of the bin itself. Note that the hopper angle required for mass flow is not a function of the flow rate, the level of powder within the hopper, or the diameter or height of the bin (as was also the case for minimum outlet size).

Since the wall friction angle generally increases with lower normal pressures, a steeper hopper is often required to achieve mass flow at smaller scales (smaller outlets). For example, assume that a specific powder discharges in mass flow from a bin with a certain outlet size. A second bin with an equal or larger outlet size will also discharge in a mass flow pattern for this powder, provided that the second bin has an identical hopper angle and surface finish. This is true regardless of the actual size of either bin; only the outlet size needs to be considered. The reverse, that is, using the same hopper angle with a bin with a smaller outlet, will not always provide mass flow.

Of course, mass flow is highly dependent on conditions below the hopper that can retard flow; a throttled valve, a lip or other protrusion, or anything that can initiate a zone of stagnant powder can convert any hopper into funnel flow, regardless of the hopper angle or surface finish.

In scaling the flow behavior of powders, it is better to rely on first principles and measured material flow properties as opposed to reliance on observations or data gleaned from the initial scale.

SCALING SEGREGATION

Although basic concepts are understood, equations based on the physics of segregation within bins are not well described. At best, a list of relevant variables can be described, but such a list would likely be incomplete. Even the process of mathematically describing a segregated powder bed beyond a "mixing index" is not well defined. After all, in addition to quantifying the variability, the spatial arrangement of the different zones is also significant. These limitations make even simple dimensional analyses of segregation within bins impossible at this time. Instead, for the pharmaceutical scientist seeking guidance during scaling, there is heavy reliance on empirical considerations, experience, and judgment and on conservative design approaches. This may also put the scientist into a "hope-and-see" or reactionary position, an uncomfortable position, given the repercussions of product uniformity failure.

AVOIDING SEGREGATION

There are three basic approaches to defeat segregation (8):

1. Modify the powder in a way to reduce its inherent tendency to segregate.
2. Modify the equipment to reduce forces that act to segregate the powder.
3. Remedy segregation that takes place by reblending the powder during subsequent transfer.

Modify the Powder to Reduce Its Tendency to Segregate

There are several ways to change the powder to reduce its tendency to segregate. One way is to change the particle size distribution of one or more of the components. If the components have a similar particle size distribution, they will generally have a lesser tendency to segregate. Another option is to change the particle size, such that the active segregation mechanism(s) become less dominant. For instance, one way to reduce fluidization segregation is to make the particles sufficiently large that the powder cannot fluidize. However, one must be careful in this approach not to activate a new segregation mechanism.

Another option is to change the cohesiveness of the powder, such that the particles in a bed of powder are less likely to move independently of each other. Increasing the tendency of one component to adhere to another will also reduce segregation. This is referred to as an ordered, adhesive, or structured blend. Granulation, whether wet or dry, is also implemented to, among other reasons, reduce segregation tendencies and improve powder flow. Bear in mind that, even if each particle is chemically homogeneous (which is rarely the case, even with granulations), segregation by particle size can result in variations that affect the end product, such as tablet weight or hardness.

Change the Equipment to Reduce the Chance of Segregation

Forces exerted on particles can induce segregation by many mechanisms. When handling a material where segregation is a concern, the designer must minimize these forces. Unfortunately, there are no scaling criteria available for guidance. Worse yet, when scaling up, forces acting on the particles increase significantly, as well as distances across which the particles can separate.

Here are some general guidelines:

- *Minimize transfer steps.* With each transfer step and movement of the bin or drum, the tendency for segregation increases. Ideally, the material would discharge directly from the blender into the tablet press feed frame with no additional handling. In-bin blending is as close to this as most firms can practically obtain and is the best one can ask for—so long as a well-mixed blend can be obtained within the bin in the first place.
- *Minimize drop height.* Drop height serves to aerate the material, induce dust, and increase momentum of the material as it hits the pile, increasing the tendency for each of the three segregation mechanisms described earlier.
- *Control dust generation.* Dust can be controlled by way of socks or sleeves to contain the material as it drops from the blender to the bin, for example. Some devices are commercially available specifically for this purpose.
- *Control fluidization of powder.* Beware of processes, such as pneumatic conveying, that increase the potential for the material to become aerated.
- *Restriction.* Slowing the fill rate can reduce fluidization and dusting segregation tendencies, in many cases.
- *Venting.* Air that is in an otherwise "empty" bin, for example, must be displaced from the bin as powder fills it. If this air is forced through material in the V-blender, perhaps sealed tight in the interest of containment, this can induce fluidization segregation within the blender. To avoid this, a separate pathway or vent line to allow the air to escape without moving through the bed of material can reduce segregation.
- *Distributor.* A deflector or distributor can spread the material stream as it enters the bin. Instead of forming a single pile, the material is spread evenly across the bin. This reduces sifting segregation but may cause additional dust generation, potentially making dusting segregation worse.
- *Proper hopper, Y-branch design.* Press hoppers, transfer chutes, and Y-branches must be designed correctly to avoid stagnant material and to minimize air counterflow.
- *Operate the valve correctly.* Butterfly valves should be operated in full open position, not throttled to restrict flow. Restricting flow will virtually ensure a funnel flow pattern, which is usually detrimental to uniformity.

Change the Equipment to Provide Remixing

The concept of knowingly letting materials segregate and then counting on material transfer to provide reblending is frankly quite scary to pharmaceutical scientists, as well as to regulatory personnel. Make no mistake however—this is a better approach than letting materials segregate and doing nothing about it. The following concepts are not radical and, in fact, have been used for many decades in the pharmaceutical and other industries.

- *Use mass flow.* In a mass flow pattern, material that has segregated in a side-to-side segregation pattern because of sifting or air entrainment will be

reblended during discharge. In most applications, this reblending is sufficient to return the blend to its initial state of uniformity. However, a mass
flow pattern will not remedy a top-to-bottom segregation pattern, such as
that caused by fluidization segregation; the top layer will discharge last.
Note that if top-to-bottom segregation occurs, funnel flow will simply result
in the top layer discharging at some point in the middle of the run, and also
will not provide any reblending.

- *Beware of velocity gradients.* With mass flow, all the material is in motion
  during discharge, but the velocity will vary. The material will always be
  somewhat slower at the walls than at the center of the bin (assuming a
  symmetrical bin with a single outlet in the center). In critical applications,
  the velocity profile could affect uniformity, with the material at the walls
  discharging at a slightly slower rate than that from the center. While far
  superior to a funnel flow pattern, a mass flow pattern with high velocity
  gradients may not be desired. To remedy this, either a hopper that is
  designed well into the mass flow regime is needed, or a flow-controlling
  insert, such as a Binsert®, must be used. Velocity profiles, and their effect on
  blending material, can be calculated a priori, given the geometry of the bin
  and measured flow properties. As a point of interest, velocity profiles can be
  carefully controlled to force a bin to behave as a static blender, as used in
  other industrial applications.

The scientist seeking to scale blending processes must be well aware of the
limitations of the state of science in this area. Equal consideration must be given
to the state of the blend in the blender, as well as the effects of subsequent
handling.

REFERENCES

1. Carson JW, Marinelli J. Characterize bulk solids to ensure smooth flow. Chem Eng 1994; 101(4):78–90.
2. Prescott JK, Barnum RA. On powder flowability. Pharm Technol 2000; 24(10):60–236.
3. Standard Shear Testing Method for Bulk Solids Using the Jenike Shear Cell. ASTM Standard D6128-06. ASTM International, 2006.
4. Jenike AW. Storage and flow of solids. Bulletin 123 Utah Eng Exp Station 1964; 53(26); revised 1980.
5. Standard Practice for Measuring Sifting Segregation Tendencies of Bulk Solids. Standard D6940-10. ASTM International, 2010.
6. Standard Practice for Measuring Fluidization Segregation Tendencies of Powders. ASTM Standard D6941-10. ASTM International, 2010.
7. Prescott JK, Garcia TP. A solid dosage and blend uniformity troubleshooting diagram. ASTM Standard D6941-10. ASTM International, 2010 2001; 25(3):68–88.
8. Prescott JK, Hossfeld RJ. Maintaining product uniformity and uninterrupted flow to direct-compression tableting presses. Pharm Technol 1994; 18(6):98–114.

9.1 Batch size increase in dry blending and mixing

Albert W. Alexander and Fernando J. Muzzio

BACKGROUND

In the manufacture of many pharmaceutical products (especially tablets and capsules), dry particle blending is often a critical step that has a direct impact on content uniformity. Tumbling blenders remain the most common means for mixing granular constituents in the pharmaceutical industry. Tumbling blenders are hollow containers attached to a rotating shaft; the vessel is partially loaded with the materials to be mixed and rotated for some number of revolutions. The major advantages of tumbling blenders are large capacities, low shear stresses, and ease of cleaning. These blenders come in a wide variety of geometries and sizes, from laboratory scale (<16 qt) to full size production models (>500 ft^3). A sampling of common tumbling blender geometries includes the V-blender (also called the twin-shell blender), the double-cone and the in-bin blender, and the rotating cylinder.

There are currently no mathematical techniques to predict blending behavior of granular components without prior experimental work. Therefore, blending studies start with a small-scale, try-it-and-see approach. The first portion of this chapter is concerned with the following typical problem: a 5-ft^3-capacity tumble blender filled to 50% of capacity and run at 15 rpm for 15 minutes produces the desired mixture homogeneity. What conditions should be used to duplicate these results in a 25-ft^3 blender? The following questions might arise:

1. What rotation rate should be used?
2. Should filling level be the same?
3. How long should the blender be operated?
4. Are variations to the blender geometry between scales acceptable?

Unfortunately, there is no generally accepted method for approaching this problem; therefore, ad hoc approaches tend to be the rule rather than the exception.

Further complicating the issue is that rotation rates for typical commercially available equipment are often fixed, obviating question (1) and suggesting that, under such conditions, true dynamic or kinematic scale-up may not be possible.

GENERAL MIXING GUIDELINES
Defining Mixedness

Before specifically addressing scale-up of tumbling blenders, this section discusses some general guidelines that cover the current understanding of the important issues in granular blending. The final objective of any granular mixing process is to produce a homogenous blend. But even determining mixture composition throughout the blend is a difficulty for granular systems. As yet, no reliable techniques for online measuring of composition have been developed; hence, granular mixtures are usually quantified by removing samples from the mixture. To determine blending behavior over time, the blender is stopped at fixed intervals for sampling; the process of interrupting the blend cycle and repeated sampling may change the state of the blend. Once samples have been collected, the mean value and sample variance are determined and then often used in a mixing index. Many mixing indices are available; however, there is no "general mixing index," so the choice of index is left to the individual investigator (1). Once a measure of mixedness has been defined, it is then tracked over time until suitable homogeneity is achieved. Ideally, this minimum level of variance would stay relatively constant over a sufficiently long window of time. This procedure is simple in concept, but many problems have been associated with characterization of granular mixtures (2).

One dangerous assumption is that a small number of samples can sufficiently characterize variability throughout the blend. Furthermore, sample size can have a large impact on apparent variability. Samples that are too small can show exaggerated variation, while too large a sample can blur concentration gradients. Unlike miscible fluids, which, through the action of diffusion, are continually mixing on a microscale, granular blends only mix when energy is inputted into the system. Hence, it is paramount that a sufficient number of samples is taken that represents a large cross-section of the blender volume.

Another concern is thinking that standard sampling techniques retrieve samples that are truly representative of local concentration at a given location. Thief probes remain the most commonly employed instrument for data gathering. These instruments have been demonstrated to induce sometimes large sampling errors as a result of poor flow into the thief cavity or sample contamination (carryover from other zones of the blender) during thief insertion (2). Care and skepticism have to be employed whenever relying on thief probes data. One method to assess blend uniformity and blend sampling error is given in PDA Technical Report No. 25 (3).

Finally, the degree of mixedness at the end of a blending step is not always a good indicator of the homogeneity to be expected in the final product. Many granular mixtures can spontaneously segregate into regions of unlike composition when perturbed by flow, vibration, shear, etc. Once a good blend is achieved, the mixture still must be handled carefully to avoid any "demixing" that might occur. The second half of this chapter deals with the scaling of flow from blenders, bins and hoppers, and the effect of segregation during handling.

Mixing Issues in Tumbling Blenders

Mixing in tumbling blenders takes place as the result of particle motions in a thin cascading layer at the surface of the material, while the remainder of the material below rotates with the vessel as a rigid body. Current thinking describes the blending process as taking place by three essentially independent mechanisms: convection, dispersion, and shear. Convection causes large groups of particles to move in the direction of flow (orthogonal to the axis of rotation) as a result of vessel rotation.

Dispersion is the random motion of particles as a result of collisions or interparticle motion, usually orthogonal to the direction of flow (parallel to the axis of rotation). Shear separates particles that have joined due to agglomeration or cohesion and requires high forces. While all mechanisms are active to some extent in any blender, tumbling blenders impart very little shear, unless an intensifier bar (I-bar) or chopper blade is used (in some cases, high shear is detrimental to the active ingredient and is avoided). While these definitions are helpful from a conceptual standpoint, blending does not take place as merely three independent scaleable mechanisms. However, attentive planning of the blending operation can emphasize or deemphasize specific mechanisms and have significant impact on mixing rate.

Most tumbling blenders are symmetrical in design; this symmetry can be the greatest impediment to achieving a homogeneous mixture. The mixing rate often becomes limited by the amount of material that can cross from one side of the symmetry plane to the other (4–8). Some blender types have been built asymmetrically (e.g., the slant cone, the offset V-blender), and show greater mixing proficiency. Furthermore, by rocking the vessel as it rotates, the mixing rate can also be dramatically increased (9). Asymmetry can be "induced" through intelligent placement of baffles, and this approach has been successfully tested on small-scale equipment (7,10–12) and used in the design of some commercial equipment. But, when equipment is symmetrical and baffles unavailable, careful attention should be paid to the loading procedure as this can have an enormous impact on mixing rate.

Nonsystematic loading of multiple ingredients will have a dramatic effect on mixing rate if dispersion is the critical blending mechanism. For instance, in a V-blender, it is preferable to load the vessel either through the exit valve or equally into each shell. This ensures that there are nearly equal amounts of all constituents in each shell of the blender. Care must be taken when loading a minor ($\sim$1%) component into the blender—adding a small amount early in the loading process could accidentally send most of the material into one shell of the blender and substantially slow the mixing process. Smaller blenders entail shorter dispersal distances necessary for complete homogeneity, and thus may not be as affected by highly asymmetrical loading. As a final caution, the order of constituent addition can also have significant effects on the degree of final homogeneity, especially if ordered mixing (bonding of one component to another) can occur within the blend (13).

Intershell flow is the slowest step in a V-blender because it is dispersive in nature while intrashell flow is convective. Both processes can be described by similar mathematics, typically using an equation such as

$$\sigma^2 = Ae^{-kN} \tag{1}$$

where σ^2 is the mixture variance, N the number of revolutions, A an unspecified constant, and k is the rate constant (6,14). The rate constants for convective mixing, however, are orders of magnitude greater than for dispersive mixing. Thus, unequal loading across the symmetry plane places emphasis on dispersive mixing and is slow compared with top-to-bottom loading, which favors convective mixing.

Process Parameters

When discussing tumbling blender scale-up, one parameter consideration that arises is whether rotation rate should change with variations in size. Previous studies on laboratory scale V-blenders and double cones have shown that, when far from the critical speed of the blender, the rotation rate does not have strong effects on the mixing rate (6,7) (the critical speed is the speed at which tangential acceleration due to rotation matches the acceleration due to gravity). These same studies showed that the number of revolutions was the most important parameter governing the mixing rate. An equation was derived by assuming that the mixture went through a specific incremental increase in mixedness with each revolution (either by dispersion or by convection). While this approach has been shown to be successful at modeling increasing in-mixture homogeneity, no scaling rules have been determined for the rate constants that govern this equation, and it remains an open question for further inquiry.

Given a geometrically similar blender and the same mixture composition, it would seem obvious that the fill level should also be kept constant with changes in scale. However, an increase in vessel size at the same fill level may correspond to a significant decrease in the relative volume of particles in the cascading layer compared with the bulk—this could accompany a large decrease in mixing rate. It has been shown in 1-pt V-blenders that running at 40% fill brings about a mixing rate that is nearly three times faster than at 60% fill (6). Thus, although fill level should be kept constant for geometric similarity, it may be impossible to match mixing rate per revolution across changes in scale if the depth of the flowing layer is a critical parameter.

SCALE-UP APPROACHES

In the literature, the Froude number ($Fr = \Omega^2 R/g$; where Ω is the rotation rate, R the vessel radius, and g is the acceleration from gravity) is often suggested for tumbling blender scale-up (15–18). This relationship balances gravitational and inertial forces and can be derived from the general equations of motion for a general fluid. Unfortunately, no experimental data have been offered to support the validity of this approach. Continuum mechanics may offer other dimensionless groups if a relationship between powder flow and powder stress can be determined. However, Fr is derived from equations based on continuum mechanics, but the scale of the physical system for blending of granular materials is on the order of the mean free path of individual particles, which may invalidate the continuum hypothesis. A less commonly recommended scaling strategy is to match the tangential speed (wall speed) of the blender; however, this hypothesis also remains untested (Patterson-Kelley, personal communication, 2000).

We now look at our general problem of scaling the 5 ft^3 using Fr as the scaling parameter: the requisites are to ensure geometric similarity (i.e., all angles and ratios of lengths are kept constant), and keep the total number of revolutions constant. With geometric similarity, the 25-ft^3 blender must look like a photocopy enlargement of the 5-ft^3 blender. In this case, the linear increase is ($5^{1/3}$) or a 71% increase. Also, for geometrical similarity, the fill level must remain the same. To maintain the same Fr, since R has increased by 71%, the rpm (Ω) must be reduced by a factor of $(1.71)^{-1/2} = 0.76$, corresponding to 11.5 rpm. In practice, since most blends are not particularly sensitive to blend speed, and available blenders are often at a fixed speed, the speed closest to 11.5 rpm would be selected. If the initial blend times were 15 minutes at 15 rpm, the total revolutions of 225 must be maintained with the 25-ft^3 scale. Assuming 11.5 rpm was selected, this would amount to a 19.5-minute blend time. Although this approach is convenient and used often, it remains empirical.

Common violations of this approach that can immediately cause problems include the attempt to scale from one geometry to another (e.g., V-blender to in-bin blender), changing fill level without concern to its effect, and keeping blending time constant while changing blender speed.

The lack of first-principle, reliable scale-up criteria can have major impacts on development time and costs. Nonsystematic means of scale-up can often lead to excessively long processing times and inefficient use of existing capacity. Long processing times can lead to unwanted side effects, such as particle sintering, heat build up, attrition, or excessive agglomeration. The advantages of rigorous scale-up include decreased process uncertainty, as we "know" what is going on. It also cuts down on the development time and experimental failures because experiments are done in a systemic manner that is based on science (not art).

NEW APPROACH TO THE SCALE-UP PROBLEM
IN TUMBLING BLENDERS

Herein, we offer a first step toward the definition of rigorous scale-up rules for tumbling blenders. We begin by proposing a set of variables that may control the process. The driving force for flow in tumbling blenders is the acceleration from gravity, which must be included in our analysis. Vessel size is obviously a critical parameter, as is the rotation rate, which defines the energy input into the system. These variables define the system parameters (i.e., the driving forces) but do not cover the mixture response. In the case of Newtonian fluids, fluid viscosity connects the driving force (pressure gradients, gravity, and shear) to the fluid response (velocity gradients). For granular mixtures, no similar parameter has been derived; hence, we will define particle size and particle velocity as our "performance variables." Particle size plays a large role in determining mixing (or segregation) rates because dispersion distance is expected to vary inversely with particle size. For granular processes, individual particles drive bulk mixture behavior and we have assumed particle velocity to be an important variable. Because all transport and mixing phenomena are driven by the motions of individual particles, it is a priori impossible to scale transport phenomena without first scaling the velocities of individual particles. Although previous studies have indicated that rotation rate (and hence probably particle velocities) do not affect mixing rate, these experiments were done in very small blenders. It is conceivable that, at larger scales, these variables could become important. Given these assumptions, we can now address the development of nondimensional scaling criteria.

Applying Rayleigh's Method

Our hypothesized set of the variables that are believed to govern particle dynamics in tumbling blenders is shown in Table 1.

Using these variables and the Rayleigh method, the resulting equation is

$$V = k\Omega^a R^b d^c g^e \tag{2}$$

TABLE 1 Variables Important to Scaling Particle Velocities in Cylinders

Variable	Symbol	Dimensions
Particle velocity	V	L/T
Vessel rotation rate	Ω	$1/T$
Vessel radius	R	L
Acceleration from gravity	g	L/T^2
Particle diameter	d	L

Abbreviations: L, length; T, time.

Applying the rule of dimensional homogeneity and making c and e the unrestricted constants leads to

$$V = k\Omega^{1-2e}R^{1-c-e}d^c g^e \tag{3}$$

To solve Eq. (3), a correlation relating particle velocities to vessel radius and rotation rate is discussed in the following sections.

Correlating Particle Velocities to Vessel Rotation Rate and Radius

To determine particle velocities, an empirical approach is taken. A digital video camera was used to record the positions of individual particles on the flowing surface in clear acrylic, rotating cylinders of 6.3-, 9.5-, 14.5-, and 24.8-cm diameter filled to 50% of capacity. Experiments were performed using nearly monodisperse 1.6-mm glass beads (Jaygo, Inc., Rahway, NJ, USA) that are dyed for visualization. The displacement of particles from one frame to the next was converted into velocities. To calculate velocity, only the motion down the flowing layer was used, and all cross-stream (i.e., dispersive) motion was ignored. Figure 1 shows an example of the data obtained from a typical experiment. Top-to-bottom in the rotating cylinder is equivalent to left-to-right on this graph (19).

Figure 2 shows the mean cascading velocity versus distance down the granular cascade for experiments run at the same tangential velocity (TV).

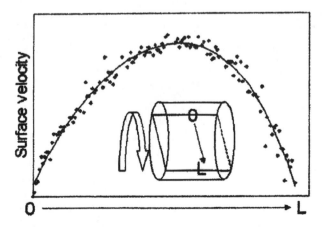

FIGURE 1 A typical velocity profile. Moving from top to bottom (0–L) in the rotating cylinder (*inset*) is equivalent to moving from left to right in the graph.

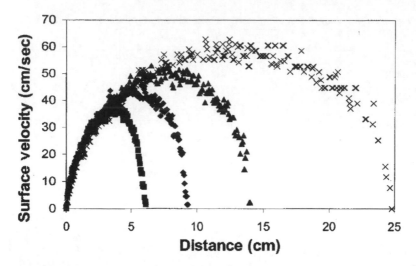

FIGURE 2 Velocity profiles for a series of experiments run at the same tangential velocity (26.4 cm/sec) in cylinders with inner diameters of 6.3 (:), 9.5 (._), 14.4 (↗), and 24.8 cm (×), which correspond to rotation rates of 40, 26.5, 17.4, and 10.2 rpm, respectively.

Despite a nearly fourfold difference in diameter, the velocity data all fall on nearly the same curve over the first 3 cm down the flowing layer. This agreement indicates that initial particle accelerations may be nearly equivalent, regardless of vessel size. Scatter in the experimental data shown in Figure 2 precludes direct calculation of accelerations, so least square polynomials were fit to the experimental data.

By differentiating the polynomial fit, we obtain an estimate of the downstream acceleration, shown in Figure 3. Over the initial or upper third (0–1/3 L) of the flowing layer, the acceleration profiles for all cylinders are nearly identical

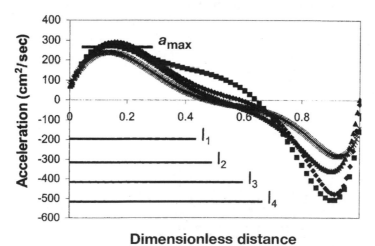

FIGURE 3 Acceleration profiles for experiments run at the same tangential velocity (13.2 cm/sec); *l* marks the distance to reach zero acceleration. The velocity profiles are shown in Figure 2.

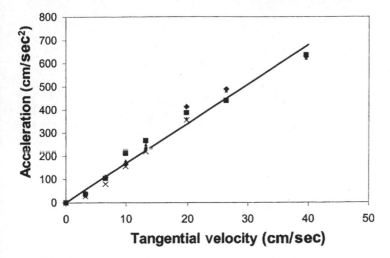

FIGURE 4 A plot of the maximum acceleration against the tangential velocity for all experiments; a near linear relationship is noted. Data is calculated from experiments in 6.3- (⋮), 9.5- (◻), 14.5- (╱), and 24.8-cm (×)-diameter cylinders.

with only minor variations in magnitude. Although the qualitative trend is the same for all curves, the distance taken to reach zero acceleration is very different, nearly two-thirds of the vessel diameter in the 6.3-cm cylinder, as opposed to only half the diameter in the 24.8-cm cylinder.

In Figure 3, maximum accelerations are nearly equal, implying that TV may be proportional to maximum acceleration. Maximum accelerations were determined for all experiments; the results are plotted against the TV in Figure 4. An approximate linear fit is

$$a_{\max} = a \times \text{TV} \tag{4}$$

where TV is the tangential velocity ($= 2\pi R\Omega$) and $\alpha = 17/\text{sec}$, is seen relating acceleration and TV for all cylinders and rotation rates. While the data clearly displays curvature, this linear fit is used as a first order approximation for scaling purposes.

In Figure 3, the distance to reach zero acceleration varies greatly among the four different velocity profiles. This parameter, denoted l, is quantitatively measured as the distance at which the relative change in velocity drops below a preset limit. However, by itself, the value of l has little meaning; it is the parameter l/r, where r is the cylinder radius, that has a quantitative effect on the velocity profile and maximum velocities. When all values of l/r were compiled, a strong correlation to rotation rate was noted. As most pharmaceutical blenders are run at low rotation rates, we restrict the remaining discussion to vessel rotation rates below 30 rpm. Figure 5 plots l/r against $\sqrt[3]{\Omega}$, showing a nearly linear relationship below ~ 30 rpm. An equation for l/r becomes

$$l/r = \beta\sqrt[3]{\Omega}, \ \Omega \leq 30 \tag{5}$$

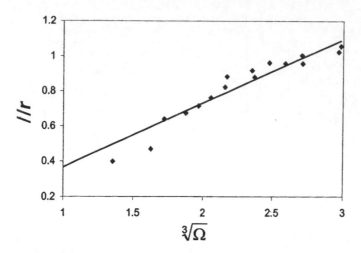

FIGURE 5 The value of l/r is plotted against the cube root of rotation rate, showing a linear relationship.

where $\beta = 0.37$ second$^{1/3}$. As l/r determines the shape of the velocity profile, experiments run at the same rotation rate should show qualitatively similar velocity profiles, regardless of cylinder size.

Developing a Model

The simplest possible model for particle velocity relates velocity and distance when acceleration is constant.

$$V^2 = V_0^2 + 2ax \tag{6}$$

where V_0 is the initial downstream velocity and x is the downstream coordinate. Acceleration has been shown, though, to vary along the length of the flowing region. Also, the distance to reach zero acceleration depends on the rotation rate. It may be possible, however, to scale peak velocities using Eq. (6) subject to some simplifying assumptions.

1. Particles emerge into the flowing layer with zero initial downstream velocity ($V_0 = 0$)
2. Peak acceleration is proportional to TV, Eq. (4)
3. Particles accelerate over the distance l
4. Acceleration (a) is not constant over the distance l, but the rate of change in acceleration scales appropriately with the value of l [i.e., $a = a_{max} f(x/l)$, x is the distance down the cascade]

   Using these assumptions and Eqs. (4–6), a new relation for particle velocity would be

$$V = R\Omega^{2/3}\sqrt{2\pi\alpha\beta} \tag{7}$$

   Equation (7) relates particle velocities to the rotation rate and the radius and can be used as the basis for scaling particle velocities with changes in cylinder diameter and rotation rate.

Returning to Dimensional Analysis

Equation (7) gives a relationship between velocity, rotation rate, and cylinder radius that can be used to complete the dimensional analysis discussed earlier. Applying dimensional homogeneity and solving leads to

$$V = kR\Omega^{2/3}\left(\frac{g}{d}\right)^{1/6} \tag{8}$$

To test the scaling criteria suggested by Eq. (8), we will look at velocity profiles between 10 and 30 rpm. Figure 6A shows the scaled velocity profiles [i.e., all data is divided by using $V = KR\Omega^{2/3}(g/d)^{1/6}$ and the distance down the cascade is divided by the cylinder diameter] for experiments run between 10 and 30 rpm (the unscaled data is shown in Fig. 6B). We see very good

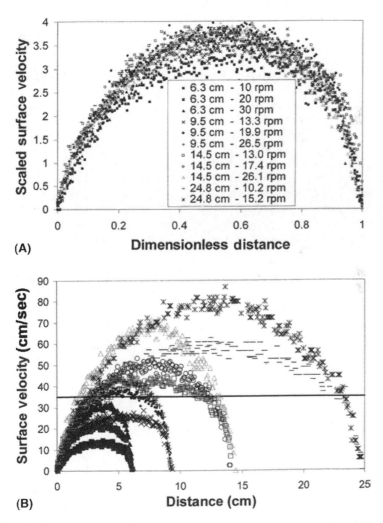

FIGURE 6 (**A**) Scaled velocity profiles for all experiments run between 10 and 30 rpm and in (**B**) the unscaled profiles.

agreement in velocity magnitudes across all rotation rates and cylinder sizes (which incorporate a 4× range in vessel radii and a 3× range in rotation rates).

Equation (8) indicates that particle size has an independent and measurable, although small, effect on particle velocities, which is further discussed elsewhere (19).

Returning to our example of scaling from 5- to 25-ft^3 blender, again the relative change in length is 71%. This time, to scale surface velocities using this approach, the blending speed (Ω) must be reduced by a factor of $(1.71)^{-3/2} = 0.45$, corresponding to 6.7 rpm (assuming the particle diameter, d, remains constant). Again, the total number of revolutions would remain constant at 225 for a blend time of 33.6 minutes.

TESTING VELOCITY-SCALING CRITERIA

Experimental work has not validated the scaling procedure above with respect to scale-up of blending processes. Since this approach also relies on empirical work, this model should not be favored over other approaches currently in use, though it may provide additional insights.

However, recent work has indicated that particle velocities may be critical for determining segregation dynamics in double-cone blenders and V-blenders (20,21). Segregation occurs within the blender as particles begin to flow in regular, defined patterns that differ according to their particle size. Experimental work demonstrates how this occurs. In a 1.9-qt-capacity V-blender at fixed filling (50%), incrementally changing rotation rate induced a transition between two segregation patterns, as seen in Figure 7A. At the lower rotation rate, the "small-out" pattern forms; the essential feature of the small-out pattern is that the smaller red particles dominate the outer regions of the blender while the larger yellow particles are concentrated near the center. At a slightly higher rotation rate, the "stripes" pattern forms, in this case, the small particles form a stripe near the middle of each shell in the blender. Both patterns are symmetrical with respect to the central vertical symmetry plane orthogonal to the axis of rotation.

To validate both the particle velocity hypothesis and our scaling criteria, similar experiments were run in a number of different capacity V-blenders. Vessel dimensions are shown in Table 2, along with a schematic, shown in Figure 8.

All the vessels are constructed from clear plexiglas, enabling visual identification of segregation patterns.

For these experiments, a binary mixture of sieved fractions of 150 to 250 mm (nominally 200 mm) and 710- to 840-mm (nominally 775-mm) glass beads was used. A symmetrical initial condition (top-to-bottom loading) is implemented. The blender is run at constant rotation rate; a segregation pattern was assumed to be stable when it did not discernibly change for 100 revolutions. In many pharmaceutical operations, the mixing time is on the order of 100 to 500 revolutions, and experiments are run with regard to this timeframe.

The transition speeds (rotation rates) were determined for the change from the small-out pattern to stripes at 50% filling for all the blenders listed in Table 2 (Fig. 7 shows results from the 1.9- and 12.9-qt blenders). As discussed earlier, the most commonly accepted methods for scaling tumbling blenders have used one of two parameters, either the Fr or the tangential speed of the blender. Earlier, we derived $V = KR\Omega^{2/3}(g/d)^{1/6}$ and showed that it effectively scales particle

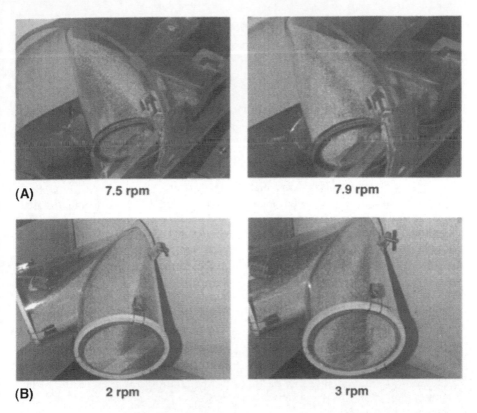

(A) 7.5 rpm   7.9 rpm

(B) 2 rpm   3 rpm

FIGURE 7 Changes in segregation pattern formation in the (**A**) 1.9- and (**B**) 12.9-qt V-blenders.

TABLE 2 Vessel Dimensions

Nominal capacity	Vessel volume (qt)	L (cm)	R (cm)	D (cm)	θ
1P	0.8	10.5	7.9	6.7	80°
1Q	1.9	13.9	10.6	9.2	80°
4Q	6.5	21.2	14.6	13.8	75°
8Q	12.9	24.7	18.8	17.6	75°
16Q	26.5	33	24.2	21.6	75°

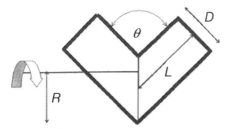

FIGURE 8 A sketch of the relevant dimensions for a V-blender; the actual values for the five blenders used are shown in Table 2.

TABLE 3   Parameter Values at Transition rpm

Blender size	Transition rotation rate	Froude number (Fr), $\Omega^2 R/g(\times 10^5)$	Tangential velocity, ΩR (cm/sec)	$R\Omega^{2/3}(g/d)^{1/6}$ (cm/sec)
1P	9.5	20	7.9	9.9
1Q	7.7	18	8.5	11.5
4Q	3.5	5	5.4	9.4
8Q	2.5	3	4.9	9.6
16Q	1.7	2	4.3	9.6

velocities when the rotation rate is below 30 rpm. We note that all three of these criteria indicate an inverse relationship between rotation rate and blender size. Table 3 shows the parameter values at the transition rotation rate for $R\Omega^{2/3}$ $(g/d)^{1/6}$, Fr, and the TV. $V = KR\Omega^{2/3}$ parameter gives much better agreement than either Fr or TV; the relative standard deviation (RSD) for $V = KR\Omega^{2/3}(g/d)^{1/6}$ is 8.5%, compared with 89% for Fr and 30% for TV.

THE EFFECTS OF POWDER COHESION

A substantial problem that remains open is how to account for the effect of cohesion of powder flow and scale-up, in particular for mixing operations. The problem is extensive, and only a brief discussion is provided here.

In simple terms, a cohesive powder can be defined as a material where the adhesive forces between particles exceed the particle weight by at least an order of magnitude. In such systems, particles no longer flow independently; rather, they move in "chunks" whose characteristic size depends on the intensity of the cohesive stresses.

The effective magnitude of cohesive effects depends primarily on two factors: the intensity and nature of the cohesive forces (e.g., electrostatic, van der Waals, capillary) and the packing density of the material (which determines the number of interparticle contacts per unit area). This dependence on density is the source of great complexity: cohesive materials often display highly variable densities that depend strongly on the immediate processing history of the material.

In spite of this complexity, a few "guidelines" can be asserted within a fixed operational scale.

1. Slightly cohesive powders mix faster than free flowing materials.
2. Strongly cohesive powders mix much more slowly.
3. Strongly cohesive powders often require externally applied shear (in the form of an impeller, an intensifier bar, or a chopper).
4. Baffles attached to vessels do not increase shear substantially.

Lacking a systematic means to measure cohesive forces under practical conditions, the effects of cohesion on scale-up have been rarely studied. The most important observation is that cohesive effects are much stronger in smaller vessels, and their impact tends to disappear in larger vessels. The reason is simple: while cohesive forces are surface effects, the gravitational forces that drive flow in tumbling blenders are volume effects. Thus, as we increase the scale of the blender, gravitational forces grow faster, overwhelming cohesive forces. This can also be explained by remarking that the characteristic chunk size of a cohesive powder flow is a property of the material, and thus to a first approximation, it is independent of the blender size. As the blender grows larger, the ratio of the chunk size to the blender size becomes smaller.

Both arguments can be mathematically expressed in terms of a dimensionless "cohesion" number Π_c.

$$\Pi_c = \frac{\sigma}{\rho g R} = \frac{s}{R}$$

where σ is the effective (surface-averaged) cohesive stress (under actual flow conditions), ρ the powder density under flow conditions, g the acceleration of gravity, and R is the vessel size. The group $s = \sigma/\rho g$ is the above-mentioned chunk size, which can be more rigorously defined as the internal length scale of the flow.

Thus, as R increases, Π_c decreases. This is illustrated in Figure 9, which shows the evolution of the RSD of a blending experiment in a small V-blender for three mixtures of different cohesion. Three systems were studied: a low cohesion system composed of 50% Fast-Flo Lactose and 50% Avicel 102; a medium cohesion system composed of 50% regular lactose and 50% Avicel 102, and a high cohesion system composed of 50% Regular Lactose and 50% Avicel 101. In all cases, an aliquot of the system was laced with 6% micronized acetaminophen, which was used as a tracer to determine the axial mixing rate in V-blenders of different capacities (1Q, 8Q, and 28Q).

Core sampling was used to gather 35 to 70 samples per experimental time point from three cores across each half of the blender. Samples were quantified using NIR spectroscopy, which was shown to be an accurate and efficient method for quantifying mixture quality. A simple model was used to determine mixing rates for both top/bottom and left/right loaded experiments. Variance measurements were split into axial and radial components to give more insight into mixing mechanisms and the separate effects of cohesion and vessel size on these mechanisms.

Convective mixing rates for radially segregated (top/bottom) loading were nearly constant regardless of changes in vessel size or mixture cohesion. Measured variances at short mixing times (i.e., five revolutions) were highly variable. These variations were attributed to unpredictable cohesive flow patterns during the first few rotations of the blender. An important conclusion was that scale-up of radial mixing processes could be obtained by simply allowing for a few (fewer than 10) "extra" revolutions to cancel this variability. As longas the shear limit was reached, the mixing rates was the same for all mixtures and vessel sizes, indicating that required mixing times (in terms of revolutions) needed to insure process outcome could be kept constant regardless of mixture cohesion or mixer size.

However, for axially segregated (left/right) loading, the scale-up factors depended on cohesion, indicating that scale-up is a mixture-dependent problem. As shown in Figure 9A, the most cohesive system mixed much more slowly in the smaller (1Q) blender. However, all three systems mixed at nearly the same rate in the larger (28Q) vessel (Fig. 9B).

The conclusion from these results is that lab scale experiments for cohesive powders are of questionable validity for predicting full-scale behavior. Behavior at small scales is likely to be strongly affected by cohesive effects that are of

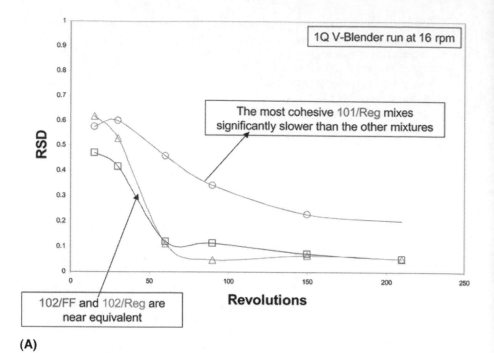

(A)

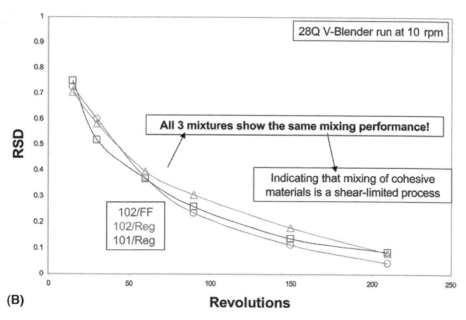

(B)

FIGURE 9   (**A**) RSD measured for axially segregated blends of different cohesion in a 1-qt V-blender. As cohesion increases, blending becomes slower. (**B**) RSD measured for axially segregated blends of different cohesion in a 28-qt V-blender. In a large vessel, the effects of cohesion become unimportant. *Abbreviation*: RSD, relative standard deviation.

much less intensity in the large scale. Moreover, the density of the powder, and therefore the intensity of cohesive effects, might also depend on vessel size and speed. An additional important comment is that the discussion presented in this section does not address another important cohesion effect: API agglomeration. As particles become smaller, cohesive effects grow larger. At some point, agglomeration tendencies become very significant.

The critical factor in achieving homogeneity becomes the shear rate, which is both scale and speed dependent.

In summary, scale-up and scale-down of blenders for cohesive powders is a risky enterprise. Caution is strongly advised.

RECOMMENDATIONS AND CONCLUSIONS

The analysis of particle velocities provides a good first step toward the rigorous development of scaling criteria for granular flow, but it is far from conclusive. For free flowing systems, while particle velocities may control the development of segregation patterns in small capacity V-blenders, velocity may not be the most important dynamical variable affecting the mixing rate. If we regard mixing and segregation as competing processes, however, then knowing that one is velocity dependent and the other is not could be significant. Earlier, we discussed that mixing rate shows little change with rotation rate but large variation with changes in fill level. These results may indicate that a proportionality factor such as $\frac{(\text{mass of contents in motion})}{(\text{total mass})}$ may be important for scaling the mixing process. It is important in granular systems to first determine the dynamical variable that governs the process at hand before determining scaling rules—the basic caveats that particle size, particle velocities, flowing layer depth, or the relative amount of particles in motion may all play a role in a given process, making it important to identify the crucial variables before attempting scale-up.

A systematic, generalized approach for the scale-up of granular mixing devices is still far from attainable. Clearly, more research is required both to test current hypotheses and to generate new approaches to the problem.

Still, we can offer some simple guidelines that can help the practitioner wade through the scale-up process.

1. Make sure that changes in scale have not changed the dominant mixing mechanism in the blender (i.e., convective to dispersive). This can often happen by introducing asymmetry in the loading conditions.
2. For free-flowing powders, number of revolutions is a key parameter but rotation rates are largely unimportant.
3. For cohesive powders, mixing depends on shear rate, and rotation rates are very important.
4. When performing scale-up tests, be sure to take enough samples to give an "accurate" description of the mixture state in the vessel. Furthermore, be wary of how you interpret your samples; know what the mixing index means and what your confidence levels are.
5. One simple way to increase mixing rate is to decrease the fill level—while this may be undesirable from a throughput point of view, decreased fill level also reduces the probability that dead zones will form.
6. Addition of asymmetry into the vessel, either by design or the addition of baffles, can have a tremendous impact on mixing rate.

Until rigorous scale-up rules are determined, these cautionary rules are the "state of the art" for now. We offer a first step toward rigorous scaling rules by scaling particle surface velocities but caution that this work is only preliminary in nature. The best advice is to be cautious—understand the physics behind the problem and that statistics of the data collected. Remember that a fundamental understanding of the issues is still limited and luck is unlikely to be on your side, hence frustrating trial and error is still likely (and unfortunately) necessary to be employed.

REFERENCES

1. Poux M, Fayolle P, Bertrand J, et al. Powder mixing: some practical rules applied to agitated systems. Powder Technol 1991; 68:213–234.
2. Muzzio FJ, Robinson P, Wightman C, et al. Sampling practices in powder blending. Int J Pharm 1997; 155:153–178.
3. PDA Technical Report No. 25. Blend uniformity analysis: validation and in-process testing. PDA J Pharm Sci Technol 1997; 51(suppl):S1–99.
4. Carstensen JT, Patel MR. Blending of irregularly shaped particles. Powder Technol 1977; 17:273–282.
5. Adams J, Baker A. An assessment of dry blending equipment. Trans Inst Chem Eng 1956; 34:91–107.
6. Brone D, Alexander A, Muzzio FJ. Quantitative characterization of mixing of dry powders in V-blenders. AIChE J 1998; 44(2):271–278.
7. Brone D, Muzzio F. Enhanced mixing in double-cone blenders. Powder Technol 2000; 110(3):179–189.
8. Weidenbaum SS, Corson RC, Miller DP. Mixing of solids in a twin shell blender. Ceramic Age 1963; 79:39–43.
9. Wightman C, Muzzio FJ. Mixing of granular material in a drum mixer undergoing rotational and rocking mogions I. Uniform particles. Powder Technol 1998; 98:113–124.
10. Carley-Macauly KW, Donald MB. The mixing of solids in tumbling mixers-I. Chem Eng Sci 1962; 17:493–506.
11. Carley-Macauly KW, Donald MB. The mixing of solids in tumbling mixers-II. Chem Eng Sci 1964; 19:191–199.
12. Sethuraman KJ, Davies GS. Studies on solids mixing in a double-cone blender. Powder Technol 1971; 5:115–118.
13. Lacey PMC. Developments in the theory of particle mixing. J Appl Chem 1954; 4:257–268.
14. Sudah O, Coffin-Beach D, Muzzio FJ. Quantitative characterization of mixing of free flowing granular materials in Tote(Bin)-blenders. Powder Technol 2002; 126(2):191–200.
15. Wang RH, Fan LT. Methods for scaling-up tumbling mixers. Chem Eng 1974; 81 (11):88–94.
16. Lloyd PJ, Yeung PCM, Freshwater DC. The mixing and blending of powders. J Soc Cosmet Chem 1970; 21:205–220.
17. Roseman B, Donald MB. Mixing and de-mixing of solid particles: part 2: effect of varying the operating conditions of a horizontal drum mixer. Br Chem Eng 1962; 7 (1):823.
18. Wiedenbaum SS. Mixing of solids, in advances in chemical engineering. In: Drew TB, Hoopes JW, eds. New York: Academic Press, 1958:209–324
19. Alexander AW, Shinbrot T, Muzzio FJ. Scaling surface velocities in rotating cylinders as a function of vessel radius, rotation rate, and particle size. Powder Technol 2002; 126(2):174–190.
20. Alexander AW, Shinbrot T, Muzzio FJ. Segregation patterns in V-blenders. Chemical Engineering Science 2003; 58(2):487–496.
21. Alexander AW, Shinbrot T, Muzzio FJ. Granular segregation in the double-cone blender: transitions and mechanisms. Phys Fluids 2001; 13(3):578–587.

9.2 Scale-up of continuous blending

Aditya U. Vanarase, Yijie Gao, Atul Dubey, Marianthi G. Ierapetritou, and Fernando J. Muzzio

BACKGROUND

Continuous processing is a relatively new area for manufacturing of solid dose pharmaceutical products. This option is attractive because processes including tabletting, roller compaction, and capsule filling are already carried out in continuous mode (1), while mixing, granulation, and coating are performed largely in batch mode; this mixture of batch and continuous steps is a frequent source of inefficiencies. To convert the current batch based manufacturing into continuous, increasing process understanding of continuous blending is critical. Continuous blending offers many advantages over batch blending including smaller equipment size, reduced in-process inventory, less solid handling such as filling and emptying the blenders (potentially reducing undesirable effects like segregation), better control, and higher uniformity of shear application. However, continuous blending has some limitations, including higher initial cost, difficult implementation for low volume products, and decreased robustness with respect to changes in material properties. Continuous blending has been applied for pharmaceutical materials, which can be found in the recent literature (2,3). Continuous blender design typically consists of an impeller rotating inside a horizontal cylindrical shell. The Gericke GCM 250 (Regensdorf, Switzerland) and the GEA Niro mixer (Columbia, MD, USA) are examples of a few commercially available convective continuous blenders.

The idea of scale-up in continuous mixers is slightly different than batch. In batch mixers, scale-up is carried out by increasing the size of the equipment whereas in continuous mixers scale-up simply by the extension of time is possible. However, if the product demands are high, scale-up by size or by flow rate could be necessary. Design of continuous mixing operations requires evaluation of a large parametric space, including selection and design of mixing and feeding equipment; evaluation of operating parameters such as impeller rotation rate and flow rate; and characterization of the effects of material properties such as particle size distribution and powder cohesion (often as a function of density and moisture content). Environmental variables include relative humidity, electrostatic charging, and temperature. This large number of variables (and their interactions), and the fact that material properties are poorly understood, make it difficult to implement the process for a new entity without detailed studies. Typical questions in developing a continuous mixing process are: What should be the size of the continuous mixer for a given material at a certain flow rate? If the process needs to be scaled-up from one flow rate to another, can mixing be carried out in the same unit? What should be the impeller rotation rate? In the context of pharmaceutical manufacturing where production volumes are relatively low, scale-up can be performed just by changing the flow rate. Depending of the size of the continuous mixer and the range of the impeller rotation rates, it can be operated over a range of flow rates. This section will focus mainly on the scale-up by flow rate case.

In this section, a case study will be presented wherein residence time distribution (RTD) measurements were performed in the continuous powder mixer for different operating conditions. Taylor dispersion model was applied to calculate the axial dispersion coefficient and axial velocity from the RTD data. Also, the behavior of integrated feeder and mixer system was examined at different flow rates.

The remainder of this chapter is organized as follows. In section "Methods, Materials, and Experimental Set-Up," materials and methods used in the case study will be presented. In section "Taylor Dispersion Model," RTD modeling methodology will be presented. In section "Effect of Flow Rate," experimental results of RTD modeling and holdup measurements will be presented. In section "Filtering Ability of the Continuous Mixer Under Different Flow Rates," Danckwerts approach applied to assess the filtering ability of the mixer under different throughputs will be presented. Summary and conclusions will be presented in section "Conclusions."

METHODS, MATERIALS, AND EXPERIMENTAL SET-UP

A commercial continuous mixer manufactured by Gericke was used in the present case study. The design of the mixer is illustrated in Figure 1B. The continuous mixer (model GCM 250) is 0.3 m long and 0.1 m in diameter. The impeller consists of 12 triangular-shaped blades, equally spaced along the axis rotation. The first and the last blade of the impeller are designed differently because of their position close to the end walls of the mixer vessel. The angle of

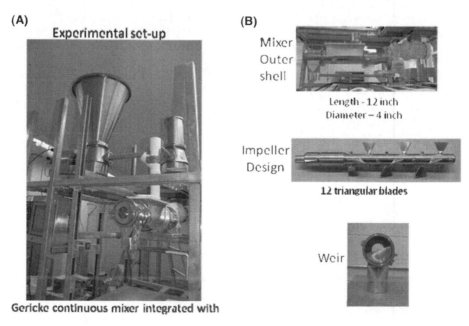

(A)

Experimental set-up

Gericke continuous mixer integrated with

(B)

Mixer Outer shell

Length - 12 inch
Diameter – 4 inch

Impeller Design

12 triangular blades

Weir

FIGURE 1 (**A**) Experimental set-up. (**B**) Equipment.

the blade with the shaft was always directed forward (in the direction of net flow).

The experimental set-up is shown in Figure 1A. Loss-in-weight (LIW) feeders manufactured by Schenck AccuRate (Whitewater, WI, USA) were used in the experiments. For LIW feeders, the size of the discharge opening, screw design, and hopper design were selected on the basis of manufacturer's recommendation.

Pharmaceutical powders including Acetaminophen and microcrystalline cellulose (Avicel PH200) were used in the experimental investigation. Concentration of the tracer (acetaminophen) in the powder samples was measured using NIR spectroscopy.

RTDs in the mixer were measured by the impulse response method. Initially, the bulk material was fed in the mixer until steady state flow was reached. Tracer was inserted manually in the inflow stream as an "instantaneous" pulse. Samples were subsequently collected at various times from the outlet of the mixer. The tracer used was acetaminophen. The samples collected were analyzed by NIR spectroscopy to determine the concentration of acetaminophen in them. Thus, for each experiment, a dataset of concentration versus time was collected. Using this data, RTD function $E(t)$ and mean residence time (MRT, τ) were calculated. RTDs were computed using the relationships given below.

$$\text{Residence time distribution } E(t) = \frac{c(t)}{\int_0^\infty c(t)dt} \tag{1}$$

$$\text{Mean residence time } \tau = \int t.E(t).dt \tag{2}$$

TAYLOR DISPERSION MODEL

In the literature, RTD is often considered for continuous blender scale-up (4–6). It characterizes the axial flow and the dispersion which can be conveniently measured using impulse response tests. Herein, we offer a methodology for scale-up of continuous mixers using RTD measurements from a case study of pharmaceutical powder blending.

The Taylor dispersion model was used to characterize the RTD in the continuous powder mixer:

$$\frac{\partial C}{\partial \theta} + \frac{\partial C}{\partial \xi} = \frac{1}{Pe} \frac{\partial^2 C}{\partial \xi^2} \tag{3}$$

$$C(\xi, \theta) = \frac{C_0 Pe^{1/2}}{(4\pi\theta)^{1/2}} e^{\frac{-Pe(\xi-\theta)^2}{4\theta}} \tag{4}$$

Equation (3) illustrates the Fokker-Planck equation (7). A simplified solution, shown in Eq. (4), is the Taylor dispersion model. $\theta = t/\tau$ and $\xi = z/l$ are the dimensionless time and location, and Pe is the Peclet number which is the dispersion efficiency of the flow system.

$$Pe = \frac{vl}{E} \tag{5}$$

v and E are the axial velocity and the axial dispersion coefficient of the system elements. At the outlet of the continuous mixer, concentration $C(\xi = 1, \theta$ is only a function of θ, which provides the RTD in the mixer. The parameters Pe, C_0, and τ in Eq. (4) are determined by minimizing the mean sum of square (MSS) error between the model-fitted and experimentally determined values of the impulse response test.

EFFECT OF FLOW RATE
Experimental RTD Measurements and Taylor Dispersion Modeling Results

To examine effect of flow rate on RTD, the above fitted parameters were used. Then on the basis of Eq. (5), Axial velocity (v) and dispersion coefficient (E) were derived at two flow rates (30, 45 kg/hr).

Figure 2 illustrates the effect of flow rate on the characteristics of the RTDs, as obtained experimentally for the materials considered. The Taylor dispersion model and nonlinear regression procedure were applied in the RTD fitting process. RTDs were found to be more sensitive to the impeller rotation rate rather than the flow rate. The effect of flow rate and rotation rate on the MRT is shown in Figure 4A. MRT is higher for lower flow rates. This effect is more significant for the cases of lower rotation rates, while at higher rotation rates the curves are hardly affected.

To analyze these effects in detail, v and E were investigated. In general, an increase in the flow rate or a decrease in the rotation rate leads to higher powder fill levels in the mixer. The dispersion coefficient (E) at different operating conditions is shown in Figure 3A. It shows a nonmonotonic effect with respect to

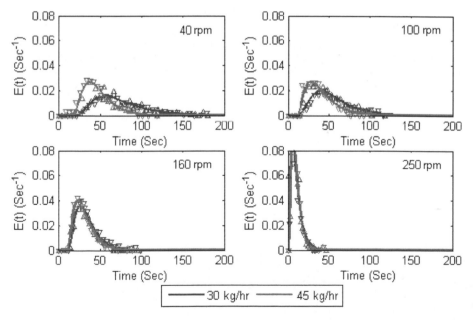

FIGURE 2 Experimental and fitted residence time distribution curves at different operating conditions.

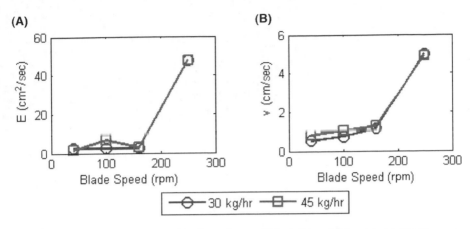

FIGURE 3 Effect of flow rate on (**A**) dispersion coefficient (*E*) and (**B**) axial velocity (*v*).

flow rate. Increase in the flow rate increases dispersion coefficient at an intermediate speed (100 rpm), but makes almost no difference when the speed is larger (160 rpm) or smaller (40 rpm). At moderate blade speed (100 rpm), the fill level increases significantly at higher flow rate (45 kg/hr), in which more powder is pushed by the blades. This behavior is not observed at 250 rpm, at which particles are fluidized in the mixing chamber, and increase in the flow rate does not change the flow conditions significantly. Similarly, at lower rotation rate (40 rpm), flow rate does not influence dispersion coefficient. This is not surprising because limited particle movement severely hinders dispersion; under such conditions the influence of fill level is not significant.

The effects of operating conditions on axial velocity are shown in Figure 2B. Between 40- and 160-rpm impeller rotation rates axial velocity was found to be higher for higher flow rates (45 kg/hr). These trends are complementary to the trends of MRT. At 250 rpm, because of the fast fluidized dispersion, axial velocity is not affected.

Effect of Flow Rate on Blade Passes
The number of blade passes which the powder undergoes as it travels through the mixer is proportional to the applied mechanical energy. The energy provided by the rotating impeller is dissipated in many ways, including the convective transport of the powder, random fluctuations of the velocity of the particles (granular temperature), and friction between the impeller and the powder and the mean strain (shear stresses in the powder). Since the impeller rotation rate has an effect on the residence time, the strain is proportional to the product of the shear rate and the residence time, which is essentially the number of blade passes in the mixer [blade passes — shear rate (rpm)*residence time (sec)/60]. Using the residence time measurements, number of blade passes at various experimental conditions was calculated.

The effect of flow rate and rotation rate on the number of blade passes in the mixer is shown in Figure 4. The number of blade passes is higher for lower flow rates. Again, this effect is significant under low rotation rates. At intermediate rotation rates, the number of blade passes was found to be maximum,

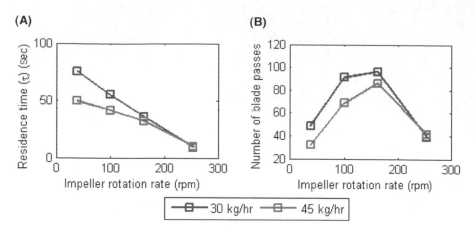

FIGURE 4 Effect of flow rate on (**A**) residence time and (**B**) number of blade passes.

entirely because of the significant change in holdup at higher speeds. Number of blade passes can be used as a scale-up criteria. When the flow rate is changed, the impeller rotation rate can also be changed so that the number of blade passes is kept constant. However, there could be a risk of changing the flow conditions completely (fluidization from a dense powder flow) while changing the rotation rate.

To clarify the effect of flow rate on residence time, holdup was measured for a wide range of flow rates (5–60 kg/hr) at a range of rotation rates (39, 162, and 254 rpm). Holdup is basically the powder mass present in the continuous blender under steady state operation. The bulk residence time (holdup/flow rate) was calculated. The results are presented in Figure 5. Remarkably, bulk residence time is not affected by the flow rate at very high rotation rates (254 rpm), which means that under these conditions, mixing performance (such as it might be) is independent of throughput. However, residence time decreases with increasing flow rate at lower rotation rates (39 and 162 rpm).

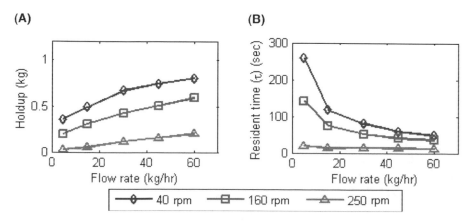

FIGURE 5 Effect of flow rate on (**A**) holdup and (**B**) bulk residence time.

Sudah et al. (8) also found similar results for rotary calciners; MRT was found to be not a function of feed rates up to 10% fill levels. In the present case, at high rotation rates (254 rpm), fill level is well below the capacity of the mixer, which yields similar results.

Effect of Flow Rate on Blend Homogeneity

The relative standard deviation (RSD), which is the most common mixing index used in industry, was computed. For each experimental run, 20 samples were collected from the outlet. Concentration of acetaminophen in each sample was measured using a NIR spectroscopy analytical method. RSD between the acetaminophen concentrations was calculated using the usual relationship.

$$\text{RSD} = \frac{s}{\overline{C}}, s = \sqrt{\frac{\sum_{1}^{N}(C_i - \overline{C})^2}{N-1}} \tag{6}$$

In Eq. (6), $\overline{C}$ is the average concentration of the total samples (N) collected in each mixing run and C_i is the concentration of each sample. s is the standard deviation between the sample concentrations. As depicted in Figure 6, the smallest RSD was observed at intermediate rotation rates (100–162 rpm). At intermediate rotation rates, the maximum number of blade passes (strain) is exerted on the powder, which leads to better mixing performance. In this case, the flow rate did not affect the mixing performance. Increase in total flow rate has an impact on fill level in the mixer and also on the input variability. Increasing the flow rate improves feeder performance, which leads to lower variance in the input concentration. Variance at the input decreases from $s_i^2 = 1.12$ to $s_i^2 = 0.41$ for the increase in flow rate from 30 to 45 kg/hr. However, the RSD at the discharge is unaffected by this large change in input variability.

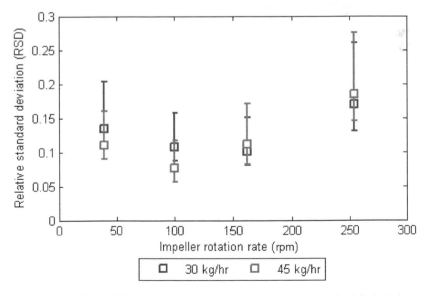

FIGURE 6 Effect of flow rate on blend homogeneity (relative standard deviation).

Thus, the conclusion, for this particular case, is that the variability contributed from feeding is almost completely filtered out by the continuous mixer, provided that enough residence time is available. The final RSD of the mixture is largely dominated by the sample size and the inherent material properties, and how the shear exposure in the mixer affects them. Equal number of blade passes scale-up criteria was not tested in this case study, because the RSDs did not seem to get affected in the flow rate range of 30 to 45 kg/hr.

FILTERING ABILITY OF THE CONTINUOUS MIXER UNDER DIFFERENT FLOW RATES

In continuous blending, feeding equipments are inherently integrated to the continuous blender. To ensure efficient operation of the integrated process, it is important to identify the key bottlenecks between feeders and the continuous blender. Using the RTD function $E(\theta)$, Danckwerts (9) defined the dynamic output concentration $(C_0 = \overline{C} + \delta_0)$ as a function of input concentration $(C_i = \overline{C} + \delta_i)$. The relationship is given in Eq. (7).

$$C_0(t) = \int C_i(t - \theta)E(\theta)d\theta \qquad (7)$$

Using the RTD and incoming feed rate variability measurements, Danckwerts' approach (9–12) can be applied to compute the remaining component of input fluctuations in the final output variance. In the literature (13,14) role of the RTD has been indicated as a high-pass filter to the feeding variability. While scaling up the continuous blending process, change in flow rate influences both the RTD (Fig. 2) as well as in coming feed rate variability (Fig. 7), which further

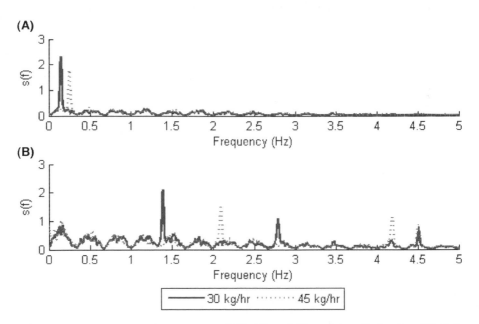

FIGURE 7 Feeding fluctuation spectrum of (A) API and (B) excipient. Notice the shift of the fluctuation to higher frequencies at 45 kg/hr flow rate.

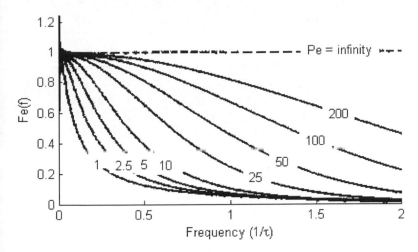

FIGURE 8 Filtering ability $Fe(f)$ of the Taylor dispersion model under a range of Peclet numbers $(1-\infty)$. The maximum value of $Fe(f)$ is unity in the case of plug flow reactor.

affects the remaining fluctuations in the output stream and hence the performance of the continuous mixer.

On the basis of the Fourier analysis (13), the filtering ability $Fe(f)$ of the RTD computed using the Taylor dispersion model was derived for a range of Peclet numbers (Pe). The results are shown in Figure 8. These plots indicate that filtering ability of the mixer is better for smaller Pe because of lower and narrower $Fe(f)$ curve. On the other hand, the model acts more like a plug flow reactor (PFR) when Pe is large, in which no smoothing takes place in the mixer. $Fe(f)$ is unity for all frequency components in the PFR, while for all other profiles with finite Peclet number are below it. Notice that the x-axis is $1/\tau$, indicating better overall filtering ability at large MRTs.

An example of the feeding fluctuation attenuation is illustrated in Figure 9 using the experimental data shown in section "Methods, Materials, and Experimental Set-Up." The mixer operates at a rotation rate of 250 rpm and 30 kg/hr flow rate. In Figure 9A the RTD function $E(t)$ is fitted using the Taylor dispersion model, characterized by the optimized parameters $Pe = 1.86$ and $\tau = 9.51$ seconds. The filtering ability profile $Fe(f)$ is computed and shown in Figure 9D. It was found that the fluctuations at frequencies higher than 0.25 Hz are almost completely filtered out, while the fluctuations below 0.1 Hz were not filtered efficiently. In Figure 9B, C, dashed lines represent the input mass flow rate $C_{in}(t)$ and the solid lines represent the output mass flow rate $C_{out}(t)$, derived by applying Eq. (7). A detailed variance reduction profile is shown in the continous variance spectrum $s(f)$ in Figure 9E, F. It was observed that the output varince component is negligible at frequencies larger than 0.25 Hz in this case study. For both excipient as well as API, peaks of fluctuations are significant at 0.05 Hz in the input feed rate, while as much as 40% of the peaks survive through the mixing process. In this perspective the system is not in its optimal set. Either shifting the peaks of feeder fluctuations to a frequency higher than 0.25 Hz or

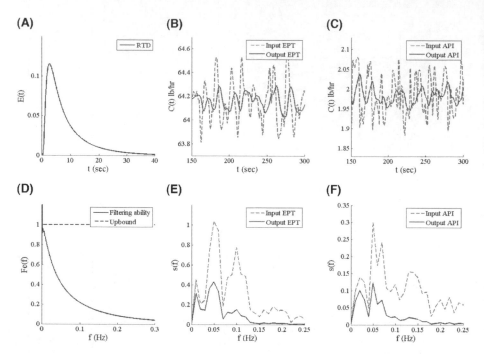

FIGURE 9   Summary of a case study. (**A**) Fitted RTD curve, representing the mixer performance at 30 kg/hr flow rate and impeller rotation rate 250 rpm. (**B**) Mass flow rate fluctuation of the excipient (EPT) at input and output streams. (**C**) Mass flow rate of the API. (**D**) Filtering ability $Fe(f)$ of the fitted RTD curve. (**E**) Continuous variance spectrum $s(f)$ of the excipient. (**F**) Continuous variance spectrum $s(f)$ of the API. *Abbreviation*: RTD, residence time distribution.

increasing the filtering ability below 0.1 Hz or both would improve the efficiency of the system on the basis of the profile of $s(f)$ and $Fe(f)$.

A typical scale-up study involves a number of experimental trials to gain insights into the response of the system to a change in the processing conditions. Studies such as the one described in the previous section form a basis of a successful scale-up operation. However, often it is expensive to carry out an entire set of trials because of material wasteage, time, labor, and environmental concerns. In recent times there has been a tremendous growth in the computing industry in both hardware and software arena. Latest computing techniques literally bring supercomputing to a user's desktop without the need for large and expensive clusters (15). There have been developments in computing algorithms that have made them highly efficient and able to make use of the multithreaded computing environment. Mechanistic modeling is thus becoming not only easier to perform but is also providing information that is difficult or expensive to garner experimentally. Mechanistic modeling tools such as discrete element method (DEM)-based simlations can greatly help reduce the number of experiments needed to perform a scale-up operation. DEM, which owes it existence to a seminal piece of work done by Cundall and Strack (16), has been used to study a number of different processes including pharmaceutical unit operations (17).

DEM is a technique for simulating the behavior of granular materials with each particle treated as a discrete unit. The motion of each particle is tracked on the basis of the calculated positions and velocities which are a result of the forces experienced by it. Forces on particles are of two types—contact forces and body forces. The contact forces are due to interparticle or particle-boundary collisions while the force due to gravity is a body force. The boundary can be any physical object in the system, such as the walls, and baffles. The particulate forces are resolved into normal and tangential components that are independent of each other. Using Newton's law the position of a particle i that has j number of contacts with its surroundings is related to the resultant force by Eq. (8).

$$m_i \ddot{x}_i = \sum_j [F_{ij}^n + F_{ij}^t] + \sum_k F_{body}, \; where$$
$$I_t \ddot{\theta}_i = \sum_j [R_i \times F_{ij}^t] + \sum_l \tau_{body}$$

(8)

In Eq. (8), m_i is the mass of the particle of radius R_i, x_i is its position, $\ddot{x}_i$ its acceleration, and I_i is its moment of intertia. F_{ij}^n and F_{ij}^t are the normal and tangential components of the contact force on particle i due to its jth contact, respectively. The term $\sum_k F_{body}$ accounts for all body forces acting on the particle using a summation index k. In this study, gravity is considered to be the only source of the body force on the particles ($k = 1$, $\sum_k F_{body} = m_i g$). The rotational components of motion are the angular displacement θ, angular acceleration $\dot{\theta}$, and sum $\sum_l \tau_{body}$ of all torques due to body forces using summation index l.

To perform this scale-up study, a computer-aided drawing of the Gericke blender with 1:1 size ratio were created using Pro/Engineer software (Fig. 10). They were imported into a commercial simulation program called EDEM™. At the inlet of the blender were two feeders providing a continuous supply of particles on either side of the impeller at a uniform feed rate. The two streams were completely segregated from each other. At the other end of the blender, a semicircular weir was placed to increase the holdup and facilitate back mixing. The weir was placed such that its straight edge made a 45° angle with the horizontal. The impeller rotation was clockwise when viewed along the axis of rotation from the outlet end. The impeller blade pattern was designed to be similar to the one used in the experimental study.

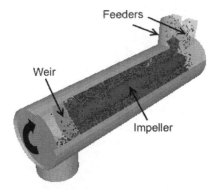

FIGURE 10 A model of the Gericke continuous mixer used in the discrete element method simulations.

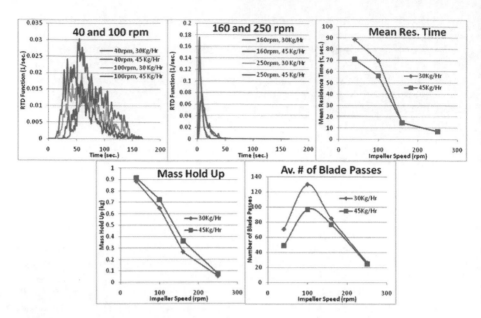

FIGURE 11 In the discrete element method simulations, the residence time distribution function shows more sensitivity to change in flow rate at lower impeller speeds (40 and 100 rpm). The mean residence times are also affected more prominently at these speeds, with higher residence times at lower feed rate. The mass holdup was higher for the higher feed rate. The average number of blade passes was highest at intermediate speeds for both flow rates with higher values for the lower feed rate.

With an aim to show the applicability of DEM in a scale-up study, this model was used to simulate the blending process and to extract some of the same information as the experiments. The effect of increase in flow rate from 30 to 45 kg/hr on properties such as MRT, RTD, material holdup and the average number of blade passes experienced by the powder show good qualitative agreement with the experimental findings (Fig. 11). When using low impeller speeds (40 and 100 rpm), an increase in the feed rate causes the RTD function to show higher peaks and lower MRT values. However this effect is diminished at the higher impeller speeds (160 and 250 rpm). Since these findings are in agreement with the experimental ones, this shows that the method is able to capture the process dynamics to a great degree of accuracy. The MRT provides another way to look at this effect; with MRTs being considerably higher at low feed rate for low impeller speeds while not being affected by the change in flow rate at higher speed. This knowledge can guide a process engineer such that if blending can be performed at high speeds then it may be safe to increase the flow rate. The mass holdup was higher at higher flow rate and the number of blade passes experienced by the powder were higher at the lower feed rate. Another important piece of information is that the number of blade passes peaks at an intermediate speed and the flow rate does not affect them at high speed. So not only does the powder spend nearly the same amount of time in the blender, it also experiences similar amount of shear at both flow rates. When there is such a degree on confidence in the model, such a model can be used to study other aspects of the process such as the effect of the change in flow rate on the forces experienced by particles, the stress on the material in different areas of the blender, emergence of any dead zones, etc. The studies can be extrapolated to other scenarios such as if a change in material or composition is desired. Mechanistic modeling is gaining importance in process design and control and as this study has shown, it can be applied in a scale-up study as well.

CONCLUSIONS

Scale up of continuous mixers can be carried by either increasing the equipment size or by increasing the flow rate. It is important to identify the capacity of the mixer while doing the scale-up by flow rate. Capacity of the mixer is decided by its capability to convey and mix the given powder at the desired rate. A blender should be selected such that it provides the minimum required residence time. Minimum required residence time (rather RTD) is a function of the incoming variability in the feed rate. At the same time, flow conditions in the mixer should be such that minimum required amount of shear application also occurs. For instance, if the minimum required residence time leads to fluidization in the mixer, blending performance could be poor. On other hand if the materials tend to form agglomerates, even if the required RTD is provided in the blender, blending performance could still be poor.

In the case study, RTDs were measured at different operating conditions by varying the flow rate and the impeller rotation rate. Between 100 and 160 rpm, number of blade passes was found to be maximum which provided better blend homogeneity. Equal number of blade passes scaling criteria could be one possible approach to scale-up continuous blending. Increasing the flow rate decreased residence time in the mixer but that did not change the mixing performance significantly. This indicates that once the minimum possible RSD is reached, it does change even if any further blade passes are applied.

The Taylor dispersion model was applied to fit the RTD data to extract model parameters (axial velocity and axial dispersion coefficient). This RTD model along with the Danckwerts approach was used to assess the filtering capability of the mixer under different feeding conditions. In the case study, it was found that incoming fluctuations in the concentration are not filtered below 0.25 Hz. Hence, 250-rpm rotation rate under these flow rates was not optimal. While doing the scale-up, caution should be taken so that the incoming feed rate variability is filtered to the maximum possible extent.

A DEM-based model was used to study the effect of change in flow rate and it found good agreement with the experimental results. This modeling technique can be employed to not only gain better process understanding for a successful scale-up but to also reduce the number of experimental trials thus reducing the cost of the operation.

REFERENCES

1. Plumb K. Continuous processing in the pharmaceutical industry: changing the mind set. Chem Eng Res Design 2005; 83:730–738.
2. Portillo PM, Ierapetritou MG, Muzzio FJ. Characterization of continuous convective powder mixing processes. Powder Technol 2008; 182:368–378.
3. Marikh K, Berthiaux H, Gatumel C, et al. Influence of stirrer type on mixture homogeneity in continuous powder mixing: a model case and a pharmaceutical case. Chem Eng Res Design 2008; 86:1027–1037.

4. Abouzeid A-M, Fuerstenau DW, Sastry KV. Transport behavior of particulate solids in rotary drums: scale-up of residence time distribution using the axial dispersion model. Powder Technol 1980; 27:241–250.
5. Ziegler GR, Aguilar CA. Residence time distribution in a co-rotating, twin-screw continuous mixer by the step change method. J Food Eng 2003; 59:161–167.
6. Sherritt RG, Chaouki J, Mehrotra AK, et al. Axial dispersion in the three-dimensional mixing of particles in a rotating drum reactor. Chem Eng Sci 2003; 58:401–415.
7. Risken H. The Fokker-Planck Equation: Method of Solution and Applications. 2nd ed. Berlin, Heidelberg, New York: Springer-Verlag, 1996.
8. Sudah OS, Chester AW, Kowalski JA, et al. Quantitative characterization of mixing processes in rotary calciners. Powder Technol 2006; 126:166–173.
9. Danckwerts PV. Continuous flow systems. Distribution of residence times. Chem Eng Sci 1953; 2:1–13.
10. Williams JC, Rahman MA. Prediction of the performance of continuous mixers for particulate solids using residence time distributions: part II. Exp Powder Technol 1972; 5:307–316.
11. Ralf Weinekötter LR. Continuous mixing of fine particles. Part Part Syst Char 1995; 12:46–53.
12. Marikh K, Berthiaux H, Mizonov V, et al. Flow analysis and markov chain modelling to quantify the agitation effect in a continuous powder mixer. Chem Eng Res Design 2006; 84:1059–1074.
13. Smith OJ, Graham DR, Palamara JE. Temporal mixing. AICHE J 2006; 52:1780–1789.
14. Pernenkil L, Cooney CL. A review on the continuous blending of powders. Chem Eng Sci 2006; 61:720–742.
15. Kirk DB, Wen-mei W Hwu. Programming massively parallel processors: a hands on approach, paperback, ISBN: 978-0-12-381472-2.
16. Cundall PA, Strack ODL. A discrete numerical model for granular assemblies. Geotechnique 1979; 29(1):47–65.
17. Moakher M, Shinbrot T, Muzzio FJ. Experimentally validated computations of flow, mixing and segregation of non-cohesive grains in 3D tumbling blenders. Powder Technol 2000; 109(1–3):58–71.

Scale-up in the field of granulation and drying

Hans Leuenberger, Gabrielle Betz, Marc Allen S. Donsmark, and David M. Jones

INTRODUCTION

The scale-up procedure of the wet agglomeration process is one of the most challenging tasks. This is due to the fact that there is often a lack of detailed understanding of this process. In this context, the granulation end point, which is often cited, plays a major role. Unfortunately, a rigorous, scientific definition of this granulation end point is missing. In praxis, it is generally referred as the time to stop the granulation process after the addition of the needed amount of granulating liquid and sufficient massing to create a snowball consistency of the wetted powder mass. It is however, on the other hand, possible to determine the necessary amount of granulation liquid by the analysis of the power consumption profile of the mixer motor during the wet agglomeration process. The characteristics of the power consumption profile depends on the formulation and on the type of granulating liquid such as water or alcohol.

The corresponding author of this chapter is involved in the topic of scale-up of the wet agglomeration process for more than 25 years (1). The key parameter is the determination of the correct amount of granulating liquid. This can be achieved by measuring the power consumption profile of the mixer/kneader during the addition of the granulating liquid. In this respect, it is mandatory that the amount of granulating liquid is added by a pump. The resulting power consumption profile can be used for determining the optimal amount of granulating liquid. Most of the mixers/kneaders, which are today available, are equipped with a possibility to monitor the wet agglomeration process. In many cases such a profile is part of a batch documentation, but it nothing more. In this context, it surprising that the resulting profile is in not more exploited for a much better understanding of the specific formulation. In fact the power consumption profile is a "fingerprint" of the composition and of the wet agglomeration process. A prerequisite for exploiting the power consumption profile as an analytical tool is the use of a low-viscous granulating liquid added slowly to the powder mass. The power consumption profile is sensitive to the type of binder, to the amount of swelling and soluble substances, to the type of mixer, etc. Such fingerprint profiles reveal a lot about the behavior of the powder mass and is a very important tool for transforming the "art of granulation" into a science (1). Specific experience is needed for a orrect interpretation of these power consumption profiles. Such a detailed knowledge about the wet agglomeration process facilitates the scale-up exercise. This approach fulfills at the same time the requirements of FDA's PAT initiative requesting a better understanding of the involved unit operations.

The production of pharmaceutical granules, using the wet agglomeration process with a subsequent drying step, is based on the batch concept. In the early stage of the development of a solid dosage form, the batch size is small, for example, for first clinical trials. In a later stage, the size of the batch produced in the pharmaceutical production department may be up to a 100 times larger. Thus, the scale-up process is an extremely important one. Unfortunately, in many cases, the variety of the equipment involved does not facilitate the task of scale-up. During the scale-up process, the quality of the granules may change. A change in the granule size distribution, final moisture content, friability, compressibility, and compactibility of the granules may strongly influence the properties of the final tablet, such as tablet hardness, tablet friability, disintegration time, dissolution rate of the active substance, aging of the tablet, etc. In the following sections of this chapter, the scale-up process is analyzed taking into account mathematical considerations of the scale-up theory (1,2), the search for scale-up invariants (3–6), the establishment of in-process control methods (7–10) as well as the design of a robust dosage form (11–14). In this respect, new concepts such as the percolation theory (11–14) play an important role. A new concept concerning a quasi-continuous production line of granules is presented (15–19). This concept permits the production of small-scale batches for clinical trials and of production batches using the same equipment. Thanks to this concept, scale-up problems can be in principle avoided in an elegant and cost-efficient way. Finally, the scale-up of the conventional fluidized bed spray granulation process is discussed because of its common use for spray granulation and/or drying as a step subsequent to some type of wet granulation. The combination of reproducibility and batch size flexibility results in a highly efficient manufacturing method.

THEORETICAL CONSIDERATIONS
The Principle of Similarity
The Definition of Similarity and Dimensionless Groups
The important concept for scale-up is the principle of similarity (1–7). When scaling up any mixer/granulator (e.g., planetary mixer, high-speed mixer, pelletizing dish, etc.), the following three types of similarity need to be considered: geometric, kinematic, and dynamic. Two systems are geometrically similar when the ratio of the linear dimensions of the small-scale and scaled-up systems are constant.

Two systems of different sizes are kinematically similar when in addition to the systems being geometrically similar, the ratio of velocities between corresponding points in the two systems are equal. Two systems of different size are dynamically similar when *in addition* to the systems being geometrically and kinematically similar, the ratio of forces between corresponding points in the two systems are equal.

Similarity criteria. There are two general methods of arriving at similarity criteria:

1. When the differential equations or in general the equations that govern the behavior of the system are known, they can be transformed into dimensionless forms.

2. When differential equations or in general equations that govern the behavior of a system, are not known, such similarity criteria can be derived by means of dimensional analysis.

Both methods yield dimensionless groups, which correspond to dimensionless numbers (1–3), for example,

REYNOLDS number Re,
FROUDE number Fr,
NUSSELT number Nu,
SHERWOOD number Sh,
SCHMIDT number Sc, etc. (3).

The classical principle of similarity can then be expressed by an equation of the form:

$$\pi_1 = F(\pi_2, \pi_3, \ldots) \tag{1}$$

This equation may be a mechanistic (case A) or an empirical one (case B):
  A. $\pi_1 = e^{\pi_2}$ with the dimensionless groups:

$$\pi_1 = \frac{P(x)}{P(0)} \tag{2}$$

where $P(x)$ is the pressure at level x and $P(0)$, the pressure above sea level $(x = 0)$.

$$\pi_2 = \frac{E(x)}{RT} \tag{3}$$

with $E(x) = Mgx$.
  $E(x)$ is the molar potential energy; M, the molecular weight; g, the gravitational acceleration; x, the height above sea level; and RT, the molar kinetic energy.
  B. Empirical general equation

$$\pi_1 = a(\pi_2)^b \cdot (\pi_3)^c \tag{4}$$

The unknown parameters a, b, c are usually determined by nonlinear regression calculus.

Buckingham's Theorem
For a correct dimensional analysis, it is necessary to consider Buckingham's theorem, which may be stated as follows (3,4):

1. The solution to every dimensionally homogeneous physical equation has the form $F(\pi_1, \pi_2, \pi_3, \ldots) = 0$, in which $\pi_1, \pi_2, \pi_3, \ldots$ represent a complete set of dimensionless groups of the variables and the dimensional constants of the equation.
2. If an equation contains n separate variables and dimensional constants, and these are given dimensional formulas in terms of m primary quantities (dimensions), the number of dimensionless groups in a complete set is $(n - m)$.

THE DRY-BLENDING OPERATION

To obtain a high degree of mixing, cohesive powder components have to be disagglomerated. For this purpose, it is often advantageous to proceed as follows:

1. Dry blending of the powder components
2. Sieving of the blend through a sieve through an appropriate mesh for disagglomeration
3. Final dry-blending step

The shear forces at work during the sieving step are important for disagglomeration of the finer cohesive material and/or favoring contacts between finer and coarser particles.

In the case of an active substance at very low dose, that is, requiring a high dilution with the auxiliary substances (e.g., 1:100), the blending operation may be divided into two steps: primary 1:10 dilution and then a secondary 1:10 blending step to obtain the final dilution.

The content uniformity that can be obtained depends, according to established theoretical considerations, on the particle size of the active substance (20,21). As a rough estimate for the obtainable relative standard deviation S of the content of the active substance, the following rule can be applied based on Poisson statistics:

$$S_{rel}(\%) = \frac{1}{\sqrt{N}} \cdot 100\% \tag{5}$$

where N is number of particles of the active substance in a unit dose such as a tablet.

Thus for a relative standard deviation of 1%, at least 10,000 particles of the active substance have to be distributed randomly in the tablet (see Examples 1a and 1b).

Example 1a:
Schematic representation of 1 mg active substance of density 1 g/cm^3 distributed as 49 particles in a tablet.
  The calculated particle diameter is equal to 273 μm.

$N = 49$ particles
$s^2 = 49$
$s = \pm 7$
$S_{rel} \pm 14.3\%$
$d = 273 \ \mu$m

Example 1b:
Schematic representation of 1 mg active substance of density 1 g/cm^3 distributed as 10,000 particles in a tablet.
  The calculated particle diameter is equal to 4.6 μm.

$N = 10,000$ particles
$s^2 = 10,000$
$s = \pm 100$
$S_{rel} \pm 1\%$
$d = 4.6 \ \mu$m

SCALE-UP AND MONITORING OF THE WET GRANULATION PROCESS

Dimensionless Groups

As the behavior of the wet granulation process cannot be described so far adequately by mathematical equations, the dimensionless groups have to be determined by a dimensional analysis. For this reason, the following idealized behavior of the granulation process in the high-speed mixer is assumed:

- The particles are fluidized
- The interacting particles have similar physical properties
- There is only a short-range particle-particle interaction
- There is no system property equivalent to viscosity, that is,
    a. there are no long-range particle-particle interactions and
    b. the viscosity of the dispersion medium air is negligible.

According to Buckingham's theorem, the following dimensionless groups can be identified as:

– Power number:

$$\pi_1 = \frac{P}{r^5 \omega^3 \rho} \tag{6}$$

– Specific amount of granulation liquid:

$$\pi_2 = \frac{qt}{V\rho} \tag{7}$$

– Fraction of volume loaded with particles:

$$\pi_3 = \frac{V}{V^*} \tag{8}$$

– Froude number (centrifugal/gravitational energy):

$$\pi_4 = \frac{r\omega^2}{g} \tag{9}$$

– Geometric number (ratio of characteristic lengths):

$$\pi_5 = \frac{r}{d} \tag{10}$$

List of symbols

P = Power consumption
r = Radius of the rotating blade (first characteristic length of the mixer)
ω = Angular velocity
ρ – Specific density of the particles
q = Mass (kg) of granulating liquid added per unit time
t = Process time
V = Volume loaded with particles
V^* = Total volume of the vessel (mixer unit)
G = Gravitational acceleration
D = Diameter of the vessel (second characteristic length of the mixer)

In principle, the following scale-up equation can be established as:

$$\pi_1 = a(\pi_2)^b \cdot (\pi_3)^c \cdot (\pi_4)^d \cdot (\pi_5)^e \tag{11}$$

In general, however, it may not be the primary goal to know exactly the empirical parameters a, b, c, d, e of the process under investigation, but to check or monitor pragmatically the behavior of the dimensionless groups (process variables, dimensionless constant) in the small- and large-scale equipment. The ultimate goal would be to identify scale-up invariants.

Experimental Evidence for Scale-up Invariables

In the case of the wet granulation process in a mixer/kneader, the granulation process can be easily monitored by the determination of the power consumption (7–10) (Fig. 1).

The typical power profile consists of five different phases (Fig. 2). Usable granulates can be produced in a conventional way only within the plateau region S3–S4 according to the nomenclature in Figure 2. As Figure 3 indicates, changing the type of mixer has only a slight effect on the phases of the kneading process.

However, the actual power consumption of mixers of different type differs greatly for a given granulate composition.

The important point is now that the power consumption profile as defined by the parameters $S3$, $S4$, Ss is independent of the batch size. For this, investigation mixers of the planetary type (DOMINICI, GLEN, MOLTENI) were used.

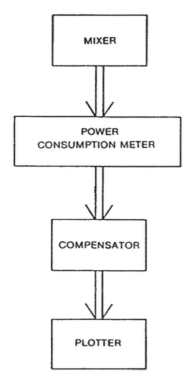

FIGURE 1 Block diagram of measuring equipment. *Source*: From Ref. 1.

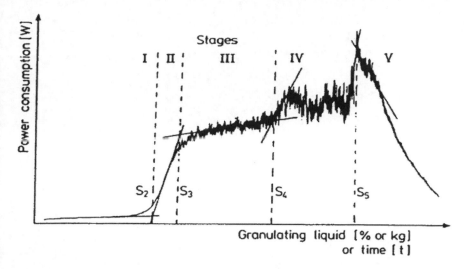

FIGURE 2 Division of a power consumption curve. *Source*: From Refs. 1, 7–10.

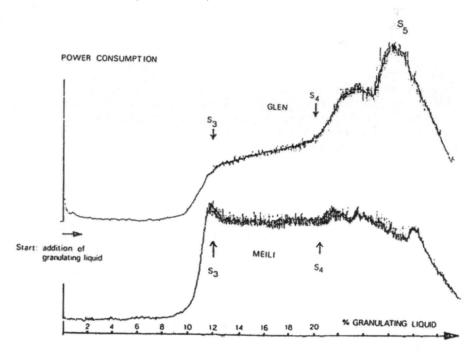

FIGURE 3 Power consumption profiles of two types of a mixer/kneader. *Source*: From Ref. 1.

The batch size ranged from 3.75 to 60 kg. To obtain precise scale-up measurements, the excipients that were used belonged to identical lots of primary material [10% (w/w) cornstarch, 4% (w/w) polyvinylpyrrolidone as binder, and 86% (w/w) lactose]. As can be seen from Figure 4, the amount of granulating liquid is linearly dependent on the batch size. During the scale-up

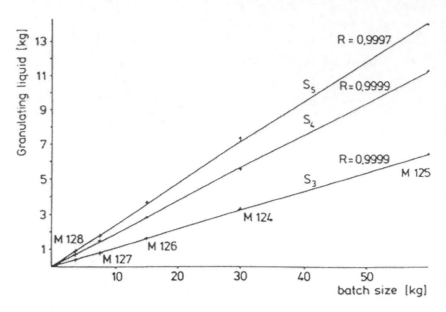

FIGURE 4 Scale-up precision measurements with identical charges. *Source*: From Ref. 1.

exercise, the rate of addition of the granulation liquid was enhanced in proportion to the larger batch size. Thus, the power profile, which was plotted on the chart recorder, showed the characteristic S3, S4, Ss values independent of batch size within the same amount of time since the start of the addition of granulation liquid. This fact is not surprising as in terms of scale-up theory, the functional dependencies of the dimensionless group numbers ~1 and ~2 were measured:

$$\pi_1 = F(\pi_2) \tag{12}$$

The other numbers π_3, π_4, π_5 were kept essentially constant. From these findings one can conclude that the correct amount of granulating liquid per amount of particles to be granulated is a scale-up invariable (6–9). It is necessary, however, to mention that during this scale-up exercise only a low-viscous granulating liquid was used. The exact behavior of a granulation process using high-viscous binders and different batch sizes is unknown. It is evident that the first derivative of the power consumption curve is a scale-up invariant and can be used as an in-process control and for a fine-tuning of the correct amount of granulating liquid (Fig. 6).

Mechanistic Understanding of the Wet Agglomeration Process and the Power Consumption Profile

The following statements refer to the situation where a well-soluble binder is added in a dry state or where the binder is dissolved in the granulating liquid showing a low viscosity. Because of environmental protection and other issues such as preferred wettability with water, a high interfacial tension, distilled or demineralized water is the granulating liquid of choice. As modern mixers/granulators are today often instrumented to measure the power consumption during the moist agglomeration process, emphasis is put on the interpretation of power consumption profiles and on the experiences obtained so far with this method. For the better understanding of the power consumption profiles, the following theoretical considerations are a prerequisite.

Liquid Bridge Force and Cohesive Stress

According to models described by Rumpf (22) and by Newitt and Conway-Jones (23), the cohesive forces that operate during the moist agglomeration process result from liquid bridges that are formed in the void space between the solid particles. The strength of the cohesive stress σ_c depends on the surface tension γ of the granulating liquid, the wetting angle δ, the distance a between the particles and the particle diameter x. In an idealized situation with $a = 0$ (contact) and $\delta = 0°$, the cohesive stress σ_c of the powder bed, consisting of isometric spherical particles with diameter x, where the void space is only partly filled up with granulating liquid (degree S^* of saturation $< \sim 0.3$) is equal to:

$$\sigma_c = \frac{1 - \varepsilon}{\varepsilon} \frac{A \pi \gamma}{x\{1 + tg(\theta/2\}} \tag{13}$$

with ε is the porosity of the powder mass, A^*, the proportionality constant depending on the geometry of packing of the particles.

Tensile Strength of Moist Agglomeration, That Is, Green Granules

Because of the principle of action = reaction the cohesive strength σ_c is equal to the tensile strength σ_t of the moist particulate matter. The tensile strength σ_t of limestone particles with diameter $x = 71$ μm forming a powder mass with the porosity $\varepsilon = 0.415$ was measured as a function of liquid saturation S^* by Schubert (24), illustrating the relationship between σ_t and S^* for lower and higher degree S^* of saturation (Fig. 5).

In a first approximation, the specific power consumption per unit volume dN/dV of the moist powder in a mixer is equal to:

$$\frac{dN}{dV} = \mu \sigma_c \kappa \tag{14}$$

with μ, the apparent friction coefficient; σ_c the cohesive strength of the moist powder bed; and κ, the shear rate.

For a fixed coefficient of friction μ and a fixed dimensionless shear rate κ, the measurement of the power consumption per unit volume of the moist powder mass is proportional to the cohesive stress σ_c. Thus, if the granulating liquid is added to the powder mass at a constant rate, the power consumption profile describes in a first approximation the cohesive stress σ_c as a function of the relative saturation S^* of the void space between the particles (Fig. 6).

The Use of Power Consumption Method in Dosage Form Design

With respect to FDA's PAT and QbD initiatives, respectively, the regulatory issues of FDA and EMEA (25) concerning ICH8 (Pharmaceutical Development) robust formulations are today an absolute prerequisite. Concerning the production of granules, the granule size distribution should not vary from batch to

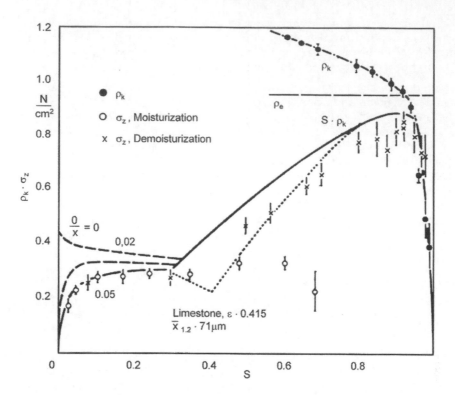

FIGURE 5   Tensile strength σ_t of a limestone powder bed as a function of the liquid saturation S^* of the void space between the particles. *Source*: From Ref. 24.

batch. The key factors are the correct amount and the type of granulating liquid. The interpretation of the power consumption profile can be very important for an optimal selection of the type of granulating liquid. The possible variation of the initial particle size distribution of the active substance and/or excipients can be compensated in case of an intelligent in-process control method, for example, based on the power consumption profile (Fig. 2). However, the formulation may not be very robust if the volume-to-volume ratio of certain excipients such as maize starch and lactose correspond to a critical ratio or percolation threshold.

With dosage form design, it is often necessary to compare the performance of two different granule formulations. These two formulations differ in composition and as a consequence vary also in the amount of granulating liquid required.

Thus, the following question arises: how can the quantity of granulating liquid be adjusted to achieve a correct comparison?

The answer is not too difficult as it is based on identified physical principles. A correct comparison between two formulations is often a prerequisite as the dissolution process of the active substance in the final granulate or tablet can be affected both by the amount of granulating liquid and by the qualitative change (excipients) in the formulation. To calculate corresponding, that is, similar amounts of granulating liquid in different compositions, it is

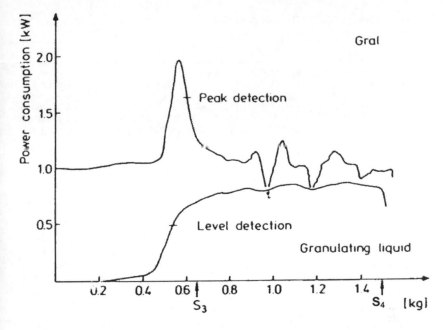

FIGURE 6   Power consumption profile of a high-speed mixer (Collette-Gral 751) with peak and level detection. Source: From Refs. 1, 8.

necessary to introduce a dimensionless amount of granulating liquid π. This amount π can be defined as degree of saturation of the interparticulate void space between the solid material (Fig. 2).

$$\pi_6 = \frac{S - S_2}{S_5 - S_2} \tag{15}$$

where S is the amount of granulating liquid (in liters); S_2, the amount of granulating liquid (in liters) necessary, which corresponds to a moisture equilibrium at approximately 100% relative humidity; and S_5, the complete saturation of interparticulate void space before a slurry is formed (amount in liters).

Power consumption is used as an analytical tool to define S values for different compositions. In fact, the power consumption profile, used as an analytical result, fulfills in an excellent way the requirements of FDA's PAT initiative. As an example, the granule formation and granule size distribution of a binary mixture of excipients can be analyzed as a function of the dimensionless amount of granulating liquid π. This strategy allows an unbiased study of the growth kinetics of granules consisting of a single substance, or binary mixture of excipients. Thus, it is important to realize that the properties of the granule batches are analyzed as a function of the dimensionless amount of granulating liquid (1,8,26–32).

If the properties of a formulation with a fixed drug load, but different amounts or qualities of different auxiliary substances (type of filler, type of

TABLE 1 The Tablet Property "Crushing Strength" Could be Well Explained by the Factors Studied

Model	GFF-MLP	SOFM-MLP	RSM
Crushing strength (N): R^2 results for the tablet compression study			
R^2 without factor batch	0.9113	0.8504	0.8970
R^2 with factor batch	0.9313	0.9246	0.9054

If the factor batch, that is, batch number, is introduced as a dummy variable, the R^2 values are not improved significantly. The "batch number" plays the role to quantify the effect of unknown factors, not taken into account during the tablet compression study. *Source*: From Ref. 33.

binder, type of disintegrant, varying amounts of excipients, different particle distributions of the starting material, etc.) are studied in a wet agglomeration process, it is extremely important to keep constant the dimensionless amount of granulating liquid π_6. If the absolute amount S of granulating liquid is kept constant instead of π_6, apples are compared with pears! In this context, it is important to realize that the statement in a standard operating procedure (SOP) of a wet agglomeration process to add as much granulating liquid as necessary is not precise at all and is one of the main source of scale-up problems. Equation (16) is the only rigorous definition of the necessary amount of granulating liquid for a correct standard operation procedure. The formerly used definition "to add a constant amount or an amount of granulating liquid, which is satisfying" to reach snowball consistency of the wet powder mass is the origin of the myth of the granulation end point (32).

FDA's PAT and EMEA's QbD initiatives (25) request a clear understanding of the unit operations involved in the manufacturing process. In this context, it is mandatory to identify key parameters responsible for the final properties of the solid dosage form such as crushing strength and drug dissolution profile of a tablet. The latter property is extremely sensitive to changes in the manufacturing process. In the publication of Bourquin et al. (33) based on response surface methodology (RSM) and on two types of artificial neural network analysis (GFF-MLP and SOFM-MLP), it was shown that only the resulting tablet crushing strength could be very well explained by the process parameters studied (Table 1). In case of the drug dissolution profile, extremely poor squared correlation coefficients R^2 were found. Interestingly, when the factor batch is included for the model development, the corresponding fitting R^2 coefficients increase (Table 2). According to the authors of paper (33), some missing parameters (factors) have already influenced the dissolution responses at a preceding fabrication step, which corresponded to the moist agglomeration and drying process.

Materials
The physical characteristics of the starting materials are compiled in Table 3. Polyvinylpyrrolidone was added in a dry state to the powder mix of lactose and cornstarch at a level of 3% (w/w). As a granulating liquid, demineralized water was used and pumped to the powder mix at constant rate of 15 g/min kg.

TABLE 2 The Tablet Property "Drug Dissolution" Could Not be Well Explained by the Factors Studied

Model	GFF-MLP	SOFM-MLP	RSM
Percentage of drug dissolved after 15 min (%): R^2 results for the tablet compression study			
R^2 without factor batch	0.2589	0.1040	0.1366
R^2 with factor batch	0.8809	0.8775	0.8679
Time to 50% drug dissolution (min): R^2 results for the tablet compression study			
R^2 without factor batch	0.3411	0.2942	0.2739
R^2 with factor batch	0.8709	0.8536	0.8449

The factor batch, that is, the batch number, contributes significantly to reach higher R^2 values. It is evident that the batch number does not improve process understanding. However, according to the conclusions of the paper, the batch number is hiding important factor(s) during the preceding granulation step.
Source: From Ref. 33.

TABLE 3 Physical Characteristics of the Starting Material

	Lactose	Cornstarch
Bulk density (g/cm^3)	0.58	0.49
Tapped density (g/cm^3)	0.84	0.65
True density (g/cm^3)	1.54	1.5
S_m (mass specific surface) (cm^2/g)	3055	
Mean diameter (μm)	40	25

Sources: From Ref. 28.

Methods

The principle of power consumption method was described in detail in the publications (8,22–27). As a high-shear mixer a Diosna V 10 was used keeping constant impeller (270 rpm) and chopper speed (3000 rpm) during the experiments.

To reduce the possible effects of friability or second agglomeration during a drying process in dish dryers, on the granule size distribution as a function of the amount of granulating liquid added, the granules are dried for 3 to 5 minutes in a fluidized bed (Glatt Uniglatt) and subsequently for 15 to 25 minutes in a dish dryer to obtain moisture equilibrium corresponding to 50% relative humidity of the air at ambient temperature (20°C). The particle size distributions were determined according to DIN 4188 using ISO-norm sieve sizes (28).

The Myth of the Granulation End Point (32)

The process of manufacturing of granules or granulation process is not well understood for the following cases, which has a direct influence on the power consumption profile:

1. The granulating liquid is non-Newtonian, that is, has a high viscosity, for example, corresponding to a paste (28)
2. The granulating liquid dissolves an important amount of the powder formulation

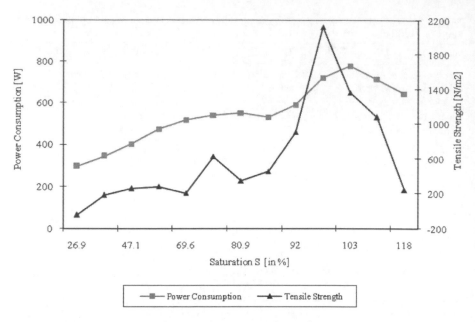

FIGURE 7 Comparison of power consumption and tensile strength measurements. *Source*: From Ref. 30.

3. The granulating liquid induces a hydration process
4. Because of a too high grade of filling ($\pi_3 = V/V^*$), the temperature (31) in the powder mix rises to such an extent that in the presence of, for example, water and starch an unwanted additional gelation processes may occur.

In an ideal case, as a binder material a very well water-soluble excipient should be added in a dry state to the powder mix and as a granulating liquid pure water should be used. In fact, the only function of the water is to form liquid bridges between the particles creating the desired attractive forces for the granulation process.

On the basis of the study of Schubert with limestone (24), the influence of the amount of liquid present in the granular material (% saturation) on power consumption and tensile strength measurements at different stops during the agglomeration process is shown in Figure 7 (30). The maxima of power consumption were determined at 100% saturation, whereas the maxima of tensile strength measurements occurs at 90% saturation as expected (24,30). The tensile strength expresses the cohesiveness between the powder particles, which is dependent on saturation and capillary pressure. The measured tensile strength σ (N/m^2) equals to the volume specific cohesion (J/m^3). The obtained results proved that the power consumption measurement is an alternative, simple, and inexpensive method to determine the cohesion of powder particles.

Thus if the cohesivity of the moist powder mass is monitored, for example, by torque or power consumption measurement a typical profile

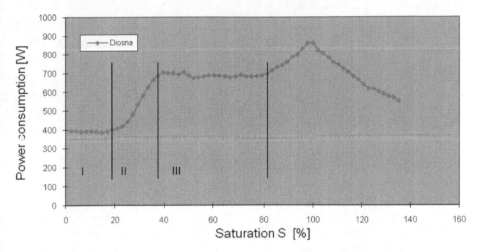

FIGURE 8 Power consumption profile of the high-shear mixer Diosna (vertical high-shear mixer).

(Fig. 8) is obtained (30,31). The Figure 8 shows the power consumption profile for a composition with 86% (w/w) lactose 200 mesh, 4% (w/w) polyvinylpyr-rolidon (as a binder in a dry state in the powder mixture, the only component that will be completely dissolved), and 10% (w/w) cornstarch. The granu-lating liquid is demineralized water, which is added by a pump with constant speed.

The different phases can be easily interpreted: *I. Water up take by corn-starch; II. start of formation of liquid bridges; III. filling-up of the interparticular void space by the granulating liquid.* Granules with a reproducible granule size distribution can be manufactured for amounts of granulating liquid, which correspond to a well-defined point of the plateau. There is no granulation end point, however there is a possibility to control the granulation process by the detection of the steepest ascent in the power consumption profile (level or peak detection method, see Fig. 6) and adding a constant amount of liquid. As an alternative, the inflexion point of the S-shaped curve of the power consump-tion profile can be determined for this "fine-tuning" process (8,15,30). The peak in Figure 6 describes a certain cohesiveness of the moistened powder bed at the beginning of the plateau phase. The peak (=first derivative of the power consumption curve) is a signal provided by the powder mass and has a self-correcting property as the signal appears at an earlier time for a slightly coarser starting material, later for a slightly finer material, i.e. taking into account the initial moisture content of the primary material, which depends on seasonal effects.

In this respect, the automated controlled mode leads to a higher homoge-neity of the granule size distribution (Table 4) than in the case of adding manually a predetermined constant amount of granulating liquid. Thus, the variability of the yield could be reduced by understanding the process.

TABLE 4   Yield and Size Distribution of Granules After a Manual and Automatic Granulation

Type of mode	Yield (% w/w) 90–710 μm	% Undersize <710 μm	% Undersize <90 μm
Manual mode n = 20 batches	81.03 ± 2.42	88.30 ± 2.05	6.80 ± 0.51
Automatic mode n − 18 batches	91.45 ± 0.36	96.80 ± 0.31	5.40 ± 0.35

Source: From Refs. 9, 10.

Practical Experiences in Scale-up using High-Shear Mixers (M.D.)

In the following practical, scale-up experiences related to high-shear mixers are reported. To study the behavior of the formulations, the power consumption pattern of the mixer/granulator is measured during the addition of granulating liquid. Thus, the power consumption level is used as a parameter to minimize batch-to-batch quality variations by keeping constant the factor "cohesional behavior" of the wet powder system.

Granulation is often considered as an art as it is a complex process and especially the transfer from a small scale to a larger scale can lead to several time-consuming unexpected events. Several issues are considered to be critical, such as the quantity of added granulating liquid, because the new mixer could require less granulating liquid as it produces a better distribution. Eventually, this could lead to a variation in the characteristics of the final tablet, such as disintegration time or the dissolution profile of the drug substance.

Two types of high-shear mixers are used in the industry, which refer to the position and direction of the mixer shaft holding the blades, that is, vertical (Fig. 9) or horizontal (Fig. 10) high-shear mixers.

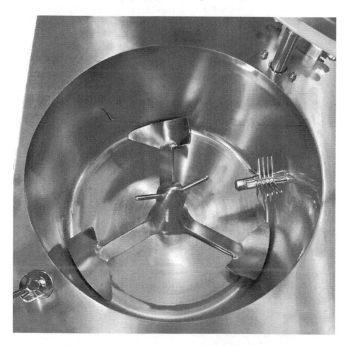

FIGURE 9   Vertical high-shear mixer type with one chopper.

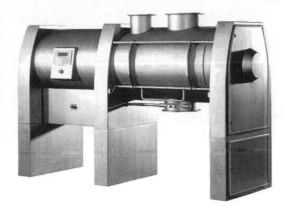

FIGURE 10 Horizontal high-shear mixer type.

The following points are considered to be crucial when working with upscaling (34–36):

1. Radius of the rotating blade and filling level
2. Swept volume (i.e., the amount of mass being moved per unit time) should always stay within an in-line ratio from one mixer to the next size up
3. Volume/force also having an in-line ratio
4. Energy input, with respect to energy input per time (i.e., power consumption)
5. Liquid saturation
6. Power consumption measurement being the tool for process control

In this chapter, practical experiences and typical problems are described together with their practical solutions/rules.

1. A typical problem that was observed several times and places was that machines, once acquired, were set out to be as versatile as possible meaning that having a mixer with a given maximum batch size, then the minimum batch size was stretched to the extreme with the result that the filling level often did not even reach the level of the chopper causing an unstable situation and result that could not be reproduced in a larger scale—*so rule number 1: Always stay within the filling level given by the producers of the mixer.* This recommendation is typically within 30% to 80% filling level (*maximum 80% and minimum being 40% out of maximum*). Again one should also here look at the position of the choppers and ensure that this is always covered with material, that is, always check bulk density and compare batch weight with volume. The point of peripheral speed was quite obvious and was not questioned.
2. The swept volume was found to have a significant impact moving from one size mixer and up. The more out of line the more out of control.
3. The volume-to-force concept was easy to comprehend, and it took only one test to establish that one would need to find a minimum size mixer that could facilitate a batch size big enough from where to make an uncomplicated scale-up.

4. Another thing that caused some curiosity was that the horizontal mixer apparently performed better than the vertical mixer producing better granules and even more controlled. In the work of Kristensen and Schaefer et al. (35,36), the idea that the shape and size of the impellers of the horizontal mixer were within the in-line ratio from one size to the next one was described. Another reason might be the *mechanically generated fluid bed*, as it visually looks as if the particle flow is easier to control. The shape of the bowl is always the same whereas the vertical mixers vary in shape from one brand to another. But there is as yet no in-depth evidence to prove this—one could only suggest that this could be a subject for a more detailed study.

Different Volumes of Horizontal High-Shear Mixers

In the beginning, mainly the vertical version of the high-speed/high-shear mixer was used for pharmaceutical applications, and some years later, experiences were also made with the horizontal type.

The Lödige horizontal mixer with a volume of 130 L was used for the upscaling experiments with a given filling level between 40% and 70%. Endless number of trials had verified this decision and for many years (decades), it had been possible to perform an uncomplicated upscaling, based on the results in the 130 L mixer and using the Froude equation, up to batch sizes of 4000 L (in the pharmaceutical industry) and furthermore also up to huge batch sizes such as 50,000 L (not within the pharmaceutical industry). The same physics and theory prevailing.

However, there is always a "but," and this represents the fourth point in the basic thoughts in upscaling: *Energy input*. A few years ago it was observed that excellent granulation results with certain specific materials (here phrased *"formulations B+"*) obtained in pilot scale could not be reproduced in production scale. This came as a complete surprise. We were used to "success" with most materials (here phrased *"formulations A+"*), that is, powder compositions with active and auxiliary substances A+, and we speak of very big numbers of formulations and over so many years there were no problems.

An investigation was initiated in order to know the effect of the size and the number of choppers of the 130 L (pilot plant) and 600 L (production plant) mixer. It was found that the only or main difference besides the volume was a 130-L mixer that had one chopper, whereas 600 L mixer had two. A simple calculation unveiled that if a 130-L mixer had one chopper then, with the same ratio to volume, a 600-L mixer should have four choppers. So a 600-L mixer was rebuilt and fitted with four choppers. The following test with formulations B+ showed that we were now having the comparable results as in pilot scale! This was a conclusion of practical experience, most surprising, as so many products had undergone the normal and basic upscaling procedure with success. In this context, a question remains, which would need a further investigation: Is the reason for the different behavior the increased energy input by the additional choppers or is it a question of the behavior of the material composition of formulations B+, showing different wet cohesion properties, which are related to the special flow characteristics of non-Newtonian fluids?

Liquid Saturation S

We realized that there is a common misunderstanding in the industry as to what relation there is between power consumption measurements and granulation end point. We saw several places where a simple ammeter was connected to the controls of a mixer and that this was expected to be the function to detect granulation end point. It is the impression of the author of this subchapter (M.D.) that despite heavy emphasis of the importance of the liquid saturation parameter, as stated in the literature, it has been widely neglected in the industry.

In many formulations, it is necessary to add the binder dissolved together with water at a higher temperature. The binder is a solid and thus a fixed parameter in the formulation, whereas water is a variable and precisely this variable is suggested to be used.

To always achieve the same level of liquid saturation from one batch to another, it is important to dose the "right" amount of liquid—which is not necessarily the same amount—during the liquid addition phase —and how is this done when one could not change the amount of binder? If the binder is added into the mass and premixed before the liquid addition there would be no problem. The pure water could be added in whatever quantity required. So we had to think differently in designing a dosing system, depicted in Figure 11.

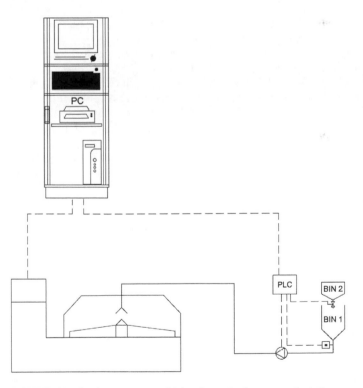

FIGURE 11 Dosing system, which allows to keep constant the amount of binder in the formulation and to "fine-tune" the required amount of "granulating liquid" by adding pure water into the vertical mixer/granulator.

It consisted of a programmable logic (PLC) controlling the pump and two bins to contain the water. The PLC was to communicate with the computer receiving load input (power consumption) from the main motor. One bin was placed on top of the other. The lower bin would contain liquid and binder, however, in a slightly more concentrated form to cater for the situation, should less liquid than usual be necessary to reach saturation level.

Why is it necessary to add different amounts of liquid to achieve the saturation level in the same formulation?

In storage, there are days of high relative humidity and days of almost zero relative humidity. Over time this one parameter can change the moisture content of the starting materials, unless the storage is humidity controlled. Other points also play an important role such as particle size distribution. Even within a given specification from a raw material supplier, when it comes to size distribution, there is room for enough variation that can cause a different surface area for the mass in total. This again would require a different amount of liquid.

Back to the description of the dosing system: When the lower bin has been emptied completely for binder/water, pure liquid/water will continue to be dosed from the upper bin down through the lower bin to wash possible residues of binder in the lower bin and the inside of the hose. When the saturation level is approaching, the pump speed can be reduced (if necessary) to whatever speed needed to ensure that liquid addition is discontinued in time. This would be determined by the technician and programmed into the recipe. On some products, this little feature had proved to be of great value.

The process recorder containing an industrial computer with a special signal amplifier made it possible to obtain a detailed graph (profile) of every product so that each process phase could clearly be detected. This signal amplifier was important to compensate for typically too powerful motors in the mixers, but also to obtain a "clean" signal where irrelevant signals such as loads coming from the gearbox were filtered away. Then we could have a pure signal related to the mass.

The power consumption was expressed in terms of load on the main motor in percentage of the capacity of the motor. At 0% of load, the motor is switched off and 100% should express the motor having reached the end of its capacity. A typical power consumption profile is shown in Figure 12.

When working in pilot scale only the recording part of the system was active to obtain the product profile, that is, to establish the product behavior as well as the saturation level. With the curve obtained in pilot scale one could set the same load levels (% load related to the capacity of the motor) to the full system when working in production scale. We could load up to 250 recipes in the database and set all values and parameters individually for each product.

This system described in the preceding text has now been in use for over 10 years both in pilot and in production, looking back the main conclusion is that the system so far has proved its function. However there are limits of course. It does not function, of course, where materials adhere to the walls during the wet massing phase. But over the years, we have made an interesting observation. In a 300-L high-shear mixer with a batch size of 120 kg, we have experienced that the system has dosed liquid with a difference of up to 7 L before the same saturation level was reached.

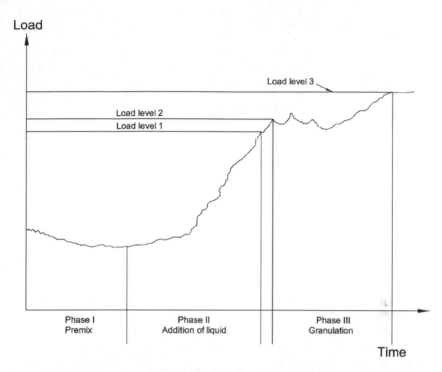

Load

Load level 3

Load level 2

Load level 1

| Phase I | Phase II | Phase III |
| Premix | Addition of liquid | Granulation |

Time

FIGURE 12 Power consumption profile (Load) as a function of time: After premixing of the powder components (API, auxiliary substances) in a dry state, the granulating liquid is added, which can consist of a binder solution and/or pure water if all binder is already in the wet powder bed (see also Fig. 11) or if the well water–soluble binder was added in the premix as a dry component. The necessary amount of granulating liquid is controlled by load levels 1 and 2, which defines the end of phase II. The end of phase III is determined by the load level 3. During phase III, that is, period of "massing" no more granulating liquid is added.

This shows that certain products really can behave differently pending environmental conditions as well as physical condition of the starting materials. Furthermore, we believe that using such a system also will be a good input to PAT initiative. Finally, it also illustrates how difficult this process can be and it is important to get the critical parameters right. What makes powder technology so interesting is that despite many years of experiences, we can still expect situations in unknown territory and several surprises.

Some General Hints Concerning the Wet Agglomeration Process in a High-Shear Mixer to Avoid Problems
According to the results described in the sections "Dimensionless Groups " to "Practical Experiences in Scale-Up Using High-Shear Mixers (M.D.)," the following hints should be helpful to reduce problems.

The production of granules consists of the following steps in general:

1. Dry blending of the primary powder material, that is, active substance and auxiliary substances in a mixer. Preference should be given to demineralized

water as granulating liquid and the excipients and the drug should show relatively low water solubility with the exception of the binder. The binder should be added preferably in a dry state as part of the powder components.

2. For disagglomeration of cohesive fine powder or for security reasons (e.g., screws left in!), a sieving step should be included. Thus for an optimal homogeneity of the powder mix, it is important to apply the following rule: blending, sieving, blending. It is evident that an appropriate mixer equipment is used such as a high-shear mixer. In case of a very potent drug, the content of the drug is low and there is a need to use micronized drug particles.

3. Wetting of the particles by adding granulating liquid, preferably pure water. If the binder is dissolved in the granulating liquid the binder solution should be Newtonian, that is, should show a low viscosity. It has to be kept in mind that the fine-tuning of the amount of granulating liquid that is optimal can only be done if the binder is a part of the dry premix. Thus, in modern high-shear mixers, the required amount of granulating liquid is often pumped into the mixer at a continuous constant rate. To avoid an over-wetting of the powder mass, a power consumption profile should be measured. In an optimal case, that is, if the formulation is suitable, the power consumption profile can be used to control the amount of the granulating liquid, which is necessary (Table 4).

4. Depending on the formulation and on the properties of the components in the powder it may be necessary to mass the moistened powder for some time before screening. However, it has to be checked whether the massing process can be avoided if the granulating liquid is pumped into the powder bed at a reasonable rate.

5. Final drying step: After the screening step, which may in certain cases have narrowed the original native granule size distribution, the granules may be preferably dried in a fluidized bed equipment using, for example, a temperature end point of the granulate temperature to define the final moisture content (1). Depending on the properties of the dried material, a final screening operation may be necessary.

ROBUST FORMULATIONS AND DOSAGE FORM DESIGN
The Effect of Percolation Theory

In the case of binary mixtures consisting of different substances, which, individually, may have a considerable effect on the physical properties (e.g., electrical conductivity) of the final product (granules, tablets, etc.), the ratio of components is essential. Thus, with a mixture between Al_2O_3 (an electrically insulating material) and copper powder, electrical conductivity of the Al_2O_3/copper tablet is only observed if the copper powder forms an electrical pathway between the electrodes attached to the surface of the tablet produced. The critical ratio where conductivity is measured corresponds to the so-called percolation threshold p_c (11). In the case of a fixed normalized amount π of granulating liquid, it is interesting to note that the granules obtained from a lactose/cornstarch powder mixture lead to granule size distributions equivalent either to the granule size distribution of lactose or to cornstarch. This result can be interpreted on the basis of percolation theory (Fig. 13); that is, the properties

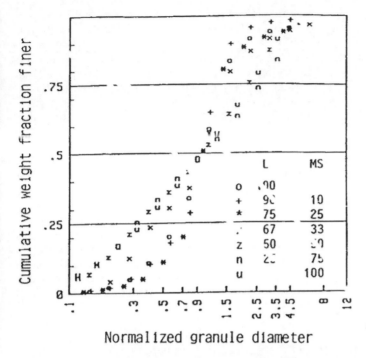

FIGURE 13 Cumulative particle size distribution of the agglomerates at a fixed normalized amount π_6 (=0.62) of granulating liquid for different ratios of the binary powder mixture lactose/cornstarch. *Source*: From Ref. 13.

differ for compositions below or above a critical ratio p_c of components between lactose and cornstarch.

A QUASI-CONTINUOUS GRANULATION AND DRYING
PROCESS (QCGDP) TO AVOID SCALE-UP PROBLEMS
Continuous Processes and the Batch Concept

In the food and chemical industry continuous production lines play an important role, whereas the pharmaceutical industry production is mainly based on a batch-type procedure. Only in case of high-volume pharmaceutical products with a production of, for example, more than 1000 kg/day, dedicated fully continuous production lines have been installed. It is important to take care of the QbD initiative as fully continuous processes need to be controlled tightly to avoid dynamic instabilities. In specific cases, the patent DE 196 39579 C 1 such a dynamic instability of the real granulation process can be used as an advantage (see patent DE 196 39579 C 1). Concerning the safety of a dosage form and quality assurance, the batch concept is very convenient. Thus, a well-defined batch can be accepted or rejected. With the upcoming *personalized medicine* in case of a specific disease linked to a specific genome of a smaller number of patients, the pharmaceutical production will rely on the batch concept.

In the case of a continuous process, a batch has to be defined somehow artificially, that is, the amount of product, for example, amount of granules produced within six to eight hours. On the other hand, continuous processes such as the dry agglomeration of particles based on a compaction process (37,38) offer two important advantages: (*i*) there is no difficult scale-up exercise necessary for larger batches, (*ii*) a 24-hour automatic production line should be possible. For this reason, the dry agglomeration process is not a topic of this scale-up chapter. It is evident that the dry agglomeration process is preferentially applied in case of water-sensitive drugs. On the other hand, it is important to realize that the compressibility and compactibility of the resulting dry granules depend on the crystalline properties of the primary material. In fact, the brittleness or the plastic behavior under stress of the primary particles are a function of the number of crystalline defects (39). Thus, a variability of the quality of the primary material can directly affect the quality of the final product. In this context, it is of interest to know that the wet agglomeration process often improves the compressibility and compactibility of the primary material. It is also well known that the wet agglomeration process improves the wettability of the drug substance, which has a direct influence on its dissolution profile in a tablet or capsule formulation (40). A survey of continuous granulation processes has been published by Vervaet and Remon (41). A fully continuous wet agglomeration process has been realized with the concept of the Glatt ProCell Equipment (42), which is used in the area of food, nutraceuticals, and pharmaceuticals (43) (Fig. 14).

The Quasi-Continuous Production Line for Granules as a Rigorous Concept to Achieve Six Sigma Quality in Scale-up

The performance of a process in terms of quality can be quantified on the basis of its sigma value. A value of six sigma means that the number of defects manufactured is as low as 3.4 ppb. Such a performance is outstanding and is reached by the chip manufacturers to ensure the functioning of computers, etc. In case of the pharmaceutical industry, the sigma value of ca. 2 has been estimated, which is low and prompted FDA's PAT and QbD initiatives and new regulatory issues (25). Many factors contribute to this low sigma value (44) and as a remedy PriceWaterhouseCoopers (PwC) has published a series of books under the topic Pharma 2020 (45). One of the conclusions and suggestions of PwC consists in replacing as much as possible expensive lab work by in silico work. The goal is to save money and to increase the quality of the work, as already realized in the aircraft industry (46,47).

In the early development of a dosage form only small batches are produced for the first clinical trials. At a later phase larger batch sizes are needed, which are produced with a different equipment of larger size. Because of the fact that the similarity criteria are in general not fulfilled, scale-up issues can become critical and may contribute significantly to a low sigma value. This is an intrinsic difficulty. A straightforward solution is to install an identical quasi-continuous production line in the R&D and production department. Thus, the desired batch size B consists of a number n of subunits b, that is, $B = nb$. The size of the subunit b can be as low as 7 kg, with $n = 1$, $B = 7$ kg, and with $n = 100$, $B = 700$ kg (16–19). In this case, the "scale-up" process is not a function of the physical size of the equipment but is translated into the time dimension (19). A larger batch size just needs a longer process time. Such a process can be automated and controlled using appropriate IPC tests.

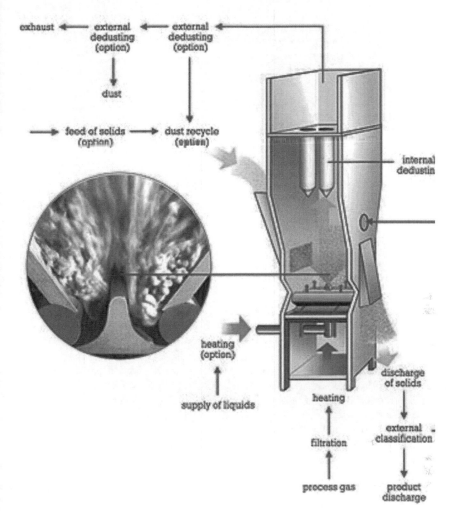

exhaust ◄─── external ◄─── external ◄───
                dedusting   dedusting
                (option)   (option)

                    ↓
                  dust

─────► feed of solids ───► dust recycle
          (option)   (option)

                                                    internal
                                                    dedustin

heating
(option)

                                                    discharge
                                                    of solids

supply of liquids   heating

                                                    external
                           filtration   classification

                        process gas   product
                                                   discharge

FIGURE 14 Scheme of the Glatt ProCell 5 spouted bed process chamber (42), which can be used as a continuous production unit equipped with a zig-zag discharge, allowing to achieve a narrow granule, respectively pellet size distribution (43).

With this concept, it is possible to combine the advantages of a batch-type and continuous production (16–19,48–51). The principle of this quasi-continuous production line developed by Glatt is based on a semicontinuous production of minibatches in a specially designed high-shear mixer/granulator that is connected to a continuous multicell-fluidized (Glatt Multicell®) bed dryer (Fig. 15).

To study the feasibility of such a quasi-continuous production line, different formulations were tested and compared with a conventional batch process.

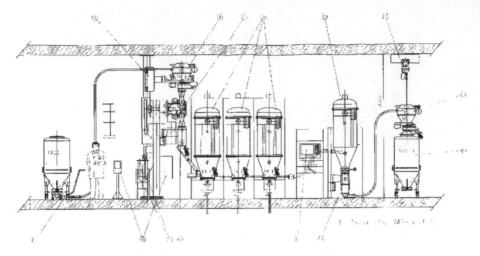

FIGURE 15 A quasi-continuous production line for granules with three drying cells (Patent EP 1 157 736 A1, Glatt AG, CH-4133 Pratteln).

The weighing system that is available on the market was not involved in the first experiments. Thus, a prefixed amount of powder of the placebo formulation was added to the specially designed high-shear mixer and thoroughly mixed. Subsequently, this amount of powder is granulated by continuously adding granulating liquid up to a fixed amount. The ideal amount of granulating liquid can be defined according to the results of a power consumption measurement (7–10,26–32). Afterward the moist granules are discharged through a screen into the first cell of the multicell-fluidized bed dryer unit to avoid any formation of lumps. Thus, the quasi-continuous production of granules can be described as a train of minibatches passing like parcels the compartments of dry mixing, granulation, and drying. The multicell dryer consists, in general, of three cells that are designed for different air temperatures, that is, in the first cell the granules are dried at a high temperature, for example, 60°C, and in the last cell ambient air temperature and humidity can be used to achieve equilibrium conditions. If appropriate more cells can be added.

Because of this principle, a batch defined for quality control purposes consists of a fixed number of n minibatches. Thus, a tight in-process control of the mixing/granulation (7–10) and drying step (1,15) provides an excellent batch record of the quasi-continuous production of granules and an excellent opportunity for a continuous validation of the process and the equipment (15–19,48–51).

Thus, based on the positive results obtained with the thesis work of Schade (16) and Dörr (18), a new plant for quasi-continuous wet granulation and multiple-chambered fluid bed drying was developed by Glatt AG CH, Pratteln, in cooperation with F. Hoffmann-La Roche Ltd. Basel and the Institute of Pharmaceutical Technology of the University of Basel. For this achievement, the Institute of Pharmaceutical Technology received the Innovation Award of the Cantons Basel-City and Basel-Country in 1994.

The system gives a new possibility for industrial manufacturing and galenical development of pharmaceutical solids specialties and has following purposes:

Automatized unattended production, withdrawing from scale-up experiments and thus a shorter development time for new specialties, with the aim of a shorter time to market. Manufacturing procedures can be simplified, validated faster, and the quality of granules, tablets, and kernels compared to common production is equal until better. Different solids specialties have been tested and validated.

Goals of the Quasi-Continuous Granulation and Drying Line

Unattended production. One of the general aims of quasi-continuous granulation and fluid bed drying is unattended production. The production of small subunits of 7 to 9 kg instead of a whole batch allows an automatized, iterative granulation and drying procedure. The division of the process into different compartments (mixing, sieving, and drying compartments) guarantees the reproducibility of the galenical properties of each subunit.

No necessity for scale-up experiments. The granulation and drying of subunits of 7 to 9 kg instead of a whole batch gives the possibility to use the plant for laboratory and production scale, because the batch size is no more characterized by the machine size but by the number of produced subunits. Using the same plant in galenical research, development and production may shorten the time to market for new solids specialties.

Simplification of manufacturing procedures. Existing manufacturing procedures can be taken over from common equipment without changing components. In certain cases, it is possible to simplify the procedures. The small mixer size and the geometry of the mixing elements allow to add the binders into the premixture and just to granulate with water.

Identical or better quality of granules and tablets. The quality of the produced granules and tablets has to be equal or better and fulfills the product specifications.

Results

Constant values and reproducibility of the process are important facts of quasi-continuous granulation. The tests could also show equal until better quality of granules and tablets compared to common granulation equipment (Diosna $\sim$ P-600 high-speed granulator).

Compression force/hardness profile. The compression/hardness profile of a granule batch is an important property. Different subunits were selected of two formulations (Figs. 16 and 17) and compressed using different compression forces to obtain tablets. The tablets were tested for hardness as a function of different subunit numbers (Figs. 16 and 17). From experience, it is well known that certain formulations show an excellent compression profile as small batches but do not keep this property on increasing batch size (Fig. 18). This is another advantage of the quasi-continuous production concept as, in principle, the quality of the small batch is not changed by the repetitive procedure.

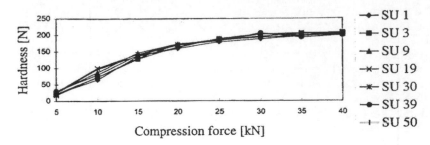

FIGURE 16 Compression force/hardness profile (formulation 1).

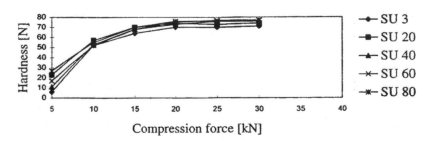

FIGURE 17 Compression force/hardness profile (formulation 2).

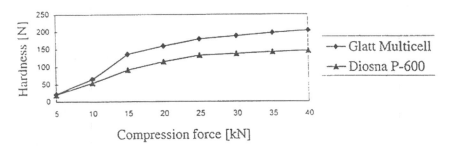

FIGURE 18 Scale-up effect showing a different compression/hardness profile of the same formulation, being manufactured in a small scale with the quasi-continuous production unit of Glatt Multicell® and conventionally in a 600-L Diosna P-600 high-shear mixer/granulator. *Source*: From Refs. 16 to 19.

Description of the Production Plant

The Glatt Multicell unit for quasi-continuous granulation and fluid bed drying consists of the following elements: a transport and dosage system for mixer filling (1); a horizontal high-speed plough-share mixer (subunits of 4–9 kg of premixture can be granulated) with an airless spray pump for the granulation liquid (2); rotary sieving machines for wet and final sieving (3); a three-chambered fluid bed dryer for predrying, final drying, and cooling down to room temperature (4); a transport system to collect the granulated subunits in a container (5); and an integrated washing-in-place (WIP) system (Fig. 19).

The Glatt Multicell Equipment

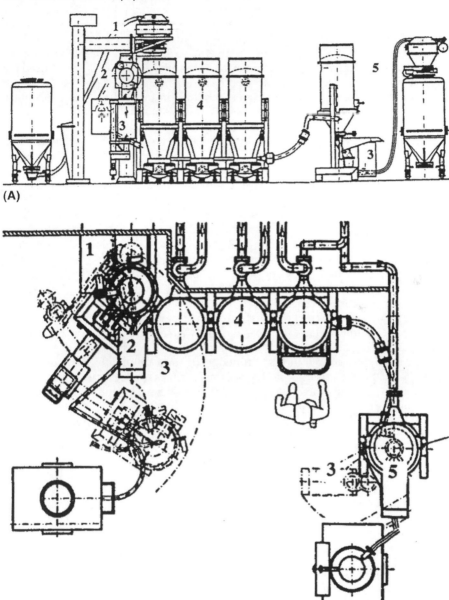

(A)

(B)

FIGURE 19 (**A**) Side view of the Glatt Multicell. 1 = transport and dosage system for mixer filling, 2 = horizontal high-speed plough-share mixer, 3 = rotary sieving machines for wet and final sieving, 4 = three-chambered fluid bed dryer, 5 = transport system. (**B**) Top view of the Glatt Multicell equipment: 1 = transport and dosage system for mixer filling, 2 = horizontal high-speed plough-share mixer, 3 = rotary sieving machines for wet and final sieving, 4 = three-chambered fluid bed dryer, 5 = transport system.

Advantages of the Quasi-Continuous Granulation and Drying Line
The production line can be fully automated and equipped with a cleaning-in-place (CIP) system. The moist agglomeration process can be monitored for each subunit by a power consumption in-process control device. Because of the three different cells of the Glatt Multicell drying equipment, a gentle drying of temperature-sensitive drug substances are possible. According to the needs, a "just-in-time production" of the desired batch size B can be implemented. Early, small-sized batches can be already considered as production batches of identical quality. Thus, these early batches can be put on a long-term stability test already at the beginning of the development of the dosage form. As the early clinical batches are produced on the exactly same equipment as the large production batches, no bioequivalence test between early clinical batches and later production batches is needed. Because of these facts no scale-up development is necessary. Thus, the development time and the time needed to market can be reduced.

Interestingly according to the studies of Schade (16) and Dörr (18), the majority of the existing formulations, manufactured separately with a wet agglomeration process in a high-shear mixer and dried conventionally in a fluidized bed equipment, can be transferred without changing the formulation to the above-described quasi-continuous production line. Totally 30 formulations were tested with a positive result of 28 out of 30. This is an excellent result, as a transfer of a formulation working fine with batch process needs in general a reformulation for a successful transfer to a real continuous process.

Unfortunately, scale-up experiments, which lead to surprising effects (Fig. 18), are not uncommon. In addition, the wet agglomeration process is still not fully understood and is a function of the formulation and equipment used (Table 2). For these reasons, the only solution to reduce "surprising" effects during the scale-up processes as a result of the type of equipment and of a nonrobust formulation is the following procedure:

1. It is absolutely important that an identical equipment of a quasi-continuous production line is available in the R&D and in the manufacturing department.
2. It is important that the formulation is optimized to be robust already in the early development phase, that is, clinical phase I.
3. To reduce the amount of laboratory work in this early development phase, new techniques need to be employed similar to the aircraft industry, that is, to introduce virtual R&D reality in the development of solid dosage forms (45–47).

For the implementation of such a rigorous concept, a close connectivity (51) between the involved departments is a prerequisite. A "standing-alone" solution of a single equipment in one of the departments is not sufficient and does not allow a return on investment.

So far, such a comprehensive concept has not yet been realized by any company. This concept allows to produce with the identical equipment small and large volumes of the desired formulation. Thus, it is possible to avoid scale-up problems and to improve the quality by design leading to a higher sigma value. This concept permits together with a reduction of the necessary amount of laboratory work to perform a paradigm change, that is, to develop already for clinical phase I a robust high-quality dosage form ready for the market (47).

SCALE-UP OF THE CONVENTIONAL FLUIDIZED BED SPRAY GRANULATION PROCESS (D.J.)
Introduction
The batch-type fluidized bed process is widely used in the pharmaceutical industry for spray granulation and/or drying as a step subsequent to some type of wet granulation. Batches produced in high- or low-shear granulators, or by the fluidized bed spray granulation process, may be dried rapidly owing to the superior heat and mass transfer capabilities of this technique. Granules produced by the wet granulation methods (high and low shear) and by fluidized bed spray granulation typically differ in structure, and possibly behavior. The force applied and the absence of evaporation during high-shear granulation tends to produce denser granules. The fluidized bed is a low-shear process in which granule properties are determined by process parameters, and the resulting granules are porous. The two processes generally do not produce equivalent products, and, in most cases, product formulations may need to be adapted to the chosen method. In high-shear granulation, the list of process variables is comparatively short—main impeller configuration and speed; chopper speed; liquid addition method and droplet size (if atomized); and finally, kneading time and power consumption or torque for end-point determination. The list is considerably longer in fluidized bed spray granulation, and these will be elucidated later. Although there are many process variables, and there is interaction among them, in general, they are well understood and repeatable. Batch-type fluid bed equipment is tailored to batch size, which may range from a few hundred grams to more than one metric ton. The combination of reproducibility and batch size flexibility results in a highly efficient as a manufacturing method.

Equipment Considerations
Figure 20 shows a fluidized bed dryer vertically integrated with a high-shear granulator, a wet mill, bottom discharge, and a dry mill. The basic components of the machine will be described beginning with the entrance of the process air. The lower plenum acts as a transition piece, conducting the process air from the round duct from the air handler (where the air is heated and may be humidity controlled) to the bottom of the product container. Within this region, a probe is located for measuring the temperature of the incoming process air. The plenum is typically open but may contain components for an agitator, which may be used for types of products that are resistant to moving by only the air stream. The product container itself is conical to enhance mixing and allow a high velocity to be used where the air enters the product bed. The base of the product container is multipurpose. Typically, a perforated plate acts as an air distribution device to assist the air, which enters the lower plenum at a right angle to the product container, to spread evenly across the bottom of the product bed. Above the distributor plate, there is a fine screen that acts as a product retention device. The type and porosity of this screen may be product dependent. The most porous screens are those as defined in the ASTM E-11 specification (used in the U.S. Standard or Tyler series). The openings are roughly square, with the

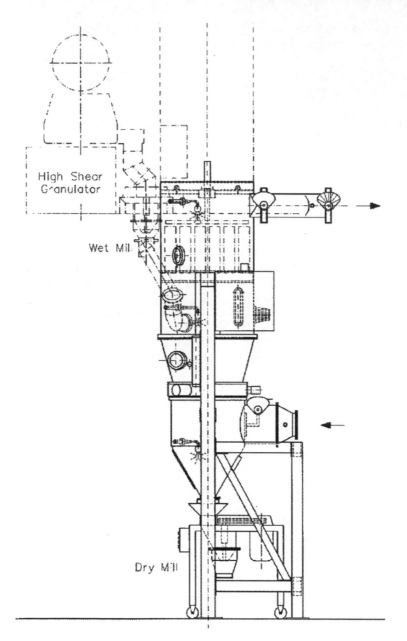

FIGURE 20 Example of a vertically integrated high shear granulator/fluidized bed dryer, including a wet mill for de-lumping and a dry mill for granule "sizing." *Source*: Courtesy of Glatt Air Techniques, Inc.

number per linear inch specified. With a defined wire diameter, the size of the opening is then identified (e.g., a 100 mesh screen has 100 openings per inch which are 150 μm). An advantage is that this type of screen is very porous (high percentage of open area) and not as subject to occlusion as other types of screening. A potential disadvantage is that they are thin and hence comparatively weak, and the square opening does not allow retention of relatively fine material (possibility of product loss in the lower plenum). For this reason, a more commonly used type is referred to as a Dutch Weave screen. This variety has the wires tightly packed in one direction, creating openings that are a more tortuous path for product to travel through to the lower plenum. The porosity of this screen is referred to in microns, and this may be the dimension of the longest portion of the opening. For instance, a 150-μm Dutch Weave screen would have an opening of 150 μm in one direction with the other dimension equal to the diameter of the wire. This results in a screen with better product retention characteristics, but lower permeability (which is not necessarily a problem). These screens are also stronger, and as such have a longer life in a manufacturing operation.

The use of screens for product retention in fluidized bed driers is not universal. In some applications, both product retention and air distribution are handled by a low-permeability perforated sheet or plate that contains relatively small openings. In the gill plate or Conidur® sheet, high fluidization air velocity through the plate may be sufficient to avoid significant material loss into the lower plenum, in spite of the fact that it is likely that some of the product is finer than the openings in the distributor plate. This type of plate may be more commonly used in applications where CIP (for product change) or WIP (a somewhat less stringent requirement) is considered in the machine design. In some plate designs, the perforations impart a horizontal flow to the air and product. The distributor plate is a composite of directed flow segments, which may be used in conjunction with side discharge. When processing is completed, the product is withdrawn (with vacuum assistance) through an opening at the perimeter of the product container. The directional nature of air flow is not manifested during processing. However, as the batch is evacuated and the bed depth decreases, the residual material begins to rotate in the product container. As it approaches the opening, it is drawn out into a receiving vessel.

Other components may be housed in the product container. First, product temperature is often a critical control parameter for the spray granulation and/or drying process. A temperature probe is located in the product container such that it is in contact with the flowing product. Within a short distance above the base of the product container, heat is exchanged for moisture, and evaporative cooling depresses the product temperature to a value well below the inlet air temperature. Above this critical distance, the bed may be considered to be isothermal—rapid motion of material creates a condition whereby the temperature is the same throughout a large region because of the rapidly fluidizing batch. As such, the location of the product temperature probe is not critical. It may be placed in an area above the product container, in the lower segment of the expansion chamber. Provided that the product continues to wash over it, the temperature response will be a consequence of conduction (solid to solid contact), not convection, which is a slower process, and therefore less responsive.

Another common component is a device for withdrawing a product sample during the process for monitoring product attributes such as particle size (and distribution), density, and, most importantly, moisture. There is debate as to how representative the sample is, and its reliability may be product dependent. If particle size distribution in the drying granulation is reasonable, it is a good method of in-process monitoring, and its use is strongly encouraged.

Moisture-laden air exits the batch, passing through a filter (sock-type fabric or a type of cartridge). A third temperature probe may be located in the exhaust duct of the machine, measuring the exiting air temperature. At some distance from the product itself, it measures exit air temperature, which may be subject to heat loss to the surrounding metal mass. Also, the change in temperature is the result of convection, and the consequence is that it is likely to be less responsive than the product temperature probe—it reacts more slowly and to a lesser degree because of the fact that it is not in direct contact with the solid product. It is therefore suggested that the exhaust temperature be used only as a backup to the product temperature probe, especially if temperature is used to aid in moisture end-point determination.

Process Variables

Table 5 lists variables to be considered when developing the fluidized bed spray granulation process:

As shown in the Table 5, the variables are typically divided into two categories—major: those typically expected to significantly influence product properties and minor: those that will have minimal impact. There are also interactions between variables. The major variables can be divided into two significant categories: those impacting the drying rate (inlet air temperature, volume, and dew point), and spraying (solution spray rate, atomizing air volume/pressure). For instance, process air volume affects not only the amount of heat energy delivered to the bed but also the fluidization pattern and particle velocity. Spray rate affects not only the droplet size (and the resultant granule size) but also the product moisture profile during spraying. When basic feasibility studies have been conducted, it is recommended that the list be narrowed, and that further experiments be carried out within the context of a design of experiments to quantify their impact on the properties of the finished product. The domain for the process variables must be selected carefully to assure that

TABLE 5   Major and Minor Process Variables to be Considered in Fluidized Bed Spray Granulation

Major	Minor
Inlet air temperature	Nozzle port size
Inlet air volume	Nozzle height (with respect to static bed surface)
Inlet air dew point	Nozzle spray cone angle
Product/exhaust temperatures (dependent variables)	Spray liquid temperature (viscosity)
Solution spray rate	Outlet filter type
Product moisture content during spraying (dependent variable)	Outlet filter shake (pulse) interval/time
Atomizing air volume/pressure	
Batch size	

the resulting effects are measurable. The success of scale-up from the lab to the manufacturing equipment strongly depends on the robustness of the product and process as well as a good understanding of which variables have the greatest impact in small-scale machines.

Scale-up Considerations

Planning for scale-up is already a part of the development process. A formulation that is a challenge to produce or reproduce in the laboratory will be an even larger problem in the manufacturing equipment. In production, batch size will increase substantially, and there will be a consequential mass effect. Fluidized bed granules or agglomerates are by nature porous, and there are both surface and interstitial pores. These generally enhance compressibility, disintegration, and dissolution. However, porosity and tensile strength are inversely related, and the influence of mass with respect to the larger batch size is that compaction may reduce porosity and/or enhance attrition (loss of granule structure). It is understandable that there is an influence of a larger batch size and increased bed depth on the granules. Granules in a batch of 500 kg are exposed to considerably more force than those in a laboratory scale batch of 5 kg. Although the magnitude of the impact is probably not predictable, in general, an increase in bulk density of approximately 20% as a function of scale-up in large machines may be expected. However, another key granule property, particle size and distribution, is related to droplet size, and as long as this is preserved in scale-up, the granule size and distribution of the larger batch should be comparable.

Scale-up Considerations: Drying—Process Air Volume

Irrespective of the method used to produce the granules and the consequent batch size, a significant factor in scale-up is the increase in drying capacity in the larger equipment. The heat delivered to the bed of fluidizing granules comes from a combination of inlet air temperature and volume, and, to a lesser extent, inlet air dew point. As previously mentioned, the process air volume is also responsible for fluidization behavior, and this will be the first variable to be considered.

All products require a volume and velocity of air to break the cohesive bonds between particles, wet or dry, to permit the batch to become fully fluidized. Laboratory trials will yield values for process air volume for the various stages of the process. Using this volume and the dimensions of the product container, a "face" velocity through the distributor plate can be estimated (permeability of the plate is not considered). It is reasonable to assume that approximately the same velocity will be needed in scale-up. In Table 6, estimates for process air volume are derived from the cross-sectional areas of the base of the product container for various sizes of fluid bed dryers.

The derived values for process air volume in the Table 6 should be used as starting points in the larger equipment, and adjusted depending on the observed fluidization behavior and performance of the outlet air filter (excessive pneumatic transport of fines into the filter may affect the ability to maintain the process air volume). Other factors may influence the response of the product. Larger product containers may be geometrically similar, and reasonably preserve the aspect ratio of the batch (bed depth to diameter) to permit axial (vertical) rotation or mixing of the fluidizing particles. Products that consist of

TABLE 6   Estimations of Process Air Volume in Scale-up as a Function of Product Container Distributor Plate Dimensions

Machine model	GPCG-5	GPCG-60	GPCG-300
Product container volume	22 L	220 L	1060 L
Cross-sectional area of bottom screen	0.042 m^2	0.42 m^2	1.04 m^2
Velocity of air through bottom screen	1.0 m/sec	1.0 m/sec	1.0 m/sec
Volume of air required to maintain velocity	151 m^3/hr[a]	1512 m^3/hr	3744 m^3/hr

[a]Assume that this value was determined by experimentation and that the velocity (above) was calculated using bottom screen or distributor plate cross-sectional area. Values for process air volume in the remaining product containers are estimates based on maintaining the same face velocity.

Source: Equipment dimensions courtesy of Glatt Air Techniques, Inc.

materials that are coarse in particle size (large substrates or granules for drying) or are high in density will react strongly to the increased bed depth common in manufacturing equipment. If the bed depth is excessive, bubbles of air will have difficulty in making their way through the mass. They will coalesce into very large bubbles, and this may result in slugging, where a large mass of product emerges from the bed as a unit before collapsing back into the product container. This fluidization regime is generally considered to be undesirable. While this behavior may be inconsequential to a drying process, it is unwelcome for spray granulation because of the adverse influence on droplet distribution in the bed. A second consequence of an overly deep bed is that the product container wall is conical, and viscose product may not funnel downward at the wall, resulting in regional bed stalling. In this condition, a significant quantity of wet product remains at the wall, unable to be exposed to the heated process air for drying. The distribution of moisture in the completed batch will be compromised. There may be consequences to the finished product properties, particularly if the granulation will be used for tableting. On the machine control panel, fluidization behavior may be seen in the response of the product differential pressure—a smoothly fluidized bed will yield a narrow range from peak to trough, whereas a slugging bed will reveal broad swings from the average. For purposes of illustration, the example in Figure 21 shows the evolution of fluidization behavior in a top spray–fluidized bed layering and coating process, where a large quantity of solid material is applied. As both the batch size and the particle size of the product increase, the range (peak to trough values) in product differential pressure is broader. The early stages of the process illustrate the behavior of a batch with a comparatively shallow bed depth, and the latter stages indicate the behavior of a considerably deeper bed.

Scale-up Considerations: Drying—Process Air Dew Point and Dry Bulb Temperature

Prior to a discussion on the impact of processing air dew point and temperature on the drying rate behavior of a product, it is necessary to consider heat and mass transfer. Water will move from the granule to air in an attempt to reach an equilibrium, or saturated condition, determined by thermodynamics, which can be read from a phase diagram or psychrometric chart. The rate at which water will move from liquid in the granule to vapor in the air increases, the further away the system is from equilibrium. When the water evaporates, it requires an

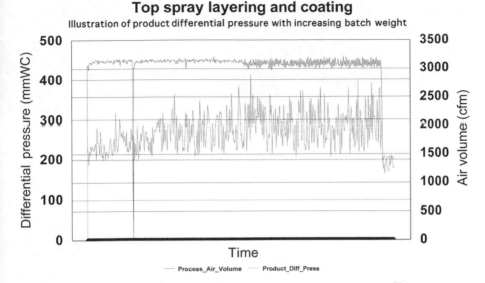

FIGURE 21 Influence of increasing batch size on product differential pressure and process air volume for a pilot scale top spray layering and coating process. *Source*: Courtesy of Glatt Air Techniques, Inc.

amount of energy, the heat of vaporization, to change from liquid to vapor. Because of this, we must also consider transfer of heat as well as movement of material. These concepts can be described by equations shown in Table 5.

It is obvious that changes in the driving force change the rate at which material and heat is removed. In addition, the proportionality constant is dependent on the surface area, temperature, drying air velocity, and the properties of the material such as porosity, density, morphology, etc.

Equations for heat and mass transfer in a wet granule are as follows:

Heat transfer $$\frac{\Delta Q}{\Delta t} = h(T_2 - T_1) \tag{16}$$

Mass transfer $$\frac{\Delta M}{\Delta t} = K(C_2 - C_1) \tag{17}$$

Relation between equations $$\frac{\Delta Q/\Delta t}{\Delta H_{\text{vap}}} = K(C_2 - C_1) \tag{18}$$

Where Q = heat
$\quad t$ = time
$\quad T_1$ = inlet air temperature
$\quad T_2$ = product temperature
$\quad h$ = heat transfer coefficient
$\quad M$ = mass

C_1 = moisture in ambient air
C_2 = capacity of the heated air
K = mass transfer coefficient
ΔH_{vap} = heat of vaporization

A major component in the delivery of heat energy to the product is the temperature of the process air. A lesser contributor, but one that should not be ignored, is the dew point of the air for processing. When warm air of a given moisture content (absolute humidity) interacts with a water-wetted batch, the heat is exchanged for moisture, and the temperature of the air drops (by evaporative cooling). The product temperature closely approximates this air temperature. If water moves freely within the substrate, the resulting temperature will represent a dew point. In other words, the air leaving the product and the machine tower is completely saturated with moisture, or is at 100% relative humidity.

If the process is developed such that a comparatively low incoming air temperature is used, variations in incoming air humidity may dramatically impact both the product temperature and the drying rate. For illustration, assume that the process air volume and liquid spray rate are held constant. In the first example, ambient air, with a dew point of 10°C, is heated to 60°C for processing. Assuming free movement of water in the substrate, air passing through the product bed will result in a product temperature of 26°C. From psychrometry software (Winmetrix v.4.5, Drying Doctor, Inc., Verdun, Quebec, Canada), the incoming air contains 7.62 g of water per kg of dry air. Exchange of heat for moisture results in 21.22 g of water per kg of dry air in the exiting air stream, for a net drying rate of 13.60 g/kg. The temperature difference between the inlet and product (60–26°C) is 34°C, and reflects a moderate drying rate. In the second example, the only change is the ambient air dew point, now elevated to 20°C. When heated to the process air temperature set point of 60°C and passed through the bed of wet product, the air again leaves saturated, containing 26.89 g of water per kg of dry air, but at a product temperature of 29.8°C. The nearly 4°C rise in the product temperature is the consequence of reduced evaporative cooling because of the increased absolute humidity in the ambient air (14.68 g/kg at 20°C dew point vs. 7.68 g/kg at 10°C dew point). The smaller difference between the inlet and the product temperatures (60–29.8°C) of 30.2°C is reflective of a decreased drying rate. In real terms, the drying rate is 12.21 g/kg in the second example and 13.60 g/kg for the first scenario, for a difference of 1.39 g/kg or 11.4%. In a simple drying application, this translates to a longer drying time when the ambient air is more humid. However, if spray granulation is taking place, there is a larger concern. In most processes, the spray rate is held at a fixed value. In this set of examples, there would be a significant difference in wetting rate, or the rate at which the batch accumulates moisture. At the higher dew point, the batch would accumulate moisture faster, and would have a higher moisture profile for the entire batch, particularly at the end of spraying. If granule properties are related to this moisture profile, which is a common characteristic, it is evident that the product could be significantly impacted simply by the variation in ambient air dew point when using a relatively low inlet air temperature.

Dew point of the process air is a concern in scale-up. In small laboratory machines (up to about 2 kg in batch capacity), the air for processing may be drawn from the room in which it is being operated. A facility air handling system typically controls the humidity of the lab areas in a comparatively narrow range throughout the year, in absolute and relative terms. In a sense, it is tantamount to having humidity control on the fluid bed. However, larger machines (pilot, production scale) require increased air volumes and must draw their air from outside of the building, making their processes subject to seasonal variation in ambient humidity. The aforementioned problem may be addressed in a number of ways. First, high inlet air temperatures should be explored, because very hot air has a much greater capacity for water. Repeating the previous examples with the process air temperature elevated to 90°C will illustrate the point. Ambient air with a 10°C dew point, heated to 90°C and passed through a bed of wet product will yield a product and exit air temperature of 32.1°C. The exit air will contain 30.68 g water per kg of dry air, and subtracting 7.62 g/kg initial absolute humidity will yield a drying rate of 23.06 g/kg. Ambient air with a 20°C dew point, heated to 90°C and passed through a bed of wet product will yield a product and exit air temperature of 35.1°C. In this case, the exit air will contain 36.80 g water per kg of dry air. Subtracting the 14.70 g/kg absolute humidity in the ambient air yields a drying rate of 22.10 g/kg, a difference of 0.94 g/kg, or only 4.1%. It is evident that there will still be an impact of the variation in ambient air dew point, but the magnitude is considerably smaller.

Ideally, all sizes of the fluid bed equipment should be equipped with inlet air dew point control. In the northern climates, this would include dehumidification in the summer months and humidification during the cold, dry winter months. In this manner, the inlet air dew point becomes a recipe-managed set point, and there is no seasonal influence of ambient dew point, irrespective of the selected inlet air temperature (high or low).

Irrespective of the possibility of dew point control, high inlet temperatures should be explored because of the influence on productivity (considerably shorter process times). Additionally, a high inlet air temperature may help to counter a factor typically only seen in scale-up: the so-called "mass effect," or the influence of the weight of the larger batch size on itself. Fluidization of a heavy batch may cause compaction of the porous granules, as mentioned previously. In general, granule porosity is related to temperature—the higher the temperature, the greater the porosity, and the lower the resulting tensile strength. This influence is critical for products requiring rapid dispersibility characteristics in their end use—those packaged into sachets and intended to be stirred into water before use, for instance. If laboratory experimentation has found that the process air temperature strongly impacts product properties, it is advisable to use the same value in scale-up. However, if compaction in the larger machine causes an increase in density (lower porosity), and the porosity was a desirable product attribute, to an extent, a higher inlet air temperature may offset the mass effect seen in the production scale equipment. A second benefit is the probability that the moisture content during spraying may be very close to the desired residual maximum value, essentially eliminating a drying step. Once spraying is completed, the process is stopped and the batch immediately discharged.

Scale-up Considerations: Spraying—Spray Rate and Droplet
Size of Sprayed Liquids

A major consideration in the scale-up of a fluidized bed spray granulation process relates to liquid delivery. As stated previously, granule size and structure is strongly related to droplet size of the binder or water being sprayed into the fluidizing substrate particles. It is imperative that the larger equipment is capable of delivering the liquid to the bed at a rate that is compatible with the available drying capacity, and at a droplet size that is essentially equivalent to that used in the laboratory. In other words, if the spray rate in the laboratory was 100 g/min at 200 m³/hr process air volume, and the production equipment operated at 4000 m³/hr, the starting point for spraying in the production equipment would be 2000 g/min, or a rate equal to 20 times that used in the laboratory machine, irrespective of batch size (Fig. 22). The spray nozzle (or nozzles) in the production machine would need to be of a size such that this increased spray rate is within its performance envelope (similar droplet size, uniform in distribution), or equivalence in granule size would be impossible. Figure 15 illustrates the concept that atomizing air pressure must be adjusted to attain similar average droplet sizes in all three scales of process equipment at the desired spray rate (data from Düsen-Schlick, GmbH, Dresden, Germany). The 970 series is typically found in laboratory inserts; the 940 series, also a single-headed nozzle, is used in pilot scale machines; and the 937 is a three-headed nozzle, typically fitted in production equipment. In very large machines, multiple wands may be used with several multiheaded nozzles to spread the liquid

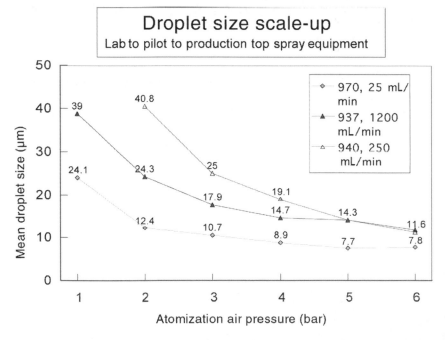

FIGURE 22 Average droplet sizes as a function of spray nozzle type (lab, pilot, and production), spray rate, and atomizing air pressure. *Source*: Data courtesy of Gustav Schlick.

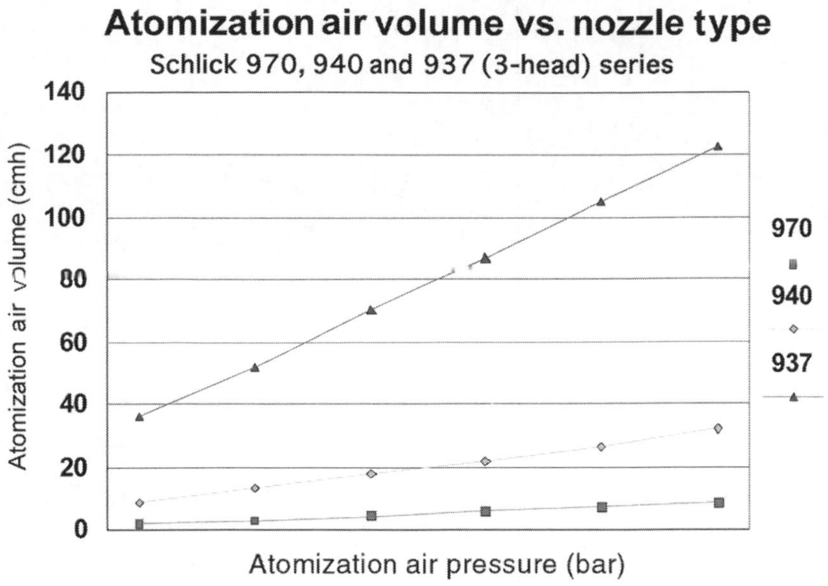

Atomization air volume vs. nozzle type
Schlick 970, 940 and 937 (3-head) series

FIGURE 23 Atomizing air volume and nozzle type for laboratory, pilot, and production scale nozzles.

over as much of the fluidizing product bed surface area as possible (typically to improve productivity).

The three different nozzles have slight differences in the configuration of the liquid insert and air cap (the path for the atomizing air), but the largest difference is in the size of the annulus between these components to permit the higher volume of compressed air to flow at the same atomizing pressures for atomization of the liquid stream (Fig. 23).

Scale-up Considerations: Product Moisture Content During Spraying

In combination with the drying rate (inlet temperature, volume, and dew point), the spray rate influences the rate of moisture build-up in the batch. In the example shown in Figure 17, the water addition rate exceeds the drying rate; the binder itself has an affinity for moisture, and is building in the product bed; and granule size is increasing with time. The change in slope begins at the 60-minute time point, when a slight increase in process air volume is enacted to ensure that the bed remains fully fluidized as it increases in weight and granule size. The rapid rate of moisture loss, beginning at the 105-minute data point, is due to an increase in the inlet air temperature for drying. This moisture profile was developed in small-scale equipment, and the example shown is for a large production batch. Product attributes such as granule size and distribution; bulk densities; and tablet properties such as hardness, friability, and disintegration time are reproduced when this moisture profile is duplicated in routine manufacture (Fig. 24).

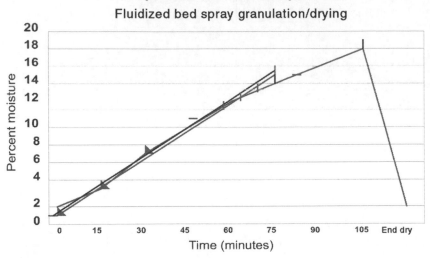

FIGURE 24 Representative in-process moisture profile for a fluidized bed spray granulation. *Source*: Courtesy of Glatt Air Techniques, Inc.

Scale-up Considerations: Minor Process Variables

The list of minor process variables includes several items with respect to the spray nozzle (port size, nozzle height above the static bed surface, and the spray cone angle). Figure 18 shows the relationship between nozzle port size and spray rate for a three-headed production scale nozzle. With a typical atomizing air pressure operating range of 2 to 5 bar, it can be seen that the port size has almost no influence on droplet size except for the high spray rate and small port size combination. Even at 4 bar and above, again, there is no influence. It is recommended that nozzle port size is selected on the basis of the viscosity of the liquid to be sprayed. Low viscose liquids can use small ports, and thicker solutions somewhat larger orifices, to allow some back pressure to build in the spray nozzle. In this manner, if a port should become clogged, increasing the spray rate through the remaining ports, the total liquid line pressure will rise. An operator can intervene to correct the problem before the larger droplet size results in an increased granule size (Fig. 25).

Droplet size is also typically impacted by liquid viscosity. In general, viscose liquids produce large droplets, resulting in coarse granules. In the case that the binder solution viscosity varies with temperature, the liquid temperature must be controlled in order that viscosity and droplet size can be reasonably reproduced.

Nozzle height above the static bed and the (spray pattern) cone angle impact the zone of contact between the droplets and the fluidizing substrate. In general, the maximum contact volume is desired (spreading the droplets over the largest product bed surface area). Experimentation has shown that this typically results in a narrow granule size distribution by minimizing the possibility of a locally high droplet/moisture concentration. In practical terms, this relates to adjusting the nozzle cone angle to its largest value. In lab and pilot

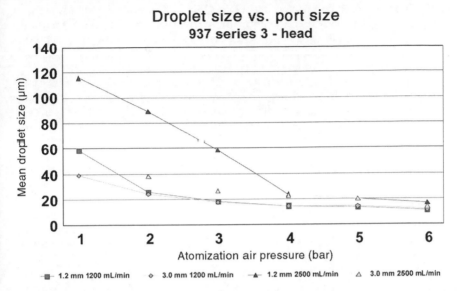

FIGURE 25 Droplet size as a function of 1.2 and 3.0 mm nozzle ports; spray rates of 1200 and 2500 mL/min using water. *Source*: Data courtesy of Gustav Schlick.

scale nozzles, this is adjustable; in production nozzles, it is fixed. Nozzle height above the static is the only way to impact the contact area in large equipment. In many spray granulation applications, the process air leaving the product bed is at or near saturation, therefore, spray drying of the binder material with the spray nozzle mounted well above the static bed is not a concern.

As mentioned previously, process air volume is selected on the basis of material properties. Fine materials are easily transported above the product bed into the outlet air filter. If the process air volume and velocity are excessive, material will be retained in the filters. Fines may become imbedded in the filter material, causing a high pressure, and a resultant loss in air volume. Filter selection is based on two criteria—porosity (the size of the pores in the fabric), and permeability (the number of opening per unit area). Filters are often selected with a porosity value that matches the particle size of the unprocessed substrate materials. In general, small porosity yields reduced permeability. The practical implications are that low permeability requires reduced process air volume, and this may impact productivity. Periodically, materials collected in the filters should be returned to the bed. This is accomplished by shaking the filters. Contemporary equipment that has a split filter housing should have each filter half shaken at least every 30 seconds such that building filter pressure does not interfere with control of process air volume, a key parameter. If the machine is constructed with cartridge type filters, the filter "pulse" should be frequent such that the fines are returned to the product bed to be exposed to the spray liquid.

SUMMARY

In the pharmaceutical industry, the production of granules is based on a batch concept. This concept offers many advantages in respect of quality assurance, as a batch can be accepted or rejected. However, the scale-up of the batch size may lead to problems. The variety of the equipment involved often does not facilitate the scale-up process. The theory of scale-up is reviewed, taking into account mathematical considerations and the search for scale-up invariants to establish an in-process control for validation purposes.

The scale-up procedure of the wet agglomeration process is the most challenging task. This is due to the fact that there is often a lack of detailed understanding of this process. In this context, the so-called "granulation end point" plays a doubtful role, as this end point is not well defined in literature and in praxis. In fact, a rigorous, scientific definition of this granulation end point is missing. It is generally referred as the time to stop the granulation process after the addition of the needed amount of granulating liquid and sufficient massing to create a snowball consistency of the wetted powder mass. It is however, on the other hand, possible to determine the necessary amount of granulation liquid by the analysis of the power consumption profile of the mixer motor during the wet agglomeration process. The characteristics of the power consumption profile depends on the formulation and on the type of granulating liquid such as water or alcohol.

As the concept of a pharmaceutical formulation includes not only the pharmaceutical unit operation such as "granulation" but also the composition (active pharmaceutical ingredient, auxiliary substances) problems concerning a robust dosage form design have to be considered in addition. For this purpose, new concepts such as percolation theory have to be taken into account. Such an approach complies with FDA's Process Analytical Technology (PAT) and Quality by Design (QbD) initiatives.

It is important that theoretical concepts are supported and can be validated by experimental findings. In this context, the corresponding author thanks the contribution of Marc Donsmark (M.D.) concerning the experimental scale-up exercises with high-shear mixers/granulators [sect. "Practical Experiences in Scale-up Using High-Shear Mixers (M.D.)"].

A solution for scale-up problems is the use of continuous processes as an alternative. For quality assurance purposes, it is however also necessary to define a "batch size" that could correspond to the amount of goods produced at a certain date during a certain time, for example, to fill a specific container of goods. Thus, it is possible to trace back the production event (time, running time, equipment, staff, in-process control charts, etc.) as a "batch" documentation for quality control purposes. Pure continuous productions have in general the problem that during the start-up phase of the production, a certain time is needed to reach equilibrium conditions. Thus, this part of the initially produced material cannot be used. For this reason, a quasi-continuous production line is presented, which combines the advantages of the batch production with the advantages of the continuous processes. Such a concept permits the production of small-scale batches, for example, for clinical trials and for large-scale batches using the same equipment.

Finally, the scale-up of the conventional fluidized bed spray granulation is discussed because of its wide use in the pharmaceutical industry for spray granulation and/or drying as a step subsequent to some type of wet granulation. Mass effects and drying capacity are key concerns in scale-up for drying of granulates produced in the separate steps of high- or low-shear granulation. A broad range of process variables exist in the fluidized bed spray granulation process, and some may have a significant impact on product properties. Experimentation should be conducted at the laboratory scale to determine the robustness of the formulation and process; thus, scale-up activities result in product with equivalent performance. The corresponding author thanks Dave Jones (D.J.) for his contribution concerning the section "Scale-up of the Conventional Fluidized Bed Spray Granulation Process."

REFERENCES

1. Leuenberger H. Scale-up of granulation processes with reference to process monitoring. Acta Pharm Technol 1983; 29(4):274–280.
2. Zlokarnik M. Dimensional analysis, scale-up. In: Flickinger MC, Drew SW, eds. Encyclopedia of Bioprocess Technology: Fermentation, Biocatalysis and Bioseparation. Hoboken, NJ: John Wiley & Sons, Inc. 1999:840–861.
3. Dimensionless Groups. In: Weast RC, Lide DR. Handbook of Chemistry and Physics. 67th ed. 1986–1987:307–324.
4. Pharmaceutical Manufacturers' Association 115 154th Street, NW Washington DC, 20005. Remington's Pharmaceutical Sciences. 15th ed. Mack Publisher Corporation, Easton PA, 1975:1429.
5. Johnstone RW, Thring MW. Pilot Plants, Models and Scale-up Methods in Chemical Engineering. New York: McGraw-Hill, 1957:12.
6. Leuenberger H. Pharm Technologie. In: Sucker H, Fuchs P, Speiser P, eds. Stuttgart: G. Thieme Verlag, 1978:80–92.
7. Leuenberger H, Bier HP, Sucker H. Theory of the granulation liquid requirement in the conventional granulation process. Pharm Technol Int 1979; 2–3:61–69.
8. Leuenberger H. Granulation—new techniques. Pharm Acta Helv 1982; 57:72–82.
9. Leuenberger H. Moist agglomeration of pharmaceutical powders. In: Chulia D, Deleuil M, Pourcelot Y, eds. Powder Technology and Pharmaceutical Processes, Handbook of Powder Technology. Vol 9. Amsterdam: Elsevier, 1994:377–389.
10. Dürrenberger M, Werani J. The control of granulation process by power consumption measurement in pharmaceutical industry. In: C.E. Capes, ed., Proceedings of the 4th International Symposium on Agglomeration, Toronto, June 2–5, Iron and Steel Soc., Inc., 1985:489–496.
11. Stauffer D, Aharony A. Introduction to Percolation Theory. 2nd ed. London, Philadelphia: Taylor & Francis, 1994.
12. Leuenberger H, Holman L, Usteri M, et al. Percolation theory, fractal geometry and dosage form design. Pharm Acta Helv 1989; 64(2):34–39.
13. Leuenberger H, Usteri M, Imanidis G, et al. Monitoring the granulation process: granulate growth, fractal dimensionality and percolation threshold. Boll Chem Farm 1989; 128:54–61.
14. Leuenberger H. The application of percolation theory in powder technology (invited review). Adv Powder Technol 1999; 10:323–352.
15. Leuenberger H. Design and optimization approaches in the field of granulation, drying and coating. Proceedings of the 6th International Symposium on Agglomeration, November 15–17, 1993, Nagoya Japan, pp. 665–673. Report in Japanese by Oguchi Toshio, Pharm. Technol. Jp.9,12,(1993)13–16.
16. Schade A. Herstellung von pharmazeutischen Granulaten in einem kombinierten Feuchtgranulations-und Mehrkammer-Wirbelschichttrocknungsverfahren, Dissertation Universitat Basel, 1992.
17. Schade A, Leuenberger H. Herstellung pharmazeutischer Granulate in einem kombinierten Feuchtgranulations-und Mehrkammer-Wirbelschichttrockungsverfahren. Chem Ing Technol 1992; 64(11):1016–1018.
18. Dörr B. Entwicklung einer Anlage zur quasikontinuierlichen Feuchtgranulierung und Mehrkammer-Wirbelschichttrocknung von pharmazeutischen Granulaten, Dissertation Universitat Basel, 1996.

19. Leuenberger H. Scale-up in the 4th dimension in the field of granulation and drying or how to avoid classical scale-up. Powder Technol 2003; 130:225–230.
20. Johnson MCR. Particle size distribution of the active ingredient for solid dosage forms of low dosage. Pharm Acta Helv 1972; 47:546–559.
21. Egermann H. Effect of adhesion on mixing homogeneity. II: Highest attainable degree of mixing of a polydisperse ingredient and a monodisprese diluent. J Pharm Sci 1985; 74:999–1000.
22. Rumpf H. Grundlagen und methoden des granulierens. Chem Ing Tech 1958; 30: 144–158.
23. Newitt DM, Conway-Jones JM. A contribution to the theory and practice of granulation. Trans Inst Chem Eng 1958; 36:422–442.
24. Schubert H. Kapillardruck und zugfestigkeit von feuchten haufwerken aus körnigen stoffen. Chem Ing Technol 1973; 45:396–401.
25. ICH Q8 Pharmaceutical Development. Available at: http://www.emea.europa.eu/pdfs/human/ich/16706804en.pdf.
26. Dürrenberger M, Leuenberger H. Steuerung und Überwachung konventioneller granulierprozesse. Chem Rundschau 1982; 35:1–3.
27. Usteri M, Leuenberger H. Agglomeration of binary mixtures in a high-speed mixer. Int J Pharm 1989:135–141.
28. Leuenberger H, Imanidis G. Monitoring mass transfer processes to control moist agglomeration. Pharm Technol 1986; 9:56–73.
29. Leuenberger H, Luy B, Studer J. New development in the control of the moist agglomeration and pelletization process. STP Pharma 1990; 6:303–309.
30. Betz G, Junker Bürgin P, Leuenberger H. Power consumption profile analysis and tensile strength measurements during moist agglomeration process. Int J Pharm 2003; 252:11–25.
31. Betz G, Junker Bürgin P, Leuenberger H. Power consumption measurement and temperature recording during granulation. Int J Pharm 2004; 272:137–149.
32. Leuenberger H, Puchkov M, Krausbauer E, et al. Manufacturing granules: is the granulation end-point a myth? Powder Technol 2009; 189:141–148.
33. Bourquin J, Schmidli H, van Hoogevest P, et al. Application of artificial neural networks (ANN) in the development of solid dosage forms. Pharm Dev Technol 1997; 2:111–121.
34. Donsmark MA. A device for automatic granulation control. 4th Pharmaceutical Technology Conference. Edinburgh, April 1984.
35. Schaefer T, Bak HH, Jaegerskou A, et al. Granulation in different types of high speed mixers, part 1. Pharm Ind 1986; 48:1083–1089.
36. Schaefer T, Bak HH, Jaegerskou A, et al. Granulation in different types of high speed mixers, part 2. Pharm Ind 1986; 49:297–304.
37. Shlieout G, Lammens RF, Kleinebudde P. Dry granulation with a roller compactor, part 1. Pharm Technol 2000; 11:24–35.
38. Shlieout G, Lammens RF, Kleinebudde P, et al. Dry granulation with a roller compactor, part 2. Pharm Technol 2002; 9:32–38.
39. Jetzer W, Leuenberger H, Sucker H. The compressibility and compactibility of pharmaceutical powders. Pharm Technol 1983; 7:33–48.
40. von Orelli JC. Search for technological reasons to develop a capsule or a tablet formulation, 2005, PhD thesis, University of Basel, Faculty of Science.
41. Vervaet C., Remon J-P. Continuous granulation in pharmaceutical industry. Chem Eng Sci 2005; 60(14):3949–3957.
42. Jakob M. ProCell technology: modelling and application. Powder Technol 2009; 189(2):332–342.
43. Pöllinger N. Innovative Glatt Fluid bed pelletizing technologies. Glatt Int Times 2008; 25:2–7.
44. Leuenberger H, Lanz M. Pharmaceutical powder technology—from art to science: the challenge of FDA's PAT initiative. Adv Powder Technol 2005; 16:3–25.
45. PwC, PHARMA 2020 Virtual R&D. Available at: http://www.pwc.com/extweb/industry.nsf/docid/705B658C95033AE8852575680022FC75.

46. Boeing 777. Available at: http://www.cds.caltech.edu/conferences/1997/vecs/tutorial/Examples/Cases/777.htm.
47. Leuenberger H, Leuenberger MN, Puchkov M. Implementing virtual R&D reality in industry: in silico design and testing of solid dosage forms. Swiss Pharma 2009; 31:18–24.
48. Leuenberger H. New trends in the production of pharmaceutical granules: the classical batch concept and the problem of scale-up. Eur J Pharm Biopharm 2001; 52:279–288.
49. Leuenberger H. New trends in the production of pharmaceutical granules: batch versus continuous processing. Eur J Pharm Biopharm 2001; 52:289–296.
50. Betz C, Junker Bürgin P, Leuenberger H. Batch and continuous processing in the production of pharmaceutical granules. Pharm Dev Technol 2003; 8(3):289–297.
51. Werani J, Grünberg M, Ober C, et al. Semicontinuous granulation—the process of choicefor the production of pharmaceutical granules? Powder Technol 2004; 140(3):163–168.

11 Batch size increase in fluid bed granulation

Dilip M. Parikh

INTRODUCTION

The size enlargement of primary particles has been carried out in the pharmaceutical industry in a variety of ways. One of the most common unit operations used in the pharmaceutical industry is the fluid bed processing. The batch size increase using fluid bed granulation requires a good understanding of the equipment functionality, theoretical aspect of fluidization, excipient interactions, and most of all, identifying the critical variables that affect the process of agglomeration.

This chapter provides the essential understanding of the fluidization theory and system description that make up the fluid bed processor, and discusses the critical variables associated with equipment, product, and the process. Upon gaining this basic understanding, one can design scale-up protocols. These protocols will be able to assure that the probability of successful transition from the R&D batch sizes to the pilot size batches and ultimately to the commercial scale will be high. As in any unit operation that requires batch size increase, fluid bed process must undergo process qualification to establish the robustness of the process. If the critical process variables are identified at an early stage of the product development and then considered together with the equipment variables, tolerances, and material handling concerns, batch size increase can be made trouble-free. The fluidized bed was used only for drying the pharmaceutical granulation efficiently in the early days, but now it is employed routinely for drying. Identification of critical process parameters prior to scale-up is essential. Quality by design can be implemented to identify such parameters. A series of design of experiments will result in identification and evaluation of critical process variables and is highly recommended: agglomeration, pelletization, and production of modified-release dosage forms using air-suspension coating. Because of this, these units are normally classified as multiprocessor fluid bed units.

Fluidized bed granulation is a process by which granules are produced in a single piece of equipment by spraying a binder solution on to a fluidized powder bed. This process is sometimes classified as the one pot system.

Fluid bed processing of pharmaceuticals was first reported by Wurster, when he used the air-suspension technique to coat tablets (1,2). In 1960, he reported on granulating and drying a pharmaceutical powder suitable for the preparation of compressed tablets, using the air-suspension technique. In 1964, Scott et al. (3) and Rankell et al. (4) reported on the theory and design considerations of the process using a fundamental engineering approach and employing mass and thermal energy balances. They expanded this application to the 30-kg capacity pilot plant model designed for both batch and continuous operation. Process variables, such as airflow rate, process-air temperature, and liquid flow rate, were studied. Contini and Atasoy (5) later reported the processing details and advantages of the fluid bed process in one continuous step.

Wolf (6) discussed the essential construction features of the various fluid bed components, and Liske and Mobus (7) compared the fluidized bed and traditional granulation process. The overall results indicated that the material processed by the fluid bed granulator was finer, more free-flowing, and had homogeneous granules, which, after compression, produced stronger and faster disintegration of tablets than the materials processed by conventional wet granulation. Reviews by Sherrington and Oliver (8), Pietch (9), and a series published on the topic of "Fluidization in the Pharmaceutical Industry" (10 16) provide an in-depth background on the fundamental aspects of the fluidized bed and other granulation technologies.

Fluidization Theory

Typical fluid bed processor elements can be seen in Figure 1.

A fluidized bed is a bed of solid particles with a stream of air or gas passing upward through the particles at a rate great enough to set them in motion, this velocity, according to Kulling and Simon (17), is higher than the incipient fluidizing velocity but lower than the entrainment velocity. When the rate of flow of gas increases, the pressure drop across the bed also increases

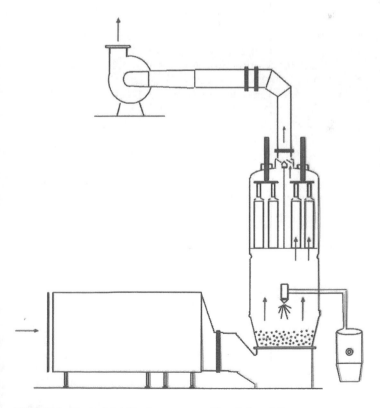

FIGURE 1 Typical fluid bed processor with solution delivery.

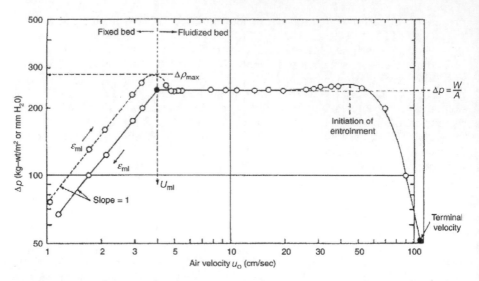

FIGURE 2 Typical pressure drop curve as a function of gas velocity. *Source*: Adapted from Ref. 18.

until, at a certain rate of flow, the frictional drag on the particles equals the effective weight of the bed. These conditions, and the velocity of gas corresponding to it, are termed *incipient fluidization* and *incipient velocity*, respectively. The relationship between the air velocity and the pressure drop is as shown in Figure 2. At low gas velocities, the bed of particles is practically a packed bed, and the pressure drop is proportional to the superficial velocity. As the gas velocity is increased, a point is reached at which the bed behavior changes from fixed particles to suspended particles. The superficial velocity required to first suspend the bed particles is known as *minimum fluidization velocity* (U_{mf}). The minimum fluidization velocity sets the lower limit of possible operating velocities, and the approximate pressure drop can be used to approximate pumping energy requirements. For agglomeration process in the fluid bed processor, air velocity required is normally five to six times the minimum fluidization velocity. At the incipient point of fluidization, the pressure drop of the bed will be very close to the weight of the particles divided by the cross-sectional area of the bed (W/A). For the normal gas fluidized bed, the density of the gas is much less than the density of the solids, and the balance of forces can be shown as

$$\Delta p_{mf} = \frac{W}{A}$$

where

$$W = (1 - \varepsilon_{mf})\rho_p \cdot \frac{g}{g_c}$$

where Δp is the pressure drop, ε_{mf} the minimum fluidization void fraction, A the cross-sectional area, W the weight of the particles, ρ_p the density of particles, and g/g_c the ratio of gravitational acceleration and gravitational conversion factor.

As the velocity of the gas is increased further, the bed continues to expand and its height increases with only slight increase in the pressure drop. As the velocity of the gas is further increased, the bed continues to expand and its height increases, whereas the concentration of particles per unit volume of the bed decreases. At a certain velocity of the fluidizing medium, known as entrainment velocity, particles are carried over by the gas. This phenomenon is called entrainment. When the volumetric concentration of solid particles is uniform throughout the bed all the times, the fluidization is termed as *particular*. When the concentration of solids is not uniform throughout the bed, and if the concentration keeps fluctuating with time, the fluidization is called *aggregative* fluidization. A *slugging bed* is a fluid bed in which the gas bubbles occupy entire cross-sections of the product container and divide the bed into layers.

A *boiling bed* is a fluid bed in which the gas bubbles are approximately of the same size as that of the solid particles.

A *channeling bed is* a fluid bed in which the gas forms channels in the bed through which most of the air passes.

A *spouting bed* is a fluid bed in which the gas forms a single opening through which some particles flow and fall on the outside.

Figure 3 shows various types of fluid beds (19).

The mechanisms by which air affects fluidization have been discussed by various researchers (11, 19, 20–23). When the fluidizing velocity is greater than the incipient velocity, bubbles of air rise through the bed causing mixing of particles. Mixing does not generally occur when the bed is fluidized at a very low or zero *excess* gas velocities, because insufficient bubbles are formed to cause bulk displacement of particles. It is the gas passing through the bed in the form

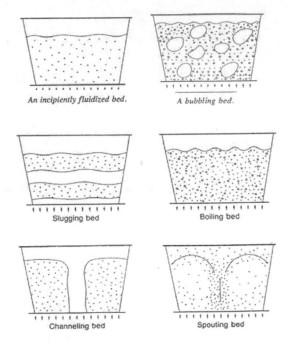

An incipiently fluidized bed.   *A bubbling bed.*

Slugging bed   Boiling bed

Channeling bed   Spouting bed

FIGURE 3 Various types of fluid beds. *Source*: From Ref. 19.

of bubbles that determines the degree of mixing. The extent of mixing appears to vary with the particle size. Mixing of particles having a mean particle size of less than approximately 150 μm decreases as the mean size approaches zero. Different types of beds, described above, are formed depending on the movement of bubbles through the bed. Bubbles play an extremely important role in the motion of particles in the fluidized bed. Solids are carried in the wakes behind rising bubbles. A number of correlations exist for estimating the bubble size in a fluidized bed (24,32). In general, bubble sizes are fairly small (2–5 cm) for powders that can be easily fluidized, while sandy powders also fluidize easily but do not show any particulate expansion, and bubbles grow with bed height to large size and can easily form slugs in a narrow diameter bed. The pattern of movement of the gas phase in and out of bubbles depends on several factors, including minimum fluidization velocity and particle size. These movements affect heat transfer between air bubbles and particles. The air distributor at the bottom of the container has a controlling influence on the uniform distribution of gas, minimization of dead areas, and maximization of particle movement. The most common reason for mixing problems, such as segregation in the fluid bed, is the particle density differences. The extent of segregation can be controlled in part by maintaining high fluidizing velocities and high bowl height to bowl diameter ratio. There are standard air velocities for various processes that can be used as guidelines. The standard velocities are based on the cross-sectional area at the bottom of the product container. Airflow velocities are normally 1.0 to 2.0 m/sec. This is calculated by using the following formula for calculating the air velocity.

$$\text{Velocity (m/sec)} = \frac{\text{airflow } \left[\text{cubic meter per hour (CMH)}\right]}{\text{area (m}^2) \times 3600}$$

where airflow in cubic meters per hour (CMH) = airflow (CFM) $\times$ 1.696.

Mass and Energy Balance

A fluidized bed is a granulator as well as a dryer. It therefore has operational limits that are defined by its ability to evaporate solvent being sprayed in. Often, the energy required to heat the granules is small compared to that required to evaporate the solvent. The exit gas and particles from the fluid bed have the same temperature as the granules in the bed due to intense mixing action of the bed. Hence, the mass energy balance limitations are quite evident.

1. The exit gas humidity cannot exceed the saturation humidity in the gas at the exit temperature. Once the exit air is saturated, no more liquid can be removed from the fluid bed.
2. The energy required to evaporate the liquid cannot exceed that available from the incoming gas.

If either of these limits is exceeded, liquid will accumulate in the bed causing bed collapse. These limits are the two constraints that must always be met.

SYSTEM DESCRIPTION
Components

A *fluid bed processor* is a system of unit operations involving heating process air, a system to direct it through the material to be processed and have the same air

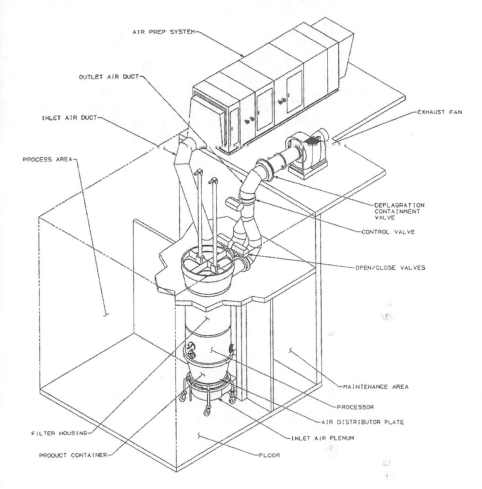

FIGURE 4 Typical components of a fluid bed processor.

(usually laden with moisture) exit the unit void of the product. Figure 4 shows a typical fluid bed processor with all the components. A more detailed description of the equipment and various components is presented by Parikh and Jones (90).

Spray Nozzle and Solution Delivery System
Two-fluid nozzles are most common nozzles used for granulation process. In the two-fluid (binary) nozzle, the binder solution (one fluid) is atomized by compressed air (second fluid) (Fig. 5). These nozzles are available as a single-port or multiport design. Generally, the single-port nozzles are adequate up to 100 kg batch, but for larger size batches, multiport nozzles, such as either a three-port (Fig. 6) or a six-port (Fig. 7) nozzle, are required. When these nozzles are air atomized, the spray undergoes three distinct phases. In the first, the compressed air (gas) expands, essentially adiabatically, from the high pressure at the nozzle to that of the fluid bed chamber. The gas undergoes a Joule–Thomson effect, and

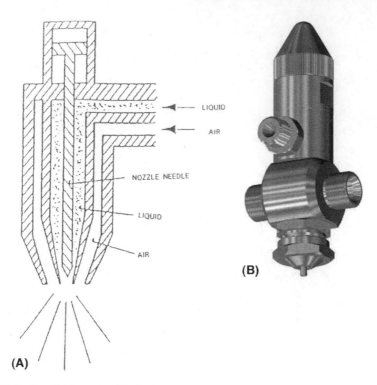

LIQUID

AIR

NOZZLE NEEDLE

LIQUID

AIR

(B)

(A)

FIGURE 5 Two-fluid nozzle with single port.

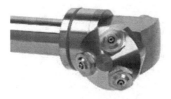

FIGURE 6 Three-port nozzle.

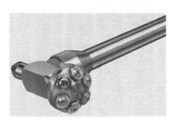

FIGURE 7 Six-port nozzle.

its temperature falls. In the second, the liquid forms into discrete drops. During this atomization, the liquid's specific surface area usually increases 1000 times. In the third, the drops travel after being formed, until they become completely dry or impinge on the product particles. During this phase the solvent evaporates and the diameter of the drops decreases. The energy required to form a drop is the product of the surface tension and the new surface area. About

0.1 cal/g is needed to subdivide 1 g of water into 1 μm droplets. The air pressure required to atomize the binder liquid is set by means of pressure regulator. The spray pattern and angle are adjusted by adjusting the air cap.

Optimum atomization is achieved by fine adjustment of the air cap and atomization-air pressure measured at the nozzle. The binder solution is delivered to the nozzle port through a spray lance and tubing. The peristaltic or positive displacement pump is commonly used to pump the binder solution. The pneumatically controlled nozzle needle prevents the binder liquid from dripping when the liquid flow is stopped. Nozzle port openings of between 0.8 and 2.8 mm in diameter are most common and are interchangeable.

The two-fluid nozzle in its simplified model is based on energy transmission as shown below.

Energy + liquid - - - - - - two-fluid nozzle - - - - - - droplets + heat

The ratio of energy dissipation by heat and by the droplet-making process is difficult to measure. Masters (25) suggested that less than 0.5% of applied energy is utilized in liquid breakup. Virtually, the whole amount is imparted to the liquid and air as kinetic energy.

PARTICLE AGGLOMERATION AND GRANULE GROWTH

Agglomeration can be defined as the size enlargement process in which the starting material is fine particles and the final product is an aggregate in which primary particles can still be identified. The granules are held together with bonds formed by the binder used to agglomerate. Various mechanisms of granule formation have been described in the literature (26–28). Three mechanisms for granule formation have been suggested by the researchers. These are as follows:

1. Bridges due to *immobile liquids* form adhesional and cohesional bridging bonds. Thin adsorption layers are immobile and can contribute to the bonding of fine particles under certain circumstances.
2. *Mobile liquids*, where interfacial and capillary forces are present.
3. *Solid bridges* formed due to crystallization of dissolved substances during drying.

Most of the fluid bed granulated products require an amount of wetting much less than the high-shear granulation. In the fluid bed granulation process, the particles are suspended in the hot air stream and the atomized liquid is sprayed on it. The degree of bonding between these primary particles to form an agglomerated granule depends on the binder used, physicochemical characteristics of the primary particles being agglomerated, and process parameters.

Schaefer et al. (29) and Smith and Nienow (30) have reported a description of the growth mechanisms in the fluid bed where the bed of particles are wetted by liquid droplets in the spray zone. During the granulation, the two particles posses a relative velocity U_o that ensures collision at some point on their trajectory and possible sticking under appropriate conditions. It is essential that some binder be present at the point of contact. Atomized liquid from the nozzle tends to spread over the particle surface as long as there is an adequate wettability of the particle by the fluid (31). The rate of granule growth by agglomeration is proportional to the collision frequency between the particles present in the granulator and the fraction of collisions that are successful, that is, the fraction of collisions that lead to coalesce rather than rebound (32). Wet particles on impact form a liquid bridge and solidify as the agglomerate circulates throughout the remainder of the bed. The type of bonds formed approaches through four transition states, described by Newitt and Conway-Jones (26) and Maroglou and Nienow (36,37) as (*i*) pendular, (*ii*) funicular, (*iii*) capillary, and (*iv*) droplet (normally happens during spray drying).

Solid bridges then hold particles together. The strength of the binder determines whether these particles stay as agglomerates. These binding forces should be larger than the breakup forces and, in turn, depends on the size of the solid bridge. The breakup forces arise from the movement of the randomized particles colliding with each other and are related to the excess gas velocity and particle size. Liquid bridges between particles critically influence the behavior of the bulk and the granulation characteristics of a powder binder system. The appropriate amount of binder can be determined by measuring the yield strength of granules or performing the granule friability test.

Granulation Mechanisms

In the fluid bed granulation, the binder introduction is usually concentrated in the so-called "spray zone," and the process of growth is not instantaneous or rapid. Hence, agglomeration and granule growth occur in the granulator while the binder is introduced, and the prevailing growth mechanisms will be locally determined by the amount of liquid present in the spray zone or in the bed. Four key mechanisms or *rate processes* contribute to granulation, as originally outlined by Ennis (33,34) and later developed further by Litster and Ennis (35). These include *wetting* and nucleation, *coalescence* or growth, *consolidation*, and *attrition* or breakage. Initial *wetting* of the powders and existing granules by the granulating fluid is strongly influenced by spray rate or fluid distribution as well as product formulation properties, in comparison with mechanical mixing. Wetting promotes nucleation of fine powders, or coating in cases where product particle size is greater than the droplet size. Often wetting agents such as surfactants are carefully chosen to enhance poorly wetting powders. In the *coalescence* or growth stage, partially wetted primary particles and larger nuclei coalesce to form granules composed of several particles. The term nucleation is typically applied to the initial coalescence of primary particles in the immediate vicinity of the larger wetting drop, whereas the more general term of *coalescence* refers to the successful collision of two granules to form a new larger granule. In addition, the term of *layering* is applied to the coalescence of granules with primary particles of powders. Nucleation is promoted from some initial distribution of moisture, such as a drop or from the homogenization of a fluid feed to the bed, as with high-shear mixing. The nucleation process is strongly linked with the wetting stage. As granules grow, they are consolidated by compaction forces due to bed agitation. This *consolidation* stage strongly influences *internal* granule voidage or granule porosity, and therefore, end-use properties such as granule strength, hardness, or dissolution. Formed granules may be particularly susceptible to *attrition* if they are inherently weak or if flaws develop during drying.

These mechanisms or rate processes can occur simultaneously in all processes, ranging from spray drying to fluidized beds to high-shear mixers. However, certain mechanisms may dominate in a particular process. For example, fluidized bed granulators are strongly influenced by the wetting process, whereas mechanical redispersion of binding fluid by impellers and particularly high-intensity choppers diminish the wetting contributions to granule size in high-shear mixing. On the other hand, granule consolidation is far more pronounced in high-shear mixing than fluidized bed granulation. These simultaneous rate processes taken as a whole and sometimes competing against one another determine the final granule size distribution and granule structure and voidage resulting from a process, and therefore, the final end-use or product quality attributes of the granulated product.

If the binding forces are in excess of the breakup forces, either in the wet state or in the dry state, uncontrolled growth will proceed to an overwetted bed or production of excessive fines, respectively. If a more reasonable balance of forces is present, controlled agglomeration will occur, growth of which can be controlled. Maroglou and Nienow presented a granule growth mechanism in the fluid bed by the use of model materials and scanning electron microscope (36).

Figure 8 shows the various paths a liquid droplet can take and its consequences on the particle growth.

Figure 9 shows the growth of the granule relative to the liquid added. In the beginning of the spraying stage, primary particles form nuclei and are held together by liquid bridges in a pendular state. The size of these nuclei depends on the droplet size of the binder solution. As the liquid addition continues, more and more nuclei agglomerate and continue the transition from the pendular state to the capillary state.

The uniqueness of the fluid bed agglomeration process is how the liquid addition and drying (evaporation) steps are concurrently carried out. When the granulation liquid is sprayed into a fluidized bed, the primary particles are wetted and form together with the binder, relatively loose and very porous agglomerates. Densification of these agglomerates is brought about solely by the capillary forces present in the liquid bridges. It is therefore important that the quantity of liquid sprayed into the bed should be relatively large compared with that used in high-shear granulation.

Drying a wet product in a fluid bed is a separate topic, but during the fluid bed granulation process it becomes an integral part of the process; hence, understanding fluid bed drying is important as we review the agglomeration process.

FLUID BED DRYING

Drying is an integral part of fluid bed granulation process. The removal of moisture from the granulated particles to a desired end point is critical for the stability and further processing of the granulated product. Efficient heat and mass transfer during processing is elemental to the control of particle morphology and moisture content of the final product. Heat is transferred to the product to evaporate liquid, and mass is transferred as a vapor in the surrounding gas; hence, these two phenomenon are interdependent. During the drying, standard air velocities are based on the application. Low air velocities such as 0.8 to 1.4 m/sec are required for drying. The velocities are higher during the early stages of drying because of the wet mass present in the bowl, but will be reduced when the product loses its moisture. The objective is to have good particle movement but to keep the material out of filters. Particle movement and quick drying are

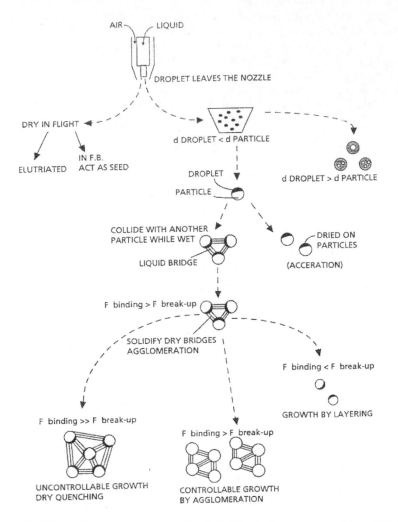

FIGURE 8 Mechanism of granulation in fluid bed. *Source*: Adapted from Ref. 37.

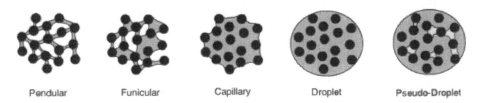

Pendular   Funicular   Capillary   Droplet   Pseudo-Droplet

FIGURE 9 States of liquid saturation. *Source*: Adapted from Barlow CG. Granulation of powders. Chem Eng (Lond) 1968; 220:CE 196–CE 201.

important during the agglomeration process. An indication of good fluidization is a free downward flow of the granulation at the sight glass of the fluid bed container. However, improper fluidization can also be detected by monitoring the outlet air temperature. Every product has a unique constant rate of drying in which the bed temperature remains relatively constant for a significant length of time. Therefore, if the outlet temperature rises more rapidly than anticipated, it will indicate an improper fluidization and the process may have to be stopped and manual or mechanical intervention may be required to assist the fluidization. The drying rate is determined by the factors affecting the heat and mass transfer. Rates of drying are usually faster in the initial stages where the water activity is higher, followed by a slower diffusion limited drying period. Amount of water that is "trapped" by diffusion limitations could be critical to chemical stability depending on the drug substance characteristics. The transfer of heat in the fluid bed takes place by convection. Convection is the transfer of heat from one point to another within a fluid (gas, solid, liquid) by the mixing of one portion of the fluid with another. The removal of moisture from a product granulated in the fluid bed granulator or in other equipment essentially removes the added water or solvent (free moisture). This *free moisture content* is the amount of moisture that can be removed from the material by drying at a specified temperature and humidity. The amount of moisture that remains associated with the material under the drying conditions specified is called the *equilibrium moisture content* (EMC).

The evaporation rate of liquid film surrounding the granule being dried is related to the rate of heat transfer by the equation:

$$\frac{dW}{dT} = h \cdot \frac{A}{H} \cdot \partial T$$

where dw/dt is the mass transfer rate (drying rate), h is the heat transfer coefficient, A is the surface area, H is the latent heat of evaporation, and ∂T is the temperature difference between the air and the material surface.

Because fluid bed processing involves drying of a product in suspended hot air, the heat transfer is extremely rapid. In a properly fluidized processor, product temperature and the exhaust-air temperatures should reach equilibrium. Improper air distribution, hence poor heat transfer in fluidized bed, cause numerous problems such as caking, channeling, or sticking. The capacity of the air (gas) stream to absorb and carry away moisture determines the drying rate and establishes the duration of the drying cycle. Controlling this capacity is the key to controlling the drying process. The two elements essential to this control are inlet-air temperature and airflow. The higher the temperature of the drying air, the greater its vapor holding capacity. Since the temperature of the wet granules in a hot gas depends on the rate of evaporation, the key to analyzing the drying process is psychrometry (38–40).

Psychrometry is defined as the study of the relationships between the material and energy balances of water vapor–air mixture. Psychrometric charts (Fig. 10) simplify the crucial calculations of how much heat must be added and how much moisture can be added to the air. The process of drying involves both heat and mass transfer. For drying to occur, there must be a concentration gradient that must exist between the moist granule and surrounding environment. As in heat transfer, the maximum rate of mass transfer that occurs during drying is proportional to the surface area, turbulence of the drying air, the driving force between the solid and the air, and the drying rate. Because the heat of vaporization must be supplied to evaporate the moisture, the driving force for mass transfer is the same driving force required for heat transfer, which is the temperature difference between the air and the solid.

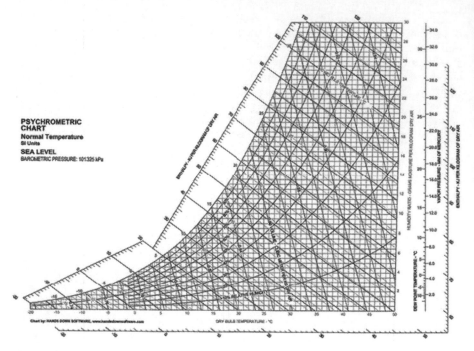

FIGURE 10   Psychrometric chart.

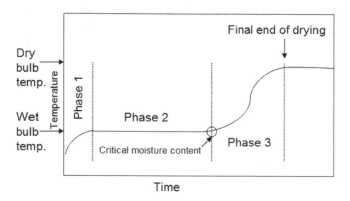

FIGURE 11   Product temperature changes during drying in a fluid bed processor. *Source*: From Ref. 19.

Schaefer and Worts (41) have shown that the higher the temperature differences between incoming air and the product, the faster the drying rate. Therefore, product temperature should be monitored closely to control the fluidized bed drying process. During fluid bed drying, the product passes through three distinct temperature phases (Fig. 11). At the beginning of the drying process, the material heats up from the ambient temperature to approximately the wet-bulb temperature of the air in the dryer. This temperature is maintained until the granule moisture content is reduced to the critical level. At this point, the material holds no free surface water, and the temperature starts to rise further.

The drying capacity of the air depends on the relative humidity (RH) of the incoming air. At 100% RH, the air is holding the maximum amount of water possible at a given temperature, but if the temperature of the air is raised, the RH drops and the air can hold more moisture. If air is saturated with water vapor at a given temperature, a drop in temperature will force the air mass to relinquish some of its moisture through condensation. The temperature at which moisture condenses is the dew point temperature. Thus, the drying capacity of the air varies significantly during processing. By dehumidifying the air to a preset dew point, incoming air can be maintained at a constant drying capacity (dew point) and hence provide reproducible process times. A strong correlation can exist between trapped water and granule stability for batches made at various scales and product temperatures. The monitoring of humidity and temperature of the product bed is important in optimizing the drying process. The successful scale-up of granulation process hence requires robust predictions of heat and mass transfer.

PROCESS AND VARIABLES IN GRANULATION
Granulation Process
In fluid bed granulation processing, as with any other granulation system, the goal is to form agglomerated particles through the use of binder bridges between the particles. To achieve a good granulation, particles must be uniformly mixed, and liquid bridges between the particles must be strong and easy to dry. Therefore, this system is sensitive to the particle movement of the product in the unit, the addition of the liquid binder, and the drying capacity of the air. The granulation process in the fluid bed requires a binary nozzle, a solution delivery system, and compressed air to atomize the liquid binder. Thurn (42) in a 1970 thesis investigated details of the mixing, agglomerating, and drying operations that take place in the fluid bed process. Results indicated that the mixing stage was particularly influenced by airflow rate and air volume. It was suggested that the physical properties of the raw materials, such as hydrophobicity, may exert a strong influence upon the mixing stage. At the granulation stage, particular attention was paid to the nozzle, and it was concluded that a binary design (two-fluid) nozzle gave a wide droplet size distribution yielding a homogeneous granule. The need for strong binders was recommended to aid granule formation, and it was suggested that the wettability of the raw materials required particular attention. Several research papers have been published on the influence of raw material (41–58), binder-type (4,7,29,41,42,51,53,58–68) binder concentration, and binder quantity (7,29,44,49,53,55,58,60,61,64–66,69–84).

Each phase of the granulation process must be controlled carefully to achieve process reproducibility. When binder liquid is sprayed into a fluidized bed, the primary particles are wetted and form together with the binder, relatively loose and very porous agglomerates. Densification of these agglomerates is brought about almost solely by the capillary forces present in the liquid bridges. It is therefore important that the liquid binder sprayed into the bed should be relatively large in quantity compared with that used in high or low shear granulation process. During spraying, a portion of the liquid is immediately lost by evaporation, so the system has little tendency to pass beyond the liquid bridge phase. The particle size of the resulting granule can be controlled to some extent by adjusting the quantity of binder liquid and the rate at which it is fed, that is, the droplet size. The mechanical strength of the particles depends principally on the composition of the primary product being granulated and the type of the binder used. Aulton et al. (73) found that lower fluidizing-air temperature, a dilute solution of binder fluid, and a greater spray rate produced better granulation for tabletting.

Formulation and Scale-Up

Scale-up of fluid bed granulation process depends on limitations and character-istics of formulation, equipment similarity or lack thereof, and critical process parameters. As the batch size increases, formed granules are subjected to overall compression due to weight of the batch as well as are subjected to attrition due to higher airflow and the free board above the bowl. Thus, the resulting granule size distribution is a strong function of the balance between different mecha-nisms and size change, for example, nucleation, layering, coalescence attrition by erosion, and attrition by breakage.

Properties of Primary Material

Ideally, the particle properties desired in the starting material include a low particle density, a small particle size, a narrow particle size range, particle shape approaching spherical, a lack of particle cohesiveness, and a lack of stickiness during the processing. Properties such as cohesiveness, static charge, particle size distribution, crystalline or amorphous nature, and wettability are some of the properties that have impact on the properties of granules formed. The cohesiveness and static charges on particles present fluidization difficulty. The same difficulties were observed when the formulation contained hydrophobic material or a mixture of hydrophilic and hydrophobic materials. The influence of hydrophobicity of primary particles has been shown by Aulton and Banks (16), where they demonstrated that the mean particle size of the product was directly related to wettability of the primary particles expressed as $\cos \theta$ (where θ is the contact angle of the particles). It was also reported that, as the hydro-phobicity of the mix is increased, a decrease in granule growth is observed. Aulton et al. in a later publication showed that addition of a surface active agent such as sodium laurel sulfate improves the fluidized bed granulation (56). In a mixture containing hydrophobic and hydrophilic primary particles, granule growth of hydrophilic materials takes place selectively, creating content unifor-mity problems. The surface energy is a useful parameter for the description of the energetic situation on the surface of a material. High surface energies usually indicate an enhanced activity of the surface, which has direct implication on the process and product performance (85). Recently, Thielmann et al. (85) studied effect of surface properties of primary particles on their agglomeration behavior in fluid bed granulator. To keep all process conditions and material properties constant, except surface energy, they used hydrophobic and hydrophilic glass beads of uniform size. The binder liquid was 2% aqueous solution of hydrox-ypropylcellulose (HPC). They concluded that the hydrophilic particles produced narrower particle size distribution than hydrophobic ones, most likely due to the fact that granules above certain critical size cannot be formed as the kinetic energy of granules during impact cannot be dissipated within the thin binder coating layer present on the particle surface. They further concluded that better wettability does not necessarily mean better granulation because larger fraction of hydrophobic particles remain ungranulated due to lower frictional surface coverage of primary particles.

Low-Dose Drug Content: Formulation
Wan et al. (86) studied various methods of incorporating a low-dose drug such as chlorpheniramine maleate in lactose formulation with polyvinylpyrrolidone (PVP) as the granulating solution. They concluded that the randomized movement of particles in the fluid bed may cause segregation of the drug and that uniform drug distribution was best achieved by dissolving the drug in granulating solution. The mixing efficiency of drug particles with the bulk material was found to increase in the proportion of the granulating liquid used to dissolve the drug. The optimum nozzle atomizing pressure was deemed to be important to avoid spray drying the drug particles or overwetting, which creates uneven drug distribution. Higashide et al. (87) studied the fluidized bed granulation using 5-fluorouracil in concentration of 0.3% in 1:1 mixture of starch and lactose. The HPC was used as the binder. The ratios of starch and lactose contained in the granules were measured gravimetrically. The researchers found that bigger amount of the drug and starch was found in larger granules than in smaller granules. The results were attributed to the hydrophobicity of the 5-fluorouracil, starch, and the hydrophilicity of lactose.

Binder and Solvent Impact
In a fluidized bed, two particles posses a relative velocity (U_o) that ensures collision at some point on their trajectory and possible sticking under appropriate conditions. It is essential that some binder be present at the point of contact, and it should have certain depth to insure sticking instead of rebound. Different binders have different binding properties and the concentration of individual binder may have to be changed to obtain similar binding of primary particles. Thus, the type of binder, the binder content in the formulation, and the concentration of the binder have major influence on granule properties. These properties include friability, flow, bulk density, porosity, and size distribution. Davies and Gloor (88,89) reported that the types of binder such as povidone, acacia, gelatin, and HPC, all have different binding properties that affect the final granule properties mentioned above. Hontz (81) investigated microcrystalline cellulose concentration, inlet-air temperature, binder PVP concentration, and binder solution concentration effects on tablet properties. Binder and microcrystalline cellulose concentration were found to have significant effect on tablet properties. Alkan et al. (67) studied binder (PVP) addition in solution and as a dry powder in the powder mix. They found a larger mean granule size when the dry binder was granulated with ethanol. However, when the binder was in solution, the granules produced were less friable and more free-flowing. This same finding was confirmed by other researchers (83,84). Binder temperature affects the viscosity of the solution and, in turn, affects the droplet size. Increased temperature of the binder solution reduces the viscosity of the solution, reducing the droplet size and hence producing smaller mean granule size. Binder solution viscosity and concentration affect the droplet size of the binder. Polymers, starches, and high molecular weight PVP cause increased viscosity,

which in turn creates larger droplet size and subsequently larger mean granule particle size (29).

Diluted binders are preferred because they facilitate finer atomization of the binder solution, provide the control of the particle size, reduce friability, and increase the bulk density even though the tackiness or binding strength may suffer (7,60,71,74,89). In most instances, water is used as a solvent. The selection of solvent such as aqueous or organic depends on the solubility of the binder and the compatibility of product being granulated. Generally, organic solvents, due to their rapid vaporization from the process, produce smaller granules than the aqueous solution. Requirement of solvent for the binder can be eliminated by incorporating binder or mixture of binders of low melting point and incorporating it with the drug substance in the dry form. The temperature of the incoming air is sufficient to melt the binder and form the granules.

Equipment Design and Scale-Up

The availability of the fluid bed processors from different suppliers of the equipment is essentially similar. The differences in design of different suppliers sometime provide difficulty in scaling-up from the laboratory units to production units in a linear scale. Product bowl geometry is considered to be a factor that may have impact on the agglomeration process. The fluidization velocity must drop from bottom to the top rim of the bowl by more than half to prevent smaller, lighter particles being impinged into the filter creating segregation from heavier product components in the bowl. Generally, conical shape of the container and expansion chamber is preferred where ratio of cross-sectional diameter of the distributor plate to the top of the vessel is 1:2.

To address the scaling up of fluid bed processes, a number of equipment manufacturers have either modified the equipment design or suggested various criteria for scaling-up, for example, LB Bohle (Pennsylvania, U.S.) maintains the air-distributor face velocity of 2 m/sec with an opening angle of process bowl at 30°, and the ratio of lower portion and upper portion area of the conical product bowl is maintained constant at 0.5. This allows the air entering the air distributor at a face velocity of 2 m/sec to slow down toward the wider portion of the conical bowl to 1 m/sec. The GEA Pharma Systems (Wommelgem, Belgium) introduced their "Flex Stream^{TM}" to eliminate the use of various process modules and to facilitate the scaling-up. Here the nozzle is placed on the side of the container, surrounded by a passage through which a low-pressure process air, diverted from the lower plenum, enters around the nozzle and creates an area of spray pattern, eliminating the possibility of overwetting of particles and keeping the nozzle clean. This approach offers a linier scale-up of the process.

To fluidize and thus granulate and dry the product, certain quantity of process air is required. The volume of the air required will vary based on the amount of material that needs to be processed. The ratio of drying capacity of the process air and quantity of the product needs to be maintained constant throughout the scaling-up process. Proportionality of the equipment design from bench top/pilot scale to production unit must be considered as the process is being scaled up; for example, air-distributor plates to match the air velocity proportional to the increase in batch size, type of filter porosity selection so the performance of in-process filter cleaning and its impact on increased batch size is minimal. Parikh and Jones (90) described in details the various equipment variables and their impact on the granulation process.

Processing Factors and Scale-Up

The fluid bed granulation is a combination of three steps, namely dry mixing, spray agglomeration, and subsequent drying. The agglomeration process is a dynamic process where a droplet is created by a two-fluid nozzle and deposited on the randomly fluidized particle. The binder solvent evaporates leaving behind the binder. Before all of the solvent is evaporated, other randomized particles form bonds on the wet site. This process is repeated numerous times to produce desired agglomerated product. There are a number of process variables that control the agglomeration. Process variables most important to consider are listed as follows:

1. Process inlet-air temperature
2. Atomization-air pressure
3. Fluidization-air velocity and volume
4. Liquid spray rate
5. Nozzle position and number of spray heads
6. Product and exhaust-air temperature
7. Filter porosity and cleaning frequency
8. Bowl capacity

These process parameters are interdependent and can produce desirable product if this interdependency is understood. Inlet process-air temperature is determined by the choice of binder solvent, whether aqueous or organic, and the heat sensitivity of the product being agglomerated. Generally, water will enable the use of temperatures between 60 and 100°C. However, organic solvent will require the use of temperatures of 50°C and lower. Higher temperature will produce rapid evaporation of the binder solution and will produce smaller, friable granules. On the other hand, lower temperature will produce larger, fluffier, and denser granules. Gore et al. (91) studied the factors affecting the fluid bed process during scale-up. The authors found that processing factors that most affected granule characteristics were process-air temperature, height of the spray nozzle from the product bed, rate of binder addition, and the degree of atomization of the binder.

Figure 12 shows the relationship of inlet and product temperature and outlet air humidity during the granulation process.

The process of drying while applying spraying solution is a critical unit operation. This mass transfer step was previously discussed. The temperature, humidity, and volume of the process air determine the drying capacity. If the drying capacity of the air is fixed from one batch to the next, then the spray rate can also be fixed. If the drying capacity of the air is too high, the binder solution will have a tendency to spray dry before it can effectively form bridges between the primary particles. If, on the other hand, the drying capacity of the air is too low, the bed moisture level will become too high and particle growth may become uncontrollable. This will result in unacceptable movement of the product bed.

Jones (92) has suggested various process-related factors that should be considered during the scale-up of a fluid bed processing.

As previously discussed, the appropriate process-air volume, inlet-air temperature, and binder spray rate are critical to achieving proper and consistent particle size distribution and granule characteristics. There are many ways

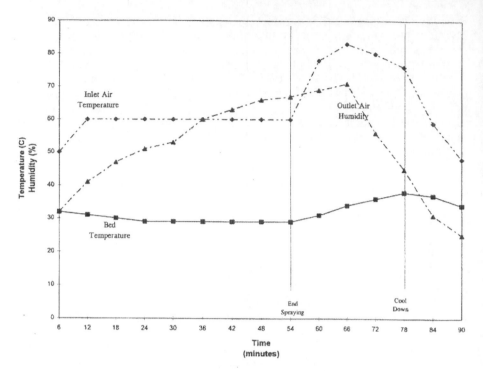

FIGURE 12 Temperature and humidity versus time for spray granulation.

to arrive at the proper operating parameters. The following procedure was found by the author to be one of the ways one can set the operating parameters when granulating with fluid bed processors.

1. Determine the proper volume of air to achieve adequate mixing and particle movement in the bowl. Avoid excessive volumetric airflow so as to entrain the particles into the filters.
2. Choose an inlet-air temperature that is high enough to negate weather effects (outside air humidity or inside room conditions). The air temperature should not be detrimental to the product being granulated. (To achieve consistent process year round, a dehumidification/humidification system is necessary, which provides the process air with constant dew point and hence constant drying capacity.)
3. Achieve a binder solution spray rate that will not dry while spraying (spray drying) and will not overwet the bed. This rate should also allow the nozzle to atomize the binder solution to the required droplet size.
4. As stated earlier, a typical air velocity used for spray granulation is from 1.0 to 2.0 m/sec. Table 1 is based on the psychometric chart that gives a first guess at determining the proper spray rate for a spray granulation process in a fluid bed processor.

Variables in the fluid bed granulation process and their impact on the final granulation was summarized by Davies and Gloor Jr. (93), where they state that

TABLE 1 Calculation of Fluid Bed Spray Rate

Given process data

Air volume range:

Minimum (1.2 m/sec) _____ m^3/hr

Maximum (1.8 m/sec) _____ m^3/hr

Inlet air temperature and humidity to be used: _____ °C_____ %RH

% Solids in sprayed solution _____ % Solids

From psychometric chart

Air density at point where air volume is measured: _____ m^3/kg air

Inlet air absolute humidity (H): _____ g H_2O/kg air

Maximum outlet air absolute humidity (H): _____ g H_2O/kg air

(Follow line of constant adiabatic conditions)

Use 100% outlet RH for spray granulator or 30% to 60% RH (as required for column coating)

Calculations for spray rate

Step 1. Convert air volumetric rate to air mass rate

Minimum _____ m^3/hr ÷ (60 × _____ m^3/kg air) = _____ kg air/min

Maximum_____ m^3/hr ÷ (60 × _____ m^3/kg air) = _____ kg air/min

Step 2. Subtract inlet air humidity from outlet air humidity

_____ (g H_2O/kg air) H out − _____ (g H_2O/kg air) H in

= _____ g H_2O removed/kg air

Step 3. Calculate (minimum and maximum) spray rate of solution:

This will provide range of generally acceptable spray rates based on the air flow used in the unit

Step 1 (minimum) _____ × step 2 _____ ÷ [1 − (____% solids ÷100)]

= _____ spray rate (g/min) at minimum air flow

Step 2 (maximum) _____ × step 2 _____ ÷ [1 − (____% solids ÷100)]

= _____ spray rate (g/min) at minimum air flow

---

the physical properties of granulation are dependent on both the individual formulations and the various operational variables associated with the process. The solution spray rate increase and subsequent increase in average granule size resulted in a less friable granulation, higher bulk density, and a better flow property for a lactose/corn starch granulation. Similar results were obtained by an enhanced binder solution, decreasing nozzle air pressure or lowering the inlet-air temperature during the granulation cycle. The position of the binary nozzle with respect to the fluidized powders was also studied. It was concluded that by lowering the nozzle, binder efficiency is enhanced, resulting in average granule size and a corresponding decrease in granule friability.

The significant process parameters and their effect on the granule properties are summarized in the Table 2.

Maroglou and Nienow (37) listed various parameters affecting the type and rate of growth in batch fluidized granulation (Table 3) and showed the influence of process parameters and material parameters on the product.

TABLE 2   Significant Variables and Their Impact on the Fluid Bed Granulation Process

Process parameter	Impact on process
Inlet air temperature	Higher inlet temperature produces finer granules and lower temperature produces larger stronger granules.
Humidity	Increase in air humidity causes larger granule size, longer drying times.
Fluidizing air flow	Proper air flow should fluidize the bed without clogging the filters. Higher air flow will cause attrition and rapid evaporation, generating smaller granules and fines.
Nozzle and position	A binary nozzle produces the finest droplets and is preferred. The size of the orifice has an insignificant effect except when binder suspensions are to be sprayed. Optimum nozzle height should cover the bed surface. Too close to the bed will wet the bed faster, producing larger granules, while too high a position will spray dry the binder, creating finer granules and increasing granulation time.
Atomization air volume and pressure	Liquid is atomized by the compressed air. This mass-to-liquid ratio must be kept constant to control the droplet size and hence the granule size. Higher liquid flow rate will produce larger droplets and larger granules and the reverse will produce smaller granules. At a given pressure an increase in orifice size will increase droplet size.
Binder spray rate	Droplet size is affected by liquid flow rate, binder viscosity, and atomizing air pressure and volume. The finer the droplet, the smaller the resulting average granules.

TABLE 3   Influence of Operating and Material Parameters on the Granulated Product

A. Operating parameters

Droplet size	NAR[a]
	Atomization air velocity
	Rheology
	Surface tension
	Nozzle position
	Nozzle type
Bed moisture content	Solution type and feed rate
	Bed temperature, fluidization velocity
	Aspect ratio
	Nozzle position and atomization velocity
	Air distributor design, jet grinding
Binder solution/suspension concentration	Bridge strength and size, rheology

B. Material parameters

Binder solution/suspension concentration	Bridge strength and size
	Rheology
Type of binder	Molecular length and weight
Wettability	Particle-solvent interaction
	Surface tension, viscosity
Material to be granulated	Average particle size
	Size distribution[a]
	Shape and porosity, drying characteristics
	Density and density differences[b]

[a]NAR is the ratio of air-to-liquid flow rates through the nozzle of a twin fluid atomizer expressed either in mass units or in volume units (air at STP).
[b]Especially important relative to elutriation and segregation.

Fluid bed processors can be one of the most uniform processes in terms of mixing and temperature. Powder frictional forces are overcome as drag forces of the fluidizing-air support bed weight, and gas bubbles promote rapid and intensive mixing. With regard to bed weight, forces in fluid beds and therefore consolidation and granule density generally scale with bed height.

As previously discussed, granule growth includes the coalescence of existing granules that have been wetted by binder spray and nucleation. As granules grow, they are simultaneously compacted by consolidation mechanisms, which reduce internal voidage or porosity. Because of this complex process, it is difficult to scale-up the granulation process based only on the process variables. The scaling-up of the fluidized granulation process from small scale to production scale is often done empirically in the pharmaceutical industry. Mehta (94) recommended the scaling-up of the process by increasing the spray rate proportionally with the inlet-air volume or the cross-sectional area of the air-distributor plate. However, this method will not always yield acceptable results, since the granule size also depends on more fundamental parameters (95), such as the droplet size (29,41) and the powder bed moisture content (96–98). Therefore, these other parameters must also be considered during scaling-up. The droplet size mainly depends on the spray rate and the nozzle settings. The powder bed moisture content depends on the balance between liquid evaporation and liquid supply. It is desirable that process variables are chosen in such a way that the fundamental variable such as droplet size and the moisture content are kept constant in the different fluid bed scales. Although the theoretical base for granule growth in the fluid bed granulation is known (99,100), few studies have been published on scaling-up of the fluid bed granulation based on the moisture content (96–98) and the droplet size (29). Various growth patterns are discussed previously; the prevailing mechanisms are dictated by a balance of critical particle level properties, which control formulation deformability, and operating variables, which control the localized level of shear or bed agitation intensity. In fluid bed granulation, some deformation takes place during granule collision. Growth is generally controlled by the extent of any surface fluid layer and surface deformability.

The amount of fluidization air required to maintain constant fluidization velocity scales linearly with the cross-sectional area of the bed. The distribution of fluidizing air in a larger fluid bed unit is a major concern, and the proper air-distributor design should be able to address this concern. Normally, the pressure drop across the air-distributor plate should be at least 20% of the total.

To obtain uniform granules, one has to start with product approaching a uniform state of mixing, which in turn will ensure equal moisture and shear levels and therefore uniform granulation kinetics throughout the bed. For scale-up, one must account for this fact where local differences will lead to a wider distribution in granule size distribution and properties in an unpredictable fashion. In fluid bed granulation, growth rate is largely controlled by spray rate and distribution, and consolidation rate by bed height and peak bed moisture. Particle growth in a fluidized bed is closely related to the particle mixing and flow pattern in the bed. This dictates that the hydrodynamics of the scaled batch should be the same as the small unit. He et al. (101) suggested scaling rules for fluid bed granulators. They are summarized as follows:

1. Maintain the fluidized-bed height constant. Granule density and attrition rate increase with the operating bed height.
2. If the bed height is kept similar, then the scaling will be dependent on the cross-sectional area of the bed.
3. Maintain superficial gas velocity constant to keep excess gas velocity, and therefore bubbling and mixing conditions similar.
4. Keep dimensionless spray flux (spray zone) constant. This is why you will need more nozzles. As you scale-up, this will facilitate increase in flow rate as the batch size is increased proportionally.
5. Keep viscous Stokes number constant. [Viscous stokes number is a dimensionless group that represents the ratio of the initial collision kinetic energy to the energy dissipated by viscous lubrication forces (35).] By adhering to the scaling rules described above, this viscous Stokes should be automatically similar in small and large scales, leading to similar consolidation and growth behavior.
6. Increase the area of the bed under the spray (spray flux) by increasing the number of nozzles. This will allow the spray rate increase and result in similar process times.

The amount of fluidization gas required to maintain constant fluidization velocity scales linearly with the cross-section of the bed. However, for large fluidized beds, one of the major concerns is the even distribution of the fluidization gas across the whole area of the bed. Thus, design of the air distributor and lower plenum modification may be required.

During the scale-up process, the quality of the granules may change. A change in the granule size distribution, final moisture content, friability, compressibility, and compactibility of the granules may strongly influence the properties of the final tablet, such as tablet hardness, tablet friability, disintegration time, dissolution rate of the active substance, aging of the tablet, etc. In order to avoid such scale-up problems, a new concept concerning a quasi-continuous production line of granules is presented (102–108).

Process Control and Scale-Up
The fluid bed agglomeration process is a combination of three steps, namely, dry mixing, spray agglomeration, and drying to a desired moisture level. These process steps are equally important. But the quality of the granules is really determined during the spraying stage, where constant building of granules and evaporation of binder solvent is taking place. Granule size is directly proportional to the bed humidity during granulation (41), and hence, control of this humidity during scale-up is essential. Gore et al. (91) studied the factors affecting the fluid bed process during scale-up. The authors found that processing factors that most affected granule characteristics were process-air temperature, height of the spray nozzle from the bed, rate of binder addition, and the degree of atomization of the binder liquid.

The atomizing air pressure and the wetness of the bed are two of the most important elements of fluid bed granulation. A higher atomizing air pressure yields a finer droplet of binder solution. Therefore, granule growth as described earlier in this section will be affected by the atomizing air pressure. A major factor that must be considered during the scale-up of fluid bed granulation process is maintaining the same droplet size of the binder for assuring successful scale-up. A recent study (109) confirmed the influence of spray nozzle set up parameters and drying capacity of the air. The study concluded that more attention should be given to the easily overlooked nozzle atomizing air pressure and volume. When considering the atomizing air pressure, attention must be paid to ensure enough air is delivered to the nozzle tip. This can be assured by placing air pressure and volume measurement devices at the nozzle. The data also shows that the drying capacity of the process air influences the final granulated particle size. Jones (92) has suggested various process-related factors that should be considered during the scale-up of a fluid bed processing. The suggestions are listed below:

Because of the higher degree of attrition in the larger unit compared to the smaller unit, the bulk density of the granulation from the larger fluid bed is approximately 20% higher than the smaller unit. He also reemphasized the importance of keeping the bed moisture level below critical moisture level to prevent the formation of larger agglomerates. Since the higher airflow along with the temperature (drying capacity) in a larger unit provide higher evaporation rate, one must maintain the drying capacity in the larger unit such that the bed temperature is similar to the smaller unit bed temperature. This can be accomplished either by increased spray rate, increased air temperature, increased airflow, or the combination of these variables to obtain suitable results. Since the ratio of bed depth to the air distributor increases with the size of the equipment, the fluidization air velocity is kept constant by increasing the air volume.

In the past, the scale-up was carried out by selecting best guess process parameters. The recent trend is to employ the factorial and modified factorial designs and search methods. These statistically designed experimental plans can generate mathematical relationships between the independent variables such as process factors and dependent variables such as product properties. This approach still requires an effective laboratory/pilot-scale development program and an understanding of the variables that affect the product properties.

In summary, when scaling up, the following processing conditions should be similar to those in the pilot-scale studies.

1. Fluidization velocity of the process air through the system.
2. The ratio of granulation spray rate to drying capacity of fluidization air volume.
3. Droplet size of the binder spray liquid.

Each of these values must be calculated based on the results of the operation of the pilot size unit. Pilot size equipment studies should also be conducted in a wide range to determine the allowable operating range for the process.

In fluid bed granulation process, moisture control is the key parameter that needs to be controlled. Faure et al. (110) have used process control for scale-up of a fluidized-bed process. They used infrared probes to monitor moisture. Since there are normally large numbers of interrelated variables, they used computerized techniques for process control such as fuzzy logic, neural networks, and models based on experimental techniques. Rambali, Baert and Massart (111) scaled up the fluid bed based on relative droplet size and the powder bed moisture content at the end of the spraying cycle.

Some of the researchers have addressed scale-up problems by adopting the semicontinuous granulation techniques (112,113). Werani et al. (114) studied quasi-continuous scale-up of a fluid bed drying after wet granulating in high-shear mixer. By using a series of fluid beds (multicell units), they transferred wet granulated product in first fluid bed dryer, when this batch was semidried, it was transferred to the next fluid bed unit in the series, while the first unit was loaded with freshly granulated batch. This continued until all the cells (fluid bed units) were full and the discharge from the last unit provided a dried product, thus providing a quasi-continuous process.

CASE STUDY

The following case study illustrates how a product is scaled up from 15 to 150 kg in an equipment supplied by Aeromatic (Niro Pharma Systems, Columbia, MD, U.S.) when one understands the critical process parameters used when scaling up.

A spray granulation process was developed in a smaller fluid bed processor for a common pharmaceutical compound. The granulation process involved the spraying of a 5% w/w binder solution onto the fluidized powder. Table 4 shows the data from the 15-kg run and resulting successful 150-kg run condition for a spray agglomeration process (115).

Airflow Calculations

To maintain the same fluidization velocity, the air volume in a larger unit must be increased based on the cross-sectional area of the product bowl. In this case, the cross-sectional area of the base of larger container was 0.77 m^2 and the smaller was 0.06 m^2. The correct airflow should be calculated as 300 × (0.77/0.06) = 3850 CMH. This number was further modified after considering the increase in bed depth in a larger unit to 4000 CMH.

Spray Rate Calculations

To maintain the same particle size, the triple-headed nozzle could spray 3 times the pilot unit spray rate at a 2.5 atomization-air pressure. However, this could result in a longer process time. Another approach to maintain the similar droplet size is to maintain the mass balance of spray rate and the atomization pressure. Thus, by increasing the atomization pressure to 5 bar, the spray rate was increased to 800 g/min, keeping the same droplet size, and hence obtaining granulation with desired characteristics.

Temperature Calculations

Finally, required inlet temperature was recalculated based on the change in ratio of air volume to spray rate. Because the air volume was increased over 13 times

TABLE 4   Scale-Up Process Parameters from a 15- to 150-kg batch

Process parameters (kg)	15	150
Air flow (m^3/hr)	300	4000
Inlet air temperature (°C)	55	50
Spray rate (g/min)	100	800
Nozzle air pressure (bar)	2.5	5
Container cross-sectional area of the base (square meters)	0.06	0.77
Number of nozzles	1	3

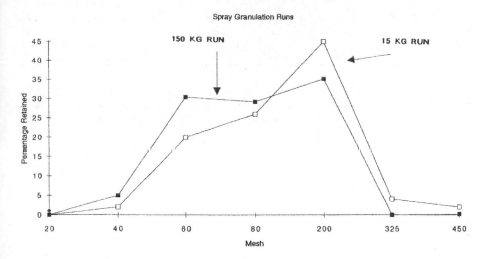

FIGURE 13 Scale-up case study and resultant particle size distribution.

but the spray rate was only increased 8 times, the inlet temperature was reduced to 50°C. This adjustment in drying capacity was necessary to avoid spray drying of the spray solution. (A three-headed nozzle used in this scale-up can be replaced by a six-headed nozzle. This would have resulted in the ability to increase the spraying rate 13 times above the pilot size unit to match the airflow. The maintenance of droplet size and temperature could have been achieved with a six-headed nozzle. The end result would be reduced process time.) Figure 13 shows the particle size distribution produced using 15-kg and 150-kg units.

Another case study conducted by Rambali et al. (95) was based on the relative droplet size. They used the same size nozzle for the small and large scale fluid bed batch with same fundamental granulation process, but produced different granule size. They proposed that the granulation process can be scaled up by regression model. By keeping the droplet size the same for the small and scale-up batch, they were able to get the same granule size. Consideration for other granule properties was not given during this scale-up. They scaled up from 5 to 30 kg and then to 120 kg with a geometric mean granule size of 400 μm.

MATERIAL HANDLING

As you scale up, the transfer of materials to and from the fluid bed processor is an important consideration. The loading and unloading of the processing bowl can be accomplished by manual mode or by automated methods.

Loading

The contemporary method for loading the unit is by removing the product bowl from the unit, charging the material into the bowl, and then placing the bowl back into the unit. This loading is simple and cost-effective. Unfortunately, it has the potential of exposing the operators to the product and contaminating the working area. To avoid the product being a dust and cleaning hazard, a dust collection system should be installed to collect the dust before it spreads. A manual process also depends on the batch size, the operator's physical ability to handle the material, and the container full of product. Furthermore, this can be time consuming since the material must be added to the product container, one material at a time.

The loading process can be automated and isolated to avoid worker exposure, minimize dust generation, and reduce loading time. There are two main type of loading systems. These systems are similar because both use the fluid bed's capability to create a vacuum inside the unit. Here the product enters the fluid bed through a product in-feed port on the side of the unit. This is done by having the fan running and the inlet-air control flap set so that minimum airflow may pass through the product container and the outlet flap is almost fully open. Once the material has been charged to the fluid bed, the product in-feed valve is closed and the granulating process started. This transfer method uses some amount of air to help the material move through the tube.

Loading can be done either vertically from an overhead bin or from the ground. Less air is required through the transfer pipe when the material is transferred vertically, because gravity is working to help the process. Vertical transfer methods do require greater available height in the process area. Loading by this method has the advantages of limited operator exposure to the product, allows the product to be fluidized as it enters the processor, and reduces the loading time. The disadvantage of this type of system is that cleaning is required between different products.

Unloading

As with loading, the standard method for unloading is by removing the product bowl from the unit. Once the bowl is removed, the operator may scoop the material from the bowl, which is the most time-consuming and impractical method, because of its potential for exposure to the product. Alternatively, the product can be vacuum transferred to a secondary container or unloaded by placing the product bowl into bowl dumping device as shown in Figure 14. This hydraulic device is installed in the processing area. The mobile product container of the fluid bed processor is pushed under the cone of the bowl dumper and coupled together by engaging the toggle locks. Subsequently, the container is lifted hydraulically, pivoted around the lifting column, and rotated 180° for discharging.

Use of the bowl dumping device or vacuum unloading device still requires that the product bowl be removed from the unit.

There are contained and automated methods for unloading the product while the product bowl is still in the fluid bed processor. The product may either be unloaded out of the bottom of the product container or from the side. Until recently, the most common contained method is to unload the material from the bottom of the unit. This requires the ceiling height high enough to accommodate or the installation becomes a multistoried installation. There are two types of bottom discharge options: gravity or pneumatic. Gravity discharge (Figs. 15 and 16) allows for collection of the product into container, which is located below the lower plenum. If the overall ceiling height limitation prevent from having the discharge by gravity, the gravity/pneumatic transfer combination can be considered. The gravity discharge poses cleaning problems, since the

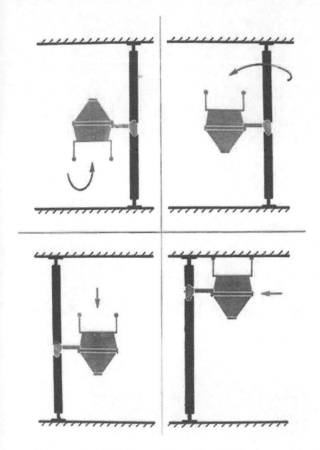

FIGURE 14 Product discharge from the fluid bed processing bowl using lift device.

process air and the product discharge follow the same path; assurance of cleanliness is always of prime concern.

The desire to limit the processing area, and the development of the overlap gill air distributor mentioned earlier in the chapter, has prompted the consideration of the side discharge as an option. The product bowl is fitted with the discharge gate as shown in Figures 17 and 18.

Most of the product being free-flowing granules flows through the side discharge into a container (Fig. 19). The remainder of the product is then discharged by manipulation of the airflow through the overlap gill air distributor. The discharged product can be pneumatically transported to an overhead bin if the dry milling of the granulation is desired.

The contained system for unloading the product helps to isolate the operator from the product. The isolation feature also prevents the product from being contaminated due to exposure to the working environment. Material handling consideration must be thought of early in the equipment procurement process. Fluid bed processing, whether used as a integral part of high-shear

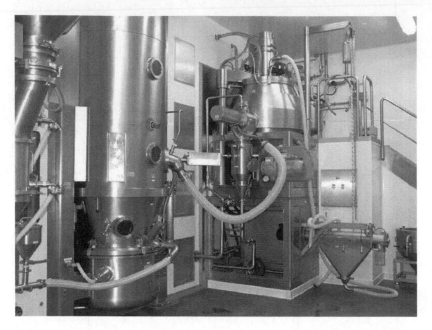

FIGURE 15   Fluid bed charging of wet granulated product from high-shear mixer.

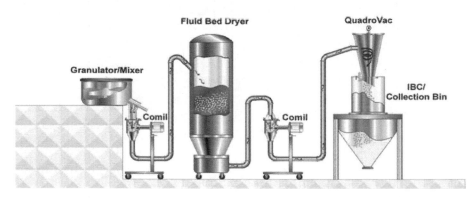

FIGURE 16   Integrated system with in-process milling and vacuum transfer. *Source*: Courtesy of Quadro Engineering.

mixer/fluid bed dryer or as a granulating equipment option, production efficiency and eventual automation can be enhanced by considering these loading and unloading options.

Number of companies has addressed scale-up challenge by introducing the smaller but continuous granulation and drying systems. Two such approaches are shown in Figures 20 and 21. The advantages in these systems is you can run this units as much or as little as you need. Hence, the process

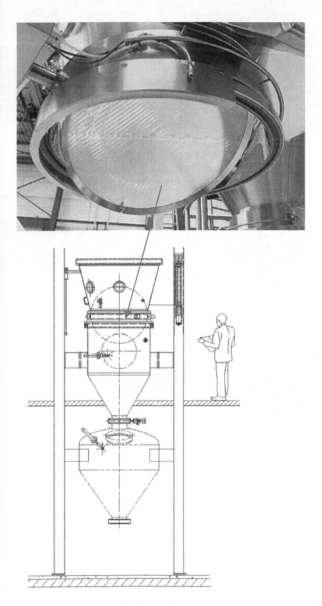

FIGURE 17 Bottom discharge from the bowl in the hopper. *Source*: Courtesy of Glatt Group, U.S.A.

variables from small-scale production to the large-scale production do not vary where you have to carry out number of runs to validate the scale-up of a batch. Obviously, it is desirable to have these systems dedicated to the single product to avoid the set up and dismantling and cleaning problems if you change the product.

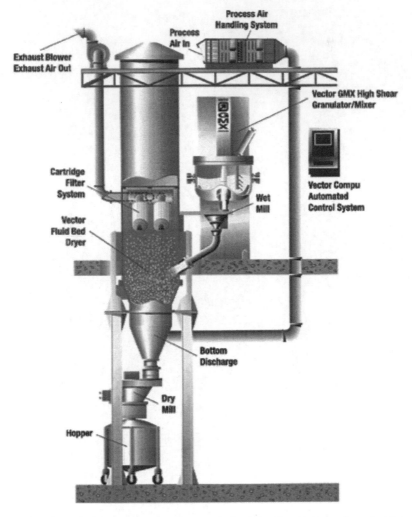

FIGURE 18 Integrated system with a gravity feed showing discharge from the high-shear mixer and from the fluid bed dryer. *Source*: Courtesy of The Vector Corporation.

REGULATORY PERSPECTIVE

Scale-up is normally identified with an incremental increase in batch size until a desired level of production is obtained. In 1991, American Association of Pharmaceutical Scientists (AAPS) with the U.S. FDA held a workshop on scale-up (116), where several speakers presented scale-up issues from an industrial and regulatory perspective. The scale-up process and the changes made after approval in the composition, manufacturing process, manufacturing equipment, and change of site have become known as Guidelines for Scale-Up and Postapproval Changes (SUPAC). The FDA since has issued various guidances for SUPAC changes designated SUPAC-IR1 (for immediate-release solid oral dosage forms), SUPAC-MR2 (for modified-release solid oral dosage forms), and

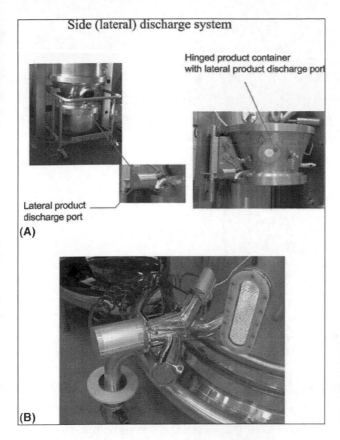

FIGURE 19 (A) Side discharge from the product bowl. (B) Side discharge from the product bowl. *Source*: Part A courtesy of The Glatt Group; Part B courtesy of GEA Pharma Systems.

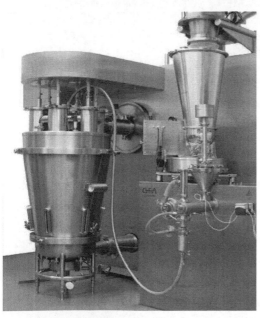

FIGURE 20 Continuous granulation and drying "consigma." *Source*: Courtesy of GEA Niro Pharma Systems.

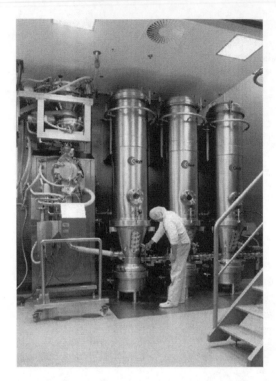

FIGURE 21 Continuous manufacturing approach with a "multicell" approach. *Source*: Courtesy of The Glatt Group.

SUPAC-SS3 (for nonsterile semisolid dosage forms including creams, ointments, gels, and lotions) (117). In 1995, FDA issued SUPAC guidance for industry (118) for immediate-release dosage forms, and in 1997, SUPAC-MR guidance was released for modified-release dosage forms (119). For current information and subsequent changes to FDA guidance, reader is advised to look up the FDA website (http://www.FDA.gov).

   Although scale-up may occur at any point in the lifetime of a product, it most often occurs after the firm has been notified that the drug product is approvable, that is, it meets all the conditions required by the FDA for marketing. With the submittal of Final Printed Labeling, a showing that the marketed product will meet the conditions for marketing as approved by the FDA (and in the case of generics, production of three consecutive scaled-up batches), and satisfactory completion of a preapproval inspection by the local FDA district office, the product is formally approved to be manufactured and sold in the United States. At this point, SUPAC begins to exert its effect.

SUMMARY
Scale-up is normally identified with an incremental increase in batch size until a desired level of production is obtained. The fluid bed process, similar to other granulation techniques, requires an understanding of the importance of characterization of the raw materials, especially of an active pharmaceutical ingredient, process equipment, limitations of the selected process, establishment of an

in-process control specifications, characterization of the finished product, and cleaning and process validation. It is equally important that the formulation and development scientists do not lose sight of the fact that the process being developed in the pilot plant will someday be transferred to the production floor. The scientists should spend enough time in the production department to understand the scale of operation that the desired process is being developed to. If the process development scientist has not spend enough time understanding the various interrelated variables then it will be difficult to have a robust process for the commercial operation.

Scaling up by maintaining the droplet size of the granulating liquid will enhance probability of uniform nucleation stage to build the granules. Similarly, scientist must think through how the material will be added and taken away from the processor on a commercial scale. Without this forethought, many a times I have seen processes that come to production are very labor-intensive. If the development scientists work with production and engineering departments from an early stage, these difficulties can be avoided.

REFERENCES

1. Wurster DE. Air-suspension technique of coating drug particles; a preliminary report. J Am Pharm Assoc Am Pharm Assoc (Baltim) 1959; 48(8):451–454.
2. Wurster DE. Preparation of compressed tablet granulations by the air-suspension technique II. J Am Pharm Assoc Am Pharm Assoc 1960; 49:82–84.
3. Scott MW, Liberman HA, Rankell AS, et al. Continuous production of tablet granulation in fluid bed I. Theory and design consideration. J Pharm Sci 1964; 53(3):314–319.
4. Rankell AS, Scott MW, Liberman HA, et al. Continuous production of tablet granulation in fluid bed I. Theory and design consideration II. J Pharma Sci 1964; 53(3):320.
5. Contini S, Atasoy K. Fluid bed granulation, a modern economic method for tabletting and encapsulation. Pharm Ind 1966; 28:144–146.
6. Wolf G. Fluidized layer spray granulation. Drugs Made Ger 1968; 11:172–180.
7. Liske T, Mobus W. The manufacture and comparative aspects of fluidized layer spray granulation. Drugs Made Ger 1968; 11:182–189.
8. Sherrington PJ, Oliver R. "Granulation" monograph. In: Goldberg AS, ed. Powder Science and Technology. London: Heyden, 1981.
9. Pietch WB. Fluidization phenomenon and fluidization technology. In: Fayed ME, Otten L, eds. Handbook of Powder Science and Technology. New York: Van Nostrand Reinhold, 1984.
10. Hersey JA. Fluidized bed technology-an overview. Int J Pharm Tech Prod Manuf 1981; 2(3):3–4.
11. Thiel WJ. The theory of fluidization and application to the industrial processing of pharmaceutical products. Int J Pharm Tech Prod Manuf 1981; 2(5):5–8.
12. Thiel WJ. Solids mixing in gas fluidized beds. Int J Pharm Tech Prod Manuf 1981; 2 (9):9–12.
13. Littman H. An overview of flow in fluidized beds. Pharm Technol 1985; 9(3):48.
14. Whitehead AB. Behavior of fluidized bed systems. Pharm Technol 1981; 2:13–18.
15. Story MJ. Granulation and film coating in the fluidized bed. Pharm Technol 1981; 2 (19):19–23.
16. Aulton MJ, Banks M. Fluidized bed granulation, factors influencing the quality of the product. Pharm Technol 1981; 2(24):24–27.
17. Kulling W, Simon EJ. Fluid bed technology applied to pharmaceuticals. Pharm Technol 1980; 4(1):79–83.
18. Gomezplata A, Kugelman AM. Processing systems. In: Marchello JM, Gomezplata A, eds. Gas - Solid Handling in the Process Industries, Chemical Processing and Engineering. Vol 8. New York: Marcel-Dekker, Inc, 1976.

19. Parikh DM. Airflow in batch fluid-bed processing. Pharm Technol 1991; 15(3):100–110.
20. Rowe PN, Patridge BA, Cheney AG, et al. The mechanisms of solids mixing in fluidized beds. Trans Inst Chem Eng 1965; T271–T286.
21. Davies L, Richardson JF. Gas Interchange between bubbles and the continuous phase in a fluidized bed. Trans Inst Chem Eng 1966; 44:T293–T305.
22. Godnichev VI, Borisov GN, Egorova VI. Parameters of the process of drying medicinal granules in apparatus having a fluidized bed. Institute of Pharm Chem, Leningrad (USSR). Translated from Russian 1974; 8:298.
23. Zenz FA. In: Kirk-Othmer, ed. Fluidization: Encyclopedia of Chemical Technology. Vol. 10, 3rd ed. New York: Wiley-Interscience Publication, 1981:548–581.
24. Kunii D, Levenspiel O. Fluidization Engineering. 2nd ed. New York: McGraw Hill, 1991.
25. Masters K. Spray Drying, an Introduction to Principles, Operational Practice and Application. 2nd ed. New York: John Wiley & Sons Inc., 1976.
26. Newitt DM, Conway-Jones JM. A contribution to the theory and practice of granulation. Int J Pharm Tech Prod Manuf 1958; 36:422.
27. Record PC. A review of pharmaceutical granulation technology. Int J Pharm Tech Prod Manuf 1980; 1:32.
28. Rumpf H. The strength of granules and agglomerates. In: Krepper W, ed. Agglomeration. New York: Interscience 1962:379–418.
29. Schaefer T, Worts O. Control of fluidized bed granulation I. Effects of spray angle, nozzle height and starting materials on granule size and size distribution. Arch Pharm Chem Sci Ed 1977; 5:51–60.
30. Smith PJ, Nienow AW. Particle growth mechanism in fluidized bed granulation. Chem Eng Sci 1983; 38(8):1223–1231; 1323–1240.
31. Aulton ME, Banks M. Fluidized bed granulation-factors including the quality of the product. Int J Pharm Tech Prod Manuf 1981; 2(4):24–29.
32. Goldschmidt MJV. Hydrodynamic Modeling of Fluidized Bed Spray Granulation [PhD thesis]. Enschede, The Netherlands: Twente University, 2001.
33. Ennis BJ. On the Mechanics of Granulation [PhD thesis]. New York: The City College of the City University of New York, University Microfilms International, 1990 (No.1416, Printed 1991).
34. Ennis BJ. Design & Optimization of Granulation Processes for Enhanced Product Performance. Nashville, TN: E&G Associates, 1990–2004.
35. Litster J, Ennis BJ. The Science & Engineering of Granulation Processes. Dordrecht, The Netherlands: Kluwer Academic, 2004.
36. Maroglou A, Nienow AW. Fourth Symposium on Agglomeration. Toronto, Canada: Iron & Steel Society Inc., 1985:465–470.
37. Maroglou A, Nienow AW. Fluidized bed granulation technology and its application to tungsten carbide. Powder Metall 1986; 29(4):195–291.
38. McCabe WL, Smith JC. Unit Operations of Chemical Engineering. New York, NY: McGraw-Hill, 1956.
39. Green Don W, ed. Perry's Chemical Engineer's Handbook, Section 20. New York, New York: McGraw-Hill, Inc., 1984.
40. Rankell RS, Liberman HA, Schiffman RF. Drying. In: Lachman L, Lieberman HA, Kanig JL, eds. The Theory and Practice of Industrial Pharmacy. 3rd ed. Philadelphia: Lea & Feabiger, 1986.
41. Schaefer T, Worts O. Control of fluidized granulation III, effects of the inlet air temperature, and liquid flow rate on granule size and size distribution. Control of moisture content of granules in the drying phase. Arch Pharm Chem Sci Ed 1978; 6(1):1–13.
42. Thurn U. Dissertation no. 4511, Eidgenossischen Technischen, Hochschule, Zurich, 1970.
43. Liske T, Mobus W. The manufacture of comparative aspects of fluidized layer spray granulation. Drugs Made Ger 1968; 11(4):182–189.
44. Schaefer T, Worts O. Control of fluidized bed granulation V, factors affecting granule growth. Arch Pharm Chem Sci Ed 1978; 6:69–82.

45. Ormos Z, Pataki K. Studies in granulation in a fluidized bed. VII. The effect of raw materials upon the granule formation. Hung J Indust Chem 1979; 7:89–103.
46. Ormos Z, Pataki K. Studies in granulalation in a fluidized bed. VIII. Effect of the raw material initial particle size upon granule formation. Hung J Indust Chem 1979; 7:105–117.
47. Banks M. PhD thesis, C.N.A.A. Leicester Polytechnic, 1981.
48. Galmen MJ, Greer W. Fluid Technol Pharm Manuf International Conference, paper 2, 1982.
49. Aulton ME. Fluid Technol Pharm Manuf International Conference, paper 3, Powder Advisory Center, London, 1982.
50. Veillard M, Benetejac R, Puisieux F, et al. A study of granule structure: Effects of the method of manufacture and effects of granule structure on compressibility into tablet form. Int J Pharm Tech Prod Mfg 1982; 3(4):100–107
51. Georgakopoulos PP, Malamataris S, Dolamidis G, et al. The effects of using different grades of PVP and gelatin as binders in the fluidized bed granulation and tabletting of lactose. Pharmazie 1983; 38(4):240–243.
52. Jinot JC, et al. S.T.P. Pharma 1986; 2(13):126–131.
53. Shinoda A, et al. Yakuzaigaku 1976; 36(2):83–88.
54. Aulton ME, Banks M, Smith DK. The wettability of powders during fluidized bed granulation. J Pharm Pharmacol 1977; 29(suppl):59P.
55. Schepky G. Die Wirbelschichtgranulierung. Acta Pharm Technol 1978; 24(3):185–212.
56. Aulton ME, et al. Proc Int Conf Powder Technol. In: Pharmacy, Powder Advisory Center, Basel, Switzerland, 1979.
57. Kocova EI. Arini S, et al. Drugs Made Ger 1983; 26(4):205–211.
58. Davies WL, Gloor WT. Batch production of pharmaceutical granulation in a fluidized bed. II. Effects of various binders and their concentrations on granulations and compressed tablets. J Pharm Sci 1972; 61(4):618–622.
59. Rouiller M, Gurny R, Doelker E. Possibilities de production avec un appareil a lit fluidise de laboratoire. Acta Pharm Technol 1975; 21(2):129–138.
60. Ormos Z, Pataki K, Stefko B. Studies in granulation in a fluidized bed. IX. Effects of concentration of various binders upon granule formation. Hung J Indust Chem 1979; 7:131–140.
61. Ormos Z, Pataki K, Stefko B. Studies in granulation in a fluidized bed. X. Effects of the relative amounts of various binders upon granule formation. Hung J Indust Chem 1979; 7:141–151.
62. Ormos Z. Studies in granulation in a fluidized bed. XI. Approximate description of the particle size distribution. Hung J Indust Chem 1979; 7:153–163.
63. Ormos Z. Studies in granulation in a fluidized bed. XII. Bed expansion of fluidized heterodisperse granule masses. Hung J Indust Chem 1979; 7:221–235.
64. Kocova El-Arini S. Pharm Ind 1981; 43(7):674–679.
65. Jager KF, Bauer KH. Acta Pharm Technol 1984; 30(1):85–92.
66. Nouh ATI. Pharm Ind 1986; 48(6):670–673.
67. Alkan H, et al. Doga Tu J Med Pharm 1987; 11(1):1–7.
68. Bank A, et al. Proc 2nd Conf Appl Physic Chem 1971; 2:687–692.
69. Davies WL, Gloor WT. Batch production of pharmaceutical granulations in a fluidized bed. III. Binder dilution effects on granulation. J Pharm Sci 1973; 62(1):170–172.
70. Ormos Z, Pataki K, Csukas B. Studies on granulation in fluidized bed. I. Methods for testing the physical properties of granulates. Hung J Indust Chem 1973; 1:307–328.
71. Ormos Z, Pataki K, Csukas B. Studies on granulation. II. The effect of the amount of binder on the physical properties of granules formed in a fluidized bed. Hung J Indust Chem 1973; 1:463–474.
72. Johnson MCR, et al. J Pharm Pharmacol 1975; 80P(suppl).
73. Aulton ME, Banks M. The factors affecting the fluidized bed granulation. Mfg Chem and Aerosol News 1978; 12:50–56.
74. Gorodnichev VI, et al. Pharm Chem J (USSR) 1980; 14(10):72–77.
75. Ceschel GC, et al. II Farmaco Ed Prat 1981; 36(6):281–293.
76. Rangnarsson G, et al. Int J Pharm 1982; 12:163–171.

77. Meshali M, El-Banna HM, El-Sabbagh H. Use of fractional factorial design to evaluate granulations prepared in a fluidized bed. Pharmazie 1983; 38(5):323–325.
78. Hajdu R, Ormos Z. Studies on granulation in a fluidized bed. XV. Establishment of steady state operation conditions in a continuously operated single cell apparatus. Hung J Ind Chem 1983; 12:425–430.
79. Devay A, Uderszky J, Racz I. Optimization of operational parameters in fluidized bed granulation of effervescent pharmaceutical preparations. Acta Pharm Technol 1984; 30(3):239–242.
80. Alkan MH, Yuksel A. Granulation in fluidized bed II—Effects of binder amount on the final granules. Drug Dev Ind Pharm 1986; 12(10):1529–1543.
81. Hontz J. Assessment of Selected Formulation and Processing Variables in Fluid Bed Granulation [PhD thesis]. Baltimore: University of Maryland at Baltimore, Dissertation Abs Int 1987; (6):1655-B.
82. Wan LSC, Lim KS. The effect of incorporating polyvinylpyrrolidone as a binder on fluidized bed granulations of lactose. S.T.P. Pharm 1988; 4(7):560–571.
83. Wan LSC, Lim KS. Mode of action of polyvinylpyrrolidine as a binder on fluidized bed granulation of lactose and starch granules. S.T.P. Pharm 1989; 5(4):244–250.
84. Grimsey I, Feeley J, York P. Analysis of the surface energy of pharmaceutical powders by inverse gas chromatography. J Pharm Sci 2002; 91:571–583.
85. Thielmann F, Naderi M, Ansari MA, et al. The effect of primary particle surface energy on agglomeration rate in fluidized bed wet granulation. Powder Technol 2007, doi: 10, 1016/ j.powtec.2006.12.015.
86. Wan Lucy SC, Heng Paul WS, Muhuri G. Incorporation and distribution of a low dose drug in granules. Int J Pharm 1992; 88:159–163.
87. Higashide F, Miki Y, Nozawa Y, et al. Dependence of drug content uniformity on particle sizes in fluidized bed granulation. Pharm Ind 1985; 47(11):1202–1205.
88. Davies WL, Gloor WT Jr. Batch production of Pharmaceutical granulation in fluidized bed II: effects of various binders and their concentrations on granulations and compressed tablets. J Pharm Sci 1972; 61:618.
89. Davies WL, Gloor WT Jr. Batch production of Pharmaceutical granulation in fluidized bed III: binder dilution effects on granulation. J Pharm Sci 1973; 62:170.
90. Parikh DM, Jones DM. Batch fluid bed granulation. In: Parikh DM, ed. Handbook of Pharmaceutical Granulation Technology. 3rd ed. New York: Informa Health, 2009.
91. Gore AY, McFarland DW, Batuyios NH. Fluid bed granulation: factors affecting the process in laboratory development and production scale-up. Pharm Technol 1985; 9 (9):114.
92. Jones DM. Factors to consider in fluid bed processing. Pharm Technol 1985; 9(4):50.
93. Davies WL, Gloor WT Jr. Batch production of pharmaceutical granulation in fluidized bed I: effects of process variables on physical properties of final granulation. J Pharm Sci 1971; 60(12):1869–1874.
94. Mehta AM. Scale-up considerations in the fluid-bed process for controlled-release products. Pharm Tech 1988; 12:46–52.
95. Rambali B, Baert L, Thoné D, et al. Using experimental design to optimize the process parameters in fluidized bed granulation on semi full scale. Int J Pharm 2001; 220:149–160.
96. Watano S, Morikawa T, Miyanami K. Mathematical model in the kinetics of agitation fluidized bed granulation. Effects of humidity content, damping speed and operation time on granule growth rate. Chem Pharm Bull 1996; 44:409–415.
97. Watano S, Fukushima T, Miyanami K. Heat transfer and granule growth rate in fluidized bed granulation. Chem Pharm Bull 1996; 44:572–576.
98. Watano S, Takashima H, Sato Y, et al. Measurement of humidity content by IR sensor in fluidized bed granulation. Effects of operating variables on the relationship between granule humidity content and absorbance of IR spectra. Chem Pharm Bull 1996; 44:1267–1269.
99. Schaafsma SH. Down-scaling of a Fluidised Bed Agglomeration Process [PhD dissertation of Rijksuniversiteit Groningen]. New York: Mercel Dekker, 2000:159.
100. Sherrington PJ, Oliver R. Granulation. London: Heyden & Son Ltd, 1981:7–60.

101. He Y, Liu LX, Litster JD, et al. Scale-up considerations in Granulation. In: Parikh DM, ed. Handbook of Pharmaceutical Granulation Technology. 3rd ed. New York, NY: Informa Health, 2009.
102. SchadeA. Herstellung von pharmazeutischen Granulaten in einem kombinierten Feuchtgranulations-und Mehrkammer-Wirbelschichttrocknungsverfahren, Dissertation Universitat Basel, 1992.
103. Schade A, Leuenberger H. Herstellung pharmazeutischer Granulate in einem kombinierten Feuchtgranulations-und Mehrkammer-Wirbelschicuttrockungsverfahren. Chem Ing Tech 1992; 64(11):1016–1018.
104. Dörr B. Entwicklung einer Anlage zur quasikontinuierlichen Feuchtgranulierung und Mehrkammer Wirbelschichttrocknung von pharmazeutischen Granulaten, Dissertation Universität Basel, 1996.
105. Dörr B, Leuenberger H. Development of a quasi-continuous production line—a concept to avoid scale-up problems. In: Leuenberger H, ed. Preprints First European Symposium on Process Technologies in Pharmaceutical and Nutritional Sciences, PARTEC 98 Nürnberg, Nürnberg Wesse, GmbH, D-90471, Nürnberg, 1998:247–256.
106. Leuenberger H. New trends in the production of pharmaceutical granules: the classical batch concept and the problem of scale-up. Eur J Pharm Biopharm 2001; 52:279–288.
107. Leuenberger H. New trends in the production of pharmaceutical granules: batch versus continuous processing. Eur J Pharm Biopharm 2001; 52:289–298.
108. Leuenberger H. Scale-up in the 4th dimension in the field of granulation and drying. 7th Int. Symposium on Agglomeration 2001, Albi, France, May 29–31, 2001:375–389.
109. Bonck JA. Spray granulation. Presented at: the AIChE Annual Meeting, November, 1993.
110. Faure A, York P, Rowe RC. Process control and scale-up of pharmaceutical wet granuation process: a review. Eur J Pharm Biopharm 2001; 52(3):269–277.
111. Rambali B, Baert L, Massart DL. Scaling up of fluidized bed granulation process. Int J Pharm 2003; 252(1–2):197–206.
112. Leuenberger H. Scale-up in the fourth dimension in the field of granulation and drying or how to avoid classic scale-up. Powder Technol 2003; 130(1–3):225–230.
113. Liedy W, Hilligardt K. Contribution to the scale-up of fluidized bed driers and conversion from batchwise to continuous operation. Chem Eng Processing 1991; 30(1):51–58.
114. Werani J, Grünberg M, Ober C, et al. Semicontinuous granulation—the process of choice for the production of pharmaceutical granule? Powder Technol 2004; 140:163–168.
115. Parikh DM, Mogavero M. Batch fluid bed granulation. In: Parikh DM, ed. Handbook of Pharmaceutical Granulation Technology. 2nd ed. New York, NY: Marcel-Dekker, 2005.
116. AAPS/FDA. Scale-Up of Oral Solid Dosage Forms. December 11–13, 1991.
117. Available at: www.fda.gov/downloads/Drugs/GuidanceComplianceRegulatory Information/Guidances/ucm070636.pdf
118. Immediate Release Solid Dosage Forms, Scale-up and Post Approval Changes: Chemistry, Manufacturing and Control, In-Vitro Dissolution Testing and In-Vivo Bioequivalence Documentation. Rockville, MD: FDA Center for Drug Evaluation and Research, November 30, 1995.
119. FDA, September 1997, 2/1999, Guidance for Industry: SUPAC-MR: Modified Release Solid Oral Dosage Forms: Scale-up and Post-approval Changes: Chemistry, Manufacturing and Controls, In vitro Dissolution Testing, and In Vitro Bioequivalence Documentation.

12 Roller compaction scale-up

Ronald W. Miller

PROLOGUE

Some elements of this chapter were described in the first and third editions of the *Handbook of Pharmaceutical Granulation Technology*, in the chapters titled Roller Compaction Technology, by the author in 1997 and 2009 (1,2). During these years a number of new equipment design features, research, roller compaction usage in the industry, and new technology advances have added to the best practices of roller compaction within the pharmaceutical unit operations (3). Since, the second edition of this book's publishing, 2006, the world's economies have slowed and capital expansion in the worldwide pharmaceutical industry, particularly in oral solid dosage forms, has suffered. A number of pharmaceutical drug companies, large and small, have had and are still reducing staffs, selling manufacturing sites, or merging (e.g., recently in 2009 Pfizer–Wyeth and Merck–Schering–Plough mergers), thus reducing costs by eliminating many duplicate jobs and ultimately rebuilding corporate cash positions. During the last three years, new drug development has slowed as well, as evident of fewer new drug approvals by the U.S. Food and Drug Administration (FDA). In spite of the apparent pharmaceutical industry economics and the innovative drug downturn trends, temporary, I do believe, the important need for dry granulation technology keeps growing in the pharmaceutical industry, as well as in other industries. Evidence is seen by roller compactor vendors still manufacturing machines for the pharmaceutical industry and bodes well for the technology. This chapter serves the abbreviated purpose of defining roller compaction scale-up in the pharmaceutical industry.

SCALE-UP BACKGROUND

This chapter does offer specific compaction process scale-up and equipment technology transfer concepts observed by the author and others, which have been published. To those who contributed and are advancing roller compaction manufacturing science, it is gratifying to see a paradigm shift and an expansion to dry granulation roller compaction technology in our industry. Additionally, with Process Analytical Technology (PAT) tools, significant opportunities to standardize roller compaction scale-up exist, and will be discussed in this chapter. My view is that PAT tools will drive roller compaction scale-up for many years to come on the likes of work established by Dr A. Gupta and others (4).

Factors of scaling-up a pharmaceutical compaction process or equipment technology transfer involve a number of issues and technologies. Numerous considerations go beyond the specific process and manufacturing science that evolve from the pilot plant to the manufacturing technical operations center. Most of these concerns are centered on the plant's current operations and its prior use or manufacture of dry granulations using roller compaction technology. See reference that cites comparative study summary (3).

Some scaling factors that go beyond specific formulation technical aspects follow: What type of equipment manufacturer support is expected? What is the reputation and reliability of the equipment manufacturer in the country? Where will the start-up occur? What is the equipment manufacturer's customer service record worldwide? How many days will it take to replace a broken or worn out part? Does the equipment manufacturer carry a reliable stock parts inventory? A pharmaceutical manufacturing survey evaluated industrial practices and preferences that addressed some of these questions (3).

Additionally, what is a company's commitment to technology and engineering support before and after start-up? Who provides the training costs? Who pays what? Is the in-process testing equipment and necessary analytical equipment operational, qualified, and ready when needed? Who will perform the validation requirements (equipment and process)? These are some of the key questions and concerns that go beyond the hardware issues and technology that need to be addressed prior to the project start-up. Discussing, planning, and financing these issues with the receiving site key personnel, equipment vendors, research, development, engineering and technology personnel well in advance of the technology scale-up will make for a much more successful process technology transition and transfer. Are the technical experts prepared and available to provide the timely support: vendor and technology? Have the following equipment, support systems, and process condition questions been asked and answered; What, Where, Why, When, How, and Who? A scale-up evaluation checklist referring to personnel training, logistical matters, engineering support, raw material delivery system, compactor design, environmental issues, raw material characterization is referenced for the interested reader (1–3).

Professionals in pharmaceutical manufacturing science understand that no single written journal article could hope to provide universal guidance on roller compaction scale-up. On the other hand, the best way to solve these types of challenges is to attack them systematically. This usually can be achieved through appropriate process qualifications and validation efforts: trial-and-error approaches before start-up, knowledge of equipment processing capabilities and limitations, and understanding the raw materials' variability. On the other hand, PAT tools and approaches will offer different pathways to better understand the scale-up and the validation process (5).

Discussion about roller compaction solid dosage form scale-up, specifically here, does not imply compliance with suggested Scale-Up and Postapproval Change (SUPAC) guidelines. The described approaches do not necessarily provide ideas/recommendations that meet tests and filing requirements for changes in manufacturing processes and equipment. Scale-up guidance for immediate-release solid dosage forms and postapproval changes have been published. Readers are suggested to familiarize themselves with the referenced material (6).

The FDA CDER (Center for Drug Evaluation and Research) has published significant new changes for good manufacturing practices for process validation when advanced pharmaceutical science and engineering principles and manufacturing control technologies provide a high level of process understanding and control capability (7). The Agency indicates that manufacturers using such procedures and controls may not necessarily have to manufacture multiple conformance batches to complete process validation (7). How times have changed!

SCALE-UP TECHNICAL ILLUSTRATIONS

The following roller compaction scale-up examples illustrate technology strategies that speak to "how to" identify equipment design features, process parameters, and evaluations defining roller compaction scale-up process parameters.

Carver Press Scale-Up to Roller Compactor

Gereg and Cappolla developed process parameters determined by a model laboratory bench-scale Carver press, model C. Carver Inc., which were translated to production-scale compactor parameters (8). Their study provided a method to predict whether a material is suitable for roller compaction. Their study objectives were to characterize properties of the material to identify process parameters suitable to achieve the necessary particle size and density using the dry granulation process and then translate laboratory information to a production-scale roller compactor. Actually, information developed from a Carver press was correlated and scaled up to a production-scale Fitzpatrick roller compactor (model IR 520 Fitzpatrick Co., Elmhurst, Illinois, U.S.). The compactor produced very similar powder granule characteristics as the Carver press. Various lactose materials, available as lactose monohydrate or spray-dried lactose monohydrate, were used as model compounds. Results indicated that a parametric correlation could be made between the laboratory bench Carver press and the production-scale compactor and that many process parameters can be transferred directly. Using the Carver press, samples were compressed by applying a force from 500 to 10,000 lb in increments of 500 lbs. The compact volume, density, and pressure were calculated. The scientists prepared regular-grade lactose compacts using the Fitzpatrick compactor from conditions determined from the Carver press. The selected compaction force value was converted to the total compaction force by multiplying the surface area of a compact by the selected compaction pressure using Eq. (1).

$$F = P \times A \tag{1}$$

Where F is the total force between rolls, P is the selected pressure, and A is the compact surface area. The total compaction force was applied to the roller compactor by converting it to pound-force per linear-inch of roll width, and ultimately converted to hydraulic pressure using the Fitzpatrick conversion table (8). The roller compactor's full axial rolls produced compacts in the form of "sticks." The unmilled compacts from both machines had the same density, 1.3 g/cm^3. The milled roller compacts produced comparative granules except for bulk density and correspondingly the Carr index values (Eq. 2).

$$\frac{\text{Tapped density} - \text{Bulk density}}{\text{Tapped density}} \times 100\% \tag{2}$$

The milled compacts generated slightly larger particles, where the round slugs produced by the Carver press produced a greater number of fines. The compactor flow rate for the milled roller-compacted material was twice as fast as that of the Carver press' granules, both flow rates were deemed acceptable. The authors concluded that both methods produced, for all practical purposes, equivalent granulated material.

Slugging Vs. Compaction Technology

A new antibiotic tablet was introduced internationally in three countries. Two countries did not have compactors to manufacture the product. Their process consisted of the following unit operations:

- Blend ingredients
- Mill blend
- Blend milled ingredients
- Slug blend
- Mill slugs
- Blend ingredients
- Compress final granulation

In the third country, roller compaction was substituted for the slugging process. While the milling of the slugs and compacts were completed on different machines, and the particle size results were not exactly the same in each situation, the tablet content uniformity results were equivalent. Content uniformity relative standard deviations of 1.5% to 2.0%, $n = 10$ tablets, were routinely achieved. For each country, the tablet dissolution profiles averaged 95% or higher within 30 minutes.

The success to manufacture the tablet formulation (with varying batch sizes of 250 to 900 kg) and achieve reproducible tablet physical results was due in part to the robustness of the formulation design and the active drug's compressibility characteristics. Illustration of the different particle size distributions observed and equipment parameters employed to achieve the desired results are noted in Tables 1 to 3 (1).

TABLE 1 Granulometry of Powder Blends Manufactured Using Slugging Technology in Country 1

| Lot no. | Mesh size (% retained accumulated) | | | | | |
	#80	#100	#140	#300	#325	Pan
1	59	64	71	78	84	100
2	51	57	65	73	82	100
3	57	62	69	74	79	100

Slugging parameters: 4 tons pressure, 0.75-in. flat-faced tooling, slug weight = 0.8–1.0 g, slug hardness = 12–18 Strong Cobb units, sized through oscillator with #16 mesh screen.

TABLE 2 Granulometry of Powder Blends Manufactured Using Slugging Technology in Country 2

| Lot no. | Mesh size (% retained accumulated) | | | | | |
	#20	#40	#60	#100	#200	Pan
1	9	28	42	60	67	100
2	9	27	41	59	66	100
3	9	27	41	58	65	100

Slugging parameters: 4 tons pressure, 0.75-in. flat-faced tooling, slug weight = 0.8–1.0 g, slug hardness = 12–18 Strong Cobb units, sized through oscillator with #1.1-mm screen.

TABLE 3   Granulometry of Powder Blends Manufactured Using Slugging Technology in Country 3

Lot no.	Mesh size (% retained accumulated)					
	#20	#40	#60	#100	#200	Pan
1	23	51	63	73	80	100

Compactor parameters: roll pressure = 62–65 bars, roll speed = 8 rpm, horizontal screw feed = 52 rpm, deaeration = −0.2 bars, sized by double rotary granulators with 4-mm and 1.2-mm screens.

Vacuum Deaeration Equipment Design Evaluation

Pilot compaction trials with an experimental compactor design were conducted to investigate the vacuum deaeration effect when compacting an antibiotic powder with 0.2 g/cm^3 density. The study determined the compact throughput, compact density, and fines (not compacted during vacuum deaeration) when using a new equipment feed design. The parameters monitored and controlled during the compaction process were vacuum deaeration pressure, roll pressure, roll and screw speeds, room temperature, and humidity.

The equipment feed design consisted of a funnel-shaped powder hopper that was located directly above the rolls (with no vacuum deaeration system). The powder hopper was retrofitted with vacuum deaeration capability. A designed high-compression feed screw, fitted inside the funnel hopper, fed the powder directly into knurled rolls. The compaction trials were conducted with and without vacuum deaeration. The compact was carefully collected directly on a #10 mesh screen. Powder particles, which were not compacted (those particles that were not attached to the compact), for example, fines bypassing roll compaction and the nonadhering compacted powder particles, were weighed and separated. The compact was not milled; the parameters are noted in Table 4.

The conclusions drawn from this trial indicated vacuum deaeration, employed in the described equipment design, increased the compaction rate, reduced the fines (noncompacted powder), and increased the compact density (R.W. Miller, unpublished notes, June 1996).

Wet Granulation Technology Vs. Slugging Technology Vs. Roller Compaction Technology

A highly water-soluble drug was incorporated at 35% into hard gelatin capsules. The active drug substance characteristics were described as small needle-shaped

TABLE 4   Compactor Parameter Settings and Compact Physical Properties

Trial no.	Vacuum deaeration (15-in. Hg)	Roll pressure (kN)	Roll speed (rpm)	Screw speed (rpm)	Compact density (g/cm^3)	Compact rate (g/min)	Fines not compacted (%)
1	No	50	4.8	27	1.05	604	7.1
2	No	50	6.8	98	1.07	1172	8.1
3	Yes	105	4.8	27	1.21	772	5.6
4	Yes	50	6.7	27	1.11	848	5.8
5	Yes	70	5.2	27	1.25	856	5.8

TABLE 5 Final Blend Physical Properties Manufactured by Slugging Process

Lot no.	#30	#50	#80	#100	#120	#200	Pan	Bulk density (g/cm³)	Tap density (g/cc³)
				Mesh size (% retained)					
N93C018C[a]	18.3	38.0	15.5	6.6	5.5	9.3	6.8	0.58	0.71
N93J071C[a]	15.8	30.0	17.1	7.1	6.2	10.9	12.8	0.56	0.72
N93M109C[a]	16.3	33.5	19.7	7.4	6.9	10.4	5.8	0.47	0.68
N94D053[a]	19.8	36.1	19.2	5.6	4.7	7.6	6.9	0.52	0.75
N94G101C[a]	8.9	40.9	19.7	6.2	4.4	8.9	11.0	0.60	0.87
N94H117C[a]	8.6	26.5	22.9	9.7	6.7	10.8	14.7	0.49	0.78
N95006[a]	11.7	31.2	19.9	8.4	5.8	8.7	14.3	0.58	0.81
N95008[a]	15.4	33.8	20.2	7.0	6.0	8.3	9.3	0.58	0.80
N95044[a]	13.6	35.5	22.4	8.9	5.7	8.8	5.1	0.51	0.73
N95134[a]	7.8	27.5	22.9	7.7	7.6	10.8	15.8	0.57	0.76

[a]Sized by oscillator equipped with #20 mesh screen.

particles, low bulk density, ≈ 0.1 g/cm³, extremely poor flow, "sticky," and highly compressible.

Initially, a conventional wet granulation process was investigated but proved not feasible due to the high solubility of the active bulk drug. When granulating, pockets of highly wetted areas formed, preventing uniform moisture distribution and granule formation. Additionally, granulating with a solution of the drug was not acceptable since the amorphous form of the compound was formed after drying.

On the basis of the encountered difficulties during the wet granulation process, the formulation scientists developed a dry slugging granulation process. This process had some deficiencies. For example, it was difficult to compress slugs to a similar consistency because of the extremely low bulk density and poor blend flow properties. Additionally, the weight and hardness of the slugs varied throughout the slugging powder process and from batch to batch. This situation created a final blend batch-to-batch nonconsistency in particle size distribution, bulk and tap densities (Table 5). Additionally, due to the extremely poor flowing powder blend, the process was not amenable to tablet scale-up; it took 10 hours to slug and size the 100-kg preblend.

Using the same active drug blend, 2×5 kg pilot compaction trials were conducted using a model AW-120 compactor (Alexanderwerk Inc., Horsham, Pennsylvania, U.S.). The compactor was fitted with deaeration capability. Results from numerous trials indicated batch-to-batch consistency in particle size distribution, bulk and tap densities (Table 6). The compaction process was scaled up to a rate of 100 to 150 kg/hr using the same compactor parameters as in the pilot trials. The granules manufactured from the compactor scale-up produced superior tablet physical properties compared to the slugging process (1). This example illustrates roller compaction technology delivering consistent predictable powder properties compared to a slugging unit operation.

Roller Compactor Pilot to Scale-Up Level

A roller compactor scale-up was conducted to show the effect of process scale-up on tablet robustness and predicted in vivo performance by Sheskey et al. (9). The effects of the scale-up from laboratory to pilot plant on granulation, tablet

TABLE 6 Physical Properties of the Blends Manufactured Using Alexanderwerk AW-120 Roller Compactor

| Lot no. | Screw speed (rpm)[a] | Roll press. (bar) | Mesh size (% retained) | | | | | | | Bulk density (g/cm^3) | Tap density (g/cm^3) |
			#30	#50	#80	#100	#120	#200	Pan		
1	45	62.5	19.4	39.9	14.0	5.7	3.8	5.7	11.4	0.60	0.69
2	38	62.5	18.8	43.2	12.9	5.2	3.3	3.9	12.6	0.60	0.72
3	38	50.0	14.2	41.2	16.2	6.3	3.9	3.4	14.8	0.60	0.72
4	38	75.0	15.1	42.2	16.1	5.8	3.5	3.8	13.5	0.60	0.70
5	30	62.5	11.6	37.7	16.2	6.8	4.2	1.7	21.8	0.60	0.72
6	53	62.5	12.6	40.6	17.4	7.0	4.4	1.5	16.5	0.58	0.70
7	38	62.5	16.4	40.7	15.2	5.4	3.6	1.6	17.2	0.58	0.71

[a]Roll speed and vacuum deaeration were kept constant at 8 rpm and 0.2 atm, respectively. Roller compactor was equipped with 5-mm primary screen. Final sizing was conducted using an oscillator equipped with #20 mesh screen.

physical properties, and drug release of samples produced with roll compaction were compared with samples produced by direct compression. The study involved a formulation containing the model drug theophylline and hydroxyl-propyl methylcellulose. The scale-up experimental protocol was established using the FDA's Guidance for Industry SUPAC-MR: Modified-Release Solid Oral Dosage Forms, Scale-Up and Post-Approval Changes: Chemistry, Manufacturing, and Controls: In Vivo Dissolution Testing and In Vivo Bioequivalence Documentation (September 1997).

The TF-Mini and TF-156 compactors (Vector Corporation, Marion, Iowa, U.S.) were equipped with concavo-convex rolls and single-flight screws. The roll speed of the TF-156 was scaled to achieve the same linear velocity 74.2 in./min as the TF-Mini model. This setting maintained a comparable dwell time for material in the compaction zone. The TF-156 roll force was scaled to 5.6 tons, which equaled a force per linear-inch approximately equal to the TF-Mini 3.1 ton/in. roll width. The authors established a feed screw speed to roll speed ratio of 1.3:1 for the trials. Table 7 gives the compactor equipment settings.

Compacts were milled from which final blends were compressed into tablets (Table 8 gives resultant powder properties). Tablets were tested for friability, thickness, hardness, and drug release.

Results of roll compaction and milling trials indicated that there were insignificant differences between pilot and plant scaling. All laboratory and pilot roller compaction trials demonstrated improved powder flowability in comparison to the non-roller-compacted original formulation (Table 8). The authors cited that all the tablets from roll-compacted granulations exhibited strong physical properties, that is, minimal chipping, no breaking, and no physical defects such as capping or lamination. Despite differences in tablet hardness and small differences in tablet properties, there were no significant differences in the rate of drug release among the direct compression ANDA product and the tablets produced by laboratory and pilot roller compactor processes. Roll compaction scaling did not affect in vitro drug release results (9).

TABLE 7 Roller Compactor Equipment Settings

Trial parameters	1	2	3	4	5	6	7	8	9	10
Compactor TF models	Mini	Mini	156	156	156	156	156	156	156	156
Roll Speed (rpm)	6	4	4	4	4	4	8	8	16	16
Throughput (kg/hr)	2	12	12	11	11	11	19	23	45	40
Linear roll velocity (in./min)	74.2	74.2	74.2	74.2	74.2	74.2	148.4	148.4	148.4	148.4
Screw speed (rpm)	17.9	5.2	5.2	5.2	5.2	5.2	10.4	10.4	20.8	20.8
Screw speed/roll speed (rpm)	3:1	1.3:1	1.3:1	1.3:1	1.3:1	1.3:1	1.3:1	1.3:1	1.3:1	1.3:1
Roll force (tons)	3	5.6	5.6	5.6	6.6	4.6	5.6	6.6	5.6	6.6
Force/linear-inch (ton/in.)	3.1	3.1	3.2	3.2	3.8	2.7	3.2	3.8	3.2	3.8
Mill design[a]	RI	RI	RB	RB	RB	RB	RB	RB	RB	RB
Granulator, U.S. standard mesh screen	12	12	16	14	14	14	14	14	14	14
Granulator speed (rpm)	500	500	117	117	117	117	117	117	117	117

[a]RI, rotating impeller; RB, rotating bar; roll diameter and width, TF-Mini: 100 mm × 25 mm, TF 156: 150 mm × 44 mm.
Source: Adapted from Ref. 9.

TABLE 8   Powder Properties from Non-Roller-Compacted Formulation and from Lab and Pilot Roller Compaction Processes

Trial description	Bulk density (g/cm^3)	Tap density (g/cm^3)	Compressibility index (%)
Original formulation (noncompacted)	0.415	0.645	36
Lab roll compaction 1	0.610	0.800	24
Pilot roll compaction 2	0.620	0.730	15
Trial 3	0.520	0.700	26
Trial 4	0.540	0.710	24
Trial 5	0.550	0.680	20
Trial 6	0.530	0.700	24
Trial 7	0.540	0.690	22
Trial 8	0.560	0.740	24
Trial 9	0.560	0.720	22
Trial 10	0.560	0.710	22

Source: Adapted from Ref. 9.

Additional efforts by Sheskey et al. completed the scaling of their work to a production-scale compactor TF-3012 (Vector Corporation) (10). Table 9 shows the settings used to scale to the TF-3012. Like the TF-Mini and the TF-156, the TF 3012 was equipped with concavo-convex rolls, a single-flighted feed screw and no vacuum deaeration. Parameters from Table 7, trial 7, were used to meet minimal feed screw speed requirements (4 rpm) to scale to the TF-3012 production machine. The roll force was scaled to 10.8 tons, which produced a force per linear-inch similar to that used with the TF-156 (3.2/in. roll width). The feed screw speed was set at 5.2 rpm to maintain a ratio of feed screw speed to roll speed of 1.3:1 equal to that used with the TF-156. These ratios provided an adequate delivery of the model drug blend to the compaction zone. Also, the TF-3012 sizing granulator was comparable to the velocity used for the TF-156 milling process (rotor bar ~ 107 ft/min).

Results generally indicated that the TF-3012 trials exhibited reduced bulk density and an increased compressibility index values compared to the TF-Mini and TF-156. The authors postulated that increased fines were caused from the milling operation, which may have occurred due to longer compact retention time in the mill chamber. All tablets manufactured from the compactors exhibited similar physical characteristics. Samples from the production-scale compactor trials showed faster drug release than did those from the laboratory compactor trials. Also, the pilot plant compactor trials' f_2 statistic (see definition below) were always larger than 80; however, production-scale compactor trials' f_2 were usually approximately 50. Thus indicating some dissolution differences between small-scale versus large-scale roller compaction processing with the modified-release matrix system studied (10):

$$f_2 = 50 \log\{[1 + 1/n_{t=1^n} \sum w_t (R_t - T_t)^2]^{-1/2} \times 100\} \qquad (3)$$

where f_2 is defined as the similarity factor, w_t an optional weight factor, n is the number of data points collected, and R_t and T_t are the percent drug dissolved at each time point for the test and reference products, respectively (10).

TABLE 9 Roller Compactor Parameters from Continued Trials

Trials and parameters	11	12	13	14	15	16	17	18	19	20
Compactor TF model	3012	3012	3012	3012	3012	3012	3012	3012	3012	3012
Roll speed (rpm)	4	4	4	8	8	8	18.4	18.4	18.4	18.4
Throughput (kg/hr)	75	75	75	130	130	135	242	228	228	228
Linear roll velocity (in./min)	148.5	148.5	148.5	297	297	297	683	683	683	683
Screw speed (rpm)	5.2	5.2	5.2	10.4	10.4	10.4	23.4	23.4	23.4	23.4
Screw speed/roll speed (rpm)	1.3:1	1.3:1	1.3:1	1.3:1	1.3:1	1.3:1	1.3:1	.3:1	1.3:1	1.3:1
Roll force (tons)	10.8	9.8	11.9	10.8	9.8	11.9	10.8	9.8	11.9	11.9
Force/linear-inch (tcn/in.)	3.1	2.8	3.4	3.1	2.8	3.4	3.1	2.8	3.4	3.4
Mill design[a]	RB	RB	RB	RB	RB	RB	RB	RB	RB	RB
Granulator, U.S. standard mesh screen	14	14	14	14	14	14	14	14	14	14
Granulator speed (rpm)	87	87	87	87	87	87	87	87	87	87

[a]RB, rotating bar; roll diameter and width, TF 3012: 300 mm × 90 mm.
Source: Adapted from Ref. 10.

Roller Compactor Development to Manufacturing Scale-Up Using Active and Placebo Blends

An initial narrow range of roller compaction parameters was established for an active 5% preblend granulation using an Alexanderwerk WP 50 roller compactor (150 mm × 75 mm roll dimensions, and granulator fitted with 4-mm and 1-mm granulating screens Alexanderwerk Inc.). No trend was noted with any of the measured compact parameters, that is, ribbon thickness for all three granulations ranged from 1.35 to 1.44 mm. Operationally, recycling of material was not required, as there was no significant powder leakage around the rolls, and the fines (particles finer than 200 mesh) were <20% (Table 10).

Additional trials developed an expanded operational range for the 5% active preblend formulation. Parameters are identified in Table 11.

The strategy to scale the AW 50 compactor parameters (Tables 10 and 11) to the AW 200 compactor was developed using a placebo blend, as it exhibited similar compaction responses as the 5% active preblend formulation. To accomplish this, the AW 50 compactor pressure per cm roll width was determined and translated to an equivalent AW 200 compactor pressure per cm roll width. This normalized the scale-up pressure of the smaller compactor's rolls to that of the

TABLE 10   Roller Compactor Operating Conditions and Particle Size Distributions for 5% Active Granulation Trials

Roll pressure (bars)	21	23	20
Roll speed (rpm)	20	20	20
Screw speed (rpm)	21	21	21
Vacuum pressure (in./Hg)	0.40	0.40	0.40
Ribbon gauge (mm)	1.42	1.44	1.35
Screen size	Trial 1 (% retained)	Trial 2 (% retained)	Trial 3 (% retained)
20	10.6	9.2	8.0
40	29.8	35.8	26.6
60	12.0	12.8	12.2
80	7.8	9.0	8.6
100	6.4	5.4	6.6
200	14.0	11.8	15.4
Pan	20.0	6.7	9.3

Note: Percent retained on screen (test performed on shaker sifter, 50-g sample).

TABLE 11   Expanded AW 50 Operating Conditions for 5% Active Granulation with Particle Size Distribution Data

Roll pressure	RP = 25	RP = 35	RP = 45	RP = 45
Roll speed	RS = 20	RS = 14	RS = 14	RS = 20
Screw speed	SS = 20	SS = 16	SS = 20	SS = 20
Screen size	Trial 1	Trial 2	Trial 3	Trial 4
20	1.3	1.5	1.3	3.1
30	25.7	26.5	28.1	30.4
40	13.5	14.9	15.4	15.9
60	12.2	12.9	13.6	12.8
140	19.1	17.6	18.4	16.4
270	26.7	24.9	22.1	20.2
Pan	1.5	1.7	1.1	1.2

Percent retained on screen (test performed on shaker-type sifter). Units: RP, bars; RS and SS, rpm.

TABLE 12   Alexanderwerk WP 50 and 200 Compactor Conversion Pressing Power

WP50 pressure (bar)	Total pressure		Pressure/cm roll length	
	kN	t	kN	t
25	30.7	3.07	4.10	0.41
30	36.9	3.69	4.92	0.49
35	43.0	4.30	5.74	0.57
40	49.2	4.92	6.56	0.66
45	55.4	5.54	7.40	0.74
WP200 Pressure (bar)				
40	26.08	2.61	3.48	0.35
50	32.57	3.26	4.34	0.43
60	39.12	3.91	5.22	0.52
70	45.63	4.56	6.08	0.61
80	52.11	5.21	6.95	0.70
90	58.66	5.87	7.82	0.78

Source: Data courtesy of Alexanderwerk Inc., Horsham, Pennsylvania, U.S.

larger compactor's rolls. The AW 50 compactor selected optimized hydraulic roll pressure range was 25 to 45 bars, (Table 11). The associated range of pressure translated to 4.10 to 7.40 kN force per cm roll width (Table 12).

The corresponding AW 200 force per cm roll width, 4.10 to 7.40 kN, translated to ~50 to 85 bars. Therefore, the optimized roller compactor-processing parameters: roll and feed screw speeds were defined within the AW 200 roll pressure range of 50 to 85 bars, while processing the placebo blend.

The compaction processing parameters selected for roll and screw feed speeds were based on the motor drives' working load capacities and equipment operating experience. The pre-crusher and final sizing granulators were fitted with 4 mm and 1 mm size screens, respectively, and were operated at determined speeds that effectively voided compacted material from each granulator (in series) and also within motor drive working load capacities. On the basis of the above criteria, the roll speed range 17 to 19 rpm and feed screw speed range 80 to 90 rpm were evaluated in a 2^4 matrix. Sixteen compactor-processing trials were determined: machine operating conditions, compact physical parameters, and retained sieve fractions. Six processing conditions were selected for repeat evaluations during a second day to confirm initial results. Ultimately, one processing condition was selected to complete the balance of the placebo scale-up trial: roll speed 17 rpm, feed screw speed 80 rpm, and roll pressure 81 bars. The resultant placebo sieve cut fractions at specific prescribed AW 200 compactor operating conditions compared favorably to the AW 50 compactor sieve cut fraction range of the 5% active granulations (Table 13).

In summary, the AW 50 to AW 200 scale-up placebo procedures, described above, successfully translated, as expected, into an active 5% granulation using the AW 200 and the parameters defined.

Roller Compaction Scale-Up Using Near-Infrared Technology

The following two sections illustrate the use of near-infrared (NIR) technology to better understand roller compaction scale-up. This first section addresses the use of NIR to evaluate roller compaction pre- and postblends. Even given the

TABLE 13   AW 200 Placebo and AW 50 Active 5% Comparative Granulometries

Screen size	AW 200, placebo granulometry (% retained)	AW 50, 5% active granulometry (% retained) (range)
20	8.3	2–12
30	26.6	11–25
40	15.9	9–16
60	13.5	11–17
100	9.4	8–21
270	17.0	17–21
Pan	9.4	10–33

stated advantages of roller compaction, there is still pharmaceutical excipient aids needed to add to a blend prior to roller compaction. These excipients aid in two important ways, internally and externally, to the formulation processing. Internally, the excipients are needed to aid formulation characteristics such as bonding, disintegration, and dissolution. Externally, specific excipients are needed to make the powder machine well during the roller compaction process; for example, lubricant to aid in powder slippage, minimize potential roll sticking, and powder flow aids to assist powder flow into the compactor hopper during processing.

Thus, the nature of the roller compaction preblend is important for a number of reasons, as stated, including the uniformity of the active pharmaceutical ingredient. The use of NIR allows monitoring roller compaction preblends in a blender to determine when a blend is uniform and ready for the next processing step. Typically, the last pharmaceutical ingredient added to a blender prior to processing the blend is a lubricant.

Usually, the pharmaceutical lubricant of choice is magnesium stearate (3). Magnesium stearate's special NIR spectral features make it easy to monitor in a blending unit operation. The minimization of the magnesium stearate spectral variance during the blending process correlates directly to the uniform distribution of the magnesium stearate in the blend. A plot of the spectral moving block variance versus the number of blender rotations (Fig. 1), developed by Dr Tim Stevens, shows the minimization of the magnesium stearate spectral variance from one rotation to the next. Figure 1 describes such a determination for NIR monitoring a preblend containing 0.25% magnesium stearate. The figure shows (a dark solid line) that between 20 and 43 rotations, the magnesium stearate reaches a minimum standard deviation (minimum spectral variability) and that one can conclude that the lubricant is uniformly blended.

Typically, after processing the roller compaction preblend into a compact, which is then sized into granules, there is a final blend step. This unit operation consists of adding some additional excipients, plus a lubricant, such as magnesium stearate as a processing aid for either tablet compression or encapsulation unit operations. Figure 1 also describes the NIR monitoring of magnesium stearate (light dotted line) in the final blend that contains an additional 0.50% magnesium stearate. In this case, it appears that minimization of the magnesium stearate spectral variance is between 20 and 22 blend rotations, suggesting blend lubricant uniformity in this region. Also observed is that subsequent blender rotations lead to more magnesium stearate spectral variance. This may suggest possible increased nonuniformity of the lubricant in the blend. However,

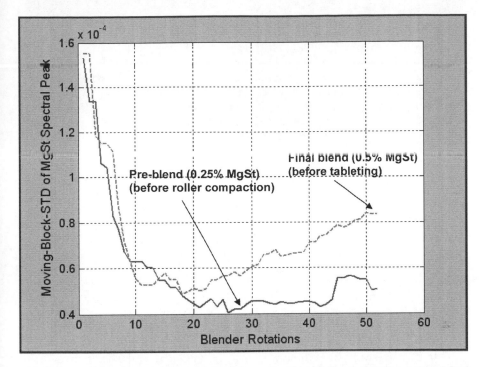

FIGURE 1 NIR blend monitoring of magnesium stearate of roller compaction pre and final blends. *Abbreviation*: NIR, near-infrared.

another possible explanation is that the additional lubricant blend time may have made the powder blend highly fluid, that is, overblended, approaching fluidlike water movement. One can imagine powder moving like water in a blender and the chaotic dynamic state. This suggests that the processing spectrometer sees varying quantities of material per rotation (different packing densities) and thereby sees differing spectral fingerprints from rotation to rotation.

In summary, it is apparent that roller compaction pre- and postblends can be NIR monitored during scale-up, independent of batch size and blender type. Using real-time NIR monitoring can advance blender unit operations knowledge and provide continuous information and assurance about specific unit operations such as roller compaction, a key FDA Process Analytical Technology interest and goal.

The second section illustrates the continuous monitoring of roller compaction to control key compact parameters such as content uniformity, moisture content, compact density, tensile strength, and postmilling particle size distribution. Understanding and controlling these attributes are desired during roller compaction to ensure consistency in the final drug product. The U.S. FDA initiative, PATs, also encourages the use of technology for "continuous real-time quality assurance" (11,12). The initiative advocates building quality into the product by "adoption of at/on/in-line measurement of performance attributes and real-time or rapid feedback controls." NIR spectroscopy makes it possible to nondestructively and simultaneously analyze multiple constituents present in any matrix. This eliminates the lag time associated with waiting for laboratory results at the end of each unit operation. NIR spectroscopy also provides the continuous real-time quality assurance as suggested by the FDA in the PAT initiative.

The use of NIR technology to monitor some of the compact parameters has been reported. Gupta et al. (13) observed a linear relationship between the compact strength and the slope of the best-fit line through the NIR spectrum. They also observed a monotonic relationship between the particle size distribution of the postmilled granules and the spectral slopes. Compacts were prepared using a Fitzpatrick roller compactor, model IR 220 (Fitzpatrick Co.), from 100% microcrystalline cellulose (MCC) as well as from a model formulation containing 10% w/w tolmetin sodium dihydrate active drug substance. In all cases, the above relationships were found to be valid for samples prepared at different roller compactor roll speed settings (Figs. 2 and 3) even when the speeds of the compactor rolls, vertical feed, and horizontal feed screws were changed simultaneously. Compacting 10% tolmetin sodium dihydrate formulation was also monitored real-time using an NIR processing spectrometer, and the spectral slope was calculated in real time. Compaction run time was four minutes at each speed setting. As evident from Figure 4, the slope of the NIR spectrum was able to track the changes in the compact's strength with changing roller compactor settings. The team also observed good agreement between the real-time slope values and the slope values obtained for the spectral data collected off-line on the same compact samples (Fig. 4).

In a later study, the authors found the above relationship between the compact's strength and the slope of the spectral best-fit line to be dependent on the moisture content of the roller-compacted powder (Fig. 5). They also found a significant influence of moisture on the physical and mechanical properties, such as density, strength, etc., of the compacts as well as on the postmilled particle size distribution. The postmilled particle size distribution was, however, found to be dependent on the tensile strength of the compacts.

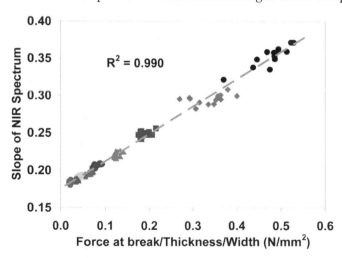

FIGURE 2 Slope of the best-fit line through the spectrum as a function of normalized force values for the 100% MCC compacts that were prepared at different roll speeds; the plot shows linear relationship between the two values. *Abbreviation*: MCC, microcrystalline cellulose.

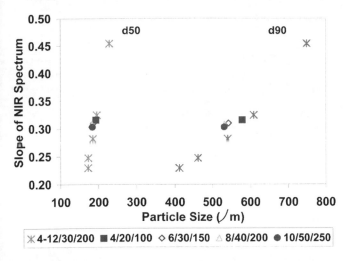

FIGURE 3 Plot of d90 and d50 values for the 10% tolmetin granules versus the slope of best-fit line showing good agreement between the values from the compacts prepared at four different sets of roller compactor roll/horizontal feedscrew/vertical feedscrew speed settings. *Abbreviation*: NIR, near-infrared.

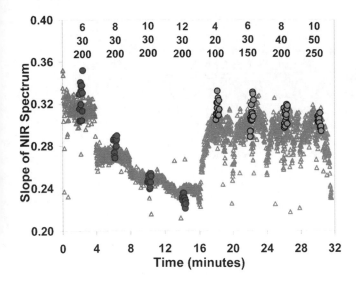

FIGURE 4 Comparison of the off-line slope values (*filled circles*) with the real-time slope values (*open triangles*) for the 10% tolmetin compacts prepared at different roller compactor settings; values on top are the roll, horizontal feedscrew, and vertical feedscrew speeds, respectively. *Abbreviation*: NIR, near-infrared.

NIR Monitoring of Roller Compaction Scale-Up

This illustration shows Dr Gupta studied the ability of NIR to monitor the scale-up from the laboratory Carver Press to the Fitzpatrick roller compactor. Since the NIR signal is influenced by changes in the physical and the mechanical properties, multivariate data analysis techniques were used to identify and

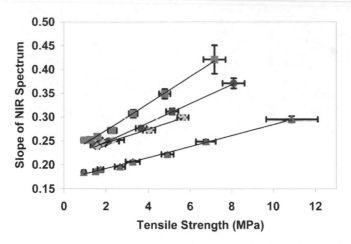

FIGURE 5 Relationship between the slope of the NIR spectrum and the tensile strength of the corresponding roller-compacted sample at different moisture contents; triangles, 3.5%; diamonds, 4.6%; circles, 5.7%; squares, 7.2% LOD samples. *Abbreviations*: NIR, near-infrared; LOD, loss on drying.

separate these contributions in the overall NIR signal. A flat-faced rectangular die and punch set, 40 × 15 mm in size, was fitted on the laboratory Carver Press to prepare tablets similar in shape and size to the roller-compacted samples (13).

Initially, 100% MCC (Avicel PH 200, FMC Corp. Newark, Delaware, U.S.) powder was used as the model compound for feasibility studies. Tablets, weighing approximately 2 g each ($n = 6$), were compressed from the MCC powder at compression pressures from 10 to 90 MPa in increments of 10 MPa. Different moisture contents were obtained by equilibrating the MCC powder under relative humidity (RH) conditions between 15% and 75% and compressing under the same RH conditions for equilibrating the powder. The RH range used represents powder moisture content from 2.5% to 8.5% w/w on wet weight basis. Key sample attributes of moisture content, density, tensile strength, and Young's modulus were measured for all tablets. Moisture content was determined by loss on drying (LOD) method; density (ρ) from sample weight and volume measurements; and tensile strength and Young's modulus using the three-point beam bending method on a TA.XT2i Texture Analyzer (Texture Technologies Corp., Scarsdale, NY/Stable Micro Systems, Godalming, Surrey, U.K.). True density (ρ_{true}) of 100% MCC powder was determined using helium pycnometer (AccuPyc 1330, Micromeritics Instrument Corporation, Norcross, Georgia, U.S.), following the manufacturer's recommended procedure. Sample densities were converted to relative densities by correcting for the contribution of water using the formula $D = 100 \times \rho/[(100-\text{LOD}) \times \rho_{true} + \text{LOD}]$. NIR spectra were also collected for all tablets.

Moisture content, density, and tensile strength of the sample are known and were found to influence the NIR spectra. Hence, multivariate data analysis by partial least squares projections to latent structures (PLS) was used to separate these confounding signals. PLS is a mathematical procedure commonly used for resolving sets of data into latent variables, that is, principle components

(PCs), whose linear combinations approximate the original data to any desired degree of accuracy. The latent variables are constructed in such a way so as to account for the maximum amount of covariance between the dependent and the independent variables. Successive components are calculated orthogonally to the preceding components with each component accounting for the maximum possible amount of residual variance in the data set, followed by cross-validation to prevent overfitting of the data (13).

Different spectral preprocessing and transformations available in SIMCA P+ (ver. 10.0, Umetrics, Sweden) were evaluated and the best approach for data handling and manipulation was determined. Data collected on the surrogate tablets were divided into a training set, to generate the PLS models, and a prediction set, to test the PLS models. MCC powder, equilibrated at different RH, was also roller compacted at different roll speeds on a Fitzpatrick IR220 roller compactor fitted with smooth rolls. Powder feed rate and roll pressure were kept constant for all experiments. The key sample attributes measured on the surrogate tablets were also measured for the samples prepared by roller compaction.

Good agreement was observed between the NIR-PLS predicted values and the values determined using the reference methods for all key attributes for the surrogate tablets as well for the samples prepared by roller compaction. A number of PLS models, generated using different data preprocessing and transformations, gave satisfactory results. However, best results were obtained when the spectral data was transformed using the multiplicative signal correction (MSC), followed by mean centering and the use of three PCs (Fig. 6). Since PCs represent the separated contribution of different sample attributes to the overall NIR signal, they were related to the sample attributes used in this study.

The first PC quantified the moisture content as evident from the strong contribution around 1930 nm region, which represents the combination band of

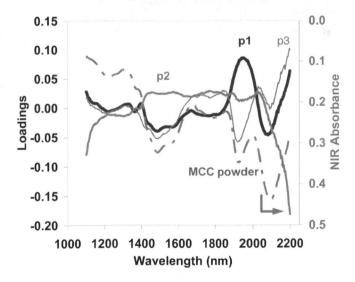

FIGURE 6 First three loading vectors of the NIR-PLS model generated on the surrogate MCC tablets; p1: very thick line, p2: thick line, p3: thin line, and NIR spectrum of 100% MCC powder: dashed line. *Abbreviations*: NIR, near-infrared; PLS, projections to latent structures; MCC, microcrystalline cellulose.

TABLE 14 Root Mean Squares Errors for the NIR-PLS Predicted Values of Different Sample Attributes for the MCC Surrogate Tablets and Roller-Compacted Samples

Data set	LOD (%w/w)	D	TS (MPa)	E (GPa)
Training set (tablets)	0.38	0.043	0.99	0.13
Prediction set 1 (tablets)	0.38	0.033	0.86	0.13
Prediction set 2 (compacts)	0.72	0.074	1.49	0.36

Abbreviations: NIR, near-infrared; PLS, projections to latent structures; MCC, microcrystalline cellulose; LOD: loss on drying; D, relative density; TS, tensile strength; E, Young's modulus.

the –OH stretching and –OH bending vibrations. The second PC quantified the baseline shift due to changing sample density as a result of changing compression pressures. The third PC quantified the changes in MCC structure as evident from its resemblance with NIR spectrum collected on the 100% MCC powder sample. The root mean square errors of prediction for different sample properties are summarized in Table 14.

The study was extended to monitor the scale-up of a pharmaceutical blend containing an active pharmaceutical ingredient. A binary mixture of acetaminophen (APAP) with MCC was selected as the model formulation. The ability of NIR spectroscopy to monitor real-time the content uniformity, in addition to the aforementioned compact attributes, during roller compaction was also tested (13).

NIR calibration curves were prepared by measuring the key compact attributes on rectangular surrogate tablets prepared on the laboratory Carver Press. The preparation of the calibration curve requires samples with attributes spanning the range of values likely to be encountered during roller compaction. Hence, drug content (for content uniformity), RH (for moisture content), and compression pressure (for density, tensile strength, and Young's modulus) were selected as the three variables for establishing the conditions required for preparing the surrogate tablets. The actual conditions of these three variables were selected using two different experimental designs, namely, the Latin square design and the extreme vertices analysis. Experiments using the Latin square design can have 3, 4, or 5 levels each, of all three variables, resulting in 9, 16, or 25 experiments, respectively, instead of 27, 64, or 125 experiments if all combination of the three variables were tested. Since the multivariate analysis of data requires more data points for higher accuracy, the Latin square design involving five levels each of all three variables was selected (Table 15).

The extreme vertices analysis, involving three variables at three levels each, was also evaluated. The extreme vertices experimental design reduced the number of experiments to 15 against 27 if all combinations of the three variables were tested. The 15 experiments represent the 8 experiments having the highest or the lowest level of each variable and 7 experiments with at least 2 variables at the middle level. Tablets, weighing approximately 2 g each ($n = 6$), were compressed from different powder blends at compression pressures according to the experimental designs outlined above. When equilibrating and compressing the above powder blends at different RH conditions (15%, 32%, 43%, 60%, and 68%), different moisture contents were obtained. No internal or external lubricant was used during the preparation of tablets. All tablet surfaces were found to be free from visible defects upon ejection (13).

TABLE 15 APAP Content, RH, and Pressure Combinations Selected Using the Latin Squares Experimental Design for Preparing Surrogate Tablets

		Relative humidity (%)				
Pressure (MPa)		15	30	45	60	75
APAP content (% w/w)	6	10	30	50	70	90
	8	50	70	90	10	30
	10	90	10	30	50	70
	12	30	50	70	90	10
	11	70	00	10	30	60

Abbreviations: APAP, acetaminophen; RH, relative humidity.

The 10% w/w APAP powder blend was roller compacted. Different moisture contents were achieved by equilibrating the aforementioned roller-compacted powder blends at 24%, 45%, and 65% RH conditions; representing 3.3%, 5.0%, and 6.3% w/w moisture content, respectively. Compacts were prepared at 5.0, 6.0, and 7.2 rpm roll speeds with the powder feed rate and roll pressure kept constant. Compaction run time was four minutes at each roll speed. Samples were also collected for off-line measurements for the key sample attributes. Real-time monitoring of roller compaction was also performed.

Data collected on the surrogate tablets were divided into the training and prediction sets. Three different PLS models with different training sets were evaluated. Data collected on surrogate tablets prepared with the Latin square experimental design, extreme vertices experimental design, and the combined data from the two experimental designs, respectively, were used as the data for the three training sets. Tablet data from the other experimental design for the first two PLS models (prediction set 1) and the data collected during real-time monitoring of roller compaction (prediction set 2) were used to evaluate the above PLS models. In all cases, data were subjected to MSC followed by mean centering before the use of PLS analysis (13).

PLS models generated using different training set data gave satisfactory results in all three cases. For all five sample attributes, good agreement was observed between the NIR predicted and measured values. However, best results were obtained with the PLS model generated on the data collected using the Latin square experimental design when four PCs were used (Fig. 7). In all models, first PC quantified the moisture content of the samples, second and third PCs together quantified the APAP concentration, relative density, tensile strength, and Young's modulus. The fourth PC accounted for the day-to-day variation in data collection and to improve the predictability of the PLS models.

The PLS model generated on samples prepared according to the Latin squares experimental design was used to predict the key compact attributes from the real-time spectral data collected for roller-compacted samples (Fig. 8). Good agreement was observed between the NIR predicted values and the values measured off-line using the reference methods (Table 16).

Very little scatter was observed in the PLS predicted values for sample LOD, (Table 16) and APAP concentration.

The advantage of NIR real-time roller compaction monitoring is that it provides instantaneous feedback and determination of environmental or process change effects. Also, it can predict the influence of such changes on key compact attributes.

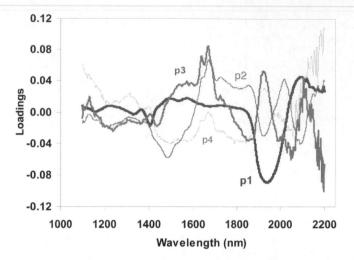

FIGURE 7 First four loading vectors of the NIR-PLS model (MSC and mean centering) generated on NIR data collected from 10% APAP surrogate tablets prepared according to the Latin square experimental design. *Abbreviations*: NIR, near-infrared; PLS, projections to latent structures; APAP, acetaminophen.

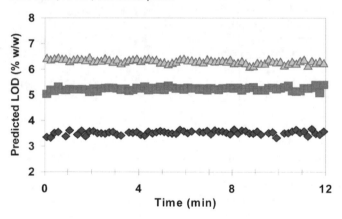

FIGURE 8 PLS predicted values of LOD from NIR data collected during real-time monitoring of roller compaction at different RH; diamonds, 24% RH; squares, 45% RH; triangles, 65% RH. Four minutes each at 7.2, 6.0, and 5.0 rpm roll speeds, respectively. *Abbreviations*: PLS, projections to latent structures; LOD, loss on drying; NIR, near-infrared.

Load Cell Technology Monitoring During Scale-Up

The compacted ribbon characteristics emerging from a roller compactor is dependent on the *force-time* profile imparted to the entering powder by the rollers. This is a critical process parameter (CPP) central to scale-up and thus important to understand and quantitatively characterize the force-loading profile across the roller width.

Knowing the force-time profile, the compact density can be determined and modeled in real time. Generating real-time compaction density provides not

TABLE 16 Comparison of the Measured and NIR Predicted Values for Different Sample Properties for Compacts Prepared at Different Roll Speeds and RH Conditions

Property	RH	Measured at roll speed			NIR predicted at roll speed		
		7.2	6.0	5.0	7.2	6.0	5.0
APAP conc. (% w/w)	24	10.1 (0.6)	10.05 (0.6)	9.8 (0.6)	10.2 (0.8)	10.7 (1.0)	9.1 (0.9)
	45	10.2 (0.5)	9.9 (0.6)	9.9 (0.6)	10.1 (0.7)	10.0 (0.7)	9.8 (0.8)
	65	9.5 (0.4)	9.3 (0.4)	9.3 (0.5)	9.5 (0.7)	9.9 (0.6)	8.8 (0.6)
Relative density	24	0.68 (0.01)	0.70 (0.01)	0.76 (0.01)	0.69 (0.04)	0.72 (0.08)	0.74 (0.10)
	45	0.72 (0.02)	0.78 (0.02)	0.79 (0.02)	0.72 (0.05)	0.77 (0.06)	0.87 (0.09)
	65	0.73 (0.02)	0.77 (0.02)	0.81 (0.03)	0.75 (0.04)	0.84 (0.07)	0.93 (0.08)
Loss on drying (% w/w)	24	3.3[a] (0.1)	3.3[a] (0.1)	3.3[a] (0.1)	3.5 (0.1)	3.5 (0.1)	3.6 (0.1)
	45	5.0[a] (0.1)	5.0[a] (0.1)	5.0[a] (0.1)	5.2 (0.1)	5.2 (0.1)	5.2 (0.1)
	65	6.3[a] (0.03)	6.3[a] (0.03)	6.3[a] (0.03)	6.4 (0.1)	6.4 (0.1)	6.3 (0.1)
Tensile strength (MPa)	24	2.9 (0.3)	3.2 (0.4)	4.9 (0.3)	3.6 (0.7)	3.4 (1.5)	5.1 (1.8)
	45	3.3 (0.2)	5.3 (0.3)	6.9 (0.5)	2.9 (0.9)	4.0 (1.3)	6.1 (1.7)
	65	2.5 (0.2)	3.9 (0.2)	5.5 (0.6)	3.0 (0.7)	5.2 (1.4)	7.4 (1.8)
Young's modulus (GPa)	24	0.56 (0.07)	0.59 (0.08)	0.87 (0.08)	0.61 (0.12)	0.72 (0.24)	0.81 (0.30)
	45	0.57 (0.05)	0.91 (0.06)	1.27 (0.07)	0.54 (0.14)	0.70 (0.20)	1.02 (0.28)
	65	0.44 (0.04)	0.64 (0.03)	0.75 (0.14)	0.56 (0.11)	0.90 (0.22)	1.20 (0.28)

[a]LOD values determined on the powder blend used for roller compaction.

Abbreviations: NIR, near-infrared; APAP, acetaminophen; RH, relative humidity.

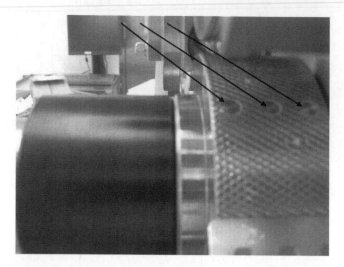

FIGURE 9   Three load cells positioned on compactor roll: Bristol Myers Squibb Proprietary Info.

only a compaction process footprint but the manufacture can initiate control with electronic signals to equilibrate compaction density, for example, by adjusting feed screw speed, roll speed, roll pressure, and roll gap. Also important, the sized compacted granulate can be modeled from the force-time profile relationship to understand and predict the granulometry and particle size distribution.

This temporal loading profile is a signature of the process that can be directly linked to the characteristics of the ribbon from the fed powder blend. Schematically, this is described in Figure 9.

Three elements, powder blend characterization, ribbon property characterization, and final blend characterization, are necessary to understand the whole physical-chemical process characterization. These sources of information are necessary to build an experimental data base that contains the information for the development of physically based models that link the properties of the input (powder blend) with the compactor output (compact ribbon and sized granules).

This type of model is desired for designing products attendant to the powder and process characteristic, and thus, central to the quality by design initiative. These models are also necessary for developing robust scaling-up guidelines using numerical simulations that account for the material characteristics as well as boundary and initial conditions, such as techniques that include discrete particle dynamics and finite element methods. The predictive capabilities of these numerical techniques rest on the accuracy of the constitutive relations for the evolving properties, in this case, the roller-compacted material, which starts as a loose powder and is transformed into solid ribbon compact and is then converted back to loose powder.

A force instrumented roll provides a new dimension in the translation from R&D to manufacturing scale-up and routine manufacturing, which is a model-independent approach. The central idea is to instrument two different rolls: one typical for R&D environments (small roll fitted on small compactors) and one for manufacturing environments (large roll fitted on large compactors).

The strategy is that once a successful roller compaction process is achieved in the R&D lab, the load-time signature is recorded as well as compact density and the sized granulometry measurements. When it comes to scale-up at the manufacturing site, the conditions of the production compactor are tuned to produce the same load-time signature using the larger instrumented roll just as previously achieved with the R&D instrumented roll. From an operational point, there is no need for constant use of the instrumented roll in the lab or in the manufacturing plant after the specific process has been validated by this technology. The sensor roll will be used only to develop and record the load-time profiles during the design of experiments. Similarly, the sensor roll on the production compactor will be used only during scale-up and validation. With modern compactors containing PLCs, process parameters are stored in the compactor's control memory for real-time process monitoring and control; thus, there is no need for the continued use of the specialized sensor rolls. Figure 9 shows pictorially an instrumented roll with small inserted load cells positioned across the roll face that measure $F = P \times A$ of the compact in real time. Real-time force information is generated by this device that enables the development of a design of experiments, modeling, and scale-up strategies to larger roll compactors (with more of the same sensors on the larger-type roll).

Wireless communication instrumented from the roll interior facilitates the sensor information to software that statistically interprets the data real time (Fig. 10). The scale-up and compaction control through real-time statistical feedback goes to a monitor where the information is processed, displayed, and stored.

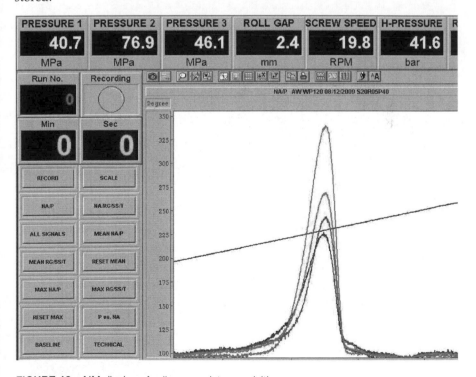

FIGURE 10   AIM display of roll sensor data acquisition.

This applied instrumented roll approach goes to the heart of *process analytical technology* by providing real-time data to expand the processing knowledge and the manufacturing science, to shorten the drug product development time, to shorten drug product scale-up time, to reduce raw material loses, and to reduce drug product manufacturing risks due to processing failures that originates from out-of-control processes.

The author and an engineering firm are currently implementing this technology on production-scale drug product R&D compactors. A paper is planned later in the year.

REFERENCES

1. Miller RW. Roller compaction technology. In: Parikh DM, ed. Handbook of Pharmaceutical Granulation Technology. 1st ed. New York, NY: Marcel Dekker, Inc., 1997:99–150.
2. Miller RW. Roller compaction technology. In: Parikh DM, ed. Handbook of Pharmaceutical Granulation Technology. 3rd ed. Boca Raton, FL: Informa Healthcare, 2009:163–182.
3. Miller RW, Sheskey PJ. A survey of current industrial practices and preferences of roller compaction technology and excipients year 2000. Am Pharm Rev 2001; 4(1): 24–35.
4. Miller RW, Gupta A, Morris KR. Roller compaction scale-up. In: Levin M, ed. Pharmaceutical Process Scale-Up. 2nd ed. Boca Raton, FL: Taylor and Francis, 2006:237–266.
5. Miller RW. Process analytical technologies (PAT) part 2. Am Pharm Rev 2003; 6 (2):52–61.
6. Guidance for Industry. Immediate Release Solid Oral Dosage Forms Scale-Up and Post Approval Changes SUPAC: Chemistry, Manufacturing, and Controls In Vitro Dissolution Testing and in Vivo Bioequivalence Documentation. Published by the Coordinating Committee (CMC CC) of the Center for Drug Evaluation and Research at the Food and Drug Administration, November 1997.
7. FDA. Pharmaceutical cGMPS for the 21st Century—A Risk-Based Approach: Second Progress Report and Implementation Plan. Available at: http://www.fda.gov/Drugs/ DevelopmentApprovalProcess/Manufacturing/QuestionsandAnswersonCurrent GoodManufacturingPracticescGMPforDrugs/UCM071836. Accessed March 12, 2004.
8. Gereg GW, Capolla ML. Roller Compaction Feasibility for New Drug Candidates Laboratory to Production Scale, Pharmaceutical Technology Tableting and Granulation Yearbook. Pittsfield, MA: Advanstar Communications, 2002:14–23.
9. Sheskey P, Sackett G, Maher L, et al. Roll Compaction Granulation of a Controlled-Release Matrix Tablet Formulation Containing HPMC, Pharmaceutical Technology Tableting and Granulation Yearbook. Pittsfield, MA: Advanstar Communications, 1999:6–21.
10. Sheskey P, Pacholke K, Sackett G, et al. Roll compaction granulation of a controlled-release matrix tablet formulation containing HPMC. Pharm Technol 2000; 24(11): 30–52.
11. PAT—A Framework for Innovative Pharmaceutical Manufacturing and Quality Assurance. 2003. Available at: http://www.fda.gov/ohrms/dockets/dailys/03/ Nov03/110303/03d-0380-c000004-01-vol1.pdf.
12. Innovation and Continuous Improvement in Pharmaceutical Manufacturing Pharmaceutical CGMPs for the 21st Century. Available at: http://www.fda.gov/ohrms/ dockets/ac/04/briefing/2004-4080b1_01_manufSciWP.pdf. Accessed September 29, 2004.
13. Gupta A, Peck GE, Miller RW, et al. Nondestructive measurements of the compact strength and the particle-size distribution after milling of roller compacted powders by near-infrared spectroscopy. J Pharm Sci 2004; 94(4):1047–1053.

13 Scale-up of extrusion and spheronization

Raman M. Iyer, Harpreet K. Sandhu, and Navnit H. Shah

INTRODUCTION

Extrusion-spheronization is a pelletization process for making pellets that are amenable for immediate and controlled release preparations. It includes the processes of blending, granulation, extrusion, spheronization, drying, screening and encapsulation or compression into tablets. The major advantages in formulating drugs as pellets include (1) the ability to incorporate a high drug loading, improved homogeneity from uniform distribution of ingredients and improved wetting/dissolution because of larger surface area than a single unit such as a tablet. From a bioavailability standpoint, pellets minimize inter- and intrasubject variability and food effects as they undergo gradual but continuous and uniform gastric emptying. While pellets have been confined to formulation of small molecules, they also offer a convenient mode of dosing for large molecules typically administred by parenteral route (2). In addition, pellets are less prone to dose dumping that is commonly associated with single unit such as a tablet. Other advantages include improved flow properties, dust control and marketing appeal. A list of marketed pellet dosage forms is shown in Table 1.

Though many types of pellet dosage forms have been introduced in the marketplace, a greater understanding is needed of the role of excipients, equipment, process variables and controls involved in the pelletization process. More research and understanding of critical factors that govern the process are needed for successful scale-up from laboratory to manufacturing. The following chapter describes critical aspects in the scale-up of extrusion-spheronization process including the influence of equipment, excipients, process conditions and controls. Finally, some aspects related to monitoring extrusion-spheronization under the FDA's PAT initiative using online process controls are also presented.

EXTRUSION-SPHERONIZATION: AN OVERVIEW

Newitt and Conway-Jones defined (3) pelletization as the process of transforming a wet, solid mass of finely divided particles into dry, spherical bodies by a continuous rolling or tumbling motion. In a broader sense, pelletization is an agglomeration event used in many powder processes either for ease of handling or to add value to the product. It spans a range of industries that process solid particles into some suitable form, such as metallurgical, chemical, plastics, fertilizer, rubber, food and pharmaceuticals (4–7). Since spheres have lowest surface/volume ratio and exhibit reproducible packing, an ideal pelletizing process should produce spheroids with the required tensile strength, density, uniformity of content, size and a narrow size distribution. In addition, for the pharmaceutical industry, such processes must meet its unique needs of safety, quality, potency, bioavailability, GMP and regulatory conformance.

TABLE 1   Examples of Multilithic Drug Products (Pellets, Spheroids, Granules)[a]

Brand name	Drug	Company	Product form	Market form
Xenical®	Orlistat	Roche	Uncoated pellets	Capsule
Nexium®	Esomeprazole Mg	Astrazenaca LP	Delayed-release pellets	Capsule
Toprol-XL®	Metoprolol succinate	Astrazeneca LP	EXR coated pellets	Tablet
Verelan PM®	Verapamil HCl	Schwarz	EXR pellets with controlled onset	Capsule
Singulair®	Montelukast sodium	Merck	Oral granules	Granule
Prevpac® and Prevacid®	Lansoprazole	TAP	Enteric granules	Capsule
Paser®	Aminosalicylic acid	Jacobus	Enteric granules	Granule
Effexor XR®	Venlafaxine	Wyeth	EXR spheroids	Capsule
Aggrenox®	Aspirin IR Dipyrimadole ER	Bohringer Ingelheim	EXR pellets + tablets	Capsule
Cymbalta®	Duloxetine	Eli Lilly	EXR pellets	Capsule
Dexedrine® Spansule®	Dextroamphetamine	GSK	SR pellets	Capsule

[a]PDR Electronic Library, 2005, Main Edition.

Webster's (8) defines extrusion (*ex* + *trudere*) as an act to expel, thrust, force or push out material, that is, to shape by forcing through dies by pressure. Simply put, extrusion is a molding or shaping process in which an irregular, shapeless mass of wet material is molded into a regular, three-dimensional, solid object with a measurable size, shape and moisture content. The extruded product is often subject to further shaping and sizing process to obtain spheroidal pellets by the process of spheronization (or also referred to as spheroidization), first invented (and patented) in Japan by Nakahara (9) in 1964. It describes a method of preparing spherical granules from a wet powder mixture. It became widely known in the United States in the 1970s after it was introduced by Conine and Hadley of Eli Lilly and Company (10,11). It is also referred to as "Marumerization" after the trade mark of the Fuji Denki Kogyo company in Japan.

Extrusion-spheronization is therefore a novel technique for making spherical pellets, the oldest of which is that of pill making (10). Traditional pill making and extrusion-spheronization begin with a wet massing stage, common to both, in which medicaments and excipients are mixed with suitable binders to form a plastic mass. The difference between the two is that in pill making, the wet mass is rolled into cylinders which are then cut and rolled into spherical balls manually. In spheronization, the wet mass is extruded into cylinders which are shaped into spherical pellets in a spheronizer. It is therefore regarded as a fast, efficient and novel pill-making process. Melt extrusion is a variant of wet extrusion in which instead of a wet mass, a molten mass is extruded.

Extrusion-spheronization can provide highly dense, spherical pellets with a smooth surface and a narrow particle size distribution and with drug loading

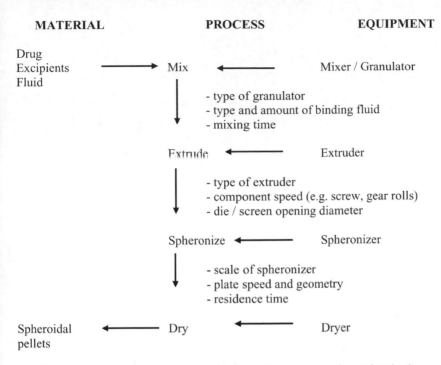

FIGURE 1   A schematic of the extrusion-spheronization process and associated unit operations.

as high as 90%. It is also amenable to batch or continuous processing (10–12). A schematic of extrusion-spheronization and associated unit operations (13,14) are shown in Figure 1.

A typical process begins with a dry blend of drug and excipient that is suitably wetted with water, a water-solvent mixture or a binder solution to form a wet agglomerated mass. The wet mass is conveyed by one or more feeder screws in a suitable configuration and forced through a perforated screen or die resulting in short, right cylindrical, rod-shaped extrudate. The extrudate are rotated at a suitable speed over a friction plate in a spheronizer (Marumerizer®). The rods are broken down into uniform lengths and rolled into spheres by frictional, centrifugal and centripetal forces during rotation in the spheronizer, within 30 seconds to several minutes depending on the formulation. A diagrammatic sketch of the process is shown in Figure 2. The key variables for successful development of the extrusion-spheronization process are as follows:

- Formulation (selection of excipients)
- Wet granulation (particularly moisture content)
- Extruder design and extrusion parameters
- Type of spheronizer and the spheronizing conditions

For the sake of clarity, the formulation and granulation aspects are discussed in tandem as they relate to the extrusion and spheronization processes rather than discussed separately.

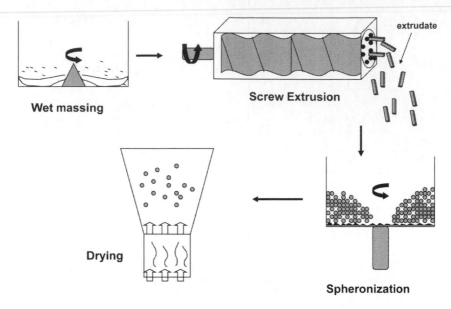

FIGURE 2   A diagrammatic sketch of the critical operations in extrusion-spheronization.

EXTRUSION

The attributes of the extrudate such as density, thickness, and moisture content are controlled by variables due to the formulation, extrusion process, and equipment design. While the moisture content of the wet mass determines its binding and lubrication during transport, the mechanical variables largely influence temperature, shear stress and throughput rates in extrusion.

Equipment Design

Extruders can be broadly classified (15,16) as screw and cylinder extruders on the basis of the feed mechanism that transports the wet mass toward the die and further on the basis of the die configuration and discharge mechanisms. Figure 3 shows extrudors of varying scales from lab to production while Figure 4 shows schematics of the various configurations of extruders used in the pharmaceutical industry. A comparison of attributes of various types of extruders is shown in Table 2.

Screw Feed Extruders

The screw extruder is simply a hollow chamber of suitable length that contains single or double rotating screws driven by a variable speed drive to move the wet mass through the cylinder. The wet mass is fed into the void space at the upstream end of the drive, transported through the cylinder and pushed through a perforated screen or die. Some shear work is required in screw extruders to generate the pressure needed for extrusion leading to a rise in temperature in the chamber. A cooling jacket around the chamber is an option to offset the heat buildup. The double-screw type has either co- or counter-rotating screws. The LCI and Gabler extruders belong to this class. On the basis of the

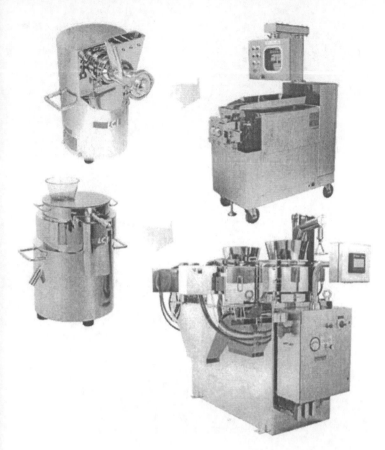

FIGURE 3 Extruders and spheronizers, laboratory scale to production. *Source*: Courtesy of LCI.

orientation of the feed screw and discharge mechanism, extruders can be further classified as follows:

1. Axial feed/axial discharge (A-A)
2. Horizontal feed/radial discharge (A-R)
3. Vertical feed (gravity)/radial discharge (R-R)

The A-A extruders are equipped with a flat perforated plate or screen combined with two flat extrusion heads. The wet mass is pressed axially through the screen parallel to the feed screws. The extrusion forces are the highest compared with other low pressure extruders resulting in hard and dense extrudate. It is commonly used in the extrusion of food, thermoplastics and other industries where a large pellet diameter and thermosetting properties are desired.

In the A-R type, the feed screws end in blades that rotate along the horizontal axis but force the wet mass through a screen placed radial or cylindrical around the blades (Fig. 5). These extruders have somewhat conical extrusion heads resulting in an "overflow," that is, a certain amount of feed

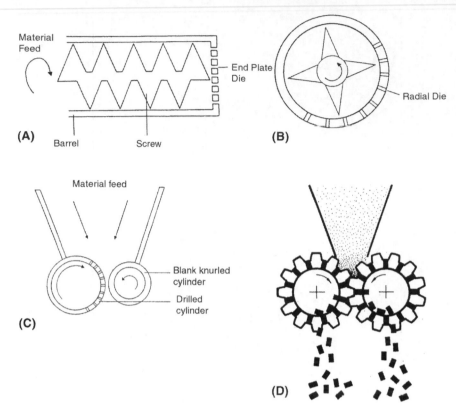

FIGURE 4 Schematics of the various configurations of extruders used in the pharmaceutical industry.

material is pushed axially between the screen and extrusion head at the front instead of radial through the screen area. A greater open area of screen results in a higher and faster throughput However, the hardness and density of resulting extrudate are medium because of lower force of extrusion.

The dome extruder is a variation of the radial extruder that uses a dome-shaped (hemispherical) screen in combination with dome-shaped extrusion heads, introduced by Fuji Paudal, Inc. in 1992 as the TDG series. This generates lower pressure than the axial and radial extruders resulting in extrudate with lower density and hardness. The dome extruder has almost no overflow resulting in higher throughput.

The R-R type, also known as a basket extruder, consists of a vertical rotating shaft with two or four extrusion blades located inside a right cylindrical screen and moving along the major axis of the cylinder. The material is fed by gravity from a hopper located above the cylindrical screen while the rotating blades press it through the screen openings. The wet mass is not under pressure except during the actual extrusion. The low heat buildup makes it amenable for thermally unstable formulations. An example of a basket extruder is shown in Figure 6. The NICA's and LCI's BR extruders belong to this class.

TABLE 2　A Comparison of Attributes of Different Types of Screw Extruders Based on Feed and Discharge Geometries

Attribute	A-A	A-R	A-A (dome)	R-R (basket)	Gear/cylinder	Roller
Feed	Axial	Axial (horizontal)	Axial	Axial (gravity)	Axial (gravity)	Axial (gravity)
Discharge	Axial	Radial	Axial	Radial	Gear axial cylinder radial	Radial
Screw/roll configuration	Single or twin	Single or twin	Single or twin	Single	Dual-toothed gears/ dual cylinders (one blank and one drilled)	Dual solid
Screen configuration	Flat screen/die with flat extrusion heads	Radial screen with conical extrusion heads	Hemispherical screen with dome-shaped extrusion heads	Vertical screw with two or more extrusion blades	No screen; extrudate size based on size of drilled holes	Radial screen with roller extrusion heads
Typical extrudate	Hard and highly dense	Medium	Medium	Soft and poorly dense	Medium	
Throughput	Low	Low	Medium	High	Medium	Medium
Energy use	++++	+++	++	+	+	+
Temperature	Up to 100°C	Up to 60°C	Up to 40°C	Up to 10°C	10–20°C	10–20°C
Screen opening	2–15 mm	0.5–3 mm	0.3–2 mm	0.5–2 mm		
Scale-up	Based on L/D ratio	Need to adjust water level	Some adjustment of water level may be needed	Straightforward	Straightforward	Some adjustment of water level needed

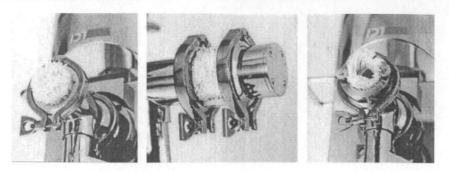

FIGURE 5   Axial, radial, and dome extrusion assembly. *Source*: Courtesy of LCI.

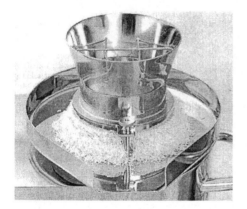

FIGURE 6   An example of extrusion through a basket extruder. *Source*: Courtesy of LCI.

Cylinder Extruders

In these extruders, the wet mass is fed either into the nip formed between two cylinders which are either rollers or a set of hollow, toothed meshing gear wheels as shown in Figure 7. In the former, the dies are in the form of a perforated cylinder while in the latter they are in the form of holes drilled between the gear teeth down to the hollow bore. In both cases, the extrudate exits from the center of the arrangement (17). A shear stress is generated only on the wet mass held either in the nip between the cylinders (rolls) or that flows through the die land (gear) instead of on the entire mass as in screw extruders. The advantages of low shear and minimal heat buildup are offset by low throughput as the heavy gears rotate at a slow speed (<50 rpm). The Caleva and Alexanderwerk extruders belong to this class. Table 3 provides an overview of extruders of varying designs and capacities available in the marketplace.

The quality of the extrudate is determined by both the characteristics of the wet mass and type of extruder. The critical variables that may be monitored to obtain desirable product attributes are addressed in the next section.

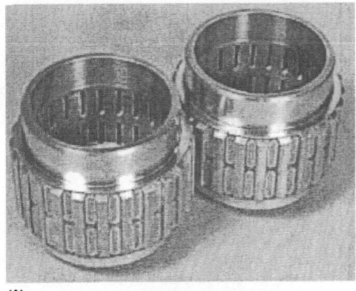

(A)

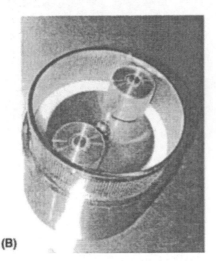

(B)

FIGURE 7 Cylinder extruder parts: (**A**) extrusion gears and (**B**) extrusion rollers. *Source*: Courtesy of Caleva.

Process Control and Scale-up
Dimensional Analysis in Scale-up of Extrusion
Dimensional analysis is a tool often used to express similarities between two scales, both geometric and dynamic. It has been applied to distributive mixing and conveying processes in compounding extruders (18–22) where the screw is segmented and composed of feed, mixing and shearing elements unlike wet extrusion that typically employs a single pitch, nonsegmented screw element.

TABLE 3 An Overview of Extruders of Varying Scales and Capacities

Configuration	Model	Capacity (kg/hr)	rpm
		LCI	
Axial	EXDF-60	50–100	
	EXDF-100	150–200	
	EXDF-130	300–400	
	EXDF-180	500–800	
Radial (twin screw)	EXD-60	30–50	19–75
	EXD-100	50–200	20–85
	EXD-130	200–500	20–85
	EXD-180	500–1200	
Dome	TDG-80	100–150	30–120
	TDG-110	200–300	40–160
	TDG-220	800–1200	
Basket	BR-150		10–90
	BR-200G	50–100	12–50
	BR-300G	100–300	12–50
	BR-450G	150–750	12–50
		Caleva	
Radial screw	Extruder 20	~ 25 kg	
Cylinder roller	Extruder 35	200	
Gear	Extruder 40C M	40–100	
	Extruder 40C A	40–100	
	Extruder 100	200	25–130
		Alexanderwerk	
Gear	GA-65 Granulator	30–50	
Basket	RFG 150D	600	
0.5–10 mm	RFG 250D	1500	
	RFG 250DL	3000	
	RFG 250DDL	4500	
		NICA	
Basket	E140	30–120	
	E200	120–480	
		Gabler	
Axial	DE-40	0.5–100	
	DE-60	5–200	
	DE-80	25–500	
	DE-120	100–1500	

However, since extrusion is similar in both cases, an example of such an analysis from melt extrusion literature is presented here.

In its simplest form, the ratio of screw diameter is the basis for scaling. The ratio of the large diameter D_2 of large scale unit to the small diameter D_1 of the laboratory unit is represented by d as shown in Table 4. The primary scaling

TABLE 4 Geometric Scaling Ratios of Primary and Secondary Variables for Screw Extruder

Variable	Small unit	Large unit	Cube rule N constant D/H constant	Square root rule $H \sim \sqrt{d}$ $N \sim 1/\sqrt{d}$
Primary variables				
Screw diameter (D, m)	D_1	$D_2 = D_1 d$		
Channel depth (H, m)	H_1	$H_2 = H_1 d^h$	$h = 1$	$h = 0.5$
Screw length (L, m)	L_1	$L_2 = L_1 d^l$		
Helix angle (ψ, radians)	ϕ_1	$\phi_2 = \phi_1 d^b$		
Screw speed (N, rpm)	N_1	$N_2 = N_1 d^v$	$v = 0$	$v = -0.5$
Secondary variables				
Shear rate (γ)	γ_1	γ_2	$\gamma_1 = \gamma_2 = \frac{\pi.D.N}{H}\gamma_1$	$\gamma_2 = \gamma_1.d$
Mean residence time (t, sec)	T_1	T_2	$T_1 = T_2 = \frac{L}{\pi.N.D.\sin\phi}$	
Power consumption (E, W)	E_1	E_2	$E_2 = E_1.d^\beta$	$E_2 = E_1.d^{2.5}$
Throughput rate (Q, kg/hr)	Q_1	Q_2	$Q_2 = Q_1.d^\beta$	$Q_2 = Q_1.d^2$
Total shear (S) = $f(\gamma_t, t)$	S			$S = \frac{L}{H.\sin\phi}$

variables are channel depth H, screw length L, helix angle ϕ, and screw speed N. The ratio of the primary variables of the two scales is then expressed as a power of the screw diameter ratio, d.

The secondary variables such as shear rate, mean residence time, power consumption, throughput rate, etc., are expressed as a function of the primary variables. For example, the shear rate (or material displacement rate) in the screw channel is a function of the primary variables D, N, and H and proportional to $1 + v - h$, a scale-up factor. For a given type of screw with fixed helix angle ($b = 0$), at fixed speed, N and fixed L/D and H/D ratios, the shear rate is constant as $1 + v - h = 0$ while at varying screw speeds across scale, the total shear S remains constant.

A constant total shear S suggests that the extrusion profiles of the material in the two different size screw extruders are similar or that the material distribution (homogeneity) in the extruder is independent of screw speed. In a similar manner, scale-up factors for power consumption, specific energy consumption, throughput rate, etc., have been compiled in the literature (22,23).

The scale-up factors depend on the specific event being scaled up in extrusion. The "cube rule" for mixing (24) states that at constant screw speed, output and power consumption increase with the cube of the diameter ratio when H/D ratio is constant. The "square root rule" for material conveying (25,26) states that when channel depth is increased and screw speed decreased with the square root of the diameter ratio, the output rate increases with square of the diameter ratio while power consumption increases 2.5 power of the diameter ratio. These relationships are shown in Eqs. (1–3) where the indices 1 and 2 represent the extruders that are scaled to and from, respectively (see Table 4 for notations). This is based on a constant helix angle and L/D ratio (27).

One could obtain scale-up factors (exponents) in a manner similar to the foregoing analysis to determine and monitor the secondary variables during scale-up.

$$Q_2 = \left(\frac{D_2}{D_1}\right)^2 * Q_1 \tag{1}$$

$$N_2 = \left(\frac{D_1}{D_2}\right)^{0.5} * N_1 \tag{2}$$

$$H_2 = \left(\frac{D_2}{D_1}\right)^{0.5} * H_1 \tag{3}$$

The notion of similarities help the reader in realizing the design attributes of extruders from smaller to larger scales for handling small to large amounts of material. However, the process still needs to be monitored at each scale using suitable criteria that are accurately and reproducibly measurable. In other words, the process chemist needs to monitor parameters that are a function of formulation, process and geometry variables during extrusion.

Process Monitoring

The goal in wet extrusion is to obtain a dense extrudate with a smooth surface and a thickness close to the diameter of the die or screen opening but also fragile enough to be broken down into short rods with an aspect ratio between 1 and 2. This is governed by the choice of formulation, process, and equipment design variables shown in Table 5. In a typical scale-up operation, the formulation is provided by pharmaceutical R&D, while the equipment manufacturer provides the geometry and performance indicators such as motor power consumption. The scale-up personnel therefore have to rely on the process variables and their control to monitor product performance. The early process parameters are often

TABLE 5   An Overview of Formulation, Process and Equipment Design Variables That Influence Extrudate Attributes

Formulation	Process	Geometry
Dry ingredients (drug, binder, filler)	Mixing	Extruder
Particle size	Mixer speed (rpm)	Screw length, pitch, and diameter
Solubility	Mixing time (min)	Screw channel depth
Crystallinity	*Extrusion*	Screw blade configuration
Melting point	Screw speed (rpm)	Die or screen configuration (radial, axial)
Thermal stability	Screen size (mm)	Number of screws (single/dual)
Hygroscopicity	Feeding rate (g/min)	Die *L/D* ratio
Percent loading	*Spheronization*	Roll diameter (mm)
	Plate speed (rpm)	Screw speed (rpm)
Wetting fluid	Residence time (min)	*Spheronizer*
Percent loading	Material load (g)	Plate diameter
Dielectric	*Drying*	Groove spacing
Viscosity (mPa·sec)	Drying time (min)	Groove pattern
	Temperature (°C)	
	Type of dryer	

derived on small laboratory scale instruments with about 1-kg batch size, thus limiting their utility. However, critical parameters such as moisture content of extrudate or process temperature could still be measured at the smaller scale. Therefore, the ability to monitor the process critical parameters should be considered during scale-up in addition to selection of the extruders and downstream processing.

Evaluation of extrusion-spheronization for drug product manufacturing has focused on two main areas.

- Mechanistic and kinetic aspects of the process using instrumented equipment
- The impact of various formulation, process, and device geometry variables on the physicomechanical properties of and drug release from dried pellets

Instrumented extruders could be used to monitor continuously changing product attributes during extrusion. An instrumented extruder is equipped with transducers that measure the forces (or stress) developed during extrusion which in turn is dependent on material properties and equipment geometry. This may be expressed as the pressure exerted by the blades or rolls at the screen or die during product exit (28) torque exerted on the screw shaft (29), shear stress in the barrel during material transport (30,31) and product temperature during exit at the screen or the die (29). These in turn are a function of the moisture (fluid), heat flow and shear rate gradients that develop during extrusion and impact the yield and properties of extrudate.

A common indicator in an extruder console is the power, E, consumed by the motor drive in transporting material from feed to product exit. Higher power consumption could mean greater friction during product movement or an overloaded chamber. The torque of extrusion is the energy expended by the motor drive in rotating the screw(s) and is expressed as

$$F = \frac{E}{N} \qquad (4)$$

where E is the power consumption to drive the screw shaft at a speed of N rpm.

Another indirect parameter is the specific energy consumption, K (32,33), which is the power normalized for throughput Q and expressed as

$$K = \frac{E}{Q} \qquad (5)$$

$$K = \frac{(FN)}{Q} \qquad (6)$$

Figure 8 shows the effect of speed on K at varying throughput rates. The value of K is similar when scaling from small (ZSK-30) to large (ZSK-53) extruders as long as the throughput rate is same across the scale. A question becomes should the specific energy remain constant across scale? Since K is directly related to screw speed and inversely related to throughput, mfg. operations would prefer to lower the speed and increase the throughput thus lowering K or the energy cost. On the other hand, since K is a measure of energy expended in bonding and densifying the extrudate, the process chemist may choose to maintain K constant, thereby increasing the speed to compensate for

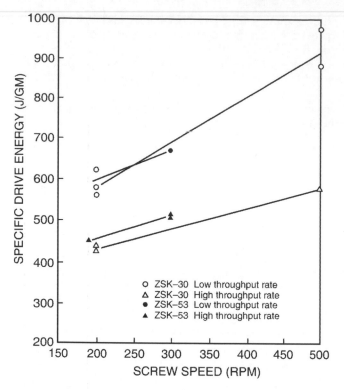

FIGURE 8 The effect of screw speed on specific energy consumption at varying throughput rates for extruders of two different scales. *Source*: From Ref. 29.

high throughput. Thus identifying an optimal value for K is desirable to monitor the extrusion process.

The torque, screen force, specific energy and power could be regarded as end point statistics and therefore, a measure of process conformance and product quality. Additional examples are shown in Table 6.

Selection of Extruders for Pharmaceuticals
Given extruders of various designs, type and geometry are available in the marketplace, let us examine some aspects that drive selection of the appropriate extruder for a product. Harrison et al. (30,34) obtained force-displacement profile during extrusion of microcrystalline cellulose (MCC) formulations using a ram extruder and resolved it into three stages as seen in Figure 9: compression, steady state, and forced flow. On the basis of surface smoothness and cohesive strength, a predominant steady-state region was found necessary for high quality extrudate while poor quality extrudate remained in the compression stage. The ejection stress based on angle of convergence from barrel to the die affects the surface smoothness of the extrudate and was found to be dependent on the moisture content.

TABLE 6 **Examples of End Point Statistics for Product and Process in Extrusion-Spheronization**

Product	Process
Moisture content (% w/w)	Mixer output (*N*, A, W) (e.g., torque of mixing, amperage, power consumption)
Particle size and size distribution (mm or μm)	Torque (force) or pressure of extrusion (N·m or Pa)
Deformation behavior (e.g., strain, viscosity)	Barrel/die temperature (°C)
Shape and shape factors	Rate of evaporation (e.g., moisture, alcohol) (mL/sec)
Density (g/cm^3) (e.g., bulk, tapped, and true)	Shear rate of extrusion
Cohesive strength (mPa) (e.g., tensile, compressive)	Throughput rate (kg/hr)
Surface morphology (e.g., smoothness)	Extruder power consumption (W)
Friability	Residence time (sec)
Porosity (volume and distribution)	Spheronizing torus volume (L)
Drug release/dissolution rate	Plate angular velocity (m/sec)

Note: Wet agglomerates, wet extrudate, or dried pellets

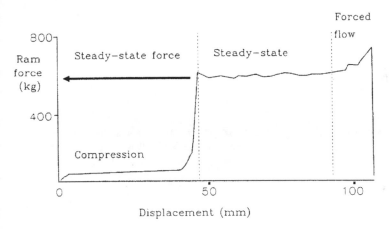

FIGURE 9 Schematic of a force-displacement profile from an instrumented ram extruder. *Source*: From Ref. 27.

The ram extruder develops high moisture and thermal gradients due to a high pressure buildup within the barrel. The product is axially compressed through a narrow die resulting in temperatures as high as 150°C, which could be unsuitable for thermally unstable compounds. Though the ram extruder is more easily scaled up than other types of extruders based on constant *L/D* ratio (*L*, barrel length; *D*, die diameter), it is not very amenable to continuous processing. The gravity (basket) feed and screw extruders enable extrusion at relatively low shear stress due to the following attributes:

• Larger open area of screen or die lowers the extrusion pressure at exit
• Lower shear within extrusion chamber due to lower effective contact area between screw surface and chamber wall than in a ram extruder

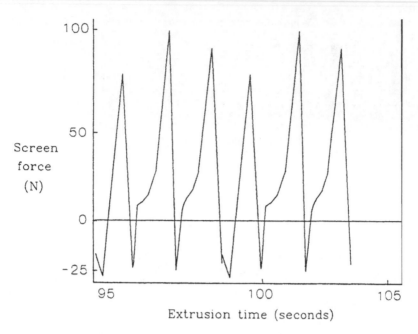

FIGURE 10 Schematic of a screen force profile from an instrumented radial screen screw extruder. *Source*: From Ref. 25.

The pressure exerted by the rotating extrusion heads on the screen as product is being pushed out in an A-R screw extruder (28) is shown in Figure 10. Each spike in the profile represents one revolution of the extrusion head while the frequency represents screw speed. On the basis of the shear stress developed during extrusion, wet mixtures of MCC-lactose had a lower yield stress in the radial screw extruder (130 kN/m^2) than in the ram extruder (250 kN/m^2), suggesting better performance of the screw extruder (35). Similarly, the basket and gravity feed roll (gear) extruders generate lower extrusion forces than axial screw extruders in which frictional forces are higher (31).

Among the formulation variables that control extrudability of a product, several studies (28,29,36–38) point to the fluid or moisture content of the wet feed material being more critical than others. The force or torque of extrusion and power consumption are often inversely proportional to moisture content of the extrudate as seen from Figures 11 and 12 (29,39–41), while the particle size of pellets increased linearly with water content when extruded with gravity feed basket and roll extruders (36). Using instrumented gravity feed and radial screw extruders, a three to fourfold decrease in the force has been noted with a 10% increase in water content of feed material (40).

The aqueous solubility of solid ingredients is inversely proportional to the water content required to obtain acceptable pellets (42) as shown in Figure 13. Screw extruders poorly extrude when proportion of water soluble compounds such as mannitol or lactose reaches 50% or higher. Such formulations are better extruded with low shear basket extruders (31). As the solubility increases from 5% to 30%, the percent water needed for extrusion could decrease by up to 25%.

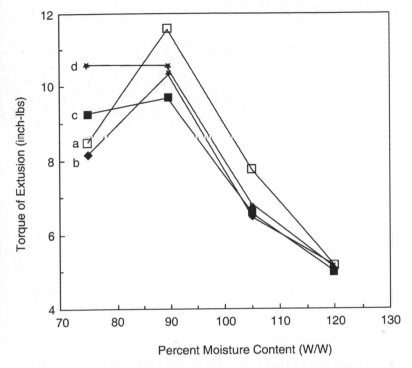

FIGURE 11 Torque of extrusion as a function of moisture content of wet mass of microcrystalline cellulose at varying screw speeds: a, 19 rpm; b, 28 rpm; c, 38 rpm; and d, 48 rpm. *Source*: From Ref. 26.

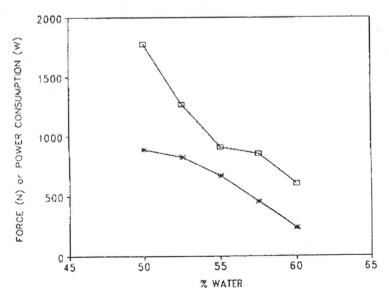

FIGURE 12 Influence of the amount of water on the extrusion forces (gravity feed extruder) and power consumption (twin-screw extruder) on extrusion of microcrystalline cellulose. ■, gravity feed extruder (N); and *, twin-screw extruder (W). *Source*: From Ref. 37.

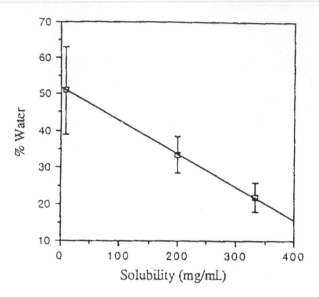

FIGURE 13 Effect of drug solubility on water required for 80% and 85% yields of pellets containing microcrystalline cellulose. *Source*: From Ref. 39.

This has implications for scale-up as early lots of API may have different crystallinity or solubility profile than pilot lots.

On the other hand, the lack of adequate liquid-solid bonding between poorly water soluble, cohesive powders with high yield stress such as calcium carbonate and calcium phosphate can also lead to high shear, temperature, and force of extrusion, resulting in fragile and low-density extrudate. Serrated extrudate with a rough surface are termed "shark skinned" and often the result of high extrusion pressures and use of elongated screens or dies with smaller openings.

The formation of moisture gradients within the material during extrusion resulting in migration of liquid from within the interparticulate spaces to surface of the extrudate has been reported (28,43). At low initial moisture content, the friction within the chamber can result in higher temperatures leading to loss of moisture of up to 12% from the extrudate surface. This effect is more pronounced with A-A extruders.

All these point to the need to optimize moisture content of the wet mass and extrudate by careful selection of formulation ingredients and type of extruder. A basket or gear/roll extruder is preferred for a very dense and moist wet mass as it generates little shear and temperature rise, while an axial or radial screw extruder that increases granule density and hardness is desirable for a wet mass that is less cohesive with poor binding. For drugs that are adversely affected by moisture, the inclusion of hydrophobic lipids such as glyceryl monostearate during extrusion has been found to improve the stability (44). The extrusion pressure could be further modulated by choice of dies or screens with appropriate L/D ratios. The pressure differential between points of die entry and exit due to viscosity for a Newtonian material moving within a cylinder is represented by Eq. (7), derived from the Hagen-Poisuille expression for pressure drop in a pipe of constant diameter as (45)

$$\Delta P = 4\tau_{\mathrm{w}} \left(\frac{L}{D} \right) \tag{7}$$

where ΔP = pressure drop between die entry to exit points, dyne/cm²; τ_{w} = die wall shear stress (viscous drag), dyne/cm²; D = die diameter, cm; and L = die length, cm.

The use of screens with a larger L/D ratio in a low shear basket extruder can provide additional pressure for wet mass with low bonding strength. A gravity feed extruder with $L/D = 2$ recorded (31) higher forces compared with power generated from a twin-screw extruder with $L/D = 0.9$ upon extrusion of mixtures of MCC with either lactose or DCP. The extrudate from basket extruder was denser with a smoother surface than from the screw extruder. Similarly, material extruded through a screen with $L/D = 4$ in a basket extruder was denser than with a $L/D = 2$ (40). However, a smaller L/D ratio is preferred in an axial extruder. An improper L/D ratio could result in a loosely bound extrudate with large surface defects (40) resulting in a formulation less amenable to extrusion as seen from Figure 14. Since the mean diameter of the pellet often approximates the diameter of the die used in extrusion, choice of the latter is also dictated by desired pellet size. In an empirical study, the size profile of pellets obtained from a ram extruder at 200 mm/min was found similar to that obtained using a screen extruder at a rotational speed of 46 rpm, for the same formulation as seen from Figure 15 (44).

Screw speed is another variable that impacts extrudate quality via residence time. The effect of screw speed on extrusion shear stress is given (23) by the expression

$$\tau_{\mathrm{w}} = m \left(\frac{V_{\mathrm{b}}}{H} \right)^{n} \tag{8}$$

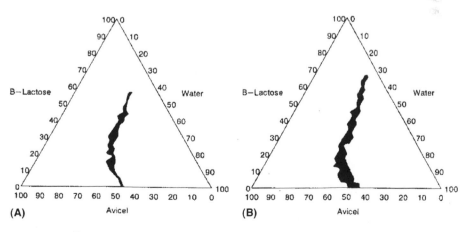

FIGURE 14 Phase diagrams indicating the zone where pellets of desired quality were obtained for lactose/microcrystalline cellulose/water mixtures. (**A**) Zone for $L/R = 2$ and (**B**) zone for $L/R = 4$. *Source*: From Ref. 38.

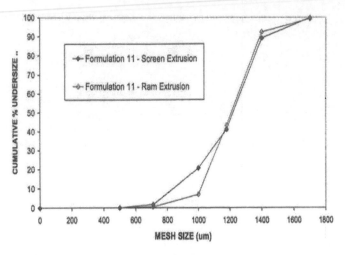

FIGURE 15 Comparison of size profile of pellets from ram and screen extruders. *Source*: From Ref. 44.

where m is the consistency index, n is the power law index, V_b is the screw velocity, and H is the channel depth of the screw.

Using a melt extruder with only feed screw elements (similar to wet extruder), a dense extrudate was obtained at 20 rpm that became soft and powdery at 50 and 100 rpm (46). At a lower speed, the material resides longer within the chamber that could lead to greater homogeneity of binding fluid (water) in the material. In addition, the slower rate of extrusion provides a more uniformly dense extrudate. In a somewhat similar study with a focus on screw design, the wet granulation of lactose monohydrate using aqueous solutions of povidone as binder was profiled in a twin-screw extruder with different types of screw elements at a screw speed of 10 rpm (47). The energy-intensive mixing elements increased granule size because of their compaction effect, while conveying elements with low energy input gave finer particles primarily because of agitation effect. This again indicates another way of modulating extrudate characteristics by the use of geometry variables, that is, selection of screw elements and design.

From a formulator's perspective, the ability to modulate the rheology of the wet mass is critical to successful extrusion. Toward this end, MCC has often been used to facilitate extrusion. It is a dry binder used in tableting because of its plastic deforming ability that imparts tensile strength to a tablet. However, MCC has been used in wet extrusion for formulations containing a high amount of soluble ingredients (e.g., lactose, mannitol) or noncohesive, poorly bonding inorganic materials such as barium sulfate (38). With soluble materials, it lowers the yield force thereby enabling uniform movement of the wet mass in the chamber while with material like calcium carbonate, it provides the required cohesive or bonding strength for the extrudate. It has also been used in a coprocessed (e.g., spray-dried) form with other polymeric binders, notably, sodium carboxymethylcellulose (Na-CMC) to increase density of the extrudate though at a high-shear stress (42,48,49), specially in the presence of soluble ingredient like lactose. Avicel RC-581®, a commercially available grade of

TABLE 7   Critical Variables in Scale-Up of Extrusion

Formulation	Process/extruder	Process monitoring
Moisture content	Configuration Screw vs. gear	Moisture content

Type and level of binder (e.g.,
  microcrystalline cellulose,
  sodium carboxymethylcellulose)
	Rotational speed of extrusion
	  head (screw or gear)
		Temperature

Soluble ingredients (e.g., drug, lactose)	Die or screen L/D ratio	Torque or force of extrusion
		Specific energy or power consumption
		Throughput (rate of product conveyance)

coprocessed MCC-Na-CMC mixture enabled extrusion at a moisture level of less than 25% with improved yield, a moisture level too low for extrusion with only MCC (50). Upon wetting, these coprocessed mixtures form colloidal dispersions that depending on the concentration and applied stress can range from a pseudoplastic sol to a thixotropic gel or a paste.

To summarize, while selection and scale-up of extruders is governed by extruder geometry, formulation and process variables, secondary variables could be used to monitor the process on a continuous basis. On the basis of the reports thus far in the literature, the variables that seem to play a critical role in scale-up of extrusion are summarized in Table 7.

SPHERONIZATION

Spheronization, simply stated, is the process of forming spheroids from a given material. In the present context, the rod-shaped cylindrical pieces of extrudate are placed in a device called the spheronizer and "formed" into spheres when subjected to a high speed rotation. The spheronizer basically consists of a grooved, horizontal friction plate rotating at a given speed within a stationary, vertical, right cylinder fitted with a door for discharge of the product. The cylinder is open at the top and has smooth internal walls. There is a clearance of about 0.25 mm between the edge of the plate and the inner wall of the cylinder. The grooves on the plate often are set to intersect at right angles to forming "cross-hatch" geometry and vary in size from 1 to 5 mm in width. Other patterns are used as shown in Figure 16. The diameter of the plate varies from 9 to 15 in. for laboratory scale equipment with an output of about 10 kg/hr to about 27 in. for a production size unit with an output of about 100 kg/hr of wet spheroids. The speed of the plate could be varied from 100 to 1200 rpm with the operation typically ranging from 200 to 800 rpm.

The success of spheronization depends on whether the extrudate can be suitably deformed into pellets. The ideal extrudate should break up into short, uniform rod-shaped pieces and have sufficient plasticity to be rolled into spheres by the action of the friction plate. So that the granules are separate and discrete throughout the process, the extrudate should not adhere to itself or the plate and retain enough cohesion so as not to break up into fine particles. Pellets typical of this process are dense and round in appearance with a narrow particle size distribution compared with granules from a conventional

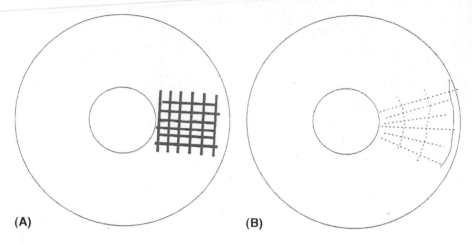

(A)   **(B)**

FIGURE 16   Geometry of friction plate in spheronizer. A cross-hatch, B radial. *Source*: From Ref. 14.

granulation process. The final pellet size and yield are dependent on such factors as diameter of the extrudate, formulation attributes such as moisture content, rotational speed of the plate and residence time in the spheronizer.

Mechanistic Aspects of Spheronization

The earliest description of mechanism of spheronization was given by Reynolds (10) and Miyake (51). Because of centrifugal acceleration and deceleration, the material rotates in an annular shape against the wall of the spheronizer, thus generating a toroidal, rope like motion. The collisions against the wall and the plate initially break the extrudate into short cylinders. The centrifugal forces generated by the moving plate and frictional forces due to the rough surface deform the broken cylinders into spheroids as shown in Figure 17. Hypotheses of this conversion based on a series of intermediates that include cylinders, cylinders with rounded ends, dumbbells, ellipsoids, spheroids with cavities and finally spheres have been proposed (15,52). The intermediates are formed by collision of pellets against each other, against the friction plate and against the wall of the spheronizer. The process is complete when the area of collision reaches a minimum.

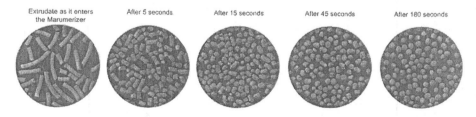

Extrudate as it enters   After 5 seconds   After 15 seconds   After 45 seconds   After 180 seconds
the Marumerizer

FIGURE 17   Illustration of deformation of extruded pellets into spheres over time.

Zhang et al. (53) developed a model for spheronization process based on second-order kinetics and predicted the half life at which the size of 50% of spheres (1:1 mix of acetaminophen-MCC) was greater than the size of a #14 mesh screen opening (1400 µm) at 36 seconds after spheronization. On the basis of this model, the process is essentially complete in less than five minutes. It has been theorized with the aid of high speed photographic imaging that shaping of pellets occurs by aggregation within 30 to 60 seconds of formation of the broken extrudate segments (54). Iyer et al. (29) obtained steady-state sphericity of pellets within three minutes of spheronization of mixtures of lactose and MCC, as shown in Figure 18, while Newton et al. (55) observed that roundness of pellets increased exponentially with number of plate revolutions. All these suggest clearly that spheronization is a fast process and the events happening in the first few minutes are critical to the quality of resulting pellets. A primary goal in scale-up would then be to optimize the formulation and process variables such that this initial "window" is prolonged as much as needed to have a more robust process. Operationally, a shorter time is often a goal in manufacturing. An optimal time of spheronization could then be identified.

The collision of the broken wet segments during spheronization can result in two effects: deformation and coalescence. The migration of moisture or soluble binders from the core to the surface of the pellets improves surface plasticity which is needed for deformation and rounding of the pellets (43,56). While deformation is desirable for shaping of the pellets, excess surface moisture could result in high degree of liquid-solid bonding that leads to coalescence or uncontrolled "growth" of spheronizing mass. An extreme case of this

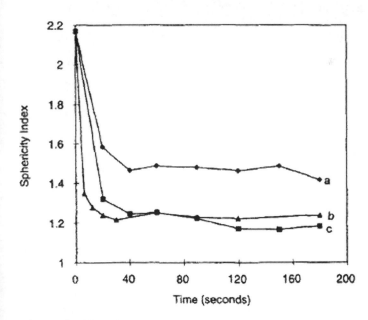

FIGURE 18 Effect of residence time on sphericity of pellets at varying plate speeds. a, 350 rpm; b, 680 rpm; and c, 830 rpm. *Source*: From Ref. 26.

phenomenon is the formation of "golf ball"–sized pellets. A limiting agglomerate size, δ, may be defined (57,58) above which the tensile forces that separate particles due to centrifugal rotation exceed binding forces due to liquid saturation and surface plasticity using a power law expression as

$$\delta = A\left(k^{2/3}\sigma_t\right) \tag{9}$$

where A = constant, k = agglomerate deformability, and σ = tensile stresses on the agglomerate.

Low values of σ could result in aggregation or incomplete separation of pellets (e.g., dumbells) as the forces may not be enough to overcome the liquid-solid bonding.

A modified expression for pellet deformation was given by Kristensen (59,60) as

$$\delta^{2/a} = \frac{(\Delta L/L)^3}{\sigma_t} \tag{10}$$

The left hand side is a compliance parameter or bulk strain normalized for the centrifugal, gravitational and inertial stresses exerted on the material during spheronization. The volume shape factor of pellets became closer to a sphere as the compliance of the extrudate increased, when measured in a creep test (61).

The challenge in spheronization is then to effect surface deformation without coalescence of wet pellets in the early stages of the process. The binding forces due to free surface liquid and saturated liquid within cause deformation and rounding of pellets, while the separating forces due to inertial and centrifugal motion retard coalescence by keeping them apart. While formulation variables such as moisture content and binder level control deformation, the process and geometry variables such as plate speed, diameter and residence time assist in retarding coalescence. A balance of these stresses is critical to obtaining discrete, spherical pellets.

Among formulation variables, the moisture content, specially, on product surface needs to be optimized. While excess surface moisture could lead to uncontrolled agglomeration, a dry extrudate can break up into fine powder. Upon spheronization for prolonged periods at high speeds, moisture gradients develop within pellets by migration from core to the surface. This is also a function of the concentration of dissolved solids and spheronizing time. The surface moisture could be lost over time because of evaporation and friction (62) unless the soluble materials migrate to the surface and form a moisture barrier that could prevent further loss. Since such phenomena are well established in the drying, that some degree of drying occurs during spheronization may be deduced.

End Point Determination

It has been described before that spheronization occurs via cutting of rod-shaped extrudate into smaller cylinders followed by deformation into spherical pellets. Since the pellet properties vary over a continuum, a mass of pellets is often defined by distribution of the properties on a suitable basis such as number, weight or volume. Limits or range of tolerance may then be assigned over this distribution and product acceptability or yield could be defined in this manner. A process end point, however, is difficult to convey as the precise moment at which deformation is complete is unclear since it involves changes in bulk properties of materials (shape, size, porosity). The latter in turn are dependent on the type of extruder, size and mass of extrudate and spheronizing conditions including residence time and plate speed (63–65). However, since deformation occurs from collision of extrudate and pellets against each other, against the plate and spheronizer wall, one or more outcomes of the collision events may be used to define the process. This could be a change in moisture content, impact force, pellet size or wall friction though techniques to measure these in a continuous manner during spheronization are not widely available.

The physical properties of pellets have been widely used to determine acceptable yield of pellets. These include shape indices, size and size distribution, different densities, pore volume and distribution, flow properties and friability. Of course, drug release from the pellets is a critical parameter to be monitored to ensure potency and uniformity of drug distribution.

Sieve analysis using standard mesh screens is commonly used to determine particle size and size distribution of pellets and the reader is referred to standard texts for further information (66). Several types of densities have been defined for pellets on the basis of interparticulate (void fraction) and intraparticulate pore volumes and include true, apparent, effective, bulk and tapped. The bulk and tapped densities may be obtained using simple devices as that used to evaluate granulations in tableting while the true and apparent densities need more complex techniques based on mercury intrusion, gas flow, powder displacement, imaging or minimum fluidization velocity (67).

Since the desired shape of a pellet is a sphere, shape factors have been used to describe the pellets. These are characterized variously as sphericity, roundness, shape coefficient, elongation index, and aspect ratio (68–72). Using the volume diameter, d_v, and projected diameter, d_p, a good measure of sphericity is the volume shape factor, α, given by

$$\alpha_v = \frac{\pi d_v^3}{6 d_p^3} \tag{11}$$

$$d_v = (6/\pi \rho_g N_s)^{1/3} \tag{12}$$

where ρ_g is the apparent granule density and N_s is the specific particle number. The density ρ_g may be obtained by mercury porosimetry at low intrusion pressures. The projected diameter d_p is a two-dimensional value obtained from microscopy. The volume shape factor equals $\pi/6$ for a perfect sphere with smaller or larger values indicating deviations from sphericity. The more accurate surface volume diameter, d_{sv}, is difficult to measure for porous, irregular spheronized pellets. A more commonly used two-dimensional sphericity is the roundness factor using microscopic imaging. Chapman et al. (73) characterized the roundness as the angle of inclination of a plane at which a particle would roll, termed as "one plane critical stability." A summary of various shape indices is shown in Table 8.

It was already noted that the presence of excessive moisture on surface of pellets during spheronization could lead to uncontrolled agglomeration. This effect could be minimized by adding adsorbents like colloidal silicon dioxide or

TABLE 8 Shape Indices of Spheronized Pellets

Index	Expression	Sphere value
Sphericity	$\phi = d_{sv}/d_v$	1
Surface shape factor	$\alpha_s = S/d_p^2$	π
Volume shape factor	$\alpha_v = V/d_p^3$	$\pi/6$
Volume form factor	$K_e = \alpha_{v\sqrt{}}/RM$	$\pi/6$
Surface volume shape coefficient	$\alpha_{sv} - Sd_p/V$	6
Shape factor	$\alpha = S/V^{2/3}$	4.837
Shape coefficient	$\alpha = (S_w\rho d_p) + (L/W)$	7
Aspect or elongation ratio[a]	$\alpha = d_{max}/d_{min}$	1
Circularity[a]	$\psi = P^2/4\pi S$	1
Roundness[a]	$K = 4S/\pi d_p^2$	1

[a]obtained by microscopy

Abbreviations: d_{sv}, surface volume diameter; d_v, volume diameter; d_p, projected diameter = $0.99\sqrt{LW}$; L or d_{max}, length (longer axis); W or d_{min}, width (shorter axis); S, surface area of pellet; V, volume of pellet; R, ratio of maximum diameter d_{max} to minimum diameter d_{min}; M, ratio of pellet width to pellet depth; S_w, specific surface area; ρ, particle density; P, perimeter.

talc to the spheronizing pellets, increasing viscosity of binding fluid and complexing soluble materials in the mixture. As in extrusion, inclusion of MCC in a formulation can provide highly dense, less friable and spherical pellets, depending on the drug loading. While elastic materials such as starch are more sensitive to moisture content during spheronization, MCC is easily deformable when its plastic limit is reached at a moisture content of 20% greater than its own weight (51,74). As in extrusion, coprocessed forms of MCC with sodium CMC enable spheronization of formulations containing a high drug loading of 50% to 80% (75). A spray-dried mixture of MCC with hydrophilic polymers was found to be less sensitive to moisture content, yielding pellets more spherical in shape compared with a physical mixture (48). The more adhesive polymers such as sodium CMC and HPMC could inhibit deformation due to surface adhesion resulting in lower sphericity values, while the more plastic and less adhesive HPC and PVP polymers provide greater roundness of pellets.

On the basis of the authors' personal experience (unpublished data) in formulating a low melting drug (melting point about 45°C), the selection of excipients was critical to both quality of pellets and scale-up of the process. In presence of a low melting, hydrophobic drug, lactose exhibited significant sticking to the plate during spheronization. The addition of MCC and a surfactant reduced this sticking effect significantly. It was theorized that MCC holds significant water during spheronization thus preventing water loss. This led to reduction in the percent fines and subsequent sticking of the fines to the low melting drug. In addition, the surfactant reduced erosion at the edges by forming a smoother surface on the pellets. The addition of a small amount of vegetable oil significantly reduced product buildup and sticking, likely due to its lubricant effect minimizing particle-plate friction and formation of fines.

In general, extrudate with high moisture content undergo greater degree of deformation providing pellets with increased roundness when spheronized for a longer time at a critical speed (64,65,72). It was observed earlier that sphere formation happens within a short time period and some moisture loss occurs during the high speed rotation. This possibly means though deformation

(sphere formation) may be complete, it may be necessary to continue spheronization so as to keep the pellets apart until surface moisture content is reduced
enough to minimize agglomeration. The particle size at this stage should
approximate the extrusion screen size. Continued spheronization repeats this
cycle resulting in spherical pellets with a smaller particle size and narrower
distribution. However, spheronization for very long time periods at very high
speeds could lead to further moisture loss and dry pellets that may disintegrate
into fine particles or a powdery mass, being unable to withstand the rotational
and frictional stresses. Under such conditions, the choice of binder and binding
strength are critical to maintain the physical integrity of the pellets

The binding fluid can weaken the binder as seen with pectin when used
with ethanol as the fluid. Ethanol reduces swelling ability of pectin making the
hydrocolloid ineffective resulting in spherical but weak pellets (68,76). The
porosity of the pellets increased with increasing fraction of 2-propanol in
water-propanol mixtures as binding fluid (77). An opposite effect was seen
with chitosan that when used in aqueous medium retarded drug release and
dissolution from the spheres (78). As in extrusion, the aqueous solubility of the
drug was inversely linear to amount of water required for optimal spheronization. Typically, poorly soluble drugs require more binding fluid and longer
residence time for spheronization.

Process Control and Scale-up

It is noteworthy to mention that all spheronizers across scales and manufacturers have only one and the same basic design component, that is, a rotating
circular metal plate. An overview of spheronizers is shown in Table 9. A fully

TABLE 9   An Overview of Spheronizers of Varying Scales and
Capacities from Various Manufacturers

Company	Model	Typical operating capacity (kg)	Maximum plate speed (rpm)
LCI			
	QJ-230	0.1–1.5	1800
	QJ-400	0.2–3.0	1280
	QJ-700	1.0–15	690
	QJ-1000	2.5–35	790
Caleva			
	Spheronizer 120	0.03–0.05	3000
	Spheronizer 250	0.1–1.0	3000
	Spheronizer 380	0.5–4	1500
	Spheronizer 500	1–11	1000
	Spheronizer 700	5–20	1000
Gabler			
	R-250	0.15–0.6	2000
	R-400	1–3	2000
	R-600	2–6	1200
	R-900	Up to 20	1200
NICA			
	S-320	0.2–1	600
	S-450	0.4–2	450
	S-700	2–10	300

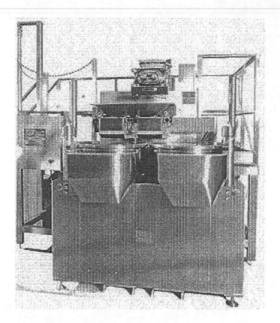

FIGURE 19 A fully automated, production scale twin spheronizer with an incorporated gear extruder assembly. *Source*: Courtesy of Caleva.

automated system as shown in Figure 19 has two plates rotating in tandem to handle large batch sizes in a continuous operation. There may be some variations such as degree of plate roughness but by far the simplicity of design makes spheronization easy to scale-up. At the same time, the wide variation in recommended batch size by manufacturers A and B for their respective spheronizers is shown in Figure 20. The range provided by vendor A is broader (0.1–15 kg) for a 700-mm-diameter plate than that given by vendor B (5–20 kg) for the same size spheronizer. Further, the range becomes wider with increasing scale suggesting that an optimal material charge needs to be developed for each application.

The two critical process variables are plate speed and residence time of pellets in spheronizer while the plate diameter is a geometry variable that increases with material load. The importance of optimizing moisture content during scale-up has already been noted.

For a given plate speed (S rpm), plate diameter (D mm), and spheronizing time (T seconds), the scale-up may be based on keeping constant the number of revolutions, rotational distance, or peripheral velocity.

a. Number of revolutions (N)

$$N = ST \tag{13}$$

b. Peripheral velocity (V)

$$V = \pi D S \tag{14}$$

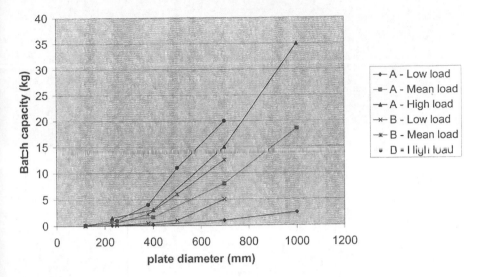

FIGURE 20 Comparison of material loads at high, low, and average values recommended by manufacturers A and B for spheronizers with varying plate diameters.

c. Rotational travel (X)

$$X = \pi DST \qquad (15)$$

Fixed Number of Revolutions
Often, spheronizers are not available with variable motor drives which means different but fixed speeds of operation. Figure 21 shows the impact of residence time for spheronizers of varying plate diameters and source when scaling based on fixed number of revolutions. The scale ratio based on output is 10× to 15×. Spheronization from source A in the larger unit at 690 rpm requires a process time of 20 minutes to maintain the same number of revolutions when scaling up from the smaller unit at 1800 rpm for 7 minutes. The effect of surface moisture on pellet quality is more apparent because of the longer residence time at the larger scale. Spheronizers from source B seem less subject to effect of residence time since the plate speed over the entire scale is within a narrow range of 1500 to 2000 rpm. With this approach, scaling based on fixed speed implies a constant residence time. This would require the batch charge to be proportional in some manner to the plate diameter.

A drawback in scaling based on fixed number of revolutions is that it does not factor in the geometry variable (plate diameter) which typically increases more than 3× for a 10× scale in batch size.

Fixed Peripheral Velocity
The peripheral velocity, on the other hand, is a function of plate speed (process) and diameter (geometry) which vary across scale and across equipment from

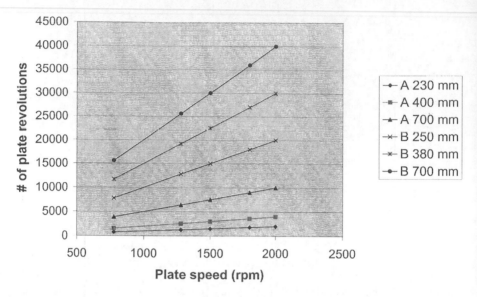

FIGURE 21 Plate revolutions simulated for varying spheronization times for three spheronizers of increasing scale from two manufacturers A and B. Each simulation at maximum recommended speed of operation. Each rpm in legend for A or B represents a spheronizer of a specific diameter (scale).

different vendors. It is analogous to the "tip speed" commonly used in granulation scale-up. Newton et al. (55) obtained pellets of similar quality while scaling up spheronization at a constant peripheral velocity across a 25× scale. A 0.2-kg batch size spheronized using a 22.9-cm-diameter plate was scaled over a 125-fold range to 25-kg batch size using a production spheronizer with a 65.6-cm-diameter plate. The plate speed was decreased from 900 rpm at smaller scale to 340 rpm at larger scale to maintain a constant linear peripheral velocity at 424 cm/sec. The "one plane critical stability" angle and mean diameter of the pellets were comparable across the scales and decreased to the same minimal value as the number of revolutions was increased as shown in Figure 22. This approach was also found to be somewhat independent of mode of extrusion prior to spheronization (79).

Figure 23 shows simulated peripheral velocities at varying speed for spheronizers of different diameters from two different sources. It is evident that this approach is independent of the manufacturer since the only scale information needed is the plate speed which is obtained from the plate diameter and the peripheral velocity at the smaller scale that was used to obtain the target pellet attributes.

The Froude number is often used as a dimensionless index to scale up a fluid whose flow field is governed by gravitational forces, among others (45). It is essentially a ratio of kinetic to inertial (gravitational) forces acting on a body. For a spheronizing particle, the kinetic parameter is the centrifugal force and

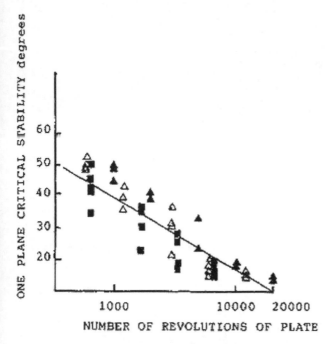

FIGURE 22 Change in the value of one plane critical stability with the number of revolutions of the spheronizer plate for granules from within the largest sieve fraction for batches spheronized on plates of varying diameter plates: △ 22.9 cm, ▲ 38.1 cm, and ■ 65.6 cm.

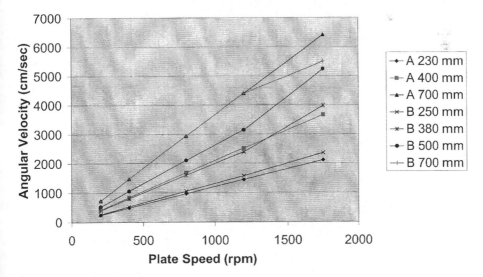

FIGURE 23 The angular velocities at varying plate speeds for three spheronizers of increasing scale from manufacturers A and B. Each simulated run is at maximum recommended speed of operation. Each number in legend represents plate diameter of spheronizer from A or B.

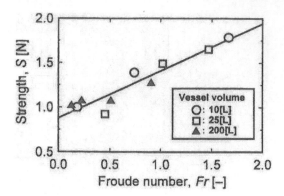

FIGURE 24 Scale-up characteristics of pellet strength by means of Froude number. *Source*: From Ref. 81.

determined by plate speed and diameter while g represents the gravity field. The Froude number is expressed as

$$Fr = \frac{U}{\sqrt{gL}} \tag{16}$$

where U is a characteristic velocity, the peripheral velocity (m/sec), g is acceleration due to gravity (m/sec^2), and L is a characteristic length, the plate diameter (m).

Since g is a constant, the scale-up factor becomes the centrifugal force as given byz

$$F^c = \frac{MS^2}{D} \tag{17}$$

with M being the material load. On the basis of this approach, using Froude number, spheronization of an ibuprofen product across a 10× ratio (80) and wet massing in a high-shear kneader across a 20× ratio were scaled up with acceptable product attributes as seen from Figure 24 (81).

PROCESS ANALYTICAL TECHNOLOGY
While the goal of PAT is to understand and control the manufacturing process, PAT itself is being defined (82,83) as a system for designing, analyzing, and controlling manufacturing through timely measurements (i.e., during processing) of critical quality and performance attributes of raw and in-process materials and processes with the goal of ensuring final product quality. The PAT instrumentation helps profile the key formation on a continuous basis, for example, sensors on the blenders that check for blend uniformity, moisture and granule size growth during granulation, and for particle size changes during manufacture of suspension, and provide valuable information to fingerprint the batch that in turn provides a means to control the process. The PAT initiative

relies on four main components: data analysis, process analytical tools, process monitoring, and continuous feedback to assure the product quality. In the foregoing discussions, we addressed the various critical variables based on mechanistic events and geometry (design) of components that influence these events. On the basis of the various online, at-line, and in-line analytical technologies available to date and the process considerations, the following aspects of extrusion-spheronization lend themselves to be evaluated under the PAT initiative.

Moisture Content and Content Uniformity

As shown in previous sections, moisture acts as a plasticizer and lubricant during the extrusion process and its control is critical to produce uniform and consistent pellets. Various online techniques that are available for measuring moisture are near-infrared (near-IR) and thermal effusivity. The near-IR spectroscopy and its several variations including near-IR chemical imaging, Solid-state acoustooptic tunable filter (AOTF)-NIR analyzers have found widespread acceptance as PAT because of its nondestructive nature, sensitivity and flexibility of implementation and analyzing range of samples (solids, liquids, powders) (84–86). The data collected by near-IR can be easily analyzed for moisture content (Fig. 25) as well as blend uniformity analysis using various chemometric algorithms and "principle component analysis," thus making it a useful quantitative tool. For moisture analysis, the near-IR can provide accurate measurement down to 0.02% while being capable of monitoring the granulation process requiring moisture as high as 50%. For blend uniformity analysis, the near-IR can be used to analyze fairly complex systems provided that material is scanned by the instruments over several lots to establish the boundary conditions or failure points. Similarly thermal effusivity, on the basis of the heat transferability of materials, can provide a mapping of material distribution in the powder mass. This nondestructive sensor is available for online monitoring

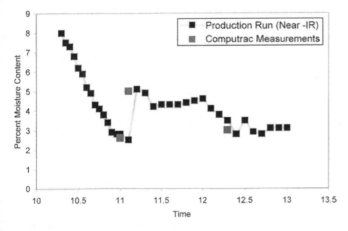

FIGURE 25 Online moisture measurements during fluid bed drying versus at-line measurement using Computrac®. *Source*: Courtesy of Lasentec.

of many processes including moisture content, density, particle size distribution and morphology (87).

The moisture determination is critical during granulation, extrusion, spheronization and drying processes. Both of these techniques have been widely used in the granulation and drying processes, however they can be easily adapted to extrusion and spheronization processes as well to provide key information needed for process control. For example effusivity sensors can be retrofitted onto the walls or covers of the processing equipment to enable comparison of the real time reading without removing samples from the process.

Particle Size and Size Distribution

The particle size and size distribution of granules (feeding material) and the pellets (dried pellets) are important process attributes that determines the process reproducibility and robustness. The measurement of wet granules (size and size distribution), extrudates size (diameter and length) and spheronized pellets (morphology, sphericity, size, and size distribution) provide a useful insight in evaluating the role of process variables or formulation changes on the final product. The online measurement techniques ranges from Focused Beam Reflectance Measurement (FBRM) and continuous in-process video microscope [Particle Vision and Measurement (PVM)] to Insitec (88,89). These techniques are being extensively evaluated for granulation process, however as indicated earlier can be easily adapted to extrusion (for rods), spheronization (for pellets) and drying steps (pellet size) processes as well. They are capable of providing consistent data in the particle size range of 0.5 to 1000 μm, however FBRM has been shown to work well for particles up to 2 mm and is one of the most widely evaluated tool because of its application in chemical processes. The FBRM measures distance as chord length, that is, distance between any two edges of the particle and does not assume any shape. The large number of measurements over given period of time provides a statistically reliable measurement of the particle size and growth. A material prerequisite for using FBRM is that material should have some degree of backscattering. Most excipients and therapeutic agents used for extrusion-spheronization generally fall in this category.

Rheology and Flow of Wet Mass

An important consideration in the extrusion process is the flow of wet mass under pressure through die. An appropriate control of granulation end point is important to assure the reproducible processing of batch during extrusion as well as spheronization. Power consumption and torque measurements are commonly used for this purpose. Measurement of current can adequately express the torque for some DC operated motors and most extruders are equipped with this functionality to provide an indirect measurement of torque (89). The flow of wet mass in extruder is generally monitored using at-line techniques such as ram extruder or torque rheometer. They provide useful information in assessing effect of process and formulation variations on the processing. The flow of granules in extruders is regarded as three step process consisting of compression, steady-state flow, and forced flow. A comparison of compression zone and steady-state flow and forced flow zones for different formulations or granulation provides valuable information in optimizing the extrusion process (30,90). A typical force-displacement curve showing the three stages as shown in Figure 9 and can be used to track the product performance from small scale to various stages of scale-up. The mixer torque rheometer is also frequently employed in characterizing the wet mass and has been useful in establishing the boundary conditions for granulations in terms of providing reproducible pellets (90).

Another parameter of interest in the extrusion process is screen pressure, and the extruder can be fitted with suitable pressure transducer to monitor the pressure drop associated with extrusion. One such device available from Heastern (Dynisco products) is shown in Figure 26, that allows the measurement of temperature and pressure. The measurement of back pressure at the extruder screen, pressure at the extruder outlet and the temperature provides an excellent opportunity for implantation of PAT. Nowadays some extruders are equipped with pressure transducer and digital indicator with high-pressure shutdown providing a safety feature as well as a continuous profiling of the extrusion process.

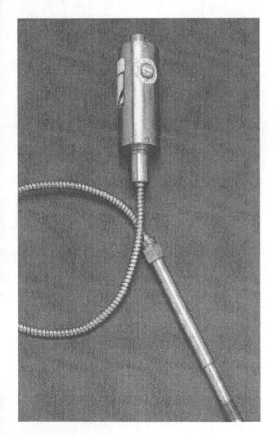

FIGURE 26 Integrated thermocouple and pressure transducer to measure temperature as well as pressure during extrusion. *Source*: Courtesy of Heaster Industries.

SUMMARY

In summary, extrusion-spheronization process has been successfully used in pharmaceutical applications and provides the formulator with range of choices to manufacture pellet dosage forms. The process consists of five unit operations, dry mixing, granulation, extrusion, spheronization and drying. While the process of extrusion and spheronization imposes stringent formulation requirements in terms of various viscoplastic processes that it has to undergo, it is somewhat easier to manage from scale-up perspective. The extrusion being continuous process process is somewhat easier to scale-up from laboratory scale to large scale equipment. The successful scale-up of spheronization can also be predicted with careful evaluation of geometry, rotation speed, load and time. Thus a good understanding of the mechanical process, formulation science and equipment geometry are essential to determine the critical variables that impact both extrudate and pellet properties.

REFERENCES

1. Ghebre-Sellassie I. Pharmaceutical Pelletization Technology. New York: Marcel Dekker, 1989.
2. Scala BJ, et al. Pellets for oral administration of low-molecular-weight heparin. Drug Dev Ind Pharm 2009; 35(12):1503–1510.
3. Newitt DM, Conway-Jones JM. A contribution to the theory and practice of granulation. Trans Inst Chem Eng 1958; 36:422–442.
4. Fenner RT, Williams JG. Some experiments on polymer melt flow in single screw extruders. J Mech Eng Sci 1971; 13(2):65–74.
5. Simonds HR, Weith AJ, Schack W. Extrusion of Plastics, Rubber and Metals. New York: Reinhold Publishing, 1962.
6. Dietrich R. Food technology transfers to pellet production. Manuf Chem 1989; 60: 29–33.
7. Senouci A, Smith A, Richmond P. Extrusion cooking: food for though. Chem Eng 1985; 417:30–33.
8. Webster's New International Dictionary. 2nd ed. Springfield: G & C Merriam Company Publishers, 1948:2422.
9. Nakahara N. Method and apparatus for making spherical granules. U.S. Patent 3,277,520, October 11, 1966.
10. Reynolds AD. A new technique for the production of spherical particles. Manuf Chem Aerosol News 1970; 41:40–43.
11. Conine JW, Hadley HR. Preparation of small solid pharmaceutical spheres. Drugs Cosmet Ind 1970; 90:38–41.
12. Gamlen MJ. Pellet manufacture for controlled release. Manuf Chem 1985; 56:55–59.
13. Newton JM. The preparation of spherical granules by extrusion/spheronization. STP Pharma 1990; 6(6):396–398.
14. O'Connor RE, Schwartz JB. Extrusion and spheronization technology In: Ghebre-Sellaise I, ed. Pharmaceutical Pelletization Technology. New York: Marcel Dekker, 1989:187–216.
15. Rowe RC. Spheronization: a novel pill-making process? Pharm Int 1985; 119–123.
16. Van doorslaer T. Introduction to Low Pressure Extrusion. Version 2.0. Sint-Niklaas, Belgium: The Fitzpatrick Company Europe NV, 1997.
17. O'Connor RE. Extrusion and spheronization. Granulation Technology for Bioproducts. Boca Raton: CRC Press, 1991:101–118.
18. Kanai T, Kimura M, Asano Y. Studies on scale-up of tubular film extrusion. J Plast Film Sheeting 1986; 2:224–241.
19. Kaiser H. Scale-up of extrusion dies for tubular film blowing. Polym Proc Eng 1987; 5 (1):1–21.
20. Nakatani M. Scale-up theory for twin-screw extruder, keeping the resin temperature unchanged. Adv Polym Technol 1998; 17(1):1, 19–22.

21. Potente H. Existing scale-up rules for single-screw plasticating extruders. Int Polym Process 1991; 6(4):267–278.
22. Bigio D, Wang K. Scale-up rules for mixing in a non-intermeshing twin-screw extruder. Polym Eng Sci 1996; 36(23):2832–2839.
23. Rauwendaal C. Scale-up of single screw extruders. Polym Eng Sci 1987; 27(14):1059–1068.
24. Carley JF, McKelvey JM. Extruder scale-up theory and experiments. Ind Eng Chem 1953; 45:985–989.
25. Maddock BH. SPE J 1959; 15:983.
26. Maddock BH. Extruder scale-up by computer. Polym Eng Sci 1974; 14(12):853.
27. Covas JA, Costa P. A miniature extrusion line for small scale processing studies. Polym Test 2004; 23(7):763–773.
28. Shah RD, Kabadi M, Pope DG, et al. Physico-mechanical characterization of the extrusion-spheronization process. Part II: rheological determinants for successful extrusion and spheronization. Pharm Res 1995; 12(4):496–507.
29. Iyer RM, Augsburger LL, Pope DG, et al. Extrusion/spheronization – effect of moisture content and spheronization time on pellet characteristics, Pharm Dev Technol 1996; 1(4):325–331.
30. Harrison PJ, Newton JM, Rowe RC. The characterization of wet powder masses suitable for extrusion/spheronization. J Pharm Pharmacol 1985; 37:686–691.
31. Thoma K, Zeigler I. Investigations on the influence of the type of extruder for pelletization by extrusion-spheronization. I. Extrusion behavior of formulations. Drug Dev Ind Pharm 1998; 24(5):401–411.
32. Agur EE. Extruder scale-up in a corotating twin-screw extrusion compounding process. Adv Polym Technol 1986; 6(2):225–232.
33. Kleinbudde P. Use of a power-consumption-controlled extruder in the development of pellet formulations. J Pharm Sci 1995; 84(10):1259–1264.
34. Harrison PJ, Newton JM, Rowe RC. Convergent flow analysis in the extrusion of wet powder masses. J Pharm Pharmacol 1984; 36:796–798.
35. Fielden KE, Newton JM, Rowe RC. A comparison of the extrusion and spheronization behavior of wet powder masses processed by a ram extruder and a cylinder extruder. Int J Pharm 1992; 81:225–233.
36. Thoma K, Ziegler I. Investigations on the influence of the type of extruder for pelletization by extrusion-spheronization. II. Sphere characteristics. Drug Dev Ind Pharm 1998; 24(5):413–422.
37. Baert L, Remon JP, Knight P, et al. A comparison between the extrusion forces and sphere quality of a gravity feed extruder and a ram extruder. Int J Pharm 1992; 86:187–192.
38. Bains D, Boutell SL, Newton JM. The influence of moisture content on the preparation of spherical granules of barium sulphate and microcrystalline cellulose. Int J Pharm 1991; 69:233–237.
39. Jover I, Podczeck F, Newton M. Evaluation, by a statistically designed experiment, of an experimental grade of microcrystalline cellulose, Avicel 955, as a technology to aid the production of pellets with high drug loading. J Pharm Sci 1996; 85(7):700–705.
40. Baert L, Remon JP, Elbers JAC, et al. Comparison between a gravity feed extruder and a twin screw extruder. Int J Pharm 1993; 99:7–12.
41. Vervaet C, Baert L, Risha PA, et al. The influence of the extrusion screen on pellet quality using an instrumented basket extruder. Int J Pharm 1994; 107:29–39.
42. Hileman GA, Upadrashta SM, Neau SH. Drug solubility effects on predicting optimum conditions for extrusion and spheronization of pellets. Pharm Dev Technol 1997; 2(1):43–52.
43. Chien TY, Nuessle NO. Factors influencing migration during spheronization. Pharm Technol 1985; 9(4):42–48.
44. Fitzpatric S, Taylor S, Booth SW, et al. The Development of a stable, coated pellet formulation of a water-sensitive drug, a case study: development of a stable core formulation. Pharm Dev Technol 2006; 11:521–528.
45. Granger RA. Fluid Mechanics. New York: CBS College Publishing, 1985:10017.

46. Nakamichi K, Nakano T, Yasuura H, et al. The role of the kneading paddle and the effects of screw revolution speed and water content on the preparation of solid dispersions using a twin-screw extruder. Int J Pharm 2002; 241:203–211.

47. Thompson MR, Sun J., Wet granulation in a twin-screw extruder: implications of screw design. J Pharm Sci 2009; 99(4):2090–2103.

48. Law MFL, Deasy PB. Use of hydrophilic polymers with microcrystalline cellulose to improve extrusion-spheronization. Eur J Pharm Biopharm 1998; 45:57–65.

49. Raines CL, Newton JM. The extrusion rheology of various grades of MCC. J Pharm Pharmacol 1987; 39(suppl 90P):90.

50. Malinowski HJ, Smith WE. Use of factorial design to evaluate granulations prepared by spheronization. J Pharm Sci 1975; 64(10):1688–1692.

51. Miyake Y, Shinoda A, Furukawa M, et al. Yakuzaigaku 1973; 33(4):161–166.

52. Baert L, Remon JP. Influence of amount of granulation liquid on the drug release rate from pellets made by extrusion spheronization. Int J Pharm 1993; 95:135–141.

53. Zhang G, Schwartz JB, Schnaare RL, et al. Kinetics of sphere growth in marumerization. J China Pharm Univ 1990; 21(2):73–76.

54. Fielden KE, Newton JM, Rowe RC. The influence of lactose particle size on spheronization of extrudate processed by a ram extruder. Int J Pharm 1992; 81:205–224.

55. Newton JM, Chapman SR, Rowe RC. The assessment of the scale-up performance of the extrusion/spheronization process. Int J Pharm 1995; 120:95–99.

56. Kristensen HG. Industrial wet granulation. Acta Pharmaceutica Suecica 1988; 25(4–5):187–204.

57. Ouchiyama N, Tanaka T. The probability of coalescence in granulation kinetics. Ind Eng Chem Process Des Dev 1975; 14:286–289.

58. Ouchiyama N, Tanaka T. Physical requisite to appropriate granule growth rate. Ind Eng Chem Process Des Dev 1982; 21:35–37.

59. Kristensen HG, Holm P, Schaefer T. Mechanical properties of moist agglomerates in relation to granulation mechanisms: part I. Deformability of moist, densified agglomerates. Powder Technol 1985; 44:227–237.

60. Kristensen HG, Holm P, Schaefer T. Mechanical properties of moist agglomerates in relation to granulation mechanisms: part II. Effects of particle size distribution. Powder Technol 1985; 44:239–247.

61. Iyer RM. A study of select rheological attributes of wet extrudate and their relationship to the design of pelleted pharmaceutical formulations, PhD thesis, Univ. of Maryland, 1994.

62. Hellen L, Yliruusi J, Merkku P, et al. Process variables of instant granulator and spheroniser: I. Physical properties of granules, extrudate and pellets. Int J Pharm 1993; 96:197–204.

63. Hellen L, Yliruusi J, Kristoffersson E. Process variables of instant granulator and spheroniser: I. Size and size distributions of pellets. Int J Pharm 1993; 96:205–216.

64. Wan LSC, Heng PWS, Liew CV. Spheronization conditions on spheroid shape and size. Int J Pharm 1993; 96:59–65.

65. Baert L, Vermeersch H, Remon JP, et al. Study of parameters important in the spheronization process. Int J Pharm 1993; 96:225–229.

66. Allen T. Particle Size Measurement. London: Chapman and Hall, 1981.

67. Geldart D. Estimation of basic particle properties for use in fluid-particle process calculations. Powder Technol 1990; 60:1–13.

68. Tho I, Kleinebudde P, Sande SA. Extrusion/spheronization of pectin-based formulations. I. Screening of important factors. AAPS Pharm Sci Tech 2001; 2(4): article 26.

69. Waddell H. J Geol 1933; 41:310.

70. Heywood HJ. J Pharm Pharmacol 1963; 15:56T.

71. Lovgren K, Lundberg PJ. Determination of sphericity of pellets prepared by extrusion-spheronization and the impact of some process parameters. Drug Dev Ind Pharm 1989; 15:2375–2392.

72. Hellen L, Yliruusi J. Process variables of instant granulator and spheroniser: III. Shape and shape distributions of pellets. Int J Pharm 1993; 96:217–223.

73. Chapman SR, Rowe RC, Newton JM. Characterization of the sphericity of particles by the one plane critical stability. J Pharm Pharmacol 1988; 40:503–505.
74. Rowe RC, Sadeghnejad GR. The rheology of mcc powder/water mixes-measurement using a mixer torque rheometer. Int J Pharm 1987; 38:227–229.
75. O'Connor RE, Schwartz JB. Spheronization II: drug release from drug-diluent mixtures. Drug Dev Ind Pharm 1985; 11(9 and 10):1837–1857.
76. Millili GP, Schwartz JB. The strength of microcrystalline cellulose pellets: the effect of granulating with water/ethanol mixtures. Drug Dev Ind Pharm 1990; 16(8):1411–1426.
77. Schroder M, Kleinbudde P. Structure of disintegrating pellets with regard to fractal geometry. Pharm Res 1995; 12(11):1694–1700.
78. Tapia C, Buckton G, Newton JM. Factors influencing the mechanism of release from sustained release matrix pellets, produced by extrusion/spheronization. Int J Pharm 1993; 92:211–218.
79. Milojevic S. Amylose coated pellets for colon-specific drug delivery, PhD thesis, University of London, 1993.
80. Chukwumezie BN, Wojcik M, Malak P, et al. Feasibility studies in spheronization and scale-up of ibuprofen microparticulates using the rotor disk fluid-bed technology. AAPS Pharm Sci Tech 2002; 3(1): article 2.
81. Watano S, Okamaoto T, Sato Y, et al. Sale-up of wet kneading in a novel vertical high shear kneader. Chem Pharm Bull 2005; 53(1):18–21.
82. Office of Regulatory Affairs, Center for Drug Evaluation and Research, Food and Drug Administration. Guidance for Industry: PAT: a framework for innovative pharmaceutical development, manufacturing, and quality assurance. Available at http://www.fda.gov/downloads/drugs/guidancecomplianceregulatoryinformation/guidances/ucm070305.pdf. Accessed September 2004.
83. Yu LX, Lionberger RA, Rawa AS, et al. Applications of Process Analytical Technology to Crystallization Processes, Center for Drug Evaluation and Research, FDA, 8, 2003.
84. Rubinovitz R. Diverse Measurements Through NIR, Pharmaceutical Formulation and Quality, 6b, May 2004.
85. Lewis EN, Schoppelrei J, Lee E. Near IR chemical imaging and the PAT initiative. Spectroscopy 2004; 19(4):26–32.
86. Bruker Optics, Near IR Analysis of Powder Moisture in a Fluid Bed Drier, AF#506E. Available at: www.brukeroptics.com.
87. Mathis N. PAT: Quality by Design, Pharmaceutical Formulation and Quality, 5a, March-April 2004.
88. Menning M, Ju TR, Kim D. Monitoring In-process Particle Behavious During High-Shear Granulation with the Lasentec D600L Focussed Beam reflectance Measurement (FBRM), Lasentec Technical Note, March 2005.
89. Kopcha M, Roland E, Bubb G, et al. Monitoring the granulation process in a high shear mixer/granulator: an evaluation of three approaches to instrumentation. Ind Pharm 1992; 18:1945.
90. Parker MD, Rowe RC, Upjohn NG. Mixer torque rheometry: a method of quantifying the consistency of wet granulations. Pharm Technol Int 1990; 2:50–62.

14.1 Scale-up of compaction and the tableting process

Matthew P. Mullarney and Jeffrey Moriarty

INTRODUCTION

Tablets and capsules are the most common oral solid dosage form for delivering active pharmaceutical ingredients (APIs). Tablets are typically composed of compacted powder cores that are often film coated for functionality and/or elegance. The powder compaction process requires the application of high uniaxial stresses (e.g., 100–500 MPa) by two punches within a die to enable powder densification and deformation with the goal of forming semipermanent bonds among the particulates of the bulk powder. There are many factors that can influence the compaction process including both material properties and manufacturing equipment designs. The design of complementary material bulk properties (e.g., flow performance, particle size distribution, mechanical properties) is key to achieving robust manufacturing performance on a tablet press. For example, it is very difficult to scale-up a tableting process for a blend with highly deficient flow performance even if it has excellent compaction properties because of the high variability in tablet weight uniformity.

The tableting process is scalable from the development laboratory through to commercial manufacturing with a high degree of success for well-designed formulations. In the simplest terms, scale-up involves a significant increase in product volume and/or throughput rate often with the goal of reducing the cost of the tablet. At the development scale, single-station eccentric presses, compaction simulators, and small rotary presses are often used to design and assess the basic compaction performance of 10 to 1000 g batches. As the process is transferred to the pilot scale, often involving 1 to 50 kg batches, moderately sized rotary tablet presses are used for manufacturing. At this scale, material properties such as powder flow and segregation become more relevant along with compaction performance. At the commercial manufacturing scale (>50 kg), both the tableting equipment design and material properties must be optimized to enable robustness for the product's manufacturability.

The objective of this chapter is to describe the key process parameters and material property attributes to consider during the compaction and tableting scale-up process. The chapter discusses the attributes and limitations of tableting equipment used at each scale, tooling design considerations, bulk powder property targets, scale-up parameters, tablet property assessments, and line measurements of performance, and illustrate the scale-up process in case studies.

TABLET COMPACTION EQUIPMENT

Scale-up of the compaction process from the development laboratory to the commercial production site requires not only the control of processing variables, such as production speed and applied stresses, but also the understanding of the scalable features of the equipment. While other texts (1) are available for the general description of the anatomy and basic operating principles of tableting equipment, this section describes the scalable features of pharmaceutical compaction equipment.

Single-Station Manual Presses

Single-station manual presses are small laboratory scale devices typically utilized to form basic compacts for early product development such as excipient compatibility studies, intrinsic dissolution experiments, and basic mechanical property assessments. These presses generally are equipped with a fixed lower punch and die assembly and apply compaction stress to the powder with a moving upper punch via a manually actuated hydraulic cylinder. This type of compaction arrangement is known as "single-sided" compaction where one punch moving and one punch fixed. With the exception of being a uniaxial compression arrangement, this process in no way emulates the time-dependent stress and strains applied during tableting on a production scale press. Powder compacts formed using single-sided compaction are often very different in their compact stress and density distributions compared to compacts formed using double-sided compaction (2). Therefore, the mechanical properties of the resultant compact, such as strength and friability, are likely to be very different, and the compaction process variables are not scalable to production presses.

Additionally, this press is not equipped to emulate pilot or production scale precompaction and postcompaction processes (e.g., powder flow, die filling, ejection, takeoff). Although single-station manual presses are often inexpensive and relatively easy to operate, they should generally only be used for preformulation assessments where the goal is to form a coherent powder compact for basic preformulation screening experiments.

Single-Station Eccentric Presses

Single-station eccentric presses are used in the development laboratory and sometimes for small-scale clinical tablet manufacturing campaigns. Like the manual presses described in the preceding text, eccentric presses utilize single-sided compaction to form tablets and, therefore, come with the aforementioned potential differences in tablet properties. The dies can be filled manually or using a gravity-enabled feed shoe that shuffles across the die prior to compaction. The feeding mechanism is not scalable to a rotary tablet press. Eccentric presses are designed with a moving upper punch that is fitted on the end of a rod that is actuated by an eccentric wheel. The cycle of the eccentric wheel imparts a sinusoidal upper punch displacement profile to compact the powders in the die against a fixed position lower punch. This profile does not enable a measurable time period at which the punch tips remain at their minimum separation, or "dwell time." Therefore, it is difficult to scale-up the tableting operation from an eccentric press to a rotary tablet press for materials that are compression speed sensitive as dwell time can be a key process parameter.

In some cases, eccentric presses are instrumented to measure and record applied punch compression forces. These forces can be used as first approximations of the forces required to achieve equivalent tableting performance on other tablet presses. However, differences in displacement profiles (e.g., shape and speed) between an eccentric press and rotary tablet press could result in the application of different force levels (3). An alternative to using compression force as a scale-up parameter would be to scale-up the tableting operation using tablet thickness as the scale-up target, assuming equivalent tooling tip design and tablet weight. For materials that are not overly compression speed sensitive, the relationship between tablet solid fraction (inversely proportional to tablet thickness) and tablet tensile strength (proportional to tablet crushing strength) should be relatively constant (4).

It is worth noting that many eccentric presses cannot be fitted with typical rotary press tooling types such as B-type or D-type and require specialized tooling designs such as F-type. Although equivalent punch tips can be manufactured for different tooling design types, the punch barrel diameters, punch barrel lengths, and punch head geometry is different. Details of these differences are summarized elsewhere (5) and examples are illustrated in Figure 1. Therefore, new tooling will likely be needed for scaling from an eccentric press to a rotary press.

Compaction Simulators

Compaction simulators are specifically designed to mimic the double-sided compaction profile of a rotary tablet press. The punches are actuated mechanically by using cams or high-speed hydraulic pistons. Compaction simulators are highly instrumented to measure punch forces, punch displacement, ejection force, and die wall force, and therefore are excellent machines for studying compaction behavior using as little as one tablet's worth of powder. Often they can be fitted with the exact tooling used on a rotary tablet press and can mimic the compaction profile of nearly any rotary tablet press (e.g., precompression, dwell time, ejection). This makes compaction simulators an ideal tool for scaling-up the compaction cycle and systematically studying the potential impact of (1) tableting profile changes on the same press, (2) press-to-press transfers, and (3) tooling design changes. A detailed description of compaction simulator designs and applications is available in the literature (6). From compaction simulator experiments, tablet compaction forces, compression dwell times, and tablet properties can be directly scaled to a rotary tablet press as these product and process targets are quantitative. Like manual and eccentric presses, compaction simulators are not designed to emulate the hopper discharge nor the powder feed mechanism on a rotary tablet press. Typically, compaction simulators are equipped with small, simple hoppers to enable consistent die filling. The other scaling limitation of compaction simulators is its relatively slow tablet cycle time. Therefore, it is sometimes not practical to assess problems associated with long compression runs such as heat buildup or cumulative sticking phenomenon.

Rotary Tablet Presses

In most cases, a rotary tablet press is used for clinical and commercial production of tablet cores. Therefore, it is the goal of most scale-up efforts to understand the behavior of powders as they move through a tablet press feed and ejection systems, rather than only in the compaction process. A bulk powder's journey typically begins in an intermediate bulk container (IBC) that is docked to a transfer chute through which the powder will charge the tablet press hopper. Gate or butterfly valves can be placed in-line with the IBC and/or hopper discharge for stopping or starting powder transfer. From the hopper, powder flows into the feed-frame that is designed to direct powder into the dies.

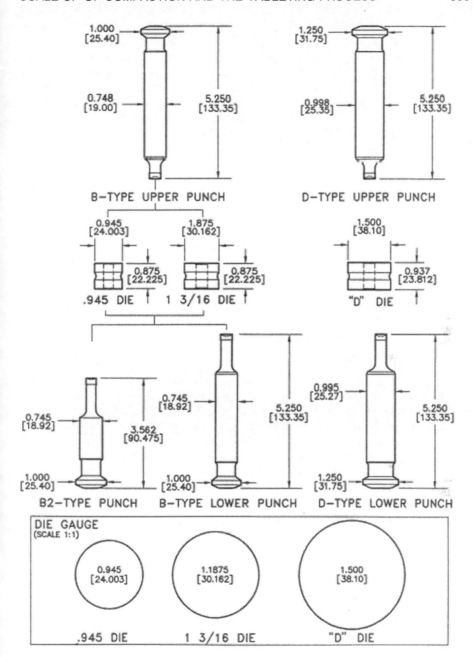

FIGURE 1   Variety of common tooling designs used in tablet production. *Source*: From Ref. 5.

Although some very good flowing powders will flow directly into the dies by gravity, force feed-frames or centrifugal feed-frames are typically used to enable die filling. Force feed-frames utilize rotating paddles to move bulk powder over the outer portion of the turret and into the dies. Centrifugal feed-frames feed the powder to the center of the turret and direct the powder through radial channels using the centrifugal force of the spinning turret to move the powder to each die.

The quantity of powder that enters the die is controlled at the fill station where the lower punch is retracted to a fixed position within the die and excess powder is scraped off to enable a constant volume for powder filling. After the filling station, the punches and filled die travel to a precompression station (if so equipped) where a moderate tamping force ($\sim 10\%$ of main compression force) is applied to the powder. The purpose of precompression is to deaerate the powder and/or increase compaction time for enhanced interparticulate bonding with the goal of improving tablet property deficiencies, such as low crushing strength or unacceptable friability. Next, the primary compaction event occurs at the main compression station (~ 5–50 kN). In both the precompression and main compression stations, the punch displacement profiles are controlled by the geometry of the punch head and the roller diameter. This will typically result in a sinusoidal-type compression and decompression profile with a fixed dwell time in between (Fig. 2). The dwell time is dictated by the turret speed and the punch head flat diameter (see sect. "Tablet Scale-up Parameters" calculations). After compression, the lower punch forces the tablet out of the die as it is raised by a sloped ejection cam. A takeoff bar directs the tablet (now resting on the lower punch and positioned at the top of the die) to a chute and bulk tablet container. See Figure 3 for a summary of a typical tablet press cycle (5).

Some rotary tablet presses are "double-sided," meaning that a second set of filling, precompression, and main compression stations are positioned around the turret. This enables two compactions in each die for each revolution of the turret. If the two sets of fill-compression-ejection stations are independent, two tablets are manufactured for each turret revolution, effectively doubling the production rate. However, if the tablet is not ejected after passing through the first half of the turret, a second powder layer can be filled and compressed in the die thus forming a bilayer tablet. It is important to note that the feed-frames of double-sided presses can be smaller than single-sided presses with a similar turret diameter. This will decrease the die's residence time in the feed-frame filling region. If the die-filling event is sensitive to this residence time when

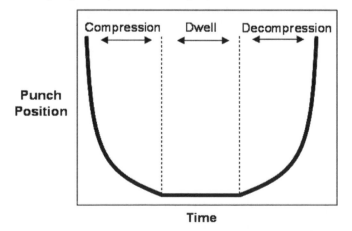

FIGURE 2 Typical rotary tablet press punch displacement profile showing compression phase, dwell time, and decompression phase.

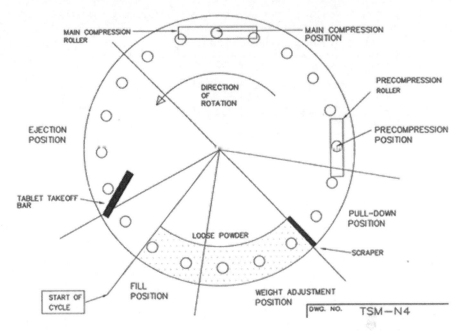

FIGURE 3 Rotary tablet press turret depicting fill position, compression stations, and ejection station. *Source*: From Ref. 5.

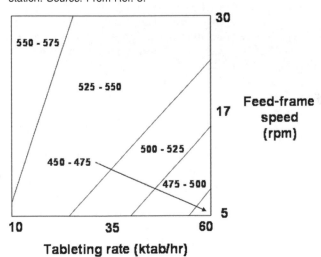

FIGURE 4 Impact of production rates and feed-frame speeds on tablet weight (tablet weight in units of milligrams).

scaling-up to a press with a smaller feed-frame, the turret speed will need to be adjusted to achieve an equivalent residence time. Figure 4 shows how turret rotation rate and feed-frame rate can significantly influence the quantity of powder in the die. This plot was generated after measuring tablet weight when feed-frame speed and tableting rate were varied while the fill height was kept constant. For this reason, bilayer tablet presses are often operated at a lower production rate than single layer tablet presses, especially for powders with marginal flow performance. For large production scale tablet presses, the turret diameter is often large enough to accommodate equivalent sized feed-frames to the smaller-scale presses.

POWDER PROPERTY ASSESSMENTS
Powder Flow
To enable an efficient tablet production process with acceptable unit dose weight uniformity, the powder flow properties of the formulation must complement the design of the manufacturing equipment. This means that the tableting blend must demonstrate adequate flow properties and the equipment must be designed to enable the uniform transport of the powder. The methodology for measuring powder flow properties and hopper design are detailed elsewhere (7); however, it is important to consider the synergistic relationship between the powder and the equipment when scaling up a tableting operation. Both the powder flow properties and the geometry and surface roughness of the IBCs and hoppers should be measured to assess the potential for flow problems, such as funnel flow discharge and arch formation at the hopper outlet (7). Additionally, an assessment of the permeability of the powder to air is prudent to determine the critical flow rate of a powder exiting a hopper. This will help to avoid erratic flow rates because of a possible negative pressure differential inside of the hopper relative to the hopper outlet (8). Because of possible differences in equipment geometry, equipment surface roughness, fill volumes, and throughput demands, one cannot assume equivalent flow performance on different tablet presses, even if they are similar in design and manufacturer. Therefore, the careful assessment of differences in equipment design and production conditions is needed for successful scale-up.

Segregation
Component segregation within a bulk powder mass requires the movement of particles relative to one another (9). Because pharmaceutical materials are generally of similar true density, segregation of components typically occurs because of a significant difference in particle size among components. Assuming a well-mixed system is achieved after blending in an IBC, there are multiple opportunities for segregation to occur as the powder travels through the tablet press—exiting the IBC, filling the hopper, discharging from the hopper, transfer through the feed-frame, and transfer within in-line tubes and chutes. Two of the most common segregation mechanisms are fluidization and sifting segregation. Fluidization segregation occurs when a countercurrent air stream of sufficient velocity carries finer particles in the opposite direction of the bulk powder flow. This can occur during transport through long vertical chutes and in pneumatic conveying. When this occurs, the receiving container can have a significant proportion of fine particles at the top and coarse particles at the bottom. This gradient can result in both particle size and potency heterogeneity in the receiving container. Often at commercial scale, charging containers are on stages above the tablet press. In these situations, the tableting process equipment should be designed or modified to minimize long drops and/or pneumatic

conveying, especially with powders with a high propensity for fluidization segregation. Even if a container were to discharge in mass flow (i.e., first in, first out), the finer particles would be tableted at the end of the batch, which could lead to significant variability in tablet mechanical properties, weight, and potency.

Another common mechanism for segregation is sifting. Sifting segregation occurs upon container filling where larger particles at the free surface of a forming pile preferentially roll to the perimeter of the pile. As a result, the receiving container may have a high proportion of coarse particles around the edge and a high proportion of finer particles in the center. If a container charged like this were to discharge in funnel flow (i.e., center of hopper discharges first) the finer particles would be tableted first. This could also lead to significant variability in tablet mechanical properties, weight, and potency. Tableting blends, charging methods, and equipment need to be carefully assessed to minimize the potential for sifting segregation if they possess this propensity. At smaller scales, segregation may not be observed because of small batches or manual manipulation of powder movement. However, upon scale-up, larger batches are handled with production equipment in closed systems and a greater risk for segregation is present. Methods for segregation assessments are detailed in ASTM standards (10,11).

Bulk Density

The importance of the blend bulk density is often overlooked in tableting operations and scale-up. Proper bulk density is essential for achieving target container filling efficiency, enabling powder flow by gravity, and efficient die filling. If a powder is too "fluffy" where it has low bulk density, it can compromise the performance of the unit operation. As production scale is increased, higher powder bulk density will enable an increase in the batch size and, therefore, can increase the product yield. Denser powders will also enable powder flow as gravitational forces will overcome interparticulate forces for larger and denser particles. Therefore, flow performance can improve. Lastly, since tableting die cavities have a limited fill volume, the powder must be dense enough to fit the target mass into the die, especially for larger tablet weights. Figure 5 describes the relationship among powder bulk density, standard round concave (SRC) tooling diameter, and tablet weight for an example tablet with a target aspect ratio of 2, solid fraction of 0.85, true density of 1.5 g/cc, and a fill cam pull-down distance of 16 mm. Simple geometric calculations can be used to identify the minimum bulk density of the powder blend required to manufacture a tablet with a desirable aspect ratio and final solid fraction. These types of calculations can help to assess the edge of failure when designing drug product formulations, selecting tableting process conditions, and assessing the suitability of a tooling design.

Compact Mechanical Properties

Like powder flow, the existing literature extensively describes methodologies for the measurement of compact mechanical properties that are relevant to compaction and the tableting operation (e.g., tensile strength, brittleness, elasticity, yield behavior) (12). However, the one property very relevant to compaction scale-up is the impact of production speed on mechanical properties because of the increased throughput demand. The mechanical properties of

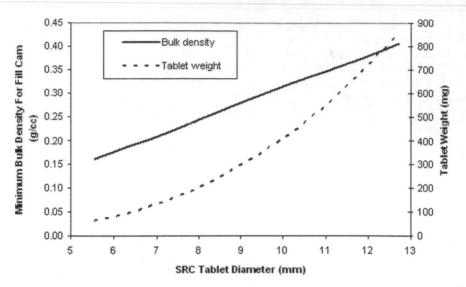

FIGURE 5 Relationship among tablet weight, blend bulk density, and SRC tooling diameter for a tablet with a target aspect ratio of 2, solid fraction of 0.85, true density of 1.5 g/cc, and a cam pull-down distance of 16 mm.

some materials are tableting "speed sensitive," which can affect their robustness (e.g., crushing strength and/or ruggedness). This means that their yield behavior and ability to form and retain interparticulate bonds affected by the applied strain rate (i.e., punch velocity). Strain rate sensitivity can be assessed for powders using techniques such as Heckel analysis (13), Hiestand's viscoelastic index (14), or tableting experiments at different compaction rates. For example, the mechanical properties of certain grades of starch powder are much more strain rate–sensitive than powder such as calcium phosphate (4). In general, powders whose particles deform plastically when compressed, like starch and microcrystalline cellulose, rather than by fragmentation, like dibasic calcium phosphate, are likely to be more speed sensitive. During decompression, however, materials that form interparticulate bonds that are relatively brittle and sensitive to internal defects like lactose are more likely to exhibit tableting deficiencies such as capping and lamination because they are not able to dissipate stresses during elastic recovery without fracturing bonds. Therefore, an assessment of the sensitivity of a blend to compaction speed is recommended prior to scale-up.

The second property worth mentioning is "sticking." Sticking is a term commonly used in the pharmaceutical industry to describe the propensity of the tableting blend to adhere to the punch tips. This phenomenon can result in compromised tablet appearance and, in severe cases, a measurable loss of tablet potency. Unfortunately, sticking may not be detected during small-scale tablet manufacturing and may only manifest during scale-up to larger production volumes or longer tableting runs as not enough tablets are made at the small scale. Although the mechanism for sticking and small-scale methods to detect sticking are still under investigation (15–17), it is likely that a combination of factors such as heat buildup on the press, microaccumulation of the powder on

TABLE 1   Tooling Used During Tooling Surface Coating Experiments

#	Manufacturer	Surface	Manufacturing process
1	A	Chrome	PVD (physical vapor deposition)
2	A	Hardened chrome	Electroplating
3	A	Textured hardened chrome	Electroplating + mechanical texturing
4	A	High gloss chrome	Electroplating + polish
5	A	Chromium nitride	PVD
6	A	Chromium nitride	PVD + polish
7	A	Nickel polytetrafluoroethylene	Electroless nickel plating
8	A	Diamond-like carbon	PVD
9	A	Steel 1	Polish
10	A	Steel 2	Polish
11	A	Stainless steel	Polish
12	B	Hardened chrome	IBED (ion beam–enhanced deposition)
13	B	Chromium nitride	IBED
14	B	Titanium nitride	IBED
15	C	Hardened chrome 1	PVD
16	C	Hardened chrome 2	PVD
17	C	Diamond-like carbon	PVD
18	C	Titanium-aluminum nitride	PVD

Source: From Ref. 18.

the punch tips, and specific properties of the punch tip and powder, such as composition, surface roughness, melting point, particle size, morphology, and adhesion behavior, contribute to different degrees of sticking. Therefore, to reduce risk for sticking upon scale-up, careful inspection of tablet tooling after each manufacturing run during development and scale-up is recommended to detect sticking problems as early in a product's life cycle as possible.

Although the use of a lubricating excipient in a tableting blend is common for managing sticking, various tooling surface treatments can also be applied to the punch tips and die wall to reduce punch tip adhesion. During development of a formulation that had shown a propensity for sticking, several different tooling coatings from three manufacturers were tested on a pilot scale tablet press (Table 1) (18). Two compression trials were conducted on a pilot scale rotary tablet with each station outfitted with a different set of modified tooling (18 total different punch tip surface types). The tablets and punch surfaces were visually evaluated after each run for evidence of sticking. Additionally, residual material adhered to the punch tips were assayed to quantify the amount of drug adhered (Fig. 6). For this particular formulation, tooling with a textured finished demonstrated the highest amount of sticking and material buildup, while tooling that contained chrome or chromium nitride performed the best. This novel technique can quickly and systematically evaluate the effect of punch surface treatments on sticking propensity and shows the benefit of studying and evaluating different tooling finishes during drug product development.

Another strategy to manage sticking and reduce ejection forces is to use external lubrication. External lubrication is a manufacturing technique where lubricant is sprayed onto the surface of the punch tips and die wall. Most external lubrication systems involve the dispersion of dry magnesium stearate delivered via compressed air. However, a system that suspends magnesium

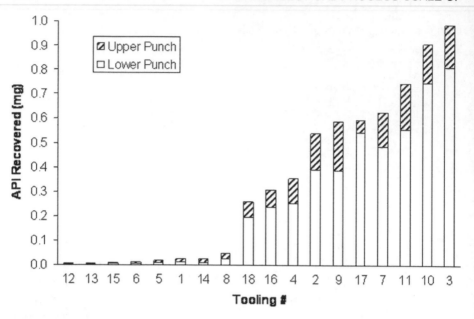

FIGURE 6 Analytical results from HPLC assay on tooling rinses to show relative sticking propensity. See Table 1 for tooling descriptions. *Source*: From Ref. 18.

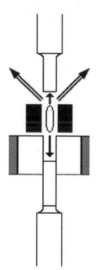

FIGURE 7 Illustration of an external lubrication system.

stearate in isopropanol has also been used (19–21). On a rotary tablet press, the spray nozzle can be positioned on the turret between the tablet takeoff and powder feeder. The spray system (black arrows in Fig. 7) applies the lubricant to the tablet punch tips and die wall, and excess lubricant can be removed via vacuum recovery ports (double arrows in Fig. 7).

Validation of the external lubrication process is necessary to demonstrate consistent application of lubricant and control of the manufacturing process. When scaling up, it is critical to determine the amount of lubricant added to the tablet during the process. Dispensing of the lubricant under gravimetric control and recovery of the excess lubricant with a vacuum system would provide sufficient data to calculate a theoretical amount of lubricant on the surface of each tablet. Other methods for determining lubricant level on the tablet surface include, but are not limited to, atomic absorption spectrometry (22) and titration (23).

When implementing an external lubrication system, it is most important to determine the optimum spray rate of the lubricant. The spray rate should provide efficient coverage of lubricant on the tooling surface but not allow buildup over time. During scale-up, a properly designed design of experiment (DOE) should define the relationship between the external lubrication process parameters, such as spray rate, air pressure, and lubricant feed rate, and the key attributes of the tablets, such as elegance and dissolution.

Impact of Bulk Material Variability

For the purpose of a simplified discussion in the remainder of this chapter, it will be assumed that the ingoing properties of the powder are equivalent at each manufacturing scale. However, it is worth briefly noting that ingoing properties of the tableting blend and even its components (APIs and excipients) can be different from batch to batch. For components whose compaction properties influence tableting performance, a shift in properties such as particle size or moisture content could significantly change product quality. Standard vendor specifications provided on the certificate of analyses (COA) for excipients are often inadequate to comprehensively assess compaction similarity among lots, due to the low relevance of compendial testing data and broad particle size targets (e.g., 90% < 100 μm). To reduce the risk for scale-up problems, an assessment of the variability in key material properties, such as particle size distribution, is recommended during scale-up and product qualification.

Compactibility, Tabletability, and Compressibility Relationships

During a compaction event, an applied compression stress is required to form a compact of a given solid fraction and tensile strength. Compression stress is the applied compression force normalized over the cross-sectional area of the tooling tip. Solid fraction is the proportion of solid material in the compact (relative to air). Tensile strength is the stress required to cause irreversible interparticulate bond failure in tension. These three properties—compression stress, solid fraction, and tensile strength—are associated with one another through three distinct relationships: compactibility (tensile strength vs. solid fraction), compressibility (compression stress vs. solid fraction), and tabletability (tensile strength vs. compression stress) (4,24). These values can be calculated using both tooling tip dimensions and tablet property measurements. Usage of these three normalized parameters enables a direct comparison of data from different tablet sizes. Methods for the calculation of tablet solid fraction and tensile strength are summarized elsewhere (12).

A systematic study of the effect of these three relationships has suggested that the tabletability and compressibility of some materials like pregelatinized starch are affected by dwell time (4). This is of particular interest as it is very common for solid dosage forms to be characterized using a tabletability profile. However, the use of the compactibility relationship for scale-up may be preferred as it appears to be more independent of dwell time. In practice for a given dosage form being scaled up using the same tooling and target tablet weight, tablets compacted to the same solid fraction or thickness should have the equivalent tensile strength and, therefore, exhibit equivalent mechanical property performance. Therefore, careful control of the compactibility-compressibility-tabletability relationships, along with an understanding of the impact of dwell time on a given formulation, will lower the risk for tableting performance problems and surprises upon scale-up.

TABLET SCALE-UP PARAMETERS
Dwell Time and Contact Time
The most common and practical method for scaling up the rotary tablet press compaction process is the use of dwell time as the key process parameter. Dwell time is the time interval over which the punch tips are at their minimum separation during the compression cycle. This constant strain state enables the formation of interparticulate bonds through time-dependent stress relaxation, and increasing dwell time usually improves tablet mechanical property performance (e.g., higher tablet crushing strength, reduced incidence of capping and lamination).

There are two common methods for calculating dwell time—*mechanically* from the known equipment geometry and *empirically* from the compression force versus time profile (25). The mechanical dwell time is calculated from the turret tangential velocity at the center of the die and the diameter of the tooling punch head flat. This method of calculation is independent of powder compression behavior and can be determined a priori when scaling-up.

$$\text{Dwell time} = \frac{\text{Punch head flat diameter}}{\text{Turret tangential velocity}}$$

Empirically, dwell time is determined from the compression force versus time profile by inspecting the measured waveform and calculating the time interval over which the compression force is not less than 90% of the maximum applied compression force (Fig. 8). This method cannot be used to determine dwell time without experimentation. However, it has been shown that the two different methods for calculating dwell time are equivalent (25) and can be independent of the particle deformation mechanism (i.e., brittle fragmentation or plastic deformation) as shown in Figure 9.

Although dwell time is the most common parameter for compaction scale-up, contact time can also be determined in a similar manner. Theoretically, the contact time is the time interval over which the powder is in contact with and being compacted with a measurable force by the punch tips. Empirically, the contact time can be estimated by determining the time interval over which the compression force is not less than 10% of the maximum applied compression force (Fig. 8). Mechanically, contact time is determined by:

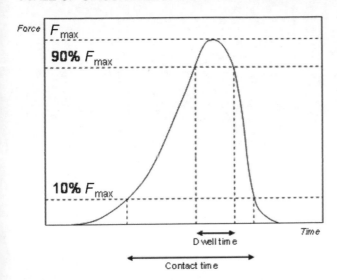

FIGURE 8   Empirical definitions of dwell time and contact time.

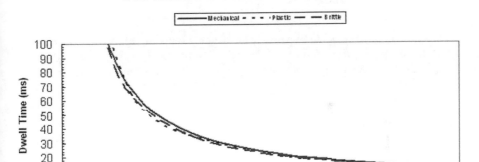

FIGURE 9   Empirically derived dwell time for brittle and plastically deforming materials and mechanical dwell time comparison. *Source*: From Ref. 25.

1. Assuming a fixed displacement over which the compression/decompression event occurs (usually 2–3 mm—corresponding to the upper punch penetration depth)
2. Determining the time interval for the compression and decompression events from the known geometry of the tablet press and tooling head configuration (26). The Rippie and Danielson model can be used to calculate

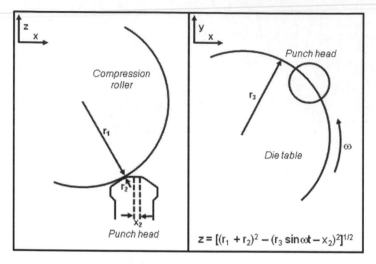

FIGURE 10 Rotary tablet press compression cam, turret, and punch head geometry used for displacement calculations. *Source*: Adapted from Ref. 26.

the compression and decompression profiles from the tablet press and tooling geometry using Eq. (1).

$$z = [(r_1 + r_2)^2 - (r_3 \sin \omega t - x_2)^2]^{1/2} \tag{1}$$

The model describes the vertical displacement (z) of the punch head as it rotates with the turret along path "B" and its radius (r_2) is in contact with the compression roller (A) of radius r_1 (Fig. 10). The decompression displacement is a mirror image of the compression displacement.

3. Summing the compression time, dwell time, and decompression time.

In general, mechanical dwell time should be appropriate as the target scale-up parameter. However, for cases when there is a significant change in tablet press roller diameter or punch head geometry, an empirical assessment of dwell and/or an assessment of contact time would be prudent.

Key Process Parameters

In general, a key process parameter is any function of the machine, materials, operators, processes, measurements, or environment that can have a potential impact on a final quality attribute of the product (e.g., tablet strength, disintegration time, dissolution performance). The key process parameters often identified for a tableting process are tableting speed, precompression force, compression force, punch penetration, fill height, and feeder paddle speed. Each of these parameters can be adjusted on most rotary tablet presses and should be given careful consideration at each scale of development.

When using the same tableting punch type, the tableting speed of a press dictates the dwell time of the compaction, which is of utmost importance if the material exhibits sensitivity to compression time. Typically, longer dwell times will improve tableting performance and equivalent dwell times are recommended during scale-up. For high-volume products, the ability to run at high

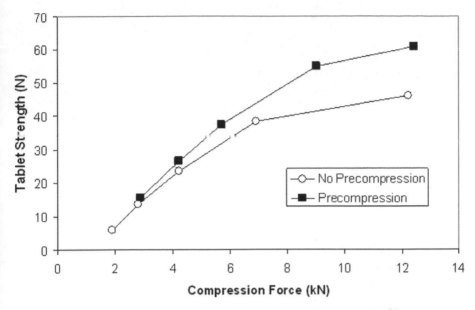

FIGURE 11 Effect of precompression on tablet crushing strength.

tableting speed can improve efficiency and reduce overall production costs, but the effect of dwell time on product quality should be investigated prior to making significant changes to tableting rates.

As summarized in a previous section, the mechanical properties of many tablet formulations benefit from the use of a precompression event prior to main compression. For example, during the development of an immediate release 100 mg tablet with microcrystalline cellulose and lactose as the primary diluents, a precompression force of 1 kN increased the maximum achievable tablet strength by approximately 40% (Fig. 11). Although precompression is not a universal solution to reducing tableting deficiencies, it is a simple and commonly available process parameter that should be considered for each product as it could be used as a "rescue option" if tableting performance changes upon scale-up or press transfer.

For a given powder and press setup, the minimum punch separation used for the main compression cycle will dictate the applied main compression force and final tablet properties (e.g., strength, thickness, friability, and disintegration behavior). Prior to manufacturing supplies on a tablet press for the first time, a tablet strength versus compression force profile should be generated by manufacturing prototype tablets at different target minimum punch separations. To minimize the likelihood of tooling damage during profile generation, it is recommended that 90% of the maximum allowable force recommended by the tooling manufacturer is not exceeded. Tablets from the compression force profile should be tested for weight, thickness, strength, friability, disintegration time, and dissolution performance. The target-tableting condition for bulk supply manufacture is selected to achieve acceptable performance while avoiding overcompression, which can lead to poor product robustness and difficulty in achieving consistent results upon scale-up.

The upper punch maximum penetration setting can be changed on some tablet presses to control the how far into the die the upper punch travels during compression. This parameter will remain constant during punch separation adjustments. When tablets exhibit a propensity for die wall sticking or when high ejection forces are observed, the upper punch penetration can be decreased to minimize the travel distance of the tablet during ejection from the die. In most cases, an upper punch maximum penetration setting of 2 to 4 mm is suitable throughout all scales of tableting scale-up. When unusually high ejection forces (e.g., >500 N) are present, the tablet may need to be compressed at a higher location in the die or tapered dies may be required.

Most commercial tablet presses are equipped with a force feeder that continually fills a die with powder as the turret rotates. To control the available die fill volume, the position of the lower punch below the die surface during the filling operation can be adjusted. On the basis of the size of the tablet and press speed, the feeder speed should be adjusted to provide for low tablet weight variation. Guidance for tablet content uniformity criteria is provided in the USP (27) but typically a tablet weight uniformity of less than 3% is indicative of suitable tablet weight control.

The residence time of a blend in the tablet press feed-frame is important because the rotation of the feeder paddles subjects the powder to additional shear and mixing. Residence time can be increased by slowing the turret rate and/or decreasing the number of compression stations used during production. If the properties of the powder such as segregation, lubrication, or attrition are sensitive to blending time or degree of agitation, the residence time in the feed-frame can be a key process parameter for the tableting operation as it affects tablet properties. Tye and coworkers demonstrated that the tablet compactibility profile (tablet tensile strength vs. solid fraction) for a model placebo blend was sensitive to feed-frame residence time (28). They found that when tableting rate was held constant, tablets with higher mass exhibited higher compactibility. The increased powder residence time in the feed-frame for the smaller tablets (i.e., lower throughput rate resulting in higher residence time) enabled a greater degree of dispersion of the lubricant that ultimately decreased the compactibility of the placebo formulation (Fig. 12). Similar compactibility profiles were attained by adjusting the tableting speed to achieve a constant powder mass throughput rate for each of the different tablet weights, thus enabling an equivalent degree of blending (Fig. 13). This demonstrates the importance of maintaining equivalent powder residence time in a tablet press feed-frame upon scale-up, especially for tablets produced using a common blend approach.

LINE MEASUREMENTS OF PERFORMANCE

During tablet manufacture, in-process tests for the control of tablet weight, thickness, strength, friability, and disintegration should be performed to ensure that drug product is within the required specifications. The number of sampling time points and sample size is dependent on the batch size and needs to be clearly documented in a sampling protocol. For a product in early development, sampling at the beginning, middle, and end of a tableting run may be sufficient, especially in the laboratory setting. Manufacture of clinical supplies on a pilot scale in a cGMP setting requires stratified sampling based on the size of the batch. For a commercialized product and process that has been carefully studied

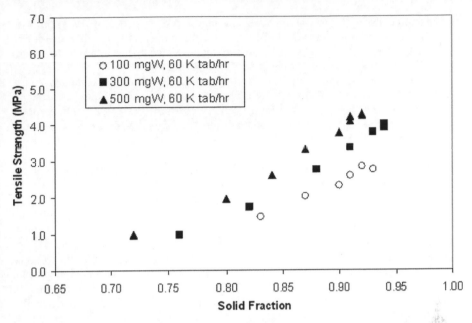

FIGURE 12 Compactibility profiles for tablet formulations produced with different tablet weights.

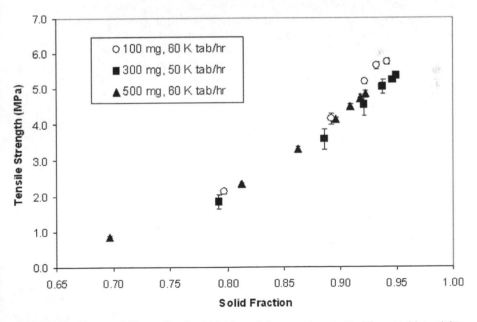

FIGURE 13 Compactibility profiles for tablet formulations produced with different tablet weights after correction for residence time in the feed-frame (to compensate for lubrication effects).

and modeled through extensive DOEs, the target tablet specifications should be well known and the process should be tightly controlled. Further guidance regarding testing procedures and standard acceptance criteria can be found in the USP Official Compendia of Standards Formulary (27).

Modern commercial tablet presses are equipped with robust control systems that can tightly control the tablet weight and strength throughout the compression run. For example, a system operating under a constant punch separation mode will reject a tablet if a high or low force is detected. This rejection is based on the assumption that the subsequent tablet will not meet the target weight specification. Automatic tablet weight and strength testers can also be utilized, which would periodically test tablets and adjust the fill height and compression force to maintain the desired properties. In-line process control units are best utilized on commercial equipment when manufacturing large batches, due to the quantity of tablet samples to measure. Smaller development and clinical batches may not have tableting runs that are long enough to fully realize the benefit of the in-line testing.

Appearance or elegance testing is a critical component of in-process testing. A representative composite sample of tablets (e.g., 100 tablets) should be visually inspected for any defects and imperfections. In addition to a composite sample, tablets should also be examined after friability testing. Magnification may aid in the examination of small tablets or tablets with logos or debossed text. Tablet imperfections fall into different categories based on the severity of the defects. A tablet with capping or lamination would be a severe deficiency, while a logo with minor erosion on the edge of the lettering may be considered minor. Minor defects may be mitigated by a process modification, like using precompression, increasing the main compression force, or reducing the lubrication blending time. Sufficient deficiencies may require reformulation or a change in excipients, if process parameter modifications do not resolve the problem.

The content uniformity of the batch can be measured through the use of stratified sampling. Stratified sampling requires samples to be taken throughout the tableting run at evenly spaced intervals either based on time (e.g., every 15 minutes) or by the percent completion of the batch (e.g., 5% intervals). Samples should be analyzed for potency, and the trend of potency throughout the tableting batch can be analyzed to determine if any segregation is taking place in the hopper or feed-frame during manufacture. For example, a spike of potency may be observed at the beginning or at the very end of a tableting run due to API preferentially sticking to interior metal surfaces or stagnant flow zones in the feed-frame.

The content uniformity of a tableting run can also be controlled through the use of process analytical technologies (PAT), such as near-infrared spectroscopy (NIR). The strength and thickness of the tablet can be a source of variability in spectrum analysis (29) even with tablets of the same potency; therefore, a carefully designed set of calibration tablets should be manufactured. A calibration set should comprise a range of tablets potencies (e.g., 75–125%), and, at each potency, the weight and strength of the tablet should be varied. For example, when developing a tablet with a target weight of 500 mg, tablets of different strengths of 480 and 520 mg could also be manufactured in addition to the target. The low and high values targeted for the weight and strength should depend on the drug load, tablet size, and target product specifications. Because of the quantity of work involved in developing an NIR model, late stage and commercial products are the best candidates, since the final tablet properties have been determined and samples from different manufacturing batches exist to test the model.

CASE STUDIES
Scaling-up a Tableting Process from the Laboratory to Commercial Scale

At the onset of tablet formulation development, there are typically very limited quantities of API available for experimentation. This necessitates the use of small-scale tableting equipment, such as a compaction simulator for manufacturability feasibility assessments. This case study shows how the compactibility of a powder blend can be evaluated at the laboratory scale prior to scaling up to larger pilot or commercial scale tablet presses.

During the development of a dry granulated immediate release tablet formulation, a compaction simulator was used to assess the tableting performance using a very small-scale development batch (<200 g). The dry granulation was prepared using small blenders, roller compaction simulation, and bottle blenders (30). The compaction simulator was set up to mimic a pilot scale tablet press with B-type TSM standard tooling operating at 45,000 tablets/ hr correlating to a mechanical dwell time of 14 milliseconds. At these conditions, tablets at a solid fraction of approximately 0.85 achieved acceptable friability (<0.2%) and disintegration performance (<15 minutes).

Both the dry granulation and tableting process for this formulation were scaled up to the pilot scale (∼5 kg batch size) and then to the commercial scale (>30 kg). To challenge the tablet performance and increase productivity at the larger manufacturing scales, both tablet presses were set up to produce tablets with a mechanical dwell time of 10 milliseconds. This dwell time was slightly shorter than the one used in the compaction simulator experiments, but considered to be of close enough to achieve similar tableting performance.

Although at first inspection the tableting profiles for tablets produced on pilot and commercial scales appeared to be superior to the compaction simulator tableting profile (Fig. 14), the equivalence of the compactibility profiles at all three manufacturing scales demonstrated a scalable tableting process (Fig. 15). It is clear that the value of compression force is useful for minimizing the risk of overcompression of the tableting blend or tooling, but compression load instrumentation often varies between equipment types and manufacturers, which makes it difficult to use as a product specific scale-up parameter. Therefore by using the tablet properties only (tensile strength and solid fraction), the manufacturing equipment–dependent measurements are removed. Ultimately, it is the final tablet properties that dictate performance and, therefore, should be used to as a first-line approach for scaling up the tableting process with equivalent dwell time.

Design Space Exploration for Immediate Release Tablet Core Manufacturing

In the later stages of product development, the design space for the tablet manufacturing process should be explicitly studied during product development to provide evidence of process understanding and product robustness. By the time a product has reached the stage where commercialization is imminent, many (10 or more) clinical and development batches have typically been manufactured and the key process parameters should be defined. The final step in tableting scale-up is to explore a range of values for every key process parameter to map the proven acceptable range (PAR) and recommend a normal operating range (NOR) for manufacturing.

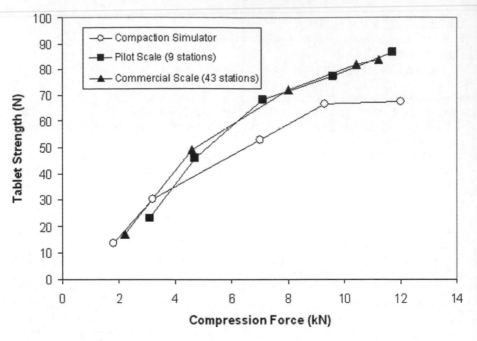

FIGURE 14 Tableting performance profile for similar formulations at different manufacturing scales.

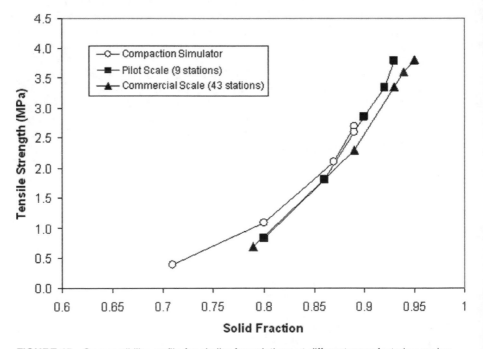

FIGURE 15 Compactibility profile for similar formulations at different manufacturing scales.

The PAR is a range of process parameters or product attributes that have been experimentally shown to produce a final product that meets all required specifications. It is mapped through a multivariate analysis of the relationships among the input and response variables. Values outside of the PAR are either unexplored or unacceptable to meet product requirements. The PAR is defined experimentally for each key process parameter and should be as broad as possible to enable manufacturing flexibility and process understanding. Once the PAR is established, a smaller region called the NOR is defined for the target-manufacturing conditions. A wide PAR and NOR for tablet press parameters allows the operators flexibility to change the process parameters depending on batch size, raw material properties, and manufacturing time constraints and still be assured of delivering drug product that meets all required specifications.

The PAR and NOR for the tableting process of a dry granulated immediate release tablet were established by studying the effect of key process parameters—tablet press speed, compression force, and lubrication blending time prior to tableting. A full factorial DOEs (Table 2) studying the impact of low, medium, and high values for each parameter was conducted, and the resulting tablet weight, thickness, strength, friability, and dissolution were evaluated. Overall, 30 experiments were performed and the run order was randomized to eliminate the effects of time related variables. Figure 16 shows an example experimental design that could be conducted on the key process parameters deemed most important to the tablet properties. In this example, lubrication blend time, compression force, and tableting speed showed criticality in early experiments and manufacturing runs and required further design space definition to establish the PAR.

The DOEs showed that tablet strength (hardness) was the property most impacted by the changes in operating parameters where faster tableting speeds with a shorter dwell time decreased tablet strength. At a lubrication time of two minutes, the tablet strength values at the low compression forces decreased when the tableting speed was increased (Fig. 17). At the highest force, the two profiles converged as the maximum compressibility of the granulation was approached. Through further data analysis, the tablet strength was found to be dependent on lubrication blend time (Fig. 18), which was attributed to the greater dispersion of the lubricant onto the blend particles thus weakening interparticle bonding. The friability and dissolution performance for all tablets within the conditions studied were within the acceptable range and no statistically significant trend was observed.

TABLE 2   Full Factorial DOE for Investigating the Effects of Lubrication, Tablet Production Rate, and Compression Force on Tablet Performance

Input variables	Units	Values
Lubrication blending time	Minutes	2
		5
		8
Tablet press speed	Tablets/hr	160,000
		210,000
		260,000
Compression force	KN	6.2
		9.0
		11.8

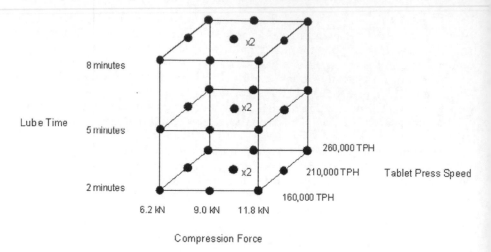

FIGURE 16 Experimental design space for tableting performance evaluations.

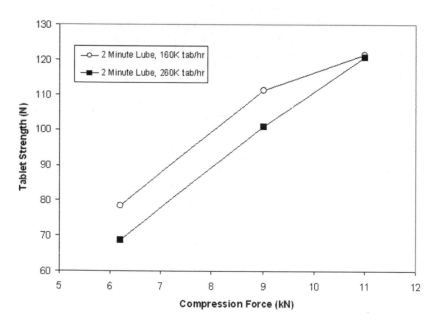

FIGURE 17 Tableting speed effects on tablet strength for low lubrication extents.

Using these data, a multivariate analysis of the key process parameters and target tablet attributes was completed to identify the PAR. Target values for the drug product included a five-minute lubrication time, strength of 100 N, friability less than 0.3%, and a dissolution extent of greater than 80% at 20 minutes. Using these target criteria and data from the DOEs, the PAR was established for this drug product. In the response plot for this study (Fig. 19), the

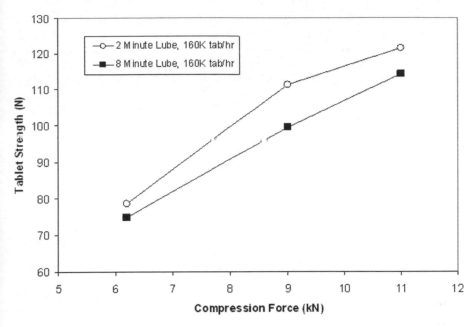

FIGURE 18   Effect of lubrication extent on tableting performance.

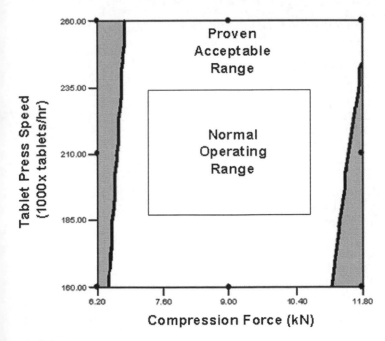

FIGURE 19   Proven acceptable range for achieving tablet critical quality attributes.

white region indicates the PAR and the gray area indicates the unacceptable operating range. The NOR for the drug product (boxed region) is defined within the PAR so that the manufacturing conditions are well within the PAR and are in-line with production capabilities and needs. This case study shows how the definition of the design space is critical to establishing a robust tableting process for a tablet dosage form.

REFERENCES

1. Gennaro A. Remington: The Science and Practice of Pharmacy. 21st ed. Baltimore, MD: Lippincott Williams & Wilkins, 2005.
2. Train D. Transmission of forces through a powder mass during the process of pelleting. Trans Inst Chem Eng 1957; 35:258–266.
3. Palmieri GF, Joiris E, Bonacucina G, et al. Differences between eccentric and rotary tablet machines in the evaluation of powder densification behaviour. Int J Pharm 2005; 298:164–175.
4. Tye CK, Sun C, Amidon GE. Evaluation of the effects of tableting speed on the relationships between compaction pressure, tablet tensile strength, and tablet solid fraction. J Pharm Sci 2005; 94:465–472.
5. Young LL. Tableting Specification Manual. 7th ed. Washington, DC: American Pharmacists Association, 2006.
6. Bourland M, Mullarney M. Compaction simulation. In: Augsburger LL, Hoag SW, eds. Pharmaceutical dosage forms: tablets. New York: Informa Healthcare, 2008: 519–554.
7. Jenike AW. Storage and Flow of Solids, Bulletin No. 123. Salt Lake City, Utah: University of Utah, Engineering Experiment Station, 1964.
8. Carlson GT, Hancock BC. Development of a material sparing method to determine powder permeability to air. In: American Association of Pharmaceutical Scientists Annual Meeting. Atlanta, GA, 2008.
9. Bates L. User Guide to Segregation. Hartford, Northwich, Cheshire, UK: British Materials Handling Board, 1997.
10. ASTM. ASTM D6941 - 05e1 Standard Practice for Measuring Fluidization Segregation Tendencies of Powders, 2009.
11. ASTM. ASTM D6940 - 04 Standard Practice for Measuring Sifting Segregation Tendencies of Bulk Solids, 2009.
12. Alderborn G, Nystrom C. Pharmaceutical Powder Compaction Technology. New York: Marcel Dekker, Inc., 1996.
13. Heckel RW. Density-pressure relations in powder compaction. Trans Metall Soc AIME 1961; 221:671–675.
14. Hiestand E, Smith DP. Indices of tableting performance. Powder Technol 1984; 38: 145–159.
15. Waimer F, Krumme M, Danz P, et al. A novel method for the detection of sticking of tablets. Pharm Dev Technol 1999; 4:359–367.
16. Wang JJ, Guillot MA, Bateman SD, et al. Modeling of adhesion in tablet compression. II. Compaction studies using a compaction simulator and an instrumented tablet press. J Pharm Sci 2004; 93:407–417.
17. Wang JJ, Li TL, Bateman SD, et al. Modeling of adhesion in tablet compression. I. Atomic force microscopy and molecular simulation. J Pharm Sci 2003; 92:798–814.
18. Polizzi M, Larsen R, Daugherity PD, et al. Evaluation of punch sticking improvement using various tooling surfaces at small scale. American Association of Pharmaceutical Scientists Regional Meeting, Rocky Hill, CT, 2011.
19. Laich T, Kissel T. Experimental characterization of an external lubrication system on rotary presses. Pharm Ind 1997; 59:265–272.
20. Laich T, Kissel T. Investigation of lubricant dependent parameters on a reciprocating tableting press equipped with an external lubrication system. Pharm Ind 1998; 60: 547–554.

21. Laich T, Kissel T. Automatic adaptation of lubricant quantity by control of an external lubrication: tests on a reciprocating and on a rotary tablet press. Pharm Ind 1998; 60:896–904.

22. Jahn T, Steffens K-J. Press chamber coating as external lubrication for high speed rotary presses: lubrication spray rate optimization. Drug Dev Ind Pharm 2005; 31: 951–957.

23. Otsuka M, Sato M, Matsuda Y. Comparative evaluation of tableting compression behaviors by methods of internal and external lubricant addition: inhibition of enzymatic activity of trypsin preparation by using external lubricant addition during the tableting compression process. AAPS PharmSci 2001; 3:1–11.

24. Joiris E, Martino PD, Berneron C, et al. Compression behavior of orthorhombic paracetamol. Pharm Res 1998; 15:1122–1130.

25. Sedlock R. Dwell time. American Association of Pharmaceutical Scientists Annual Meeting. Toronto, Canada, 2002.

26. Rippie EG, Danielson DW. Viscoelastic stress/strain behavior of pharmaceutical tablets: analysis during unloading and postcompression periods. J Pharm Sci 1981; 70: 476–482.

27. USP_32. The United States Pharmacopeia (USP 32), The National Formulary (NF 27). Rockville, MD: The United States Pharmacopeial Convention, 2009.

28. Tye K, Ingraham S. The significance of powder residence time / mass output rate in a tablet press on tablet mechanical properties and its implications to scale-up. American Association of Pharmaceutical Scientists. Los Angeles, CA, 2009.

29. Blanco M, Alcala M. Content uniformity and tablet hardness testing of intact pharmaceutical tablets by near infrared spectroscopy. Anal Chim Acta 2006; 557: 353–359.

30. Mahmoudi ZN, Alvarez-Nunez FA. Roller compaction of a poorly compressible drug substance chemically incompatible with typical functional excipients. Am Pharm Rev 2005; 8:142–145.

14.2 Dimensional analysis of the tableting process

Michael Levin and Marko Zlokarnik

INTRODUCTION

A rotating press operates in the same way as a revolver. The compressive force is generated between an upper and a lower pressure roll, so that the tablet is compressed from both sides, from above as well as from below. The pairs of punches along with their dies are mounted in a rotating die platform. Each pair of punches produces one tablet per revolution. The capacities of the rotating presses depend on the number of punch pairs and the rate of rotation.

For very high-speed presses, the persistence of the powder being fed into the dies can present problems. If the tablet press runs properly, then any perturbations of the process are limited to those related to the properties of the powder. The most important parameters that influence the tableting process and the quality of the tablets are the material properties of the powder, moisture content, and compression time ("dwell time") τ (1,2).

In introducing the dimensional analysis to the tableting process, the aim is not to lay foundation for a scale-up of a tablet press, but to examine which process and material parameters govern the output of tablets of same size and shape of a given appliance. What should be undertaken from this part to increase the capacity of the tablet press?

RELEVANCE LIST
Target Quantity

In the tableting process, we are pursuing different quality features:

1. Tensile strength (hardness) of the tablet H [M L^{-1} T^{-2}]
2. Stability of the tablet (mechanical disintegration time) θ_m [T]
3. Bioavailability (dissolution time, release of the active ingredient) θ_b [T]

Each of these target quantities (quality features) entails a separate set of variables that are not necessarily completely equal in each case. In the following, we will pursue only the first of them, the tensile strength (or tensile stress) of the tablet H [M L^{-1} T^{-2}] with the dimension of pressure.

If the test method is designed in a way that the tablet failure is a result of the application of tensile stress only, strength can be calculated by the relationship

$$H \equiv \frac{2F}{\pi d h_t} \tag{1}$$

$$H \equiv F(2F; \pi d h_t)$$

where H is the radial tensile strength, F, the force to cleave the tablet, and $\pi d h_t$, the jacket surface of the tablet (1).

Geometric Parameters

Given the cylindric shape of the tablets, the geometry of the die is described by only two geometric parameters:

Diameter of the die d [L]
Depth of fill (loading depth) H [L]

Material Parameters (Physical Properties of the Powder Mixture)

There is a wealth of material parameters that exert a big impact on the tableting process. They influence the flow behavior of the powder in the hopper (formation of bridges!) and of the feed to the dies. Too high a moisture content of the powder or too little lubrication leads to sticking, cracking, and coating. The interaction of the particle size distribution, the crystal shape (morphology), and other physical properties of the powder are the principal factors affecting the tensile strength, the disintegration time, and the release of the active ingredient (1,2).

From the viewpoint of the dimensional analysis, it is not necessary to know and list all these physical parameters, if we succeed in finding an intermediate quantity (a "lumped" parameter), which takes into consideration their influence on the process. As such we have chosen (3) the powder compressibility κ, which is easily measurable and is defined as the relative change of the powder volume (or its height within the die) with the pressure:

$$\kappa \equiv \frac{1}{V_t} \frac{\Delta V}{h_t} \equiv \frac{1}{h_t} \frac{H - h_t}{\Delta p} \quad [M^{-1}LT^2] \tag{2}$$

The subscript $_t$ relates to the tablet, κ has the inverse dimension of the pressure.

Process-Related Parameters

Besides the maximum applied pressure p [M L^{-1} T^{-2}], it is the compression rate v (linear velocity of the punch!) that affects tableting and tablet properties most (1). It is defined as the ratio of the displacement of the punch from the first application of a detectable force to the point of maximum force to the time required for this displacement to occur (1):

$$v \equiv \frac{H_t - h_t}{t_{p=max} - t_0} \, (m/s)$$

The impact of the compression rate on the tableting is understandable because it causes the frictional effect of air, rapidly escaping powder pressed between the punch and the die. Sliding and rearrangement processes of the particles are also hindered by turbulence in the powder because of rapid compression.

We have chosen the compression time (dwell time) τ (s) instead (3). It is defined as that time when the flat portion of punch head with the diameter of d_{ph} is in contact with the wheel. During this time, the powder is submitted to the highest compression. (Contrary to this, the contact time is defined as the time during which the punch head is in contact with the wheel.)

MCC (4) employed the following formula for the determination of the dwell time:

$$\tau = \frac{d_{ph}}{Dn} \, [\text{s}] \tag{3}$$

d_{ph} is the diameter of the flat portion of the punch head (mm)[a]; D, the circle diameter of the turret on which the dies are arranged (mm); n, the rotational speed of the turret $[\text{s}^{-1}]$.

The relevance list now reads as follows:

Target quantity

$\quad H \quad [\text{M L}^{-1} \text{T}^{-2}] \quad$ Tensile strength of the tablet

Influencing parameters

-Geometric
$\quad d \quad [\text{L}] \qquad\qquad$ Diameter of the die
$\quad H \quad [\text{L}] \qquad\qquad$ Depth of fill (loading depth)

-Material
$\quad \kappa \quad [\text{M}^{-1} \text{L T}^2] \quad$ Powder compressibility

-Process related
$\quad p \quad [\text{M L}^{-1} \text{T}^{-2}] \quad$ Maximum applied pressure
$\quad \tau \quad [\text{T}^{-1}] \qquad\quad$ Dwell time

$$\{H, d, H, \kappa, p, \tau\}$$

Of these six parameters three have the dimension of pressure, two of length and only one of time. The dimension of time cannot be eliminated. This situation shows that there must be one more influencing parameter having the dimension of time. This can only be the rotational speed of the turret n and τ are primarily independent of each other, because the definition formula of dwell time, Eq. (3) contains the diameter D of the turret.

We add the rotational speed of the turret to the relevance list and obtain

$$\{H, d, H, \kappa, p, \tau, n\} \tag{4}$$

GENERATION OF Pi NUMBERS

We obtain from the relevance list (4) $7 - 3 = 4$ dimensionless pi numbers. They consist of one target, two processes, and one geometric number:

$$\{H/p, p\kappa, \tau n, H/d\} \tag{5}$$

A clearer insight into the dependence $H(p)$ may be gained by separating H and p:

$$\{H\kappa, p\kappa, \tau n, H/d\} \tag{6}$$

$\Rightarrow$ At this point, it should be pointed out that the influence of the pure process number τn on the tableting process can be investigated only when different tablet presses are compared to each other. In working with only one tableting

---

[a]MCC put $d_{ph} = 12.9$ mm = constant, because this happens to be flat portion of the punch head for IBT B tooling.

press, this number remains constant, but it must be quantified and noted as such!

CARRYING OUT AND EVALUATION OF MEASUREMENTS

The measurements were executed (4) on two tablet presses:

Manesty Betapress $D = 0.178$ m; $z = 16$; $\tau n = 1.77 \times 10^{-2}$
Fette, Model PT 2090 IC $D = 0.30$ m; $z = 36$; $\tau n = 9.86 \times 10^{-3}$

Both appliances had equal die diameter: $d = 9.52$ mm
     Two different powders were applied:

Avicel PH 101 with a density of $\rho = 1.58$ g/cm^3 and $\kappa = 2.45 \times 10^{-8}$ Pa^{-1}
Emcompress with a density of $\rho = 2.34$ g/cm^3 and $\kappa = 7.58 \times 10^{-9}$ Pa^{-1}

In Figure 1, 61 measurements on both powders and both tablet presses are presented in form of the dependence $H/p \, (n\tau)^a = f \, (p\kappa)$. It is striking that no

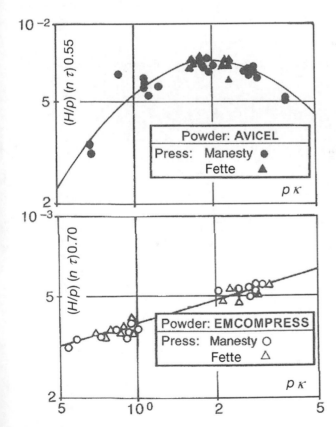

FIGURE 1   Evaluation of the measurements in the pi space {H/p, τn, $p\kappa$}.

influence of type of the tablet press is found. *All differences relate solely to different powder properties:*

1. The ordinates (H/p) for both powders differ from one another by almost one decade.
2. The type of powder determines the influence of the process numbers τn of the tablet press: The values of the exponent a in $(n\tau)^a$ are 0.55 for Avicel and 0.70 for Emcompress, respectively.
3. In both cases, the tensile strength H increases overproportionally with the applied pressure, but in case of Avicel only until $p\kappa = 2.0$ is reached.

The analytical expressions for fitting lines in Figure 1 are

Avicel:

$$[(H/p)(\tau n)^{0.55}]^{-1} = 1.46 \times 10^2 (p\kappa)^{-1.5} + 4.22 \times 10^1 (p\kappa) \quad 0.5 < (p\kappa) < 5.0$$

Emcompress:

$$(H/p)(\tau n)^{0.70} = 3.8 \times 10^{-4} (p\kappa)^{0.30} \quad 0.5 < (p\kappa) < 5.0$$

It has been mentioned that a clearer insight into the dependence $H(p)$ might be gained by separating H and p. In Figure 2, the fitting lines of Figure 1 are presented in the corresponding dimensionless frame

$$\{H\kappa, p\kappa, \tau n, H/d\}$$

One can see that the dependence of H on p for both powders is not excessively different.

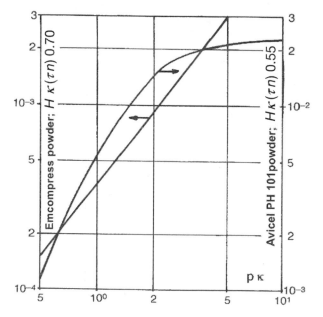

FIGURE 2   Representation of fitting curves in Figure 1 in the pi space $\{H\kappa, \tau n, p\kappa\}$.

In these correlations, an influence of the geometric parameter H/d was considered as insignificant and therefore neglected: H/d values varied depending on the type of press between $H/d = 0.73 - 0.96$.

In this examination, the goal was neither to change the size of the tablet nor to change the tablet press, but to increase the tablet output by increasing the process number τn. Therefore, different types of tablet presses will have to be examined to vary the process number more strongly.

REFERENCES

1. Leuenberger H, Rohera BD. Funamentals of powder compression. I. The compactibility and compressibility of pharmaceutical powders. Pharm Res 1986; 2(1):12–22.
2. Sommer K. Size enlargement, chapter tableting. In: Gerhards W, ed. Ullmann's Encyclopedia of Industrial Chemistry. Vol B2, 7-31/35. Germany: VCH Weinheim, 1988.
3. Levin M, Zlokarnik M. Dimensional analysis of the tableting process. In: Levin M, ed. Pharmaceutical Process Scale-Up. New York: Marcel Dekker, Inc., 2002.
4. The measurements were performed by Metropolitan Computing Corporation (MCC), East Hanover, New Jersey, USA.

15 Practical considerations in the scale-up of powder-filled hard shell capsule formulations

Larry L. Augsburger

INTRODUCTION

Hard shell capsules continue to occupy a central role in drug product development and manufacture, ranking second behind compressed tablets in frequency of utilization in drug delivery. In product development, such capsules are often the first dosage form for any orally administered drug substance. Although the final marketed form often will be a compressed tablet, firms may consider using the capsule as the first marketed form to shorten the overall development cycle.

Most drug substances are provided to the formulator in the form of dry, particulate solids, and the initial development goal typically is to produce an immediate-release oral solid dosage form. Preformulation studies will determine whether the drug substance can be filled in the form of relatively simple powder blends or must be granulated. Although hard shell capsules may be filled with a range of materials other than powders and granulations, such as pellets, liquids, semisolid matrices, and tablets, and even combinations of these, to provide modified release or, perhaps, to solve special formulation problems related to poor drug solubility or compatibility, the scope of this chapter will be limited to capsules filled with simple powder blends or granulated powders. This chapter will not discuss the issues of scaling up of blending or granulation. These unit operations are not exclusive to capsules and are treated elsewhere in this book. Similarly, the scale-up issues related to tablet compression, coating pellets and coating tablets are also discussed elsewhere. Rather, this chapter will address the issues involved in transferring simple powder blends or granulated powders from a smaller capacity filling machine to a larger-capacity filling machine.

TYPES OF FILLING MACHINES AND THEIR FORMULATION REQUIREMENTS

Any discussion of the issues of scaling up capsule filling must take into account the design and operating principle of filling machines and their formulation requirements.

Most production capsules are filled on machines that form plugs from powder or granular formulations by compression with tamping pins or pistons and then eject the plugs into capsule bodies. Although the compression/ejection events bring to mind tableting, it is important to recognize that capsule plugs are vastly different from compressed tablets. In the first place, plug height to diameter ratios are typically >1 and often as high as 5:1. This is in marked contrast to tablets where the height to diameter ratio is generally <1. Furthermore, plug compression forces, often in the range of 50 to 150 N, are about 50 to 100 fold less than typical tablet compression forces. The resulting plugs are very soft, and when they can be handled, they often exhibiting breaking strengths of less than 1 N (1). Plugs need only retain their mechanical integrity until delivered into the capsule body and often are not able to be recovered intact from the filled capsule. Interestingly, relatively high piston or tamping pin compression speeds in the range of about 100 to 500 mm/sec have been reported for several machines (2–4). These rates easily exceed the approximately 50 mm/sec range considered typical of traditional single-station eccentric tablet presses (5) and bracket of the maximum total punch speed of about 250 mm/sec reported for the double-ended compression event of a Manesty Betapress operating at 1300 tablets/min (6).

There are two main types of plug forming machines: the dosator type (e.g., MG-2, Zanasi, Matic, and Macofar machines) and the dosing disk type (e.g., Bosch GKF, Impressa, Index, and Harro Höfliger machines). Bosch GKF machines were formerly manufactured by Höfliger and Karg (H & K). Both types of machines have capsule rectification and separation operations. As empty capsules are fed in to these machines, they are first rectified, that is, oriented so that they are delivered body end down into split bushings. Separation occurs when an applied vacuum pulls the body segments down into the lower portion of the split bushing, leaving the cap segment behind in the upper bushing portion. When the split bushings are separated, the capsule bodies are exposed for filling with plugs.

The two types of filling machines have different powder handling and plug forming mechanisms that should be considered in making formulation decisions. Ideally, the type of machine chosen for routine production should dictate the properties of the formulation to be filled.

Dosator Machines

One type of machine employs a dosator. The dosator can be viewed as a hollow tube containing a moveable piston (Fig. 1). The piston is preset to a particular height in the tube so that the volume between the piston head and the open end of the dosator would contain the appropriate mass of the formulation. In operation, the open end of the dosator is plunged downward into a powder bed that had been struck off neatly at a particular height. Often, the powder bed height is as much as double the piston height. Thus, as the dosator moves down through the powder bed, the formulation enters the open end of the dosator and becomes lightly compressed against the stationary piston. While the dosator is in its lowest position in the powder bed, these machines can provide additional compression to the plug via the piston through a compression knob or cam mechanism. When plug compression is complete, the dosator bearing the plug is lifted out of the powder bed and positioned over an open capsule body segment held in a bushing. The dosator piston is then depressed via an ejection knob or cam mechanism to push the plug from the dosator to the capsule body. In certain machines, the body bushing is rotated into position under the dosator to receive the ejected plug. Plug porosity and mechanical strength (breaking force) depend on the compression force. Plug weight depends on the piston height setting (primarily) and the powder bed height.

A successful filling operation with these machines requires the quantitative retention of powder within the dosator during transfer from the powder bed to the capsule shell. As a minimum, a stable powder arch needs to be

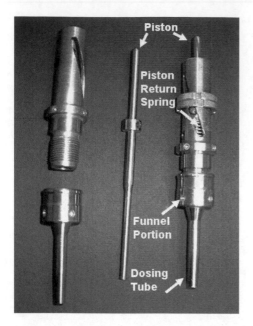

FIGURE 1   Dosator from a Zanasi LZ-64 intermittant-motion filling machine.

formed at the dosator outlet to prevent loss of material during the time that the open end of the dosator tube is exposed (7,8). This stable arch is dependent on the angle of wall friction of the powder with the dosing tube and the degree of compression applied. An optimum angle of wall friction exists for which the compression force required to ensure a stable arch is a minimum (8). Quantitative transfer also requires that the plug ideally remain intact during the actual ejection event to prevent material loss. Loose powder can be lost with the displaced air. Formulations thus require cohesiveness, and fillers that have been modified to enhance both their flowability and compactibility may be particularly advantageous. These include, for example, microcrystalline cellulose, compressible (pregelatinized) starch, and various direct compression grades of lactose. Direct-fill powder formulations for dosator machines may benefit from the higher compactibility of microcrystalline cellulose fillers. Patel and Podceck (9) noted that medium and coarse particle size grades of microcrystalline cellulose can be considered "good" excipients for capsules on the basis of studies using a Zanasi AZ5 dosator machine. Guo and Augsburger (10) demonstrated the higher compactibility of microcrystalline cellulose and silicified microcrystalline cellulose compared with Starch 1500 and anhydrous lactose at low plug compression forces.

Meeting a flowability criterion appropriate to these machines is also an important determinant of successful filling. Flowability is not only important for proper powder feed from the reservoir to the powder bed, but also to facilitate the efficient closing in of the hole left by the dosator when a plug is withdrawn from the powder bed and to reestablish the bed packing density before another plug is formed from that region of the bed. Dosator machines provide various agitation and scraping mechanisms to restore the powder bed, but proper flowability is nevertheless also required. Maintaining a uniform bed density helps assure that plugs of uniform weight will be picked up by the dosator and that plugs of uniform cohesiveness will be formed for a given compression setting. Irwin et al. (11) found that the better the rate of flow in a flow meter, the more uniform the weight of capsules filled on a Zanasi LZ-64 machine. Heda (12) found that powders exhibiting a Carr compressibility index (CI%) between 25 and 35 yielded minimum weight variation in a Zanasi LZ-64. [CI% is calculated from the loose (ρ_{Loose}) and tapped (ρ_{Tapped}) bulk densitites as follows: $CI\% = \frac{\rho_{Tapped} - \rho_{Loose}}{\rho_{Tapped}} \times 100$ (13). There is a close relationship between the CV% and the flowability of the powder. Higher values of CV% reflect greater friction and cohesiveness within the powder and thus relatively poorer flowability.] Stronger plugs with lower weight variation were produced with powders exhibiting higher CI% values, undoubtedly reflecting the greater cohesiveness in those powders. More free-flowing powders with CI% values <20 were more difficult to retain in the dosator tube. Very free-flowing powders may "flood" in the powder handling mechanism of a dosator machine. It is apparent that a proper balance must be struck between the ability of the powder to both form good plugs and to reform and maintain a uniform density in the powder bed after plug removal.

Glidants (e.g., colloidal silicon dioxide, talc) may need to be added to formulations to achieve desired flow properties, especially when the drug/filler ratio is relatively high. Usually, there is an optimum concentration of glidant for best flow, often less than 1% for the colloidal silicas (14,15). The following order of effectiveness of glidants has been reported for two powder systems: fine silica > magnesium stearate > purified talc (16).

Formulations typically also require the inclusion a lubricant for successful filling. Lubricants reduce adhesion to piston faces and other metal surfaces with which the powder comes into contact, reduce friction between sliding surfaces, and ease the ejection of plugs. The same lubricants used in tableting are used in capsule formulations. The most commonly used lubricant is magnesium stearate and the level required depends on the formulation and the machine settings. Comparing different concentrations of magnesium stearate in standard fillers filled into capsules using an instrumented Zanasi LZ-64 machine, Small and Augsburger (17) found minimum ejection forces at 0.1% magnesium stearate with pregelatinized starch, 0.5% with microcrystalline cellulose, and at 1% with anhydrous lactose. The magnitude of the ejection force depended on the setting of certain operating variables. Generally, ejection force increased with compression force, but at a given compression force, ejection force also increased with increases in either the piston height or the powder bed height (Fig. 2). On the basis of an experimental design, Tattawasart and Armstrong (18) concluded that 0.5% magnesium stearate was optimal for α-monohydrate lactose when tested in a simulator for a Macofar 13/2 dosator machine.

Dosing Disk Machines

In contrast to dosator machines, dosing disk machines form plugs in segments through a series of tamping or compression events. The dosing disk machines made by various manufacturers can vary in the number of tamping stations utilized and, in certain cases, may employ modified tamping mechanisms.

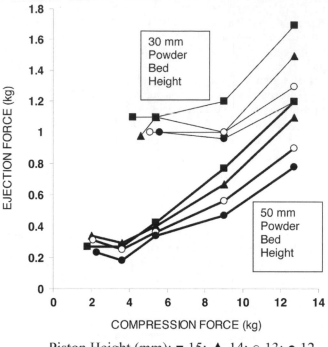

FIGURE 2 Effect of compression force, piston height setting, and powder bed height on plug ejection force of Starch 1500 (0.005% magnesium stearate) on a Zanasi LZ-64 filling machine. Piston height (mm): ◆ 15, ▲ 14, X 13, and ■ 12. Powder bed height (mm): — 30 and – 50. *Source*: From Ref. 17.

The plug forming portion of dosing disk machines may be viewed as a powder bowl the bottom of which is a plate through which sets of circular holes or perforations have been drilled (the "dosing disk"). The dosing disk rotates on a sealing plate that effectively closes off the sets of perforations to form the dosing disk cavities in which the plugs are formed. A different dosing disk is required for each capsule size (i.e., diameter). The required thickness of the dosing disk is determined by the plug length that can be achieved for the required weight of a given formulation. The appropriate thickness for a given formulation can be estimated using a plug compression tester developed by H & K in which a dose of the formulation is compressed in a die with a single stroke and the plug length is measured (19). Davar et al. (20) suggested equations and a spreadsheet calculation for predicting the required disk thickness on the basis of the formulation density and the thickness and breaking strength of trial plugs made using an Instron tester. A dosing disk whose thickness is adjustable is now available from Bosch for at least some models.

In GKF machines, sets of dosing disk cavities are arranged in equally spaced locations around the periphery of the dosing disk. Five of these locations

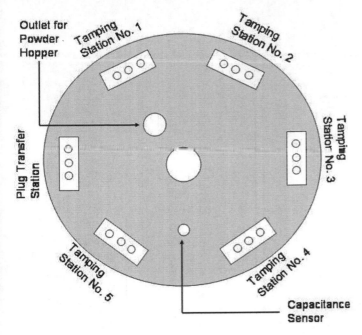

FIGURE 3 Diagrammatic representation of the dosing disk area layout of a dosing disk machine (three tamps per station).

serve as plug tamping stations, and the sixth is the plug ejection station (Fig. 3). Depending on the filling capacity of the machine, there may be as many as 18 dosing disk cavities at each location. The powder formulation is maintained at a relatively constant level over the dosing disk. The powder level is sensed by a capacitance probe and an auger feed mechanism is activated if the powder level falls below that of the sensor. Groups of tamping pins descend at each station to tamp the powder in the cavities to form plug segments. Plug segments are actually a composite of powder that enters the dosing disk cavities during disk rotation and any additional powder that enters the cavities during tamping as the pins push through the powder bed over the dosing disk (21). Most powder enters the dosing cavities by the former process (22,23). The cavities are indexed under each of the five sets of tamping pins, thus each plug is the result of five tamping events per cycle. In some applications, fewer than five tamping stations may be utilized. Shah et al. (21) reported that target fill weights could be obtained using a few as three tamping stations when filling certain lubricated fillers (Fig. 4). Excess powder is scraped off as the dosing disk indexes the completed plugs to the sixth station where the bottoms of the dosing disk cavities are exposed and the plugs are ejected by another set of pins into capsule bodies held in a bushing (the "transfer pins"). In general, the dose delivered depends on the thickness of the dosing disk (i.e., cavity depth), the powder bed depth, the tamping pin penetration setting and the number of tamping stations used, if less than all five.

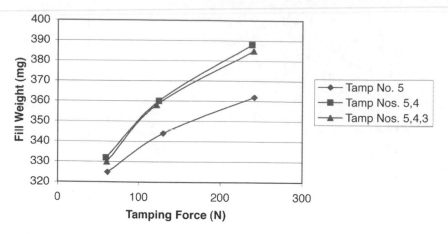

FIGURE 4 Effect of tamping force and number of tamps on fill weight of in an Höfliger and Karg GKF 330 filling machine. (Anhydrous lactose lubricated with 0.5% magnesium stearate.) *Source*: From Ref. 21.

The tamping pin block of an Harro Höfliger model KFM/3 dosing disk machine that utilizes three tamping pins in each of three tamping stations is illustrated in Figure 5. The powder in the dosing cavities is tamped twice before rotating a quarter turn to the next station.

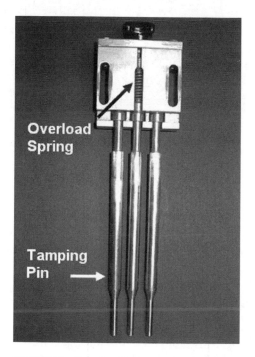

FIGURE 5 Tamping block and pins from an Harro Höfliger KFM/3 dosing disk machine.

It is easy to see from the above description how pin penetration setting or compression force contributes to fill weight in dosing disk machines. Clearly, the greater the compression at any station, the larger can be the potential volume remaining to capture powder upon rotation to the next station. At the same time, the greater the tamping pin penetration distance, the more likely powder over the disk will be pushed into the dosing disk cavity. However, it is important to recognize that the pin penetration setting is not necessarily the actual penetration distance, since overload springs at the distal end of each pin compress when sufficient resistance is encountered during plug formation. Springs made from larger diameter wire make possible the development of higher compression forces, which favor the attainment of greater fill weights (2).

In general, a successful filling operation with these machines requires formulation attributes similar to those required for dosator machines. Formulations require cohesiveness, and fillers that that have been modified to enhance both their flowability and compactibility are also likely to be advantageous. The same fillers used in dosator formulations are also used in dosing disk formulations. Meeting a flowability criterion appropriate to dosing disk machines is also an important determinant of successful filling. As with dosator machines, fillers may be selected for their flowability and an optimum concentration of glidant may be required. The same glidants and lubricants are used. Lubricants play the same role in dosing disk machines as they do in dosator machines. However, it is important to recognize that these two machine types differ in their specific requirements for flowability, compactibility, and lubrication. These differences and their possible implications for transferring formulations between these machine types will be discussed in greater detail in the sections that follow.

Continuous- Vs. Intermittant-Motion Machines

Some machines, for example, Bosch GKF, Index, Impressa, and Zanasi, are called intermittent-motion machines because they exhibit an interrupted filling sequence. That is, indexing turntables must stop at specific stations to execute the various operations described above. Continuous motion machines, for example, MG-2 and Matic, execute these functions in a continuous cycle. Eliminating the need to decelerate and accelerate from one station to the next makes possible higher machine speeds with the continuous-motion machines (24).

GENERAL FORMULATION PRINCIPLES

The development of powder formulations for hard shell capsules can present formulators with significant challenges. Just as is the case of formulations for tableting, such problems as component compatibility, powder blending and maintenance of homogeneity, flowability and lubrication are frequently encountered. The ability to measure out and transfer accurate and precise volumes of a powder or granular mass to capsule shells is the determining factor in weight variation and, to the extent that mixing is uniform, also of content uniformity. As discussed above, consideration must be given to the proper choice and use of fillers, glidants, and lubricants for successful running. Formulations must not only be designed to run successfully, but the capsule product must also exhibit appropriate drug release characteristics. Because some properties important to successful running can also adversely affect drug release and vice versa, the interplay of formulation and process variables must be carefully considered to meet both objectives. For example, to improve their dissolution rate, poorly soluble drugs are often micronized as this increases their specific surface area (surface area per unit weight). Micronization is thus expected to speed up dissolution by increasing the surface area from which dissolution can occur. However, since micronized particles have high surface-to-mass ratios, surface cohesive interactions may enhance the tendency of such particles aggregate, thus resulting is a smaller than expected effective surface area from which dissolution can occur. In one example of this phenomenon, larger particle size fractions of the poorly soluble drug, ethinamate, actually gave better dissolution from capsules of the neat drug than did smaller particle sizes when filled at equivalent porosities (Newton and Rowley) (25). The greater surface cohesive and frictional interactions of smaller particles also reduce their flowability.

For best drug release, it may be important to consider both the solubility of the filler and the drug. For instance, Newton et al. (26) long ago demonstrated that the dissolution of poorly soluble ethinamate from capsules markedly improved when the lactose in the formulation was increased to 50%. Interestingly, with the soluble drug chloramphenicol, little or no effect on dissolution was found when the formulation included up to 50% lactose, but the inclusion of 80% lactose in the same formulation markedly retarded drug dissolution from the capsules, possibly because of competition for the solvent (27).

Good running formulations generally require lubrication; however, the most effective and most commonly used lubricants are such hydrophobic substances as magnesium or calcium stearate. Indeed, magnesium stearate is the most commonly used lubricant (28,29). The level of lubricant is critical. Excessive concentrations of hydrophobic lubricants have long been known to retard drug release from capsules by making formulations more hydrophobic (26,30). Laminar lubricants like magnesium or calcium stearate shear readily and delaminate when subjected to a tangential force in the blender (31–33). Thus, if a formulation is mixed for too long a period of time after the addition of such lubricants, the net result can be the formation of an excessive hydrophobic film on particle surfaces that resists wetting, thus retarding liquid penetration into the plug matrix, deaggregation of the matrix and drug dissolution. Even a modest level of laminar lubricant can retard wetting and dissolution if the lubricant blending time is too long (34).

The presence of magnesium stearate at particle surfaces can also reduce cohesiveness and soften plugs. Mehta and Augsburger (1) found that the mechanical strength of plugs produced in a dosator machine can be reduced by the amount of lubricant used and that drug dissolution could benefit in certain cases. In a simple formulation consisting of hydrochlorothiazide, microcrystalline cellulose and magnesium stearate, plug breaking force decreased from 84 to about 2.0 g and T_{60} decreased from 55 to 12 minutes when the magnesium stearate level was increased from 0.05% to 0.75%. The capsules were filled on an instrumented Zanasi LZ-64 dosator machine using a standardized plug compression force of 22 kg. However, this phenomenon was not found when the filler was changed to anhydrous lactose. A similar phenomenon was previously reported for hand-filled rifampicin capsules (35). In this case, up to a limit, increases in the blending time of magnesium stearate led to increases in the dissolution rate, and the effect was most pronounced at lower lubricant levels. The enhanced dissolution rate appeared related to a reduced cohesiveness of the formulation that resulted from increased lubricant mixing time (35). Aside from its possible effects on drug dissolution, over lubrication, whether by over mixing or adding excessive concentrations, could lead to increased weight variation in dosator machines because of the softening effect of the lubricant on plugs and/or by reducing dosing tube wall friction.

Other excipients that may appear in capsule formulations are disintegrants, and wetting agents. At appropriate concentrations in the formulation, often 4% to 8%, super disintegrants such as croscarmellose sodium, sodium starch glycolate and crospovidone can enhance drug dissolution rate by promoting liquid penetration and capsule content dispersion or disintegration (36). This improvement in dissolution rate was much less marked when a low-dose drug was formulated using lactose as the filler, as compared with water insoluble dicalcium phosphate (37). The lactose based formulation was already a rapidly releasing system, and the soluble filler may tend to dissolve rather than disintegrate. Of possible relevance to scale-up and/or transfer across filling machine types was the observation that the beneficial effect of disintegrants was to a degree dependent on plug compression force, with dissolution tending to be enhanced at higher plug compression forces (37). Again, the effect was more apparent when the filler was dicalcium phosphate as compared with the lactose based formulation.

Capsule formulations may include wetting agents, such as sodium doc-usate and sodium lauryl sulfate. Typically used in concentrations of 0.1% to 0.5%, these excipients can help plug dispersion and drug dissolution by increasing the wettability and liquid penetration of the powder mass (25,26,38). Wetting agents can help overcome the "water-shedding" nature of hydrophobic lubricants.

Though capsules appear to be relatively simple powder-filled dosage forms, the above discussion makes clear that formulations for capsules can be complex and involve a multidimensional design space of formulation and machine operating variables. It is therefore not surprising that formulation scientists have turned to such tools as multivariate analysis and response surface methodology, expert systems and artificial neural networks to help develop successful capsule formulations. For example, Piscitelli et al. (38) carried out a multivariate and response surface analysis of the effect of formulation and process variables on piroxicam release from a capsule formulation and linked the results of that analysis to human bioavailability/bioequivalence outcomes.

Bateman et al. (39) reported an expert system for capsule formulation development that was created for Sanofi. The formulations generated by that system for three challenge drug substances were found by experienced formulators to be suitable for manufacture and initial stability evaluation. Another example of an expert system designed to support powder-filled capsule formulation is Capsugel's CAPEX® program. The latter was developed as a centralized system that incorporates a worldwide industrial experience database and original laboratory research (40). More recently, an expert system for capsule formulation support was linked with a neural net (41,42). This system consists of a *decision module* (expert system) that provides a proposed formulation and a *prediction module* (neural net) that predicts the dissolution performance of the proposed formulation. The two modules are connected by two information exchange paths to form a loop that (ideally) allows the formulator to make iterative adjustments until a formulation that has the desired dissolution performance is predicted, or the optimization is terminated by the user. This hybrid intelligent system ("expert network") was specifically designed to generate capsule formulations that meet specific drug dissolution criteria for BCS class II drugs. [Drugs that have low solubility and high permeability according to certain criteria are considered class II drugs in the Biopharmaceutcial Classification System (BCS) (43). Since such drugs are prone to exhibit dissolution rate–limited absorption, their dissolution rate may be directly linked to oral bioavailability.] In the preliminary study, a single BCS class II drug, piroxicam, was used to test proof of concept. Later, a modified and more generalized version of this system was challenged with a range of BCS class II drugs representing different solubilities and chemical classes (44). Generally, the modified hybrid network was able to predict the amount of drug dissolved within $\forall$5% for the drugs tested. Wilson et al. (45) later developed a Bayesian network (BN), a graphical probabilistic model, for the above BCS class II drugs and found that the BN could correlate the key excipient effects on dissolution performance of the drugs.

ROLE OF INSTRUMENTED FILLING MACHINES AND SIMULATION

The successful running of hard shell capsule formulations and the drug release properties of the filled capsules are dependent on a number of formulation and processing factors and their interactions. The formulators' understanding of how the interplay of these variables affects manufacturability and drug dissolution has been enhanced by the development of research instrumentation of automatic capsule-filling machines to measure the forces involved in plug formation and ejection (46). Both dosator machines (47–51, and others) and dosing disk machines (2,22,52, and others) have been successfully instrumented.

The development of instrumented capsule-filling machines has also led to capsule-filling machine simulation (3,4,53–55). The simulation of capsule filling is not nearly as well established as compaction simulation for tableting. Further development of this technology ultimately may permit the study of plug formation and ejection in the laboratory with only small quantities of material on equipment that can be programmed to simulate the action of different production machines at their operating speeds.

SCALING UP WITHIN THE SAME DESIGN AND OPERATING PRINCIPLE
Regulatory Meaning of Same Design and Operating Principle

Generally, few problems are expected when scaling up with equipment of the same design and operating principle. Indeed, the regulatory guidance on scale-up of immediate-release oral solid dosage forms (SUPAC-IR) (56) appears to recognize this point. According to SUPAC-IR, scale-up to and including a factor of 10 times the size of the pilot/biobatch is considered a level 1 change if the equipment used to produce the test batch(es) is of the same design and operating principles, Current Good Manufacturing Procedures are followed, and the same standard operating procedures (SOPs), controls, and formulation and manufacturing procedures are used. Level 1 changes are those that are not likely to cause any detectable impact on formulation quality or performance and need only be reported in the Annual report. Scale-up beyond 10 times the pilot/biobatch is only a level 2 change provided the equipment used to produce the test batch(es) is if the same design and operating principles. Similarly, the same SOPs, controls, and formulation and manufacturing procedures must be used. Level 2 changes are changes that could significantly impact formulation quality and performance and require the filing a "changes being effected supplement." It is significant that in neither case is in vivo bioequivalence data required to support the change of scale. The guidance should be consulted for a full description of the test documentation needed to be reported to FDA in these cases.

What constitutes equipment of the "same design and operating principle" was clarified in the recommendations of subsequent guidances. The current guidance "SUPAC-IR/MR: Immediate Release and Modified Release Solid Oral Dosage Forms Manufacturing Equipment Addendum" (57) applies to both immediate- and modified-release oral solid dosage forms was developed by FDA with the assistance of the International Society of Pharmaceutical Engineering (ISPE) and is an update on an earlier document. This document is organized in broad categories of unit operations (e.g., blending, drying, granulation, etc.). For each unit operation, a table is provided in which equipment is classified by class (operating principle) and subclass (design characteristic). Generally, equipment within the same class and subclass are considered to have the same design and operating principle under SUPAC-IR and SUPAC-MR. A change from equipment in one class to equipment in a different class would usually be considered a change in design and operating principle. But equipment changes to a different subclass within the same class should be carefully considered and evaluated on a case-by-case basis. By these definitions, *encapsulating*, or the "division of material into a hard gelatin capsule," is an *operating principle*. That is, all encapsulators should have in common rectification, separation of caps from bodies, dosing of fill material/formulation, rejoining of caps and bodies and ejection of the filled capsules. However, the various methods of dosing the formulation represent different design characteristics and are considered *subclasses*. Thus, a change from a dosator machine to a dosing disk machine would constitute a change in subclass, but not of operating principle.

A survey of industry practices indicated that 64% of companies develop formulations using small-scale equipment of the same design and operating principles as the production equipment (12). In that same survey, about 18% of companies responded that they use small-scale development equipment of a subclass different from the intended production equipment. Company preferences appeared about evenly divided between dosator and dosing disk machines, with about 18% using both types of machines. The following sections address some of the issues involved in scaling up or transferring formulations within and between subclasses.

Scaling Up Within the Same Subclass

In principle, scaling up within the same subclass should be subject to minimal problems. In contrast to tableting, where strain rate tends to be faster and dwell time and contact time tend to be shorter in higher-output presses, higher-output plug forming machines of the same manufacturer's series typically do not make

TABLE 1 Comparison of Three Bosch GKF Models

Model	Maximum rated output (capsules/hr)	Maximum cycle speed (cycles/min)	Powder bowl diameter (in.)	Number of tamping pins at each station
GKF 400	24,000	133	7.55	3
GKF 1500	90,000	125	13.4	12
GKF 2500	150,000	140	15.7	18

Source: From Ref. 58.

plugs any faster than the lower-output machines. This is because higher throughput is primarily achieved in these machines by increasing the number dosing units. To illustrate that point, consider Table 1 comparing three sizes of Bosch GKF machines where pin movement or dwell time are reportedly similar across machines having a broad range in output capacity (58).

The increased diameter of the powder bowl of larger machines and, therefore, of the turning radius of the dosing disk, may, however, influence the distribution of the powder over the dosing disk. For best weight variation, there may be an optimal flow criterion that should be met for dosing disk machines of this type, and that criterion may vary with the turning radius. Kurihara and Ichikawa (59) reported a minimum point in the plot of the angle of repose versus coefficient of variation of filling weight for a dosing disk machine (Höfliger Karg GKF 1000). This observation could perhaps be understood recognizing that powder is distributed over the dosing disk by the centrifugal action of the indexing rotation (baffles are provided to help maintain a uniform powder level). Kurihara and Ichikawa (59) related the relationship between the angle of repose and weight variation to the degree of acceleration that takes place in disk movement, which, in turn, is dependent on dosing disk diameter and rotational speed. Their observations suggest that powders with sufficiently high angles of repose may not have sufficient mobility to distribute well over the dosing disk via the intermittent indexing motion; whereas, powders having angles of repose that are sufficiently low may be too fluid to maintain a uniform bed. However, the interpretation of these results may need qualification since Kurihara and Ichikawa did not appear to make use of the tamping mechanism. Working with an instrumented GKF model 330, Shah et al. (21) observed that a uniform powder bed height was not maintained at the first tamping station owing to its nearness to the scrape-off device adjacent to ejection. More recent workers also have pointed to the need to properly calibrate the flow properties of formulations for this kind of filling machine. Heda et al. (60) studied model formulations having different flow properties on a GKF 400 machine and proposed that CI% values should be in the range of 18 to 30 to maintain low weight variation. More poorly flowing powders (CI% > 30) were observed to dam up around the ejection station. Podczeck (61) noted that poor flowing powders display an "avalanching behavior" in front of the ejection station in which a powder mass alternatively builds up and then collapses in the manner of an avalanche at certain intervals of time. The net effect is that the powder over stations 1 and 2 can vary dramatically, thereby causing increased capsule fill weight variation (61).

The MG-2 series of dosator machines also exhibit similar plug forming parameters across machines with different production capacities. For example, the 16 station (up to 48,000 capsules/hr) and 64 station machines (actually a double 32-station machine; up to 200,000 capsules/hr) operate at the same RPM, have the same spacing between dosators, and have similar dosator penetration and withdrawal speeds, plug compression dwell times and plug ejection speeds (62). Unlike the powder bed of dosing disk machines, the powder bed into which dosators dip to form plugs is scraped off neatly to a specific bed height. In the MG-2 continuous motion machines, the powder bed is presented in an annular ring ("powder trough") that rotates with the dosator turret (dosing head), The powder bed and dosing head rotate at slightly different speeds. Because of this difference in rotational speeds, a plug is not formed from the same location in the powder bed until approximately 8 to 10 revolutions have occurred and the bed will have been restored and stabilized (62). Maintaining a uniform powder bed density in dosator machines is essential for dosators to pick up uniform weights of powder. This difference in rotational speeds also causes the dosator to enter the powder bed at an angle, causing a furrow, rather than a vertical hole, to be formed. The axes of rotation of the annular powder bed and the dosing head are offset and the dosator turret has a smaller radius than the powder trough. Thus, as the turret rotates, dosators alternatively pass over the annular powder trough (to form plugs) and then over bushings bearing capsule bodies (to discharge plugs) (Fig. 6).

The MG-2 Futura series of machines can be fitted with different numbers of dosators to give outputs ranging from 6000 to 96,000 capsules/hr. Because turret and annular powder bed dimensions would remain the same, few problems should be expected when scaling up within this range on this machine. However, it is important to recognize that when fewer than the full complement of 16 dosators are installed, the dwell time of the powder in the feed mechanism and trough will be longer than when the machine is fully tooled.

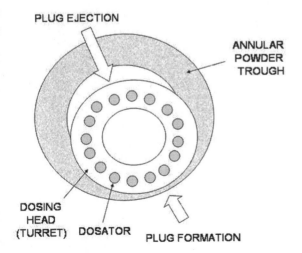

FIGURE 6 Diagrammatic representation of the plug forming and discharge stations of MG-2 continuous motion filling machine.

TABLE 2   Effect of Run Time on Dissolution from Capsules Filled on an MG-2 Machine

Drug (40 mg potency; 1% magnesium stearate)	When sampled	Percent dissolved			
		5 min	10 min	30 min	45 min
Hydrochlorothiazide	Begin of run	6.5	12.5	28.9	50.5
(solubility = 0.6 mg/mL)	After 45-min run	4.6	9.9	21.5	28.5
SQ32756 (solubility	Begin of run	9.9	20.8	58.3	70.6
= 5.0 mg/mL)	After 45-min run	9.7	20.8	49.8	69.1
Aztreonam (solubility	Begin of run	41.3	92.1	107.2	107.2
= 12 mg/mL)	After 45-min run	25.0	78.1	95.2	96.81

Source: From Ref. 63.

When filling capsules on an MG-2 Futura fitted with four dosators, Desai et al. (63) found the dissolution of three drugs of varying solubility to be slower after 30 or 45 minutes of running compared with capsules sampled at the beginning of the run (Table 2). The slow-down was greatest for the least soluble drug. The slowed dissolution was attributed to prolonged mixing by the propeller blade in the hopper leading to increased coating of particles with hydrophobic magnesium stearate (63).

To further study the problem, Desai et al. (63) conducted a simulation study in which the capsule machine was left on for up to 60 minutes without filling capsules, during which time the formulation was being constantly mixed by the propeller blade in the hopper. In this simulation, capsules were hand filled (to eliminate possible compression effects) at the beginning and at the end of a run. After a 60-minute run, dissolution from capsules filled from the hopper was significantly reduced from that of capsules filled before the start of the run.

Desai et al. (63) conducted additional studies that pointed to various formulation changes that could potentially resolve the problem. In one experiment conducted with the intermediate solubility drug and using 15-minute mixing in a Hobart mixer to simulate over mixing, no slowing of dissolution from hand-filled capsules was found when magnesium stearate (1% of formula) was replaced with an equal concentration of more hydrophilic lubricants (Stear-O-Wet or sodium stearyl fumarate). In another experiment, the MG-2 machine was turned on to allow mixing in the hopper, and machine filling was activated for 10-minute periods of time at the beginning, after 30 minutes and after an additional 60 minutes of the run. The results of this study showed no slowing of dissolution when the magnesium stearate level was reduced to 0.25%, which appeared to provide sufficient lubrication. In another approach, replacing pregelatinized starch (10% in the formula) with equal concentrations of Explotab or Primojel resulted in no slowing of dissolution, even after overmixing with 1% magnesium stearate in the formula (63).

During a trial production of 25-mg indomethicin capsules, Johansen et al. (64) reported both a segregation problem and an over mixing problem on an MG-2 model G36/4 machine. The formulation was mixed using a planetary mixer. Magnesium stearate was added separately and mixed for five minutes. Drug content and dissolution were found to vary with time during the encapsulation run. The authors concluded that the powder throughput was so

TABLE 3 Comparison of Compression Parameters

		Velocities (m/sec)		
Machine type	Output (per hr)	Dosator (dipping)	Piston/tamp (compression)	Piston/tamp (ejection)
Zanasi AZ-20	15,000	0.242	0.12	0.453
	21,000	0.350	0.16	0.653
Macofar 13/2	6,600	0.301	0.22	0.272
	12,600	0.60	0.51	0.834

Source: From Ref. 3.

slow at the hopper mixing blade rotational velocity of 1 revolution/min that over mixing occurred in the filling machine. To solve both problems, the mixing blade was removed and the hopper was fitted with an insert to convert it to a mass flow hopper.

Harding et al. (33) proposed mixing in a Turbula high-intensity mixer as a predictive stress test to determine the likelihood of encountering a dissolution problem on scale-up due to lubricant over mixing. They found a qualitative relationship between changes in the properties of a 500-g batch induced by mixing in a 2-L Turbula for six hours and the effect of a six-hour encapsulation run on a 10-kg batch of the same formulation in a Zanasi LZ-64 dosator machine.

Scaling up within the same subclass but across different manufacturers of the equipment may also entail differences that could affect the success of the outcome. Consider the data in Table 3 for two different intermittent motion dosator machines. As can be seen, there are substantial differences in the compression and ejection velocities. Working with a Macofar simulator, Britten et al. (55) found that plug ejection speed had little effect on plug properties, but higher compression speeds led to reduced plug consolidation and lower weights. Possible differences in their powder handling and mixing mechanisms and powder throughput rates also could cause formulations to perform differently. Some machines may tend more to encourage segregation of certain formulations or may be more likely to over mix magnesium stearate in the machine. A useful analysis of the relationship between bulk powder properties and the segregation tendency of powder formulations from a quality-by-design (QbD) perspective was provided by Xie et al (65).

Transferring Between Dosator and Dosing Disk Machines

Scale-up from early development may involve not only larger-capacity filling machines of the same subclass, but also machines in different subclasses. Few studies have been reported comparing the formulation requirements of dosator and dosing disk machines. As discussed in the preceding sections, there are substantial differences in the way these two types of machines handle the powder feed and form plugs. Different rates of plug compression, different dwell times, and whether the plug is formed in one stroke (dosator machines) or multiple strokes (dosing disk machines) at least theoretically could cause differences in plug bonding and densification and dissolution. The goal of this section is to provide guidance to formulators who may wish to design formulations that can be run on either type of machine or who may need to consider transferring from one machine type the other.

A Dosing Disk Machine May Be Able to Accommodate a Broader Range in Powder Properties

Bulk density and densification. The multiple tamp principle of the dosing disk machine appears more efficient at densification than the single stroke dosator machine (without vacuum densification). In a study comparing the same model formulations on an instrumented Zanasi LZ-64 and an instrumented H & K GKF-400, Heda et al. (60) found that similar fill weights could be attained on both machines, but the dosator machine required a piston height setting of 18 mm, as compared with the dosing disk height of 15 mm for the dosing disk machine.

Compactibility. Ridgway and Callow (66) long ago recognized that dosator machines would require a higher degree of compactibility due to the exposure of the plug from the open end of the dosator. Heda et al. (60) later showed that certain model formulations produced higher weight variation when run on a Zanasi machine than when run on an H & K GKF machine and related that difference to a need for greater compactibility when running on the dosator machine.

Flowability. In their analysis of the running of model formulations on a Zanasi LZ-64 and an H & K GKF 400 machine, Heda et al. (60) observed that an optimal degree of fluidity may be required for successful encapsulation on either machine. A CI% value of 20 to 30 appeared to be a suitable value for filling model formulations on both machines based on an analysis of weight variation. Highly free-flowing powders that tend to flood can cause filling problems in both types of machines. In addition, such powders often do not form plugs well enough to be transferred by a dosator. Podczeck and Newton (67) concluded that such powders could be handled in a dosing disk machine by increasing the powder bed height.

Dosing Disk Machines May Have a Lower Lubricant Requirement

When transferring a formulation originally developed on a Zanasi machine to an H & K GKF-1500, Ullah et al. (68) found that drug dissolved more slowly from the capsules filled on the dosing disk machine than from those filled on the dosator machine. They proposed that the slower dissolution was the result of shearing the laminar magnesium stearate during the tamping step in the H & K machine, thereby resulting in excessive coating of the formulation with the hydrophobic lubricant. They found that the problem could be solved by reducing the initial level of lubricant from 1% to 0.3%. This decision was based on a study using a laboratory scale mixer/grinder to simulate the shearing action of the filling machine. Satisfactory dissolution was obtained with 570 and 1100 kg (full production) size batches using this reduced level of lubricant.

Comparing model formulations at equivalent magnesium stearate levels and compression forces, Heda et al. (60) observed that plug ejection forces were lower on the H & K GKF 400 machine than on the Zanasi LZ-64. On the basis of ejectability, the dosing disk machine appeared to require about half as much magnesium stearate for the materials and conditions studied. This observation possibly reflects a greater shearing of magnesium stearate in the dosing disk machine, as proposed by Ullah et al. (68).

Formulations May Exhibit Different Dissolution Profiles

As discussed above, the same formulation run on the two types of machines may exhibit different dissolution profiles due to differences in the shearing of magnesium stearate, but conceivably, other factors could also affect dissolution. Dissolution may be affected by differences in plug density/porosity that result from differences in such variables as compression force, dwell time, and rates of compression. In a dosator machine simulator, higher piston compression speed produced a less consolidated plug (55), and plug porosity was inversely related to piston compression force (18). In dosing disk machines, the added time under pressure that already-formed plug segments can experience at additional tamping stations may lead to further densification of ductile formulations (23).

Multiple tamping, as compared with the single compression step of a dosator machine, may also affect dissolution. Using an instrumented dosing disk machine (H & K GKF 330), Shah et al. (69) found slower dissolution of hydrochlorothiazide after two and again after three tamps at a particular tamping force compared with a single tamp at the same compression force. The effect was more marked at a compression force of 200 N than at 100 N. At 100 N, mean plug pore diameter determined by Hg intrusion decreased from 12.8 μm after one tamp to 10.8 μm after two tamps. No further decrease in men pore size was noted after a third tamp at 100 N. Interestingly, the inclusion of 4% of the super disintegrant, croscarmellose, effectively eliminated the effects of multiple tamps or compression force on dissolution.

In their study of model formulations filled using both an instrumented dosator (Zanasi LZ-64) and an instrumented dosing disk machine (H & K GKF 400), Heda et al. (60) compared the dissolution profiles from capsules filled on both machines. Two compression forces were compared: 100 and 200 N. For ascorbic acid, they found two cases where the f_2 value was less than 50, suggesting that the dissolution profiles for those formulations are different when filled on the two machines with the same compression force. When dissolution profiles of hydrochlorothiazide from capsules filled on both machines were compared, the f_2 value was less than 50 for one formula at 100-N compression force. These differences in dissolution between the two machines indicated by the f_2 metric would suggest the need for a preapproval supplement, were they the outcome of a postapproval change in filling machines, since these machines belong same class, but different subclasses (56). The guidance also notes that such changes should be carefully considered and evaluated on a case-by-case basis, and places the burden on the applicant to provide the scientific data and rationale at the time of change to determine whether or not a preapproval supplement is justified. These FDA reviews such data at its discretion.

GRANULATIONS

In a survey of industry practices, Heda (12) found that as a matter of policy, 46% of the firms sampled favor direct filling of powders as a first choice over granulation prior to filling capsules. Thirty-six percent of firms allow formulators to make that decision at their own discretion; whereas, 18% of firms favor granulation of all formulations prior to encapsulation. Yet, for half of the firms responding, only 0% to 10% of their hard shell capsule products are direct-fill powder formulations, and only 27% of firms reported that more than 50% of their capsules were developed as direct-fill formulations. Although some of these non-direct-fill formulations may be controlled-release formulations, for example, barrier coated bead products, difficult direct-fill formulation problems may at least in part account for this observation.

The standard wet and dry methods used to granulate powders prior to tableting are used. When formulators granulate prior to encapsulation, they frequently do so to increase density. Thus, the weight that can be filled in a given size capsule can be increased, or a smaller capsule size can be selected. However, granulation can enhance a number of other processing characteristics and properties. Flow and compression properties of formulations can be improved, Dustiness and particle adhesion to metal surfaces can be reduced. Granulation also increases robustness by reducing variability in the physical properties of raw materials. Wet granulation may improve wettability and drug dissolution through hydrophilization (70,71). Common binders used in wet granulation such as pregelatinized starch and polyvinyl pyrrolidone are hydrophilic can be expected to deposit on particle surfaces where they may enhance wettability. Granulation can improve content uniformity by holding drug particles in granules so that the formulation can be handled without loss of blend quality. Moreover, the binder liquid phase in wet granulation provides a convenient vehicle by which to introduce and uniformly disperse a very low-dose drug throughout the mass. Among the firms sampled by Heda (12), 64% favored wet granulation for capsule formulations, 18% favored dry granulation and the remainder had "no policy."

In general, the same principles as apply to filling powders should apply to the filling of granulations, with some qualification. For instance, Podczeck et al. (67) found that an acceptable filling performance was always achieved when different granule size fractions of Sorbitol instant® were filled on both a dosing disk (Bosch GKF 400) machine and a dosator (Zanasi AZ 5) machine. However, the dosing disk machine, which depends less on forming firm plugs, seemed slightly better suited to the coarser granule size fractions than the dosator machine. On the other hand, the dosator machine invariably produced plugs that were denser than the formulation maximum bulk density, suggesting that this dosing principle might be more useful for granulations where the dose is large or where smaller capsule size is desired.

REFERENCES

1. Mehta AM, Augsburger LL. A preliminary study of the effect of slug hardness on drug dissolution from hard gelatin capsules filled on an automatic capsule filling machine. Int J Pharm 1981; 7:327–334.
2. Cropp JW, Augsburger LL, Marshall K. Simultaneous monitoring of tamping force and piston displacement (F-D) on an Hofliger-Karg capsule filling machine. Int J Pharm 1991; 71:127–136.
3. Britten JR, Barnett MI, Armstrong NA. Construction of an intermittant-motion capsule filling machine simulator. Pharm Res 1995; 12:196.
4. Heda PK, Muller FX, Augsburger LL. Capsule filling machine simulation. I. Low-force powder compression physics relevant to plug formation. Pharm Dev Technol 1999; 4(2):209–219.
5. Roberts RJ, Rowe RC. The effect of punch velocity on the compaction of a variety of materials. J Pharm Pharmacol 1985; 37:377–384.
6. Muller FX, Augsburger LL. The role of the displacement-time waveform in the determination of Heckel behavior under dynamic conditions in a compaction

simulator and a fully-instrumented rotary tablet machine. J Pharm Pharmacol 1994; 46:468–475.

7. Jolliffe IG, Newton, JM, Walters JK. Theoretical considerations of the filling of pharmaceutical hard gelatine capsules. Powder Technol 1980; 27:189–195.

8. Jolliffe IG, Newton JM. Practical implications of theoretical considerations of capsule filling by the dosator nozzle system. J Pharm Pharmacol 1982; 34:293–298.

9. Patel R, Podczeck F. Investigation of the effect of type and source of microcrystalline cellulose on capsule filling. Int J Pharm 1996; 128:123–127.

10. Guo M, Augsburger LL. Potential application of silicified microcrystalline cellulose in direct-fill formulations for automatic capsule-filling machines. Pharm Dev Technol 2003; 8(1):47–59.

11. Irwin GM, Dodson GJ, Ravin LJ. Encapsulation of clomacron phosphate I. Effect of flowability of powder blends, lot-to-lot variability, and concentration of active ingredient on weight variation of capsules filled on an automatic capsule filling machine. J Pharm Sci 1970; 59:547–550.

12. Heda PK. A comparative study of the formulation requirements of dosator and dosing disc encapsulators. Simulation of plug formation, and creation of rules for an expert system for formulation design. Ph D Dissertation, University of Maryland, Baltimore, MD, 1998.

13. Wells JJ. Pharmaceutical Preformulation: the Physicochemical Properties of Drug Substances. Chichester: Ellis Horwood Ltd., 1988:209–210.

14. Augsburger LL, Shangraw RF. Effect of glidants in tableting. J Pharm Sci 1966; 55:418–423.

15. Sadek HM, Olsen JL, Smith HL, et al. A systematic approach to glidant selection. Pharm Tech 1982; 6(2):43–62.

16. York P. Application of powder failure testing equipment in assessing effect of glidants on flowability of cohesive pharmaceutical powders. J Pharm Sci 1975; 64:1216–1221.

17. Small LE, Augsburger LL. Aspects of the lubrication requirements for an automatic capsule-filling machine. Drug Dev Ind Pharm 1978; 4:345.

18. Tattawasart A, Armstrong NA. The formation of lactose plugs for hard shell capsules. Pharm Dev Technol 1993; 2:335–343.

19. Jones BE. Powder formulations for capsule filling. Manuf Chem 1988; 59(7):28–30, 33.

20. Davar N, Shah R, Pope DG, et al. Rational approach to the selection of a dosing disk on a Hofliger Karg capsule filling machine. Pharm Technol 1997; 21:32–48.

21. Shah KB, Augsburger LL, Marshall K. An investigation of some factors influencing plug formation and fill weight in a dosing disk-type automatic capsule-filling machine. J Pharm Sci 1986; 75(3):291–296.

22. Podczeck F. The development of an instrumented tamp-filling capsule machine I.: instrumentation of a Bosch GKF 400S machine and feasibility study. Eur J Pharm Sci 2000; 10:267–274.

23. Podczeck F. The development of an instrumented tamp-filling capsule machine II: investigations of plug development and tamping pressure at different filling stations. Eur J Pharm Sci 2001; 12:501–507.

24. Cole G. Capsule filling. Chem Eng (London), 1982; 382:473–473.

25. Newton JM, Rowley G. On the release of drug from hard gelatin capsules. J Pharm Pharmacol 1970; 22:163 S–168 S.

26. Newton JM, Rowley G, Tornblom JFV. The effect of additives on the release of drug from hard gelatin capsules. J Pharm Pharmacol 1971; 23:452–453.

27. Withey RJ, Mainville CA. A critical analysis of a capsule dissolution test. J Pharm Sci 1969; 58:1120–1126.

28. Jones BE. Two-piece gelatin capsules: excipients for powder products, European practice. Pharm Tech Europ 1995; 7(10):25–34.

29. Shangraw RF, Demarest DA. A survey of current industrial practices in the formulation and manufacture of tablets and capsules. Pharm Technol, 1993; 17:32–44.

30. Samyn JC, Jung WY. In vitro dissolution from several experimental capsules. J Pharm Sci 1970; 59:169–175.

31. Shah AC, Mlodozeniec AR. Mechanism of surface lubrication: influence of duration of lubricant-excipient mixing on processing characteristics of powders and properties of compressed tablets. J Pharm Sci 1977; 66:1377–1381.
32. Miller TA, York P. Pharmaceutical tablet lubrication. Int J Pharm 1988; 41:1–19.
33. Harding VD, Higginson SJ, Wells JJ. Predictive stress tests in the scale-up of capsule formulations. Drug Devel Ind Pharm 1989; 15:2315–2338.
34. Murthy KS, Samyn JC. Effect of shear mixing on in vitro drug release of capsule formulations containing lubricants. J Pharm Sci 1977; 66:1215–1219.
35. Nakagwu H. Effects of particle size of rifampicin and addition of magnesium stearate in release of rifampicin from hard gelatin capsules. Yakugaku Zasshi 1980; 100:1111–1117.
36. Botzolakis JE, Small LE, Augsburger LL. Effect of disintegrants on drug dissolution from capsules filled on a dosator-type automatic capsule-filling machine. Int J Pharm 1982; 12:341–349.
37. Botzolakis JE, Augsburger LL. The role of disintegrants in hard-gelatin capsules. J Pharm Pharmacol 1984; 37:77–84.
38. Piscitelli DA, Bigora S, Propst C, et al. The impact of formulation and process changes on in vitro dissolution and bioequivalence of piroxicam capsules. Pharm Dev Technol 1998; 3(4):443–452.
39. Bateman SD, Verlin J, Russo M, et al. The development of a capsule formulation knowledge-based system. Pharm Technol 1996; 20(3):174, 178, 180, 182, 184.
40. Lai S, Podczeck F, Newton JM, et al. An expert system to aid the development of capsule formulations. Pharm Tech Eur 1996; 8(October):60–65.
41. Guo M, Kalra G, Wilson W, et al. A prototype intelligent hybrid system for hard gelatin capsule formulation development. Pharm Technol 2002; 26(9):44–60.
42. Kalra G, Peng Y, Guo M, et al. A hybrid intelligent system for formulation of BCS class II drugs in hard gelatin capsules. Proceedings, International Conference on Neural Information Processing (Singapore), 4, 1987–1991.
43. Amidon GL, Lennernas H, Shah VP, et al. A theoretical basis for a biopharmaceutic drug classification: the correlation of in vitro drug product dissolution and in vivo bioavailability. Pharm Res 1995; 12:413–420.
44. Wilson W, Peng Y, Augsburger LL. Generalization of a prototype intelligent hybrid system for hard gelatin capsule formulation development. AAPS Pharm Sci Tech 2005; 6(3):E449–E457. Available at: http://www.aapspharmscitech.org/view.asp?art=pt060356.
45. Wilson WI, Peng Y, Augsburger LL. Comparison of statistical analysis and Bayesian networks in the evaluation of dissolution performance of BCS class II model drugs. J Pharm Sci 2005; 94(12):2764.
46. Augsburger LL. Instrumented capsule-filling machines: development and application. Pharm Technol 1982; 9:111–119.
47. Cole GC, May G. The instrumentation of a Zanasi LZ/64 capsule filling machine. J Pharm Pharmacol 1975; 27:353–358.
48. Small LE, Augsburger LL. Instrumentation of an automatic capsule filling machine. J Pharm Sci 1977; 66:504.
49. Mehta AM, Augsburger LL. Simultaneous measurement of force and displacement in an automatic capsule-filling machine. Int J Pharm 1980; 4:347.
50. Greenberg R. Effects of AZ-60 filling machine dosator settings upon slug hardness and dissolution of capsules, Proc. 88th National Meeting, Am Inst Chem Engrs, Session 11, Philadelphia, PA, June 8–12 (Fiche 29), 1980.
51. Hauer VB, Remmele T, Sucker H. Gizieltes entwickeln und optimieren von kapselformulierungen mit einer instrumentieten dossierröhrchen-kapselabfüllmaschine I. Mitteilung: instrumentierung und einfluß der füllgut-und maschineparameter. Pharm Ind 1993; 55:509–515.
52. Shah KB, Augsburger LL, Small LE, et al. Instrumentation of a dosing-disc automatic capsule filling machine. Pharm Technol 1983; 7(4):42.
53. Jolliffe IG, Newton JM, Cooper D. The design and use of an instrumented MG2 capsule filling machine simulator. J Pharm Pharmacol 1982; 34:230–235.

54. Britten JR, Barnett MI. Development and validation of a capsule filling machine simulator. Int J Pharm 1991; 71:R5.

55. Britten JR, Barnett MI, Armstrong NA. Studies on powder plug formation using a simulated capsule filling machine. J Pharm Pharmacol 1996; 48:249–254.

56. Guidance for industry, SUPAC IR: immediate release oral solid dosage forms: scale-up and post approval changes: manufacturing and controls, in vitro dissolution testing and in vivo bioequivalenve documentation, FDA, CDER, FDA, November 1995. Available at: http://www.fda.gov/downloads/Drugs/GuidanceCompliance RegulatoryInformation/Guidances/ucm070636.pdf.

57. Guidance for Industry, SUPAC-IR/MR—Manufacturing Equipment Addendum, FDA, CDER, January 1999. Available at: http://www.fda.gov/downloads/Drugs/ GuidanceComplianceRegulatoryInformation/Guidances/UCM070637.pdf.

58. Van Tol J. Robert Bosch Packaging Technology. Minneapolis, Mn, Personal Communication, 2005.

59. Kurihara K, Ichikawa I. Effect of powder flowability on capsule filling weight variation. Chem Pharm Bull 1978; 26:1250–1256.

60. Heda PK, Muteba K, Augsburger LL. Comparison of the formulation requirements of dosator and dosing disc automatic capsule filling machines. AAPS Pharm Sci 2002; 4(3), Art. 17:1–17.

61. Podczeck F. Powder, granule and pellet properties for filling of two-piece hard capsules, chapter 5. In: Podczeck F, Jones BE, eds. Pharmaceutical Capsules. 2nd ed. London: Pharmaceutical Press, 2004:108.

62. McKee J. MG America. Fairfield, NJ, Personal Communication, 2005.

63. Desai DS, Rubitska BA, Bergum JS, et al. Physical interactions of magnesium stearate with starch-derived disintegrants and their effects on capsule and tablet dissolution. Int J Pharm 1993; 91:217–226.

64. Johansen H, Andersen I, Leedgaard H. Segregation and continued mixing in an automatic capsule filling machine. Drug Dev Ind Pharm 1989; 15:477–488.

65. Xie L, Wu H, Shen M, et al. Quality-by-design (QbD): effects of testing parameters and formulation variables on the segregation tendency of pharmaceutical powder measured by the ASTM D 6940-04 segregation tester. J Pharm Sci 2008; 97:4485–4497.

66. Ridgway K, Callow JAB. Capsule-filling machinery. Pharm J 1973; 212:281–285.

67. Podczeck F, Newton JM. Powder filling into hard gelatine capsules on a tamp filling machine. Int J Pharm 1999; 185:237–254.

68. Ullah I, Wiley GJ, Agharkar SN. Analysis and simulation of capsule dissolution problem encountered during product scale-up. Drug Dev Ind Pharm 1992; 18(8): 895–910.

69. Shah KB, Augsburger LL, Marshall K. Multiple tamping effects on drug dissolution from capsules filled on a dosing-disk type automatic capsule filling machine. J Pharm Sci 1987; 76:639.

70. Lerk CF, Lagas M, Fell JT, et al. Effect of hydrophilization of hydrophobic drugs on release rate from capsules. J Pharm Sci 1978; 67:935–939.

71. Lerk CF, Lagas M, Lie-A-Huen L, et al. In vitro and in vivo availability of hydro-philized phenytoin from capsules. J Pharm Sci 1979; 68:634–637.

16 Scale-up of film coating

Stuart C. Porter

INTRODUCTION

A comprehensive overview of pharmaceutical coating (materials, formulations, and processes) has been given by Porter and Bruno (1). It should be noted that there has been a steady transition in the pharmaceutical industry, beginning with sugar coating, moving to film coating, and finally arriving at aqueous film coating.

Sugar coating can be characterized as a relatively complex but noncritical process. Complexity stems from the multiplicity of coating formulations used during one process, and the sequencing (dosing, distributing, and drying) that must take place for each application of coating liquid; noncriticality is associated with the fact that precise control over process parameters (air volumes, temperatures, spray rates, etc.) is not a prerequisite for success in the process. In contrast, film coating is relatively simple but critical process. In this case, simplicity relates to the need to use fewer (and, sometimes, only one) coating formulations during the process, which are usually applied in a continuous but controlled manner; criticality is manifest by the need to identify, and control, a range of key processing factors, especially when applying water-based coating formulations.

Sugar coating, once dominant in the pharmaceutical industry, has been superseded for the most part by film coating, with a strong preference being shown for aqueous-based processes.

Film coating was formally introduced into the pharmaceutical industry in the middle of the last century. Initially intended to provide a means for more rapidly applying coatings to pharmaceutical tablets, it has readily been adapted for coating other types of products (such as pellets, granules, powders, and capsules). In general terms, film coating is a process during which a polymer-based coating is applied to the substrate in a manner whereby

- the rate of application of the coating fluid and the drying rate are carefully controlled;
- the coating material is uniformly applied to the surface of the substrate; and
- the quality and functionality of the applied coating are reproducibly optimized.

Although film coatings are commonly applied for aesthetic reasons, they also have an important role to play in improving product stability and robustness, masking taste, facilitating ingestion, and modifying drug-release characteristics. There is also a growing interest in using the film-coating process as a means of applying additional pharmaceutical ingredients (API) to an already formed dosage unit (such as a tablet).

The intended functionalities of film coatings are quite diverse, both in terms of their required effects on drug release as well as the potential to enhance product stability. The form in which film coatings may be applied is quite broad, including

- organic solvent based solutions of polymers (1),
- aqueous solutions or dispersions of polymers (2),
- hot-melt systems (3), and
- powder coatings (3).

Although film coatings and film-coating processes have a much more scientific foundation than sugar coatings, there is still much that remains ill-defined. Consequently, scaling up film-coating processes can pose a significant challenge, especially when the required functionality of the applied film coating becomes technically more complex.

It is one of the intriguing contradictions of film coating, especially when considering aqueous processes, that, in order to create a more robust finished product, the product being coated has to be equally robust if it is to survive a process that becomes progressively more stressful as the scale of process increases. The stressful conditions to which a product is exposed during film coating is associated with both the environmental conditions within the process and the attritional effects to which that product being coated is subjected. Failure to appreciate these issues can reduce the likelihood of achieving complete success during the scale-up process. It is also worth remembering that process scale-up is not a one-time event, rather it can be an ongoing process that is driven by the need to increase capacity, and cut operating costs, throughout the product life cycle. Under these circumstances, the need to implement process changes is ever-present. Nonetheless, there can be no question that taking great steps to confirm the robustness of both formulations (core and coating) and coating processes during the early phases of process development can pay great dividends during the subsequent scale-up process. More on this subject will be discussed later in this chapter.

Film Coating—Basic Processing Concepts

At the heart of any coating process is the coating vessel, which can exist in one of two basic forms, namely:

- Coating pans
- Fluid bed coating equipment

Initially, film-coating equipment was commonly based on that used in sugar-coating processes, namely, conventional coating pans. From its earliest beginnings, however, there was a strong appreciation for the fact that special-ized film-coating equipment was needed. The subsequent introduction of such equipment included the fluid bed coating process developed by Dale Wurster (4), which was quickly adopted for many film-coating operations. Concurrent development of the side-vented coating pan (initially in the form of the Accela-Cota) has also made a significant impact on film-coating processing technolo-gies. With the current preference shown for aqueous processes, side-vented (or perforated) coating pans are typically preferred for coating tablets, while fluid bed processes are more commonly employed for coating multiparticulates (5). While the pharmaceutical process engineer is now faced with a myriad of equipment choices, the operating principles of modern film-coating equipment (as illustrated in Figs. 1 and 2) have changed little in the last 30 years.

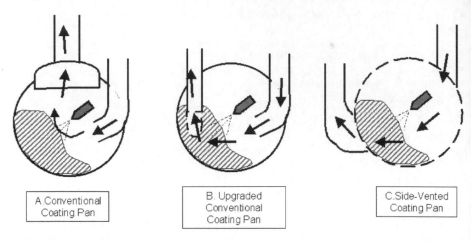

FIGURE 1   Schematic diagram highlighting the basic concepts of pan-coating equipment.

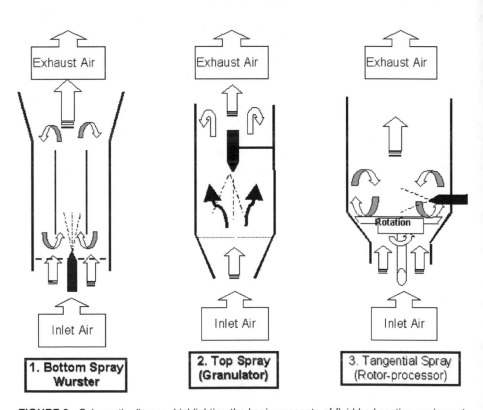

FIGURE 2   Schematic diagram highlighting the basic concepts of fluid-bed coating equipment.

While the availability of a variety of equipment has done much to expand the scope of film coating, such variety often adds an extra degree of complexity to the scale-up process. Geographical preferences in equipment selection (often as the result of a desire to source locally and take advantage of vendor support programs) often mean that the manufacturing-scale equipment selected may differ from that used during process development in another part of the world, even when the equipment used in both cases is essentially based on the "same operating principles."

As a final note, the more recent introduction of continuous coating processes has provided more options, with their attendant challenges, to be considered during scale-up.

Thermodynamics of the Film-Coating Process

At the heart of any film-coating process is the need to understand the complex interaction that takes place while the coating liquid is being applied and the volatile solvents are being removed. Never is this more true than when considering the aqueous process. The application of thermodynamic models not only allows development-scale coating processes to be fundamentally characterized, as suggested by Ebey (6) and Choi (7), but also facilitates more accurate predictions for operating production-scale processes in a manner that more closely replicates the development-scale processes.

Of course, while it would be desirable to operate all processes under constant conditions, such ideality is often beyond the practical capabilities of many film-coating operations. Application of thermodynamic concepts proposed by Ebey (6) and Choi (7), however, usually permit predictive processing adjustments to be made in order to allow for natural variation in the coating process. For example, for a process where the moisture content of the processing air varies from day to day, season to season, etc., it is possible to determine what changes, for example, in spray rates, inlet air temperatures, or inlet air volumes are required to maintain the product temperature at the predetermined set point. By way of example, the initial process conditions outlined in Table 1 represent those for an aqueous film-coating process conducted in a laboratory-scale coating pan where the inlet air has a dew point of 4.5°C. The modified conditions in the same table illustrate how the process can be adjusted, by changing the spray rate, to maintain an equivalent process when the moisture content of the inlet air has increased (as exemplified by a dew point of 15.5°C).

TABLE 1   Example of Application of Thermodynamic Model to Predict Adjustments in Process Conditions When the Inlet Air Moisture Content Is Increased

Process parameter	Initial process	Modified process
Spray rate (g/min)	75	72
Coating solution solids content (% w/w)	15.0	15.0
Inlet air temperature (°C)	70	70
Inlet air dew point (°C)	4.5	15.5
Process air volume		
(cfm)	200	200
(m³/hr)	350	350
Exhaust air temperature (°C)	43	44
Environmental equivalency factor, EE	1.761	1.761

While mathematical tools such as those described by Ebey are useful for predicting adjustments in order to maintain the equivalency of two processes, it must be remembered that these tools examine the macroenvironment within those processes. The changes that may, however, be taking place at the microscopic level (e.g., when droplets of coating liquid make contact, and begin to interact, with the surface of tablets, pellets, etc.) are much more complex and much less predictable. The use of mathematical models as suggested here, however, still have value in making predictions that can often reduce the actual number of coating trials that need to be performed, even though they cannot be used to predict empirical results such as coated tablet aesthetics.

Boundaries of the Film-Coating Process

Unlike many of the processes described elsewhere in this book, the film-coating process is inherently much more complex (see the operational boundaries highlighted in Fig. 3), since the parameters that influence the outcome are much more extensive. The existence and potential impact of these factors make achieving ultimate success more challenging.

Fundamentally, three components of the film-coating process contribute, in a very much interactive manner, to the overall success of the process:

- the core (ingredients; size; shape; surface chemistry; and physical attributes, etc.);
- the coating (ingredients; solvents; surface chemistry, rheology, tackiness, etc.); and

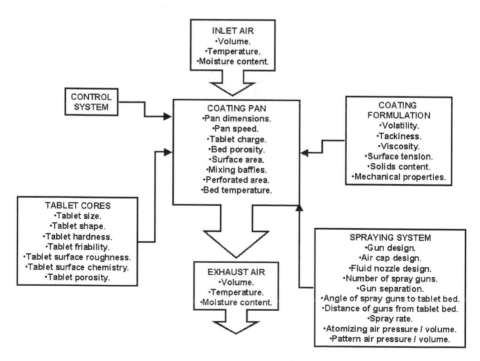

FIGURE 3 Outline of the operational boundaries of a film-coating process.

- the coating process (equipment design; process parameters employed; maintenance and calibration programs, etc.).

While the operational boundaries shown in Figure 3 relate specifically to tablet coating in a side-vented pan, the concepts are applicable to the film coating of all types of products in a wide variety of coating machines.

SCALING UP THE COATING PROCESS
General Factors to Consider

The introductory section has provided the reader with some idea of the complexities of pharmaceutical coating processes, especially those relating to the now predominant aqueous film-coating process. These complexities can be transformed into serious challenges that face the scientists and engineers charged with the responsibility for scaling up the coating process. Unlike processes associated with many other unit operations, scaling up the film-coating process involves much more than just dealing with larger batch sizes and faster throughputs. Application of coatings, often being the penultimate step prior to packaging, can leave a long-lasting impression in terms of product appearance and product performance (both in terms of functionality and stability). Additionally, once the coating stage is reached, there has already been a substantial investment (time and money) in that batch. In a somewhat simplistic way, scale-up of a coating process typically involves the following:

- Taking a laboratory-scale process (hopefully one that has been appropriately optimized) and transferring the processing technology first to the pilot scale and ultimately to full-production scale.
- Further optimizing the process on the larger scale to take into account issues whose influence could not easily be predicted during earlier process-development activities.

Irrespective of the type of coating process used, the potential process changes that commonly occur on scale-up include the following:

- Larger batch sizes
- Greater attritional effects
- Faster spray rates
- More spray guns
- Higher process air volumes
- Longer processing times (per batch)
- Different environmental conditions
- Different processing equipment (especially spray guns)

While the impact of these changes can often be quite predictable, especially when applying some of the thermodynamic concepts described earlier, the influence of some changes may be less so. For example, the impact of increased processing time, which brings with it increased exposure to stressful conditions (both mechanical and as a result of environmental conditions used in the process, especially when that process is aqueous based) is more uncertain and often leads to the need to consider making several process adjustments during the preparation of early commercial batches.

The Robustness Factor

In spite of the issues outlined in the previous section, all too often the attention spent on formulation and process design is inconsistent with the impact of the negative consequences faced when performance in the coating operation fails to meet expectations. More attention, of course, tends to be paid when the applied coating has some specialized functionality (such as improving product shelf life or modifying drug-release characteristics); however, even when the defects are aesthetic in nature and have little or no impact on product performance, failure to meet the required visual standards all too often results in batch rejection, leading to

- discarding the batch (often determined on the basis of balancing recovery costs with the inherent value of the batch),
- reprocessing the batch, and
- sorting the batch to remove defective material.

Each of these circumstances has an implicit financial impact.

Clearly, therefore, there is a strong incentive to ensure the following:

- The formulations (core and coating) are sufficiently robust to meet the needs of the operation. This requirement is all the more important when viewed in terms of the increased (but often ill-defined) stresses to which the product is subjected on scale-up.
- Critical elements of the coating process and their impact on final product quality (in the broadest sense) have been determined and taken into account during process optimization.

While these requirements seem obvious, they are often overlooked. Critical decisions with respect to design of coating formulations and processes are frequently made on the basis of data produced from small-scale processing trials. The consequences of such decisions only become apparent after product approval, thus resulting in the fact that the changes required to rectify matters are often very much constrained by regulatory issues [although these may be diminished to a degree as a result of the issuance of the Scale-Up and Post-Approval Change (SUPAC) guidances].

One of the elements of film coating that attracts much attention at technical symposia is that dealing with "troubleshooting." This very fact is a clear indication of how poorly the matters described here are considered. While it is certainly important to understand the factors that can potentially lead to problems and explore recovery options, the very idea that troubleshooting needs to be considered is clearly an admission of failure during critical stages of product and process development. The photographs shown in Figure 4 provide typical examples of problems that crop up all too often under the troubleshooting banner.

Opportunities for Process Optimization and Use of Expert Systems

Much of the data developed during product and process development is often empirically derived, and as such reflects the relative experience and preferences of those responsible for that development process. While application of prior experience should never be discounted, it is not unusual to find that each new product being developed, or process refinement being employed, has inherent

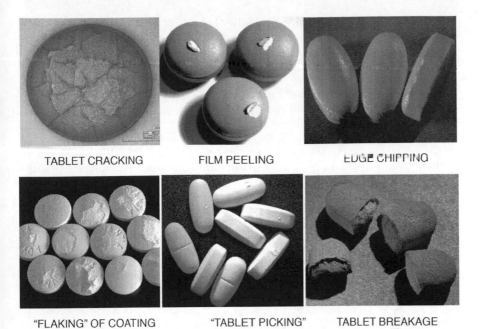

TABLET CRACKING   FILM PEELING   EDGE CHIPPING

"FLAKING" OF COATING   "TABLET PICKING"   TABLET BREAKAGE

FIGURE 4   Common examples of film-coating problems that trigger troubleshooting exercises.

idiosyncrasies for which prior experience does not provide all of the answers. In order to create a "robust" product and process, personal bias has to be removed and, instead, decisions must be made based on scientific validity.

All too often, the phrase "we have fully optimized the product and process" is used to describe a situation where decisions have been made on the basis of an iterative process where process (and formulation) variables have been studied in a "trial-and-error" manner, changing one parameter at a time. This process, often called one of "successive approximation," is followed until an acceptable process has been achieved. The problems associated with employing such techniques result in the fact that:

- A truly optimal process (or product) is rarely achieved.
- A comprehensive database, defining how critical parameters influence product quality, is rarely obtained.
- Subsequent decisions that demand further process modifications (e.g., on the basis of meeting operational requirements to improve process productivity or reduce process costs) often confound the "optimization" process.
- The need to meet the requirements of the Quality-by-Design (QbD) initiatives is compromised.

The answer to these concerns involves the employment, during the development process, of techniques that utilize statistical design-of-experiments (DoE) techniques.

The benefits of using such an approach have been well documented. For example, Porter et al. (8), in examining a side-vented pan process, were able to produce unambiguous quantitative results that defined how, inter alia, uniformity of distribution of the coating and coating process efficiency could be maximized while meeting other objectives with respect to coated product quality (e.g., gloss, smoothness, and residual moisture content). Turkoglu and Sakr (9), in studying the application of a modified-release coating to pellets in a rotary fluidized-bed process, determined that coating temperature and atomizing air pressure were key factors that influenced drug release from the pellets when applying an aqueous ethylcellulose dispersion. Finally, Rodriguez et al. (10) employed similar techniques when studying the thermodynamics of an aqueous film-coating process performed in a GS Coating Systems pan.

Ultimately, the real advantage of utilizing a DoE approach during process development and optimization is that:

- All critical process parameters can be identified in a way that removes personal bias.
- A truly optimized process can be developed, which has a sufficiently sound scientific basis to meet the requirements set by the various regulatory agencies.
- Further process refinements, particularly during scale-up, can be made in a much more predictable manner.
- The basis for defining critical process parameters can be more effectively established and used to greater effect when using the initiatives required by QbD.

Clearly then, adopting a formal, scientifically valid approach to designing and optimizing a particular coating process provides a good foundation ultimately for scaling up that process. That having been said, in these days of globalization, the scale-up process can involve technology transfer from one location to another that may be geographically remote from one another. In such a situation, the location on the receiving end of the transfer process may be in a technical void with respect to critical knowledge about that process. Under these circumstances, ready access to such technical information (on a 24-hour basis) is often of paramount importance if success in the scale-up process is to be achieved and maintained. Considering such knowledge may reside with only a few key people, the challenge is thus how to provide the necessary access. Conventional wisdom is to prepare exhaustive technical reports, either in hard copy or electronic form, than can be distributed as needs require. In the present environment, however, instant access to information, utilizing a user-friendly approach, is often demanded. One potentially effective approach involves the application of Expert Systems. Fundamentally, these systems consist essentially of a computer program that makes decisions or recommendations based on knowledge gained from experts in the field. Such programs are usually customized to fit a given situation and can utilize tools such as artificial neural networks, rule-based systems, decision trees, etc. The application of Expert Systems to pharmaceutical processes (including film coating) has been described by Rowe (11), and commercial availability of such systems has been demonstrated (12).

So far, the discussion has centered on describing the basis for typical film-coating processes, outlining some of the critical issues that need to be considered when contemplating process scale-up and identifying some useful tools that may be employed to facilitate that process. Clearly, there is no substitute for careful preparation, and the benefits of doing so can best be illustrated by reference to case studies that exemplify scale-up studies that have been successfully concluded. By way of example, two relevant case studies involve the following:

- Coating tablets in a pan process
- Coating pellets in a fluid bed process

These studies will be discussed later in this chapter.

Scaling Up a Pan-Coating Process
Introduction
It should now be quite evident that time and money spent in designing a robust process (where all of the critical process factors have been defined and their impact well documented) has potential cost benefits later on, especially during the time leading up to, and immediately after, product launch. In addition to providing a sound scientific approach to designing an optimal process, it also produces product knowledge that has great benefit in the training of process operators so that they become better informed about the critical constraints of that process.

In addition, if a particular process is applicable to a range of products that have similar characteristics, then time spent initially optimizing that process provides benefit many times over. Even when a process has been well characterized, the use of that process in a different application (such as the application of a modified-release film coating) may warrant further consideration. The challenges in these circumstances relate to the fact that the link between process characteristics and product performance may be less clear. For example, Ho et al. (13) have provided an example of the unexpected results that can occur when scaling up a coating process for the application of modified-release film coatings. In this case, they were able to demonstrate that even when great care is taken to ensure that the precise amount of coating has been applied, unidentified differences in coating process conditions that influence coating structure can create unexpected results in terms of drug-release characteristics.

Some key attributes of coated products and coating processes that may well be used to set objectives for optimizing a coating process are shown in Table 2. In some cases, the attributes as listed are very subjective and thus must

TABLE 2 Coated Product Attributes and Coating Process Characteristics That May Be Used as Objectives to Develop an Optimal Process

Coated tablet attributes		Coating process Characteristics
Aesthetic	Functional	
1. High gloss	1. Drug-release characteristics meet target requirements	1. High (and reproducible) process coating efficiency
2. Smooth coating		2. High uniformity of distribution (on a weight basis) of coating from tablet to tablet
3. Good color uniformity	2. Coated product meets stability requirements	
4. Absence of edge chipping		
5. Absence of film cracking	3. Effective taste masking is achieved (if required)	
6. Absence of logo bridging		3. High productivity
7. Absence of twinning	4. Coated tablet meets target strength requirements	
8. Absence of picking		

be defined in clearly measurable terms if they are to be used as the basis for process optimization. Additionally, meeting defined objectives may well also be influenced by formulation attributes associated with both the tablet core and the coating. Nonetheless, the information highlighted in Table 2 does provide guidelines as to the types of response that could be used as a basis for optimizing a coating process.

When optimizing coating processes, however, it is important that the critical parameters to be evaluated are carefully selected. The operating boundaries of a typical coating process (shown in Fig. 3) clearly indicate that the list of that can be considered as potentially quite extensive. Thus, in order to create a manageable DoE program, the number of variables to be studied should not typically exceed 4 or 5; otherwise the number of coating trials to be undertaken becomes prohibitive. Clearly, therefore, it is important to identify those variables that potentially have the greatest impact and would thus be considered to be critical to the success of the overall process. A useful approach to consider is to:

- Fix (as constants) those variables that are not open to change (e.g., selecting a particular type of coating pan, spray gun, mixing baffle design, pan loading, etc.).
- Utilize a preliminary screening technique, where a larger number of variables can be studied in a much more superficial manner. This approach enables the critical variables to be identified and then subsequently used as the basis for a more comprehensive evaluation.

Earlier reference was made to published articles that described the use of optimization techniques for coating processes. In particular, the one presented by Porter et al. (8) exemplifies how aesthetic, functional, and processing issues can be dealt with. The key elements of the study that formed the basis for this article are listed in Table 3, while typical results obtained in this study are

TABLE 3 Process Parameters Examined in a Study Designed to Optimize a Coating Process Based on the Use of a 24-in. Laboratory Side-Vented Coating Pan

Coating process variable	Variable range setting
A. Fixed operating parameters	
1. Pan loading (kg)	15.0
2. Drying air (cfm)	Inlet: 250, Exhaust: 300
3. Coating system	Opadry II
4. Quantity of coating applied (% w/w)	3.0 (theoretical)
5. Pattern air pressure:	
(psi)	30.0
(bar)	2.1
B. Variable operating parameters	
1. Solids content of coating suspension (% w/w)	10–20
2. Inlet air temperature (°C)	60–90
3. Spray rate (g/min)	35–75
4. Atomizing air pressure:	
(psi)	22–60
(bar)	1.5–4.1
5. Pan speed (rpm)	8–20
6. Number of spray guns used	1 or 2

TABLE 4 Typical Results Obtained in Optimization Study

Response measured	Response units	Response ranges
Uniformity of distribution of coating material	% RSD	11.88–59.59
Coating process efficiency	%	26.23–99.37
Roughness value of applied coating[a]	R_z, μm	7.76–15.90
Gloss value of applied coating[b]	G_u at 60° angle	2.60–3.78
Final moisture content of coated tablet[c]	% w/w	0.10–5.33
Exhaust temperature of coating process	°C	32.8–57.3

[a]The higher the value, the rougher the coating.
[b]The higher the value, the glossier the tablets.
[c]Initial uncoated tablet moisture content was 3.0% w/w.
Abbreviation: RSD, relative standard deviation.

summarized in Table 4. From these data, it is possible to optimize the coating process with respect to:

- Aesthetic qualities (gloss and coating smoothness) of the final coated tablet.
- Potential impact on final tablet stability (as this relates to product temperatures experienced in the process and residual coated tablet moisture content).
- Process efficiencies (with respect to actual vs. theoretical amount of coating applied and uniformity of distribution of the coating).

More importantly, on the basis of work performed as described in the article, an extensive database, relating to the coating process in question, was established, and key process variables (including their interactive effects) were identified that could provide the basis from which to begin the scale-up process.

Predicting Scale-Up Issues
Once an appropriate laboratory-scale process has been established, the critical process variables should have been determined. Some operating parameters (such as inlet air temperature, coating formulation to be used, and solids content of the coating solution/suspension) can be directly translated to the larger-scale process. Others, however, will have to change, and these include the following:

- Process (drying) air volume
- Pan speed
- Pan loading
- Number of spray guns to be used
- Gun to tablet-bed distance
- Spray rate
- Spray gun dynamics

Process (drying) air volume. Process air volume, although an easily adjustable parameter, is often selected based either on the equipment vendor's recommendations, or on the basis of conditions deemed optimal for the air-handling system that has been installed. The supply and exhaust air fan speeds should be set, based on the equipment used, to meet the negative pressure pan settings that are usually recommended. Once the appropriate drying air volume has been established, this setting becomes a driver for other key processing variables, such as spray rate (see later discussion).

It should be remembered, however, that process air volume can effectively be adjusted to offset inadequacies in other process drying factors (that might occur, for example, when the desired process temperatures cannot be attained, or when the moisture content of the process air is higher than desired).

Pan speed. Selecting the appropriate pan speed often becomes more of a challenge than is really necessary. Clearly tablet motion, a factor influenced greatly by pan speed, can be a major issue when it comes to potential tablet breakage, edge wear, and surface erosion. On the other hand, according to data established by Porter et al. (8), the uniformity of distribution of the applied coating is also greatly influenced by pan speed, with the higher pan speeds being better in this regard. Consequently, there is a great incentive to design tablet cores that can withstand high pan speeds in order to allow coating uniformity to be fully maximized.

In reality, pan speeds chosen on the production scale may well be lower simply because the tablets to be coated do not meet the robustness characteristics required of a coating process of that scale. Nonetheless, a useful "rule of thumb," based on pan speeds used on the laboratory scale and dimensions of the laboratory-scale equipment, is to calculate the linear velocity of the tablets in the coating pan, and then determine the pan speed on the larger scale, which will give an equivalent tablet linear velocity. In this way, tablet dwell time in the spray zone on the larger scale will be equivalent to that achieved on the smaller scale, and full benefit can be taken of the optimization strategies used on the smaller scale to maximize uniformity of distribution of the coating. The information shown in Table 5 illustrates how pan speed (at least as a good starting point) can be determined for scale-up purposes.

A final point to consider is the potential impact of pan speed on the effectiveness of the drying processes, even though pan speed is not, per se, a thermodynamic factor. For example, when the drying characteristics of the coating process are less than optimal, employment of high pan speeds (by shortening the dwell time in the spray zone) can reduce the potential for localized overwetting, thus reducing defects such as picking and sticking.

TABLE 5 Estimating Pan Speed on Scale-Up

Parameter	Pan size			
Pan diameter	24 in. (60 cm)	36 in. (90 cm)	48 in. (120 cm)	60 in. (150 cm)
Typical pan rotational speed ranges (rpm)	5–20	3–17	2–15	2–11
Pan circumference	75 in. (190 cm)	115 in. (290 cm)	150 in. (380 cm)	190 in. (480 cm)
Peripheral pan speed at 10 rpm	12.5 in./sec (31.8 cm/sec)	19.2 in./sec (48.8 cm/sec)	25.0 in./sec (63.5 cm/sec)	31.5 in./sec (80.0 cm/sec)
Projected pan rotational speed at a peripheral speed of 12.5 in./sec (31.8 cm/sec)[a]	10	6.5	5.0	4.0

[a]This example is based on the rotational speed of 10 rpm used in a laboratory-scale coating pan.

Pan loading. In general, defining appropriate pan loadings should be simple. A coating pan of given dimensions is designed to hold a certain charge of tablets. Unfortunately, pan loadings are usually defined in terms of *volume* fill, rather than by weight. Thus, the optimum pan loading by weight will vary from product to product depending on the *apparent density* (which takes into account the mass/volume ratio of an individual tablet, as well as the shape and size of that tablet) of that product. Even allowing for such product variation, calculating optimal pan loadings remains a simple task. There are, however, a number of factors that complicate the establishment of suitable pan loadings, namely:

- On the laboratory scale, it is not too difficult to ensure that a pan is appropriately loaded. Even when only a very small amount of product is available, this problem can be dealt with by bulking up active tablets with placebos to make a full charge.
- On the production scale, pan loading often has nothing to do with the ideal loading for the pan, but rather with the total batch weight of the compressed tablets, and how evenly these can be divided into a whole number of pan loads. For example, if the total batch weight is 750 kg and these tablets are to be coated in a pan that optimally holds 120 kg per run, then the pan-loading instructions may call for *seven* pan loads of 107 kg each to be coated (in which case, the pan will be underloaded by about 10%), or *six* pan loads of 125 kg (in which case, the pan may be overloaded by about 4.5%). While overloading by such a small amount may seem trivial and is certainly a better option than coating with an underloaded pan, care must be taken to ensure that excess tablets do not spill out as the pan rotates. Underloading the coating pan has several potential consequences, including the following:
  - The possibility that, in a side-vented coating pan, there may not be enough tablets in the pan to ensure that the exhaust air plenum is completely covered (in which case drying air will take the path of least resistance and flow directly toward the air plenum, rather than passing through the tablet bed). With some pan designs, this potential problem may be obviated by the placement of a sliding damper in the exhaust air plenum, so that the exposed part can be sealed off.
  - The potential that the side walls of the coating pan, or even baffles, become more exposed to the spray, causing coating liquid to build up on exposed metal surfaces, often with the results that tablets will stick to them. Again, with some foresight, changing the gun to bed distances, gun spacing, or indeed, the number of guns used can minimize this problem. These solutions are likely to be utilized if, for a particular product, the pan loadings are relatively constant. In situations where compression batch weights frequently vary, such corrective measures are less easily employed.
  - The likelihood that when the pan is significantly underloaded, as baffles move through the tablet bed as the pan rotates, the surface of the tablet bed moves sufficiently to change the gun to bed distance. This situation, as will be seen later, could potentially change the characteristics of the spray droplets that are impinging on the surfaces of the tablets.
  - As baffles become more exposed, and as pan speeds are constantly adjusted to keep the tablets in motion (more of a challenge in an

underloaded pan), the likelihood exists that tablets will experience increased attritional effects.

Consequently, during product and process development, the capacities of the coating pans should be kept in mind when defining compression batch weights (even when these are, as is quite common, defined in turn by blender capacities).

Number of spray guns to be used. For all film-coating processes, optimization of the spray zone should be considered with respect to these key criteria:

- Making sure that the full width of the tablet bed is covered, so that few, if any, tablets on the surface pass through the spray zone without receiving some coating.
- Setting up each gun (in terms of atomizing and pattern air) so that maximum coverage is achieved without compromising the quality (in terms of droplet size, size distribution, droplet density, and relative "wetness") of the atomized coating liquid.
- Avoiding overspray on to the pan sidewalls.

Clearly, the number of spray guns employed will be a factor in achieving these objectives, and this in turn will depend on the type of spray guns available. As will be shown later, the design features of the particular spray gun(s) being used can have a significant impact on spray dynamics (in terms of droplet-size distributions, droplet velocities, and spray coverage).

Consequently, the potential impact of spray gun design (on spray performance) can be a challenge on scale-up, since the type of spray guns available on the production-sized equipment may be different from those used on the development scale, primarily because of the following:

- The spray guns used on the laboratory scale are not capable of achieving the spray rates required or maintaining effective atomization at those higher spray rates on the larger scale.
- Scale-up may involve transfer to a manufacturing site that is geographically remote from that where process development was undertaken, and preference may have been shown for locally sourced spray guns.
- The manufacturing-scale coating equipment may well have been supplied with vendor preferred guns (although, today, most vendors are amenable to preferences expressed by their customers).

It is unfortunate that, all too often, the differences in performance exhibited by spray guns of different designs are not always appreciated, and the potential criticality of those differences may be lost on those assigned with the objective of designing a suitable coating process.

In conclusion, the main objectives are to maximize bed coverage and maintain equivalent spray dynamics. Achieving these objectives may greatly influence the choice in number of spray guns used since, as suggested in Figure 5, broader coverage per gun may well reduce the number of guns required, while more restricted coverage, often chosen in attempts to produce better-coated tablet quality (Table 6) will necessitate the use of a larger number of guns.

Gun to tablet-bed distance. There are few examples of where a truly scientific approach is taken to establish appropriate positioning of spray guns inside

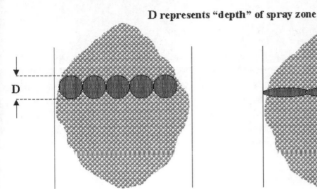

D represents "depth" of spray zone

A. 5 guns, round spray pattern

| Advantages: |
| •Smoother, glossier tablets. |
| •Denser, more uniform spray. |
| •Less risk of spray drying. |
| •Less overspray on pan walls. |
| Disadvantages: |
| •More guns required. |
| •Greater risk of localized overwetting. |

B. 3 guns, elliptical spray pattern

| Advantages: |
| •Fewer guns required. |
| •Less risk of localized overwetting. |
| Disadvantages: |
| •Greater risk of spray drying. |
| •Rougher coating on tablets. |
| •Greater risk of overspray on pan walls. |
| •Less uniform distribution of spray droplets. |

FIGURE 5 Influence of typical spray patterns on the number of spray guns used.

TABLE 6 Influence of Spray Pattern Used on Tablet Quality

Polymer concentration (% w/w)	Atomizing air pressure	Spray pattern shape	Mean coating roughness, R_a (μm)	% Tablets showing defects (picking or sticking)
9	40 psi (2.8 bar)	Elliptical	2.72	24.0
		Round	1.68	26.0
9	60 psi (4.1 bar)	Elliptical	2.53	4.5
		Round	1.44	35.0
9	80 psi (5.5 bar)	Elliptical	2.29	2.5
		Round	1.29	35.0
12	60 psi (4.1 bar)	Elliptical	3.51	2.0
		Round	2.07	9.0

coating pans (unlike with fluid bed coating machines where gun location is more often predetermined by equipment design). Typically, using simple tools, such as a ruler, the operator is often left to set up gun position by eye; modern tools, such as those that work on a laser principle, can help establish gun positioning (and gun angle) more accurately. Setting up the correct gun position is not a trivial matter, since such positioning needs to be optimized with respect to

- ensuring that optimal, and reproducible, bed coverage is achieved;
- facilitating broad coverage while providing maximum surface drying time (before tablets on the surface of the bed "fold under" and get mixed into the tablet mass); and

- achieving reproducible (from run-to-run) spray droplet characteristics as they arrive at the tablet surface (see later discussion).

It is a matter of record that spray-gun to tablet-bed distances are often different in production-scale equipment than they are in the equipment used in the laboratory. Fundamentally, however, if this parameter has been effectively optimized during process development (and it is debatable that it will have been), then, in order to maintain the same spray dynamics on the production scale (assuming the same type of spray gun is used), the same gun-to-bed distance should be used. Such an ideal rarely exists, and the rationale for why differences occur includes the following:

- On the laboratory scale, because of geometric constraints, there is often very little opportunity to optimize the gun-to-bed distance, and thus this parameter takes on a fixed setting (often defined by personal preference). This geometric constraint does not exist on the production scale.
- In production equipment, the number of spray guns supplied may well have been defined by the vendor, and the attendant "plumbing" (solution feed line and atomizing/pattern air line connections) may only support that number of guns. Consequently, in order to get effective bed coverage, the spray guns may have to be moved further away from the surface of the tablet bed.
- The required spray rate per gun, on the production scale, is likely to be substantially higher than on the laboratory scale, thus necessitating that the guns be moved further away (from the surface of the tablet bed) to prevent localized overwetting.

Clearly, careful attention must be paid to how spray guns are set up. In reality, unless spray gun positioning is optimized during process development, the same type of guns are to be used in both the laboratory and the manufacturing plant, and the spray rate per gun can be maintained (within reasonable ranges) in both cases, it is unrealistic to that the same gun-to-bed distances can be achieved independently of the scale of process used.

The result, therefore, is that gun-to-bed distances will typically be 50% to 60% greater on the production scale than those used on the typical laboratory scale (e.g., a 24-in., or 60-cm, diameter coating pan holding 12–16 kg of tablets).

Spray rate. If there are no major environmental differences (when moving from the laboratory into production) then predicting typical spray rates to be adopted during scale-up, at least as a starting point, should not be difficult. As a simple guideline, calculated predictions can be based on the relative airflows used for each scale of process, as shown in Eq. (1).

$$S_2 = \frac{(S_1 \times V_2)}{V_1} \tag{1}$$

where

S_1 is the spray rate used on the process development scale.
V_1 is the air volume used in process development.
V_2 is the air volume to be used in the larger-scale process.
S_2 is the predicted spray rate to be used as a starting point for the larger-scale process.

TABLE 7   Example of Operating Parameter Ranges Used When Scaling Up an Aqueous Film-Coating Process

| Parameter | Pan type (and size or model) | | | | | |
| | Accela-Cota | | | Hi-Coater | | |
	24 in.	48 in.	60 in.	HCT 60	HC 130	HC 170
Inlet air volume[a]:						
(a) cfm	250	1800	3800	260	900	1300
(b) m^3/hr	440	3200	6700	450	1600	2300
Exhaust air volume[a]:						
(a) cfm	300	2000	4000	280	1300	2100
(b) m^3/hr	525	3500	7000	500	2300	3700
Inlet temperature (°C)	60–80	60–80	60–80	60–80	60–80	60–80
Exhaust temperature (°C)	40–45	40–45	40–45	40–45	40–45	40–45
Spray rate (g/min)	40–70	250–500	500–1000	40–70	300–600	500–900
Pan speed (rpm)	12–14	4–7	3–6	12–14	4–7	3–6

[a]These are nominal air volumes since actual values may be different depending on the installation and whether the coating pan vendor or an independent supplier supplied the air-handling equipment.

If substantial changes in other thermodynamic parameters occur (such as environmental humidity, processing temperatures as a result of heater capabilities, etc.), then better predictions can be made using the thermodynamic principles outlined earlier (see page 447, Thermodynamics of the Film-Coating Process). It is interesting to note from these data that the drying (and exhaust) air volumes used in the production-scale Hi-Coaters (which are typical of a partially perforated pan design) are somewhat lower than those seen in an equivalent scale Accela-Cota, or, indeed, as might be predicted from studies conducted in a laboratory-scale Hi-Coater (Table 7). These differences reflect design considerations that suggest that, in the Hi-Coater, incoming air has essentially no place to go except out through the exhaust plenum and thus must pass through the coating pan (and thus, tablet bed). In other types of side-vented coating pans, particularly those that are completely perforated, incoming air is often introduced into a cabinet that surrounds the outside of the coating pan itself and must pass through the perforated section of the pan in order to gain access to the inside of the pan (and thus effectively dry the tablets). As a consequence, fully perforated pans are often operated with higher drying air volumes. These different requirements do not pose any problems unless there is a need to switch from one type of coating pan to another.

Such idiosyncrasies, in terms of airflow requirements for different styles of coating pan, complicate matters when attempting to apply the simple predictions (based on Eq. 1) for spray rates shown earlier. If the scale-up process involves switching from a laboratory-scale fully perforated pan to a production-scale partially perforated coating pan, there is a risk that the predicted spray rates will be understated. For the sake of the calculation, a useful rule of thumb is to *double* the value for the actual air volume that will be employed in the larger-scale partially perforated pan, and use that value solely for the purposes of calculation.

Spray gun dynamics. Earlier, frequent reference was made to the importance of establishing spraying conditions that are consistent from the development scale right up to that used in the manufacturing plant. Similarly, mention was also made of the scant attention typically paid to spraying dynamics and the lack of a strong understanding of what actually occurs when droplets of coating fluid emerge from a nozzle, move toward the tablet bed, and impinge upon the surfaces of tablets.

All too often, the role that spray gun design (namely, brand of gun, and features of the fluid nozzles and air caps used) can play in achieving good, and reproducible, coated tablet quality goes unrecognized. The fact that spray gun design may differ (from laboratory to production setting) is often considered to have little relevance, and accommodations for such differences are routinely made based on prior experience without the benefit of appropriate reference to scientifically derived data. A commonly held assumption, therefore, is that guns made by one manufacturer are essentially the same in terms of gun performance as those from another, and differences that exist are purely in the features presented and, ultimately, the cost.

Quality attributes of film-coated tablets that can be associated with spray-gun performance include the following:

- Appearance:
  - Coating gloss
  - Coating roughness
  - Existence of defects ("picking", edge chipping/edge wear, filling in of logos)
  - Color uniformity
- Functional:
  - Uniformity of distribution of coating
  - Coating porosity (which influences film permeability)
  - Solvent (water) penetration into the tablet cores, and hence product stability

Clearly, there is thus a great incentive to gain a better understanding of both the factors that influence gun performance, as well as the differences that exist between guns supplied from different manufacturers.

Cunningham (14) described some of the factors that can influence spray gun performance and compared the performance of spray guns from different vendors. As can be seen from the results shown in Figure 6 (where the performance of a Schlick spray gun is compared to a Spraying Systems spray gun), the influence of gun-to-bed distance and coating suspension solids content on mean droplet size is quite different for each type of spray gun. In both cases, droplet size tends to increase as distance from the nozzle increases (probably due to droplet collisions, causing size enlargement). The influence of coating suspension solids content on mean droplet size is much more pronounced, however, in the case of the Schlick gun (producing results in the range of approximately 25 to 275 µm compared to the Spraying Systems gun, which yield droplet sizes in the range of 30 to 60 µm under the same conditions). These results clearly have implications for situations where the type of gun may be changed on scale-up but also where gun-to-bed distance may be changed in the same process. Examining the data shown in Figure 7, the differences are even more pronounced when observing the influences of spray rate and atomizing air pressure on mean droplet size. Since spray rate

Fixed Settings:
Atomizing air pressure:- 30.0 psi
Pattern air pressure:- 27.5 psi
Spray rate:- 82.5 g min⁻¹

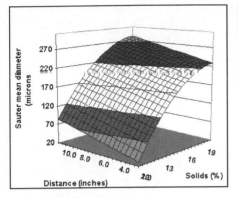
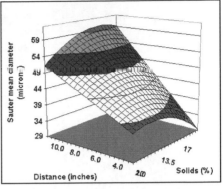

A. Schlick 930-33 Spray Gun

B. Spraying Systems VAU Spray Gun

FIGURE 6 Example of how the type of spray gun used, gun-to-bed distance, and solids content of the coating fluid can influence the size of droplets generated.

Fixed Settings:
Pattern air pressure:- 27.5 psi
Coating liquid solids:- 15.0 % w/w
Gun-to-bed distance:- 10 inches

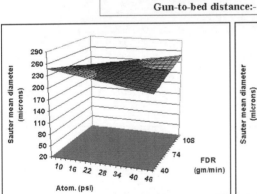
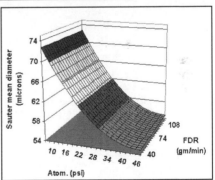

A. Schlick 930-33 Spray Gun

B. Spraying Systems VAU Spray Gun

FIGURE 7 Example of how the type of spray gun used, atomizing air pressure, and spray rate can influence the size of droplets generated.

and atomizing air pressure are commonly increased during process scale-up, it is likely that minimal change will occur when using a Schlick gun (of the type shown), but substantial changes are to be expected if a Spraying Systems VAU gun is used.

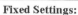

Fixed Settings:
             Pattern air pressure:-   0 psi
             Coating liquid solids:- 15.0 % w/w
             Spray rate:-   82.5 g min^{-1}

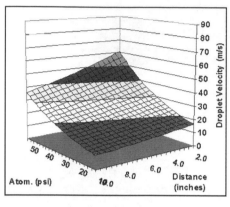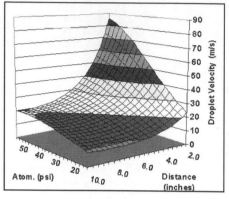

A. Schlick 930-33 Spray Gun   B. Spraying Systems VAU Spray Gun

FIGURE 8 Example of how the type of spray gun used, atomizing air pressure, and gun-to-bed distance can influence droplet velocity.

Evidently, gun design and atomizing conditions play a significant role in defining the characteristics of atomized coating liquids; the important question to be answered relates to the potential impact of such factors in the practical situation where tablets are to be coated in a typical coating pan. Certainly, the size of droplets formed can affect coating smoothness and gloss as well as have an influence on how rapidly the coating liquid dries during flight from the spray nozzle to the tablet surface.

It is also worth noting that the type of spray gun employed influences both droplet velocity (Fig. 8) and bed coverage (Fig. 9). Droplet velocity, at the moment of impact with the tablet surface, can affect:

- Wetting (velocity at impact can influence the advancing contact angle formed between the tablet surface and the droplet, and the degree to which the droplet spreads immediately after contact) and, ultimately, film adhesion. This process is often called dynamic wetting.
- Overspray, where the velocity at impact may cause droplets to be reflected (i.e., "bounce back") from the tablet surface and ultimately be deposited on exposed surfaces of the coating pan and spray equipment. This may effectively reduce coating process efficiency.

Bed coverage ultimately defines the number of spray guns that will be needed, and as the data shown in Figure 9 suggest, fewer spray guns of the Schlick type will be required to provide the same bed coverage as that achieved when using Spraying Systems VAU guns.

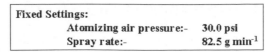

Fixed Settings:	
Atomizing air pressure:-	30.0 psi
Spray rate:-	82.5 g min^{-1}

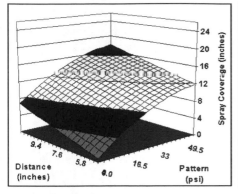

A. Schlick 930-33 Spray Gun

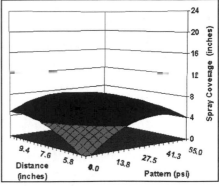

B. Spraying Systems VAU Spray Gun

FIGURE 9 Example of how the type of spray gun used, gun-to-bed distance, and pattern air pressure can influence bed coverage.

In summary, the results shown in Figures 6 to 9, while limited in scope, provide a clear indication of the potential problems that can occur if, during the scale-up process, commonly seen differences in spray-gun performance are ignored when replacing one type of spray gun with another.

Scale-Up of Pan-Coating Processes: A Case Study

From the discussion so far, there are clearly many issues to be confronted when scaling up the pan-coating process. Evidently, the more definitive data that are developed early on, the less likely that major problems will occur later on, especially problems that could inevitably delay a product launch and cost much in the way of lost revenues, particularly when dealing with a potentially "blockbuster" drug product.

In this case study, a pan-coating process designed for the application of an enteric coating to a tablet product is described, providing insight into some of the early process optimization studies that were undertaken and showing how these studies ultimately were used to create a successful manufacturing-scale process.

Process development. Initial studies were carried out using a laboratory-scale 24-in. Accela-Cota and employing a statistical DoE technique in which the operational variables examined are shown in Table 8. Although several response variables were included in this study, consideration was primarily given to achieving good functional enteric performance. Recognizing that enteric-coated products often lack sufficient robustness (exemplified by inherent brittleness of the coating, which can cause enteric failures during subsequent handling, such as

TABLE 8 Ranges of Process Variables Used During Optimization of the Enteric Film-Coating Process

Parameter studied	Ranges examined
Solids content of coating suspension (based on Sureteric® YAE-6-18108) (% w/w)	10–25
Inlet air temperature (°C)	50–70
Spray rate (g/min)	50–90
Quantity of coating applied (% w/w)	5–10
Atomizing air pressure (psi)	25–55
(bar)	1.75–3.75

emptying the coating pan, printing, packaging, etc.), an appropriate *stress test* (see later discussion) was used to determine the robustness characteristics of the coated tablets.

The two criteria used to measure enteric performance, therefore, were the following:

- *Enteric Test (ET)*: One hundred tablets were exposed to artificial gastric juice (0.1 N hydrochloric acid solution) for two hours using a modified disintegration tester. Performance was expressed in terms of *percent failure*, which was represented by the percentage of tablets showing any sign of enteric failure (such as premature disintegration, swelling, or even slight softening).
- *Stressed Enteric Test (SET)*: Essentially the same test as the ET, but in this case the 100 tablets were placed in a friability tester for four minutes at 25 rpm prior to being submitted for the enteric disintegration test in artificial gastric juice.

From this initial study and referring to the data shown in Figure 10, it is evident that good functional enteric performance can be achieved when the coating process is operated under conditions where

- the inlet air temperature is greater than 60°C and
- the coating suspension solids content is in the range of 10% to 15% w/w.

The data represented by the SET, however, tell a slightly different story (Fig. 11A). Clearly, the operating ranges of the process used, where acceptable performance (in terms of SET results) can be achieved, are quite limited. However, if a minimum quantity of 10% w/w enteric coating is applied and the coating suspension solids content is reduced to 15% w/w, then the process operating ranges capable of achieving acceptable results are expanded (Fig. 11B) to the point where an acceptable process can be obtained.

Scaling up the optimized enteric-coating process. On the basis of the results described in the previous section, an optimized coating procedure was designed and used as a platform for scaling up the enteric-coating process. Details of this optimized laboratory process, as well as the conditions used in the scale-up study, are shown in Table 9. In addition, the results for the enteric tests performed on tablets coated in these coating trials are provided in Table 10.

The fact that these results clearly meet (and in most cases, surpass) the specifications designated for the enteric testing of aspirin tablets confirms the suitability of the optimization and scale-up procedures used in this case study.

Spray Rate: 50g/min - Atomizing Air Pressure: 34psi

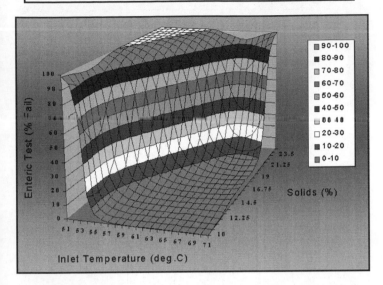

FIGURE 10 Influence of inlet air temperature and solids content of the coating suspension on enteric test performance of enteric-coated tablets.

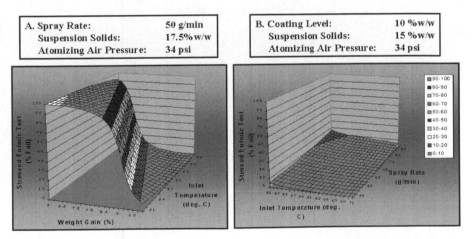

A. Spray Rate:	50 g/min
Suspension Solids:	17.5% w/w
Atomizing Air Pressure:	34 psi

B. Coating Level:	10 %w/w
Suspension Solids:	15 %w/w
Atomizing Air Pressure:	34 psi

FIGURE 11 Example of how process conditions can influence the enteric performance of tablets that have been submitted to a stress test prior to undertaking the enteric test.

Scaling Up Fluid Bed Coating Processes

Introduction

Fluid bed coating processes, although applicable for coating the full range of pharmaceutical product types, are more likely to be reserved for the coating of multiparticulates, usually with some kind of functional coating (taste masking,

TABLE 9   Coating Process Details Used in Scaling Up an Aqueous Enteric-Coating Process Using an Accela-Cota Process

	Coating process conditions for scale indicated		
Process parameter	24-in. Accela-Cota	48-in. Accela-Cota	60-in. Accela-Cota
Inlet air volume:			
(cfm)	250	1800–2000	2300–2700
(m³/hr)	425	3100–3400	3900–4600
Exhaust air volume:			
(cfm)	300	1900–2100	2400–2800
(m³/hr)	500	3200–3600	4100–4800
Inlet air temperature (°C)	75–84	70–80	70–80
Exhaust air temperature (°C)	38–41	40–45	40–45
Spray rate (g/min)	60–70	400–500	650–700
Number of spray guns (Binks 605; fluid nozzle 66SS; air cap 66SH)	2	3	5
Gun to tablet-bed distance:			
(in.)	5–7	8–12	10–12
(cm)	12–18	20–30	25–30
Atomizing air pressure:			
(psi)	35–40	60–80	50–70
(bar)	2.4–2.7	4.1–5.5	3.5–4.8
Pan loading (kg) of Aspirin 325 mg tablets	12.0	135	300
Tablet-bed prewarm temperature (°C)	45–50	45–48	45–48
Pan speed (rpm)	14	6	4
Enteric-coating suspension solids content (% w/w)	15.0	15.0	15.0
Quantity of coating applied (% w/w)[a]	10.0	10.0	10.0
Coating process time (hr)[a]	2.00	3.00–3.75	4.75–5.10

[a]This only refers to the enteric-coating layer; in addition, a subcoating (based on Opadry) applied to a level of 2.0% w/w, and a colored top coating (based on Opadry II) applied to a level of 3.0% w/w were also used.

TABLE 10   Enteric Test Results for Aspirin (325 mg) Tablets Coated in Scale-Up Processing Studies

	Disintegration test			Dissolution test	
	% Failures in 0.1 N HCl solution				% Drug released after 90 min in buffer, pH = 6.8[a]
Batch size (kg)	Enteric test (ET)	Stressed enteric test (SET)	Disintegration time in buffer, pH = 6.8	% Drug released after 2 hours in 0.1 N HCl[a]	
12	0	0	8:05 ± 0:32	0	104.5
135	0	0	7:04 ± 0:52	0	91.5
300	0	0	6:32 ± 1:00	0	105.2

[a]Compendial specification calls for: <10% dissolved in 0.1 N HCl after 2 hours, and ≥80% dissolved in buffer, pH = 6.8, after 90 minutes.

enteric, sustained release). The nature of the substrate and the purpose of the applied coating, clearly provides additional challenges during both initial process development and the scale-up process. This situation is made even more complex by the fact that with the current preference shown for employing aqueous coating formulations, functional coating formulations (that typically use polymers that are not water soluble) often require that latex, or polymer dispersion, coating systems be used. These coating systems possess complex film-forming characteristics that place extra demands on efforts to optimize the coating process in order to ensure that stable, reproducible applied coatings are obtained.

Much has already been said about scaling-up the pan-coating processes. Philosophically, many of the issues experienced in pan processes are equally applicable to the fluid bed process. There are, however, some important differences to be considered. For the most part, although there is a wide range of pan-coating equipment currently available and each brand has its specific characteristics and features, the operating principles are essentially the same. In contrast, when it comes to fluid bed coating, there are three distinct processing concepts available, as shown previously in Figure 2, and these are as follows:

- The top-spray process, which is essentially a modified fluid bed granulation process.
- The bottom spray, Wurster, process that was specifically designed for film coating.
- The tangential-spray, or rotor, process, that was originally designed as a process for producing spheronized granulates.

Each of these processing concepts, which can all be supplied by many of the major vendors of fluid bed coating equipment, has special characteristics that makes it suitable for certain tasks, as summarized in Table 11. In addition to these processing concepts (which have essentially become standards in the pharmaceutical industry), some specialized fluid bed processes have been introduced that are also worthy of note. For example, an extension of the Wurster principle is exemplified by the Precision Coater (GEA-Aeromatic Fielder, Eastleigh, U.K.), which uses a swirl actuator to modify the way processing air is introduced into the machine. Chan et al. (15) have provided

TABLE 11   Features and Uses of the Three Concepts for Fluid Bed Film Coating

Process	Advantages	Disadvantages	Uses
Top spray	• Larger batches • Easy nozzle access • Relatively simple setup • Good mixing	• Limited batch weight flexibility • Limited weight gains • Greater risk of spray drying	Application of: • Aqueous coatings • Taste mask coatings • Hot-melt coatings
Bottom spray	• Moderate batch sizes • Uniform distribution of coatings • Wide range of applications	• Poor nozzle access during coating • Requires tallest expansion chamber	Application of: • Aqueous coatings • Taste mask coatings • Modified-release coatings • Drug-layer coatings
Tangential spray	• Relatively easy setup • Easy nozzle access • Shortest processing chamber • Fast spray rates • Wide batch-weight flexibility	• High mechanical stress on product being coated	Application of: • Drug layer coatings • Modified-release coatings

a useful comparison of results that can be obtained with either a Precision Coater or a more traditional Wurster process.

A radical departure from the Wurster concept is provided by the Innojet® fluid bed process (Oystar Hüttlin, Schopfheim, Germany), while the Granurex® GRX process (Vector-Freund, Marion, IOWA, U.S.) provides an interesting approach to rotor processing.

In contrast to pan-coating processes, the characteristics of fluid bed processes that warrant careful consideration include the following:

- Nozzle positions (with the possible exception of the top-spray process) that are usually fixed and the distances between the nozzle tips and product being coated that are often quite small, both of which are unlikely to change on scale-up.
- Spray patterns that are always round, so that pattern air is not a factor in the atomizing process or in defining the spray characteristics.
- Increased batch flexibility. Although fluid bed machines have optimal operating capacities, they often have much more flexibility in accommodating a range of batch sizes within a given process (especially those based in tangential-spray units). Although there is a need to ensure that sufficient product is loaded into the machine to facilitate effective fluidization and maintain appropriate product movement, the batch flexibility of fluid bed operations is an advantage when one considers that the amount of coating material that is often applied can range from 1% to 50% (and even higher if one includes the drug-layering process, during which the API is applied to the surface of existing particles, such as pellets). Such extremes of required weight gains are rarely required in modern pan-coating operations (although drug layering onto pellets in conventional pan coaters was a technique commonly practiced in the past).
- Nozzle (atomizing) air that can contribute significantly to product movement, and thus also become a significant source of increased product attrition.
- Processing air, which has a dual purpose (one to induce appropriate product motion and the other to effect drying). Thus, the requirements for affecting both product movement and drying are not independent as they are in pan-coating processes.

Predicting Scale-Up Issues

As with pan coating, the key to successful scaling up of the fluid bed coating process involves the design of a completely optimized laboratory-scale process on which key process decisions can be based. As suggested earlier, Turkoglu and Sakr (9) provided an appropriate example of how such a fluid bed process (in this case, a tangential-spray process) might be optimized.

As with any coating process, some factors will remain unchanged on scale-up, including the following:

- Product and coating formulations
- Solids content of the coating liquid
- Inlet air and product temperatures (although these may need to be adjusted to accommodate other limitations that may arise, such as uncontrollable changes in drying air humidity and limitations on heater capacity)

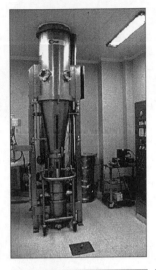 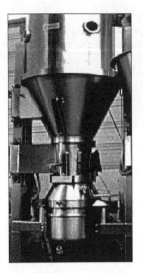 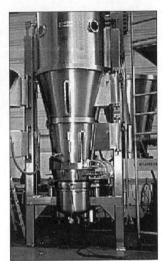

A. 7" Wurster		
Typical batch load:	4.0kg
Number of spray guns:	one
Number of partitions:	one
Partition diameter:	89mm

B. 18" Wurster		
Typical batch load:	40.0kg
Number of spray guns:	one
Number of partitions:	one
Partition diameter:	219mm

C. 32" Wurster		
Typical batch load:	180.0kg
Number of spray guns:	three
Number of partitions:	three
Partition diameter:	219mm

FIGURE 12 Photographs illustrating equipment used during the scale-up of the Wurster process.

Key factors that will change on scale-up are as follows:

- Batch size
- Drying/fluidizing air volumes
- Spray nozzle dynamics
- Spray/evaporation rate

The photographs shown in Figure 12 provide a useful example of equipment changes that can take place when scaling up a fluid bed process based on the Wurster process. One characteristic of the Wurster process, in particular, is that larger-scale machines are based on "multiples" of the 18-in. pilot-scale machine. Thus, once the appropriate pilot-scale process has been achieved, further scale-up initiatives are often simplified. Thus, the major challenges with this type of process occur when going from laboratory to pilot scale, rather than from pilot to production scale.

Determining batch size in fluid bed processes. As discussed earlier, fluid bed coaters have greater batch flexibility than their pan-coater counterparts. In the fluid bed process, the starting batch weight is often defined by two factors:

- How much coating material needs to be applied (that is, how much of the final batch weight consist of coating materials applied during the process)?

Under these circumstances, drug loading should be considered as part of the coating process for the purposes of determining starting batch weights.

- What is the minimum amount of material that can be effectively handled in the process (that is, to maintain good product flow and ensure that coating process efficiencies will be satisfactory)?

All fluid bed coating processes have a maximum batch weight defined by the interior volume of that particular machine. The ideal situation is to select a starting batch weight that will allow the process to proceed to the end point without the need to split the batch part way through because the machine capacity limit has been reached. Of course, achieving this ideal is not always possible, especially when drug loading a high dose of API and the amount of functional coating to be applied is also high. The rotor (tangential-spray) process has greater potential to facilitate the application of high weight gains without having to stop and split a batch.

Since batch size constraints may be more significant in, for example, the Wurster process, this process will be used primarily as the basis for further discussion on the subject of defining appropriate batch sizes.

For fluid bed processes, a useful limit to consider is *working capacity*, which essentially refers to the final batch weight. In the case of the Wurster process, this term refers to the volume *outside* the inner partitions. The minimum starting batch size for the Wurster process is usually approximately 40% of its working capacity. This loading is essentially a guideline, since a critical element of this process is to ensure that there will ultimately be enough material in the *up bed region* (i.e., the region inside the partition(s) when the process is in operation) to capture all of the material that is being sprayed, so avoiding low process coating efficiencies as a result of material that will either be deposited on the side walls of the inner partition(s), or material that is not captured by the product being coated and passes all the way up into the filter system. Using the 40% guideline is only suitable when the amount of coating (or drug to be layered) is substantial. When the coating level is low (<10% w/w), then the starting batch weight should be more, in the range of 60% to 70% of working capacity.

For the Wurster process, calculating batch volume on scale-up can be calculated using Eq. (2).

$$B = \frac{\pi r_1^2 L - n(\pi r_2^2 L)}{1000} \tag{2}$$

where

B is the batch volume, or working capacity (liters).
r_1 is the radius of the product (Wurster) chamber (cm).
r_2 is the radius of each inner partition (cm).
n is the number of inner partitions.
L is the length of each inner partition (cm).

If the batch volume is multiplied by the bulk density of the product to be coated, then the batch load, by weight, can be determined.

Although these examples are more specific to the Wurster process, similar guidelines can be applied to the top-spray process, although in this case, the definition for working capacity will be different. When dealing with the tangential-spray process, the quantity of product that is sufficient to ensure that the spray nozzles are completely immersed when the product is in motion will define the minimum starting batch weight.

Drying/fluidizing air volumes. As stated earlier, process air serves two purposes, namely drying and imparting motion. The key objectives in each case need not be mutually inclusive. Keeping the product moving in an appropriate manner, and the volume of air required to do that, often depends on the following:

- The mass of material inside the machine. This requirement is confounded by the fact that as more coating is applied, the mass increases, as does the requirement for fluidizing air.
- The tackiness of the coating being applied. Tacky coatings can increase both the "drag" on coated particles and agglomeration potential. When tackiness results from ineffective drying, increase in process air volume may be helpful in resolving the issue. In the case where tackiness is associated with the nature of the polymer(s) used in the coating system, the presence of other additives (such as plasticizers), or the use of latex coating systems, then any increase in process air volume may well exacerbate the problem.

In each of these scenarios, any change in air flow, because it affects the drying rate, may require a suitable adjustment in spray rate also to be made. In addition, the influence of any change in processing air volume on product movement should also not be ignored.

In general terms, the top- and tangential-spray processes may be less demanding in their requirements with respect to airflow. In the former, the fluidization pattern is quite random; in the latter, much of the burden for creating motion falls on the spinning plate so that the incoming process air is required only to

- create lift at the walls of the processing chamber;
- prevent product from dropping below the spinning plate; and
- facilitate drying.

Once again, the Wurster process presents the greatest challenge in defining optimal airflow, since it is necessary to maintain a steady and rapid movement in the up bed while also maintaining a steady gentle movement in the down bed (avoiding such problems as "rat-holing" or "bubbling"). Achieving these goals can be more challenging when working at the lower end of batch capacity. Considering the range in particle sizes of the products that may be coated in this process, some accommodation can be made in terms of specific product requirements by changing the orifice plate (which determines the relative amounts of air passing upward through the region of the inner partition(s) and also that meeting the downward moving product in the down-bed region of the processing chamber) at the bottom of the processing chamber as well as the relative height of the inner partition.

When scaling up the fluid bed process, the primary goal is to achieve product motion similar to that used on the development scale. To achieve this goal and minimize attritional effects, similar air velocities, for each size of equipment, are desirable. Thus, the overall increase in air volume required during scale-up will be related to the increase in area of the perforated base plate, and, in the case of the Wurster process, the open area of the partition plate immediately beneath each of the inner partitions.

Spray dynamics. While consideration of spray dynamics is important in pan-coating processes, such consideration can be critical in a fluid bed process because of the following:

- The product being coated is typically some form of multiparticulate, ranging in size from approximately 50 μm up to about 2 to 3 mm.
- In order to coat, in a discrete manner, each particle and avoid agglomeration, the coating fluid needs to be atomized more finely, and in a more controlled manner, than when coating tablets.
- In order to achieve effective atomization at the higher spray rates employed in the larger-scale processes, atomizing air pressures often have to be increased to levels where atomization air velocity can seriously increase product attrition.
- In order to achieve effective atomization, it is common to have to change the model of spray gun used in order to accommodate the higher spray rates required.

With the possible exception of the top-spray process (where gun adjustment is possible), gun-to-bed difference is generally fixed (since the spray gun is effectively immersed in the product being coated). However, the close proximity between the nozzle and the product being coated can potentially be problematic, since product can be drawn into the wettest part of the spray, increasing the chances of localized overwetting and agglomeration.

The use of aqueous coating systems places an added burden on the atomizing process as a result of the relatively high viscosities and surface tensions of aqueous systems. When it comes to modified-release coating applications, the common use of aqueous versions of latex, or polymer dispersion, systems places less demand on the atomization process since they generally exhibit lower viscosities, and the presence of surfactant stabilizers often reduces liquid surface tension.

The data shown in Figure 13 clearly illustrate the dilemma that one is faced with when there is a need for a substantial increase in spray rate on scale-up. For the examples shown, the Schlick 970 series gun is typical of that used on the laboratory scale, while the 940 series gun is more suitable for pilot and production-scale operations. Clearly, the 940 series gun has serious limitations when scaling up to full production requirements, since the need to maintain a fixed average droplet size (15 μm in this case) requires the use of significantly higher atomization air pressures on the production scale. The need to achieve the required droplet sizes on the manufacturing scale can be accomplished, however, by using nozzles specially designed for the task. In addition to enabling the required droplet sizes to be achieved, such specialized nozzles often enable higher spray rates also to be attained (Fig. 14) since

- higher atomizing air velocities produce smaller droplets, even at high spray rates and
- a special nozzle surround keeps product further away from the nozzle tip, thus preventing that product from being drawn into the "wet" area of the

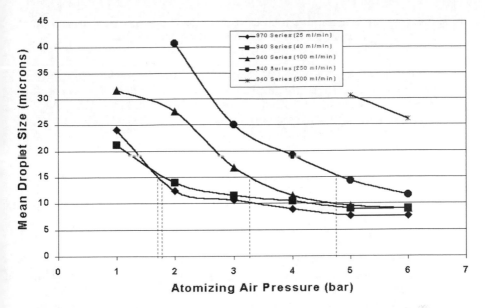

FIGURE 13 Influence of spray nozzle type and atomizing air pressure on the mean droplet size of water sprayed from guns used in a Wurster process.

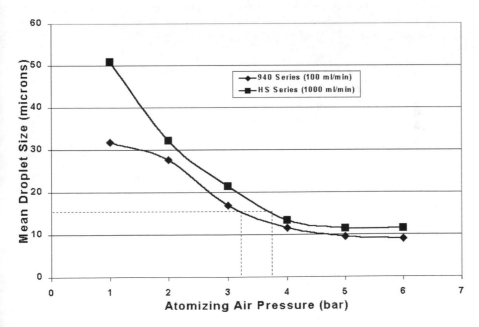

FIGURE 14 Example showing how a highly specialized nozzle (HS nozzle) can achieve equivalent atomization at high spray rates to that obtained in a more conventional nozzle when used at lower spray rates.

spray zone, and also limits the attritional effects that normally accompany the use of high atomizing air pressures and velocities.

Selecting effective spray application and evaporation rates. A relatively simple approach (as confirmed earlier through the application of Eq. 1) for defining appropriate spray rates can also be used for fluid bed coating processes; again, the caveat is that other thermodynamic factors do not change substantially. Such simple approaches can be refined further by applying appropriate thermodynamic principles. Jones (16) has described how such an approach can be applied to a fluid bed coating process.

The spray rate that can be achieved in a given process is related to the volume of air that passes through the machine, and the temperature and humidity of that air. Clearly, therefore, spray rate will be governed to some extent by the rate at which the solvent (aqueous or otherwise) can be removed. Spray rate will also be influenced by

- the behavior of the coating fluid;
- the inherent tackiness of the coating, especially during the critical time immediately after deposition onto the surface of the substrate; and
- the rate at which the product being coated moves through the spray zone. Generally, the faster that product moves through the spray zone, the lower is the "dwell time," the less coating that is captured during that time, resulting in a faster dry time for the coating. Since the rate at which the applied coating dries (a factor that influences the risk of interparticulate adhesion and thus agglomeration) has a direct influence on the ultimate spray rate that can be achieved, rapid particle movement through the spray zone enables the coating liquid to be applied faster.

Summary of scale-up issues. Scaling up the fluid bed process faces challenges similar to those faced with pan-coating processes; at the same time, additional challenges must also be faced. Differences faced in fluid bed processes are typically associated with the following fact:

- The substrate to which the coating is applied is typically relatively small, thus requiring that finer atomizing conditions be maintained.
- The smaller size of the substrate increases the risk of agglomeration, especially when the coating formulation (as is often the case) is somewhat tacky.
- The applied coating typically possesses some important functionality (such as being required to have a direct influence of drug-release rate); this places greater demands on being able to attain reproducible weight gains (of applied coating) and consistency in coating structure.

Nonetheless, achieving success in the scale-up of a fluid bed process, even one involving the application of a modified-release film coating, is not a complicated task (as long as effective process development activities have been undertaken) to which the results shown in Figure 15 are ample testament.

Statistical comparison of these data (using the f_2 factor) confirm that these drug-release profiles are essentially equivalent, although the best comparison is illustrated by the results for the coating trials performed on the pilot and

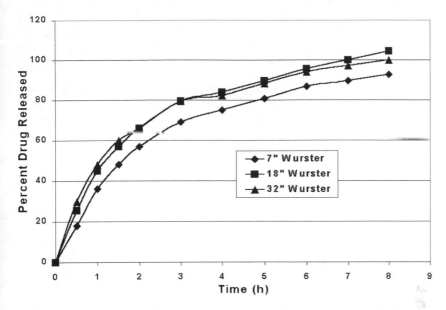

FIGURE 15 Comparison of drug release characteristics of pellets coated with an aqueous ethylcellulose dispersion using a laboratory-, pilot-, and production-scale Wurster process.

production scales, respectively (a result that is not too surprising considering the geometric similarity between these two machines, where the larger machine is factor of three multiple of the pilot-scale machine).

Scale-Up of Fluid Bed Coating Processes: A Case Study

Effective product and process optimization play a prominent role in any successful scale-up study. In this case study, the initial development, and subsequent scale-up, of a Wurster process used for the application of an aqueous ethylcellulose dispersion to drug-loaded pellets is described (Table 12). Since the

TABLE 12 Coating Process Conditions Used in the Scaling-Up of the Wurster Process for Application of an Aqueous Latex Coating to Drug-Loaded Pellets

Process parameter	Process parameter settings		
	7-in. Wurster	18-in. Wurster	32-in. Wurster
Inlet temperature (°C)	70	70	64
Inlet dew point (°C)	20	15	11
Product temperature (°C)	34	34	33
Fluidizing air volume (m³/hr)	270	1225	3740
Atomizing air pressure (bar)	2.0	2.0	3.0
Spray rate (g/min)	50	300	850
Exit air R.H. (%)	85.4	73.7	64.5
Yield (5)	99.0	96.7	98.4

coating formulation used was an aqueous polymer dispersion (of the type that exhibits special film-forming characteristics), the study also included an examination of how coating process conditions can affect behavior that is idiosyncratic of this type of coating system.

Initial process development. A preliminary study was used to establish the impact of selected processing factors on key performance attributes of the final product, especially those associated with ultimate drug-release rate (both in quantitative terms and reproducibility of the same).

On the basis of certain assumptions about formulation issues relating to the substrate being coated and the coating system being applied, the influence of the applied coating on drug-release rate was reduced to two key elements, namely

- the thickness of the coating applied and
- the structure of that coating.

Once the amount of coating to be applied and the surface area to be covered (controlled by selection of a specific size fraction of pellets to be coated) have been established, the primary factor influencing the actual amount of coating deposited is coating process efficiency. Similarly, coating structure will be influenced by

- the effectiveness of coalescence of the latex coating and
- the incidences of defects such as "pick marks" or "cracks."

Consequently, in this study, the critical factors that were examined during process development involved establishing the influence of process conditions on the following:

- Coating process efficiency
- Coalescence of the film coating (determined by means of assessing drug-release characteristics before and after imposition of a "curing" step)
- Evaluation of the impact of processing conditions on film structure (using scanning electron microscopy).

Initial process development, and ultimate process optimization, was conducted as described by Vesey and Porter (17). The study was performed in a Glatt GPCG-3 unit fitted with a Wurster insert. The process variables that were evaluated are summarized in Table 13.

TABLE 13   Process Variables Used in the Development and Optimization of a Coating Process Designed for the Application of a Modified-Release Film Coating to Drug-Loaded Pellets

Process variable	Variable ranges evaluated
Solids content of aqueous ethylcellulose dispersion (% w/w)	10.0–25.0
Inlet air temperature (°C)[a]	50–70
Spray rate (g/min)	15–45
Atomizing air pressure (bar)	1–3
Oven curing time at 60°C (hr)	0 or 24

[a]The fluidizing air volume was adjusted during each run to maintain a constant fluidization pattern; the volume of air required to achieve this was recorded in each case.

TABLE 14 Summary of Ranges Obtained For Response Variables Studied

Response variable	Variable ranges
Product temperature (°C)	22–58
Process air flow (m³/hr)[a]	61–142
Coating process efficiency (%)	79.1–97.9
T_{50}, before curing (min)	75–340
T_{50}, after curing (min)	90–320
f_2 value	56.6–95.6

[a]These ranges were used simply to maintain equivalent fluidization patterns for each coating run.

In order to assess the influence of process conditions on the coalescence efficiency of the latex coating, dissolution profiles (for samples from each coating run) were compared before and after being subjected to a curing step. Statistical analysis was undertaken using the f_2 fit factor, which is based on a logarithmic transformation of the sum of the squared error when comparing two dissolution profiles. The ultimate fit factor, expressed in terms of numerical values between 0 and 100, suggests that statistically equivalent dissolution profiles are achieved when the numeric values exceed 50.

A summary of the response variables obtained in this preliminary study are shown in Table 14, and the order ranking for the influence of process variables on the critical responses associated with coating process efficiency and drug release are provided in Table 15.

As can be seen from the summary provided in Table 14, process conditions clearly influence drug-release characteristics. Examining the data more closely, it was possible to conclude that the major causes of differences in drug-release characteristics were primarily:

- Variation in coating process efficiency, causing a significant variation in the actual amount of coating deposited.
- Overwetting, primarily seen when product temperature fell substantially below those typically observed (38–42°C) for this type of process, which substantially increases the potential for drug leaching (confirmed using elemental analysis employed during the application of scanning electron microscopy) to occur.

An optimized procedure was subsequently designed with the intent both to maximize coating process efficiency and ensure that the f_2 fit factor values exceeded 70.

Scaling up the optimized process. Employing the optimized coating process, procedures were extrapolated from the 3-kg laboratory scale to a 70-kg pilot scale, and ultimately to a 200-kg production scale. The specific coating process conditions employed are shown in Table 16, where it can be confirmed that the objectives established previously were met.

The drug-release profiles, for pellets coated on each process scale, are illustrated in Figure 16. In terms of confirming effective coalescence of the latex coating, the f_2 fit factor values achieved were 73.3, 70.6, and 75.4 (for the drug-release characteristics obtained before and after implementation of an oven-curing step) for the laboratory-, pilot-, and production-scale coating processes, respectively.

TABLE 15   Rank Order Summary of Process Variables Influencing Coating Process Efficiencies and Drug-Release Characteristics (T_{50})

Coating process efficiency		Drug release (T_{50}) before curing		Drug-release (T_{50}) after curing	
Variable	Ranking (%)	Variable	Ranking (%)	Variable	Ranking (%)
Inlet temperature	17	Spray rate	40	Spray rate	38
Spray rate × atomizing air pressure	17	Coating suspension solids	28	Inlet temp. × spray rate	21
Coating suspension solids	17	Inlet temperature	20	Coating suspension solids	19
Inlet temp. × spray rate	17	Atomizing air pressure	12	Inlet temperature	13
Spray rate × coating suspension solids	11			(Coating suspension solids)^2	9
Atomizing air pressure	11				
(Atomizing air pressure)^2	10				

TABLE 16   Details of Coating Procedures Used in Scaling Up the Wurster Process

	Coating process conditions		
Process parameter used	Glatt GPCG-3	Glatt GPCG-60	Glatt GPCG-200
Batch size (kg)	3	70	200
Fluidizing air volume			
(cfm)	83–107	800–900	N/A[a]
(m^3/hr)	140–180	1360–1530	
Inlet air temperature (°C)	64–67	60–66	72–75
Exhaust air temperature (°C)	40–45	39–41	47–51
Product temperature (°C)	41–47	40–46	43–46
Atomizing air pressure (bar)	1.5	2.0	2.0
Number of nozzles used	One	One	Three
	(Schlick 970,	(HS, 1.5-mm	(Schlick 940,
	1.2-mm orifice)	orifice)	1.5-mm orifice)
Solids content of coating	15.0	15.0	15.0
dispersion[b] (% w/w)			
Theoretical quantity of	10.0	10.0	10.0
coating applied (% w/w)			
Spray rate (g/min)	25–28	210–306	500–650
Coating process efficiency (%)	99.3	99.6	99.6

[a]Machine did not have a device monitoring airflow; fluidizing air was adjusted to maintain a fluidization pattern equivalent to those used on other scales.
[b]Surelease E-7-19010.

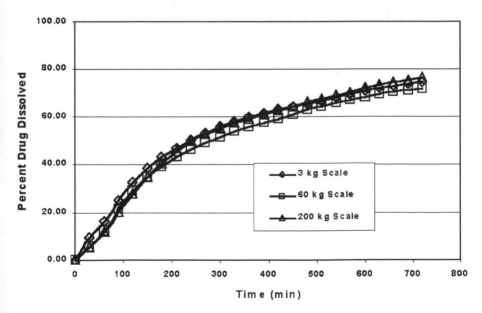

FIGURE 16   Drug release characteristics of pellets coated on various scales of the Wurster process when the laboratory-scale process, used as the basis for scale-up, has been fully optimized.

In this study, the achievement of the established objectives once again reinforces the value of taking a systematic, sound scientific approach (and one that excludes personal bias) to developing a coating process capable of facilitating a successful scale-up process.

CONTINUOUS COATING PROCESSES: AN ALTERNATIVE CONSIDERATION FOR SCALE-UP
Introduction to Continuous Coating Processes
So far, the matter of process scale-up has been dealt with in terms of moving from a small- to intermediate- to full-production-scale processes. In each case, the process has been a batch process that gets progressively larger.

While significant improvements have been made in terms of processing equipment and control systems associated with this equipment, the fundamental processing concepts have not changed substantially over the last 40 years. Since the mid-1990s, however, a significant change (at least in terms of the way coating processes are viewed) has occurred that initially had limited application, but which is now gaining more acceptance.

This change, based on continuous processing, now threatens to change our views on how scale-up of film-coating processes can be accomplished.

Certainly, until recently, these continuous coating processes have been limited to the manufacture of large-volume over-the-counter (OTC) and nutraceutical products. The process is adapted from the traditional side-vented coating pan, which is open at both ends, allowing product to be fed in at one end and exit from the other.

Mancoff (18), Pentecost (19), and Porter (20) have all described continuous film-coating processes that have been primarily designed for pharmaceutical applications. The characteristics of a typical continuous coating process are highlighted in Figure 17.

The inherent advantages exhibited by continuous processes are as follows:

* Dwell time in the coating vessel is short ($\sim$ 15–20 minutes).
* Throughput, on a continuous basis, is typically 200 to 2000 kg/hr.
* The bed depth is much shallower than typically seen in a more traditional pan.
* Coating uniformity is significantly improved, at least when viewed in terms of color uniformity.
* Stress on the product being coated is substantially reduced as a result of the shorter residence times (in the process) and the shallower bed depths used.
* Opportunities to implement the use of PAT tools (such as those associated with determining the quantity of coating applied) can be simplified, since monitoring, in many cases, can be accomplished outside the coating pan immediately after product has exited.

There is no question that using a continuous coating process can potentially simplify many of the issues traditionally associated with scaling-up of a pharmaceutical pan-coating process, especially in terms of the following:

* Deciding on appropriate pan loadings
* Defining the appropriate number of spray guns to be used
* Determining spray application rates

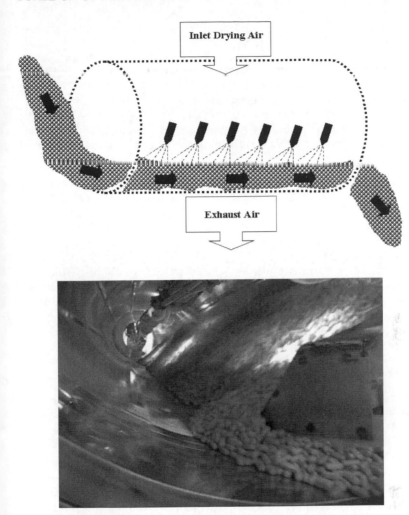

FIGURE 17 Examples of continuous pan-coating processes.

- Determining airflow volumes
- Defining appropriate gun-to-bed distances

Up until now, however, continuous processes have been limited by the fact that:

- Material produced during start-up and shutdown of the process may either have to be scrapped or reworked, since it is likely to have received less than the targeted levels of coating as a result of reduced exposure to the spray application process.
- Laboratory-scale continuous processes are essentially nonexistent, thus making process development on the laboratory scale more challenging,

since processes have to be developed on the basis of a small batch process and then transferred to a continuous process.

- The quantity of coating that can be applied in one pass is limited to about a 3.0% weight gain, thus providing a challenge when applying modified-release coatings where weight gains in the order of 2% to 10% may be required (unless the use of multiple passes is acceptable).
- The process is better suited to the coating of only large-volume products, explaining why most commercial applications of this process have been limited to those pharmaceutical and nutraceutical applications mentioned earlier.

Recent developments have addressed most, if not all, of these concerns. For example, laboratory-scale pan coaters (of a similar pan diameter to the continuous coating pan) can be used (with minor modifications to the exhaust plenums to accommodate smaller pan loadings) as a surrogate for a continuous process; in this case, the laboratory-scale coating pan functions as a segment of the continuous coating pan.

New process start-up and shutdown procedures, in which the continuous process is operated in batch mode (with suitable gun sequencing), have all but eliminated product wastage during these phases of the process. Additionally, the use of the continuous coating pan in batch mode has enabled this type of equipment to be considered as a legitimate production-scale batch process (see later discussion).

Limitations of continuous coating processes with respect to the amount of coating that can be applied have been resolved, primarily, because:

- Continuous processes generally achieve better coating uniformity (see later discussion) so that the amount of coating that needs to be applied can be reduced.
- The use of high-solids coating systems, as discussed by Porter (21), facilitates the deposition of higher amounts of coating material in a shorter period of time.

As a last point, newer coating pan designs (for continuous coaters) have been created that allow smaller volumes of product (beginning in the range of 50–200 kg/hr throughput) to be processed. This advance allows continuous coating processes to be considered as a legitimate processing option for many more pharmaceutical companies.

While some of the earliest development work in the design of continuous coaters was carried out by Coating Machinery Systems (CMS; now part of Vector-Freund,), much of the more recent pioneering work in terms of process design (primarily for pharmaceutical applications) has been carried out by both Thomas Engineering (Hoffman Estates, Illinois, U.S.) and O'Hara Technologies (Richmond Hill, Ontario, Canada). In each of these cases, product moves continuously through the equipment. A more recent development, the DRIACONTI machine (Driam USA, Spartanburg, South Carolina, U.S.) segments the coating pan into a series of chambers (in which product resides before being passed on to the next chamber); thus product flow is somewhat intermittent (defined by the programmed residence time in each segment or chamber).

Continuous Coating Processes Used in Continuous Mode

It is self-evident that continuous film-coating processes are a legitimate, although somewhat limited in application up to this point, option for scaling up coating processes. The process not only accommodates large-volume throughput, but brings other potential advantages (such as improved coating uniformity and less exposure to attritional effects) not offered by more traditional manufacturing-scale processes.

Much has been said about the potential for improved coating uniformity in continuous process. To date, most published data have been related to improvements in color uniformity; a typical example is that presented by Cunningham et al. (22). In order to achieve such improvements, certain conditions must exist within the coating process, namely:

- Product movement through the process must essentially achieve "plug flow." This means that tablet diffusion within the bed (that is, either forward or backward mixing, which causes variation in tablet residence time) must be kept to a minimum. This objective is essentially related to axial transport speed (a product of bed depth and tablet feed rate); generally, increasing tablet feed rates is likely to improve uniformity, although this will also reduce residence time and thus the amount of coating that can be deposited.
- Tablet bed perturbation (typically impacted by the atomizing air, especially when the spray guns are close to the surface of the tablet bed, as they are in continuous processes) must be minimized.

Recent advances in continuous processes are likely to increase the appeal of this type of process, not least of which (with the introduction of lower throughput machines) is the ability to marry continuous coating with the output of the tabletting process (already essentially a continuous process).

Cunningham et al. (22) have summarized the potential advances that have taken place recently with continuous coating processes and provide examples using both immediate-release and modified-release film coatings.

Typical process data, associated with continuous coating processes, are summarized in Table 17.

TABLE 17 Example of Typical Process Conditions Used in Continuous Coating Processes

Process parameter	O'Hara FC C500	O'Hara FC C1200
Coating suspension solids (% w/w)	15.0–25.0	
Number of spray guns (Schlick 930 anti-bearding)	12 (−14)	18
Pan diameter (cm)	48	72
Pan length (cm)	289.5	477.5
Process air flow (m³/hr)	2,500–8,500	8,500–20,400
Inlet air temperature (°C)	45–85	
Exhaust air temperature (°C)	40–50	
Atomizing air pressure (bar)	2.0	
Pattern air pressure (bar)	2.0	
Spray rate (g/min)	450–1500	1500–3600
Tablet throughput rate at 3% wt. gain (kg/hr)	150–500	500–1200

Continuous Coating Processes in Batch Mode

While it may seem a retrograde step to consider a continuous coater as a batch coater, the potential advantages for doing so have become more evident as a result of opportunities for starting up and shutting down continuous processes in batch mode. For example, as shown by Cunningham et al. (22), when using a continuous coater in batch mode (with a pan fill capacity of 250 kg), approximately a 3% weight gain can be achieved, with good visual color uniformity, in less than 15 minutes (determined by calculation using the data presented in the article). Conducting a similar coating trial (i.e., the same type of coating system applied at the same solids content) in a traditional batch coater, a typical coating process time is about 90 minutes.

Thus, not only does the continuous coater, in batch mode, enable the batch to be processed much faster, with potential improvements in product quality, it also provides the option of switching to continuous mode should a significant increase in production output be required, thus obviating the need for additional capital expenditure.

SCALING UP COATING PROCESSES THAT INVOLVE THE APPLICATION OF AN API IN THE COATING
Introduction

Using film-coating processes to apply an API to the surface of a core material is not new. In fact, such application, typically to multiparticulates, in fluid bed coating processes, is quite common. The challenge, however, is to achieve good content uniformity in the final dosage unit. When drug layering onto multiparticulates in fluid bed processes, these challenges tend to be minimized because of the following:

- Fluid bed processes (especially the bottom-spray Wurster process) achieve good uniformity of distribution of the coating (and API).
- The final dosage unit is made up of a multiplicity of the coated pellets, so even if acceptable, content uniformity from pellet to pellet is not completely achieved; statistically, when a large number of pellets is combined into the final dosage unit, appropriate content uniformity will be achieved.

The same story, however, cannot be told for a typical pan-coating process where the API is being applied to the surface of a single unit, such as a tablet, as indicated by Fourman et al. (23).

The Dilemma

Generally, achieving good uniformity of distribution of an applied film coating (and any API dispersed therein) in a pan-coating process is contingent on a number of factors, such as:

- Pan speed
- Solids content of the coating liquid
- The amount of coating material being applied
- Spray rate
- Mixing efficiency in the coating pan
- Uniformity of distribution of the coating material across the surface of the tablet bed

- Coating process efficiency (i.e., the actual amount of coating deposited expressed as a percentage of the amount of coating applied)

To maximize the potential for achieving uniform distribution of the coating, there are two fundamental issues to address, namely:

- Maximizing the number of times (throughout the coating process) that tablets are exposed on the surface to the coating liquid being sprayed onto that surface.
- Minimizing the amount of coating material deposited each time a tablet passes through the spray zone.

The basic issue with pan-coating processes is that it is easier to meet the required objectives when working with a small, laboratory-scale coater, but the difficulty in doing so becomes progressively greater during the scale-up process.

The reasons for this are twofold:

- In the laboratory process, the bed depth is quite shallow, so that the chances that tablets, on each revolution of the coating pan, will be exposed to the spray are potentially quite high.
- In the larger production-scale processes, as the bed depth becomes significantly deeper, tablets can easily become "trapped" in the middle of the bed, and thus see less exposure to the spray (Fig. 18).

Rege et al. (24) have evaluated the critical process variables, employing a statistical DoE technique, that need to be considered when applying an active ingredient to tablets in a laboratory 24-in. Accela-Cota. Their results show that in this laboratory-scale process, achieving content uniformity (% RSD, or relative standard deviation) values below a critical acceptance value of 6 is relatively easy to attain. By contrast, in a production-scale process of which the author of this chapter has experience, the application of approximately 5 mg of API per tablet

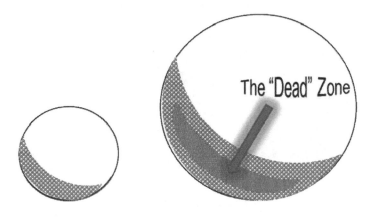

A. Laboratory-Scale Process   B. Production-Scale Process

FIGURE 18 Schematic illustration of the potential impact of increased bed depth (for a production-scale pan-coating process) on exposure of tablets to the spray application process.

required a process time in excess of eight hours, and the resultant tablets had an API content uniformity well in excess of 10% RSD; such results are not atypical.

Clearly, therefore, the dilemma is how to achieve appropriate content uniformity when transferring a process from the laboratory into production?

A useful approach is to consider some of the newer processing technologies that have been made available. Tobiska and Kleinebudde (25) and Müller et al. (26) have described process developments using a Bohle BFC 5 laboratory-scale pan coater (L.B. Bohle, Ennigerloh, Germany), in which good coating uniformity values could be obtained. This machine, designed primarily to address coating uniformity issues, possesses a rather unique helical baffle system that has been shown greatly to improve mixing efficiency within coater. More importantly, it has been demonstrated that this unique pan design can achieve equally acceptable coating uniformities on the production scale. For example, Thies (27) has shown how, using a Bohle BFC 400 production scale machine, when coating tablets with a marker active ingredient in the coating, coating uniformities in the realm of 4% RSD and better can be achieved.

While it has yet to be confirmed, on the basis of visual coating uniformity achieved so far, it is likely that the use of continuous coaters, especially in batch mode, will prove equally useful in resolving the scale-up dilemma for achieving good content uniformity when applying an API in the film coating.

SCALE-UP OF COATING PROCESSES: OVERALL SUMMARY

The characteristics of pharmaceutical coating processes sets them apart from most, if not all, other pharmaceutical unit operations not only in terms of issues that need to be understood during process development, but also when it comes to scaling up those processes. This is especially true when dealing with the number of process variables that have to be considered. Clearly, process scale-up when applied to coating processes is much more complex than just considering them in terms of geometric enlargement of the equipment concerned.

Spraying of coating liquids, ensuring that effective and consistent drying takes place, achieving appropriate uniformity of distribution of the coating, and enabling final coating structure and functionality to remain consistent with the intended purpose of that coating are all events that must be well defined if successful process scale-up is to be accomplished.

REFERENCES

1. Porter SC, Bruno CH. Coating of pharmaceutical solid-dosage forms. In: Lieberman HA, Lachman L, Schwartz JB, eds. Pharmaceutical Dosage Forms: Tablets. Vol 3, 2nd ed. New York: Marcel Dekker, 1990:77–160.
2. McGinity JW, ed. Aqueous Polymeric Coatings for Pharmaceutical Dosage Forms. 2nd ed. New York: Marcel Dekker, 1997:1–582.
3. Porter SC. A review of trends in film-coating technology. Am Pharm Rev 1999; 2:32–41.
4. Wurster DE. Method of Applying Coatings to Tablets or the Like. U.S. Patent # 2,648,609, 1953.
5. Porter SC, Ghebre-Sellassie I. Key factors in the development of modified-release pellets. In: Ghebre-Sellassie I, ed. Multiparticulate Oral Drug Delivery. New York: Marcel Dekker, 1994:217–284.
6. Ebey GC. A thermodynamic model for aqueous film coating. Pharm Technol 1987; 11(4):40.

7. Choi M. Applications of process thermodynamics in pharmaceutical coating. Tablets Capsules 2007; 5(3):12–24.
8. Porter SC, Verseput RV, Cunningham CR. Process optimization using design of experiments. Pharm Technol 1997; 21(10):60–80.
9. Turkoglu M, Sakr A. Mathematical modelling & optimization of a rotary fluidized-bed coating process. Int J Pharm 1992; 88:75–87.
10. Rodriguez L, Greechi R, Cini M, et al. Variation of operational parameters & optimization in aqueous film coating. Pharm Technol 1986; 20(4):76–86.
11. Rowe RC. Expert systems in solid dosage development. Pharm Ind 1993; 55(11):1040–1045.
12. Pharmaceutical Technologies International, inc. Information obtained from PTI website http://www.pt-int.com.
13. Ho L, Müller R, Gordon KC, et al. Applications of terahertz pulsed imaging to sustained-release tablet film coating quality assessment and dissolution performance. J Control Release 2008; 127:79–87.
14. Cunningham CR. Spray gun optimization for aqueous film-coating processes. Proceedings of TechSource® Coating Technology 99, Atlantic City, NJ, October 12–13, 1999.
15. Chan LW, Tang ESK, Heng PS. Comparative study of the fluid dynamics of bottom spray fluid bed coaters. AAPS PharmSciTech 2006; 7(2):E1–E9.
16. Jones DM. Effect of process air dew point on a top-spray fluidized bed-coating process. Presented in Session 265; Coating in the pharmaceutical industry. Proceedings of AIChE Annual Meeting, 1998.
17. Vesey CF, Porter SC. Modified-release coating of pellets with an aqueous ethylcellulose-based coating formulation: coating process considerations. Proceedings of the 13th Annual Meeting and Exposition of AAPS, San Francisco, CA, 1998.
18. Mancoff WO. Film coating compressed tablets in a continuous process. Pharm Technol 1998; 22:12–18.
19. Pentecost B. Continuous coating process. Proceedings of TechSource® Coating Technology 99, Atlantic City, NJ, October 12–13, 1999.
20. Porter SC. Continuous film coating processes: a review. Tablets Capsules 2004; 4:26–29.
21. Porter SC. The role of high-solids coating systems in reducing process costs. Tablets & Capsules 2010; 8(3):10–16.
22. Cunningham C, Hansell J, Nuneviller F III, et al. Evaluation of recent advances in continuous film coating processes. Drug Dev Ind Pharm 2010; 36(2):227–233.
23. Fourman GL, Hines CW, Hritsco RS. Assessing the uniformity of aqueous film coatings applied to compressed tablets. Pharm Technol 1995; 19(3):70–76.
24. Rege BD, Gawel J, Kou JH. Identification of critical process variables for coating actives onto tablets via statistically designed experiments. Int J Pharm 2002; 237:87–94.
25. Tobiska S, Kleinebudde P. A simple method for evaluating the mixing efficiency of a new type of pan coater. Int J Pharm 2001; 224:141–149.
26. Müller J, Knop K, Thies J, et al. Feasibility of Raman spectroscopy as a PAT tool in active coating. Drug Dev Ind Pharm 2010; 36(2):234–243.
27. Thies J. Achieving the best uniformity in functional film coating. ISPE Canada, September, 2008.

17 Virtual scale-up of manufacturing solid dosage forms

Hans Leuenberger, Michael N. Leuenberger, and Maxim Puchkov

SUMMARY

The discovery, development, and introduction of a new chemical entity as a drug substance to the market are lengthy and extremely costly processes. A large number of hurdles slows down the speed of introduction of a new medicinal product or may even prevent it. The most preferable dosage form for the majority of the companies to register is an oral solid dosage form such as a tablet. The chapter discusses the scale-up process and describes how to speed-up the development of solid dosage forms, to save money, and to improve quality. The idea is to replace expensive laboratory experiments by in silico experiments, simulating laboratory- and large-scale manufacturing equipment. Such a concept leads to a paradigm change in pharmaceutical R&D and makes it possible to *design* and *test* robust solid dosage forms for the market already in clinical phase I, as only a small quantity of the drug substance is needed to validate the in silico experiments. The in silico experiments are carried out by software and hardware packages such as F-CAD (Formulation—Computer-Aided Design) developed by CINCAP GmbH (Basel, Switzerland). However, the successful application of F-CAD should be complemented by process-specific computer models for all critical unit operations such as granulation, drying, etc. A good example of such computerized models is Virtual Equipment Simulator (VES). VES has the duty to mimic 1:1 the properties of the equipment to be used, including its look and feel. The properties of the small equipment are, in general, very well known and can be easily tested. In case of large-scale equipment, it would be very costly to manufacture batches, which cannot be sold later. On the other hand, it has to be kept in mind that key properties of the large-scale equipment can be retrieved from numerous batch records of products already manufactured or currently being manufactured. This knowledge is available but often not exploited. Thus, it is necessary to invest an additional effort to exploit such a knowledge, which is specific to the type of equipment, to the type of formulation, and to the site of the facility. The basic idea is to develop a "parallel world" of virtual equipment to be used to manufacture the robust in silico–developed, market-ready formulations developed already in clinical phase I. This is an important change of the actual paradigm. Thus, no bioequivalence testing is needed in later clinical phase(s). Scale-up problems can be reduced, thanks to in silico tests of manufacturing large-scale batches. This change of paradigm avoids a rush development in clinical phase IIb of the final formulation for the market. The risks of an insufficient quality can be reduced, as the design space according to ICH Q8 can be fully explored. An application of in silico design and testing of solid dosage forms is an innovative tool for fulfilling the requirements of PAT (Process Analytical Technology) and the Quality-by-Design initiative of FDA and EMEA.

There are additional benefits introducing a parallel world of VES: the personnel using the real equipment can be trained in silico like aircraft pilots using a flight simulator. Such training should reduce the number of rejected batches and should contribute efficiently to a faster time to market.

INTRODUCTION
Quality-by-Design and the Six-Sigma Goal

The higher cost of introducing a new medicinal product on the market is directly related to the higher attrition rate during the development of the product. Figure 1 shows the impact of this attrition rate: only one out of 10,000 molecules extensively tested in the discovery phase successfully reaches the market (1). Typical hurdles, which slow down the process of introduction of solid dosage forms, are shown in Figure 2. Because of the higher rate of attrition, the amount of experimental work

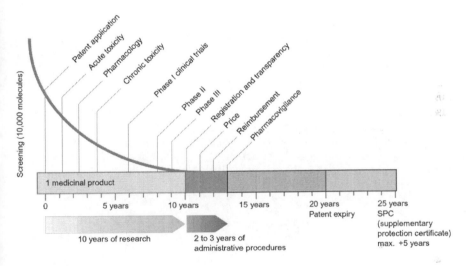

FIGURE 1   Time schedule and activities involved to introduce a new medical product on the market starting from 10,000 screened molecules (1). Courtesy of Dr. J. Werani, Pfizer Inc.

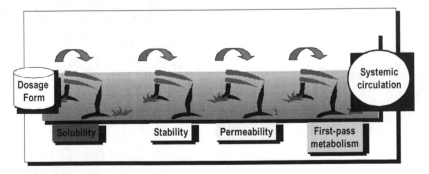

FIGURE 2   Major hurdles in the development of a solid dosage form. *Source*: According to a presentation of Dr. A. Hussain, FDA.

invested in an early phase of the development needs to be kept small. For this reason, the first dosage forms, often called "service forms" for the early clinical trials, are relatively simple dosage forms such as hard gelatin capsule formulations. The final dosage form for the market is usually designed only in the clinical phase IIb. Thus, no additional investments were effectuated in projects, which had to be sacrificed due to the attrition rate. On the other hand, the following issues have to be taken into account: The final dosage form developed for the market needs to be bioequivalent with the former service form. Thus, a *bioequivalence test* is needed. The first simple service form may not be the optimal dosage form concerning bioavailability and robustness. The development of the final dosage form for the market at later stages often suffers from time pressure, which is related to speed-up time to market. Severe problems arise if the "bioequivalence tests" are not satisfactory and if some of the clinical studies have to be repeated due to a lack of robustness of the early "service" dosage form.

From a principal point of view, it can be shown that this current concept cannot fulfill the requirement of Quality by Design (QbD) to achieve the goal of a six-sigma quality (1,2). Unfortunately, it is often necessary to apply expensive "repair actions" in the development of the final marketed dosage form (1) to achieve a bioequivalence (Fig. 3).

What happens if the earlier "service dosage form" was far from optimal? In such case, the final marketed dosage form needs to be adjusted to the quality of the dosage form tested in clinical phase II. Indeed, such problems are well known to companies developing generics: the new developed formulation has a better bioavailability than the original product. To show bioequivalence, the generic companies then need to reduce the bioavailability of their product to comply with the originator. It is generally recognized that such a situation

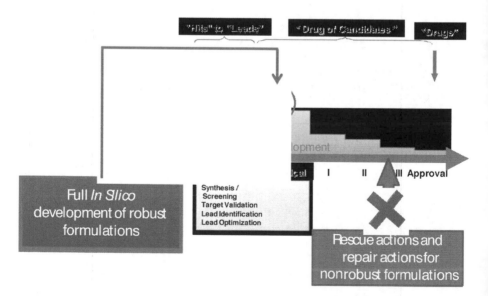

FIGURE 3   Slide based on the presentation of Dr. A. Hussain, FDA, with comments added (1) concerning an earlier development of a robust formulation for the introduction to the market.

should be an exception. However, unfortunately it is difficult to predict, if the service dosage form has been the optimal reference dosage form. On the contrary, due to the low investment in the development of the early service dosage form, it cannot be anticipated that this dosage form is the optimal one concerning bioavailability and robustness (3–5). The fact that early "service" dosage forms often have a poor quality is linked to the concept that the company is unable to invest more time and efforts in this early stage of development having 12 or more promising drug substances simultaneously in the development pipeline (Fig. 3) (1). Obviously, there are not enough resources and time slots for doing additional expensive laboratory work available. Thus, it is not surprising that the quality of earlier dosage forms is far from showing a six-sigma performance. This problem has severe consequences, as according to the regulatory point of view, the formulation concept should remain intact in a fundamental way during the forthcoming clinical trials.

A Paradigm Change Needed

To obtain six-sigma quality it is a prerequisite to develop already for clinical phase I a robust, market-ready dosage form! It has been generally accepted that the quality of pharmaceutical products has a quality of approximately two sigma. In case of a "snapshot view," that is, looking at manufacturing a single batch, a two-sigma quality corresponds to ~4.5% defectives. Looking at a sequence of batch productions over a longer period of time, the percentage of defectives of the sum of batches increases to ~20%. The higher value is due to drift of individual results because of measurements over an extensive time period. This poor quality performance and the actual knowledge applied (Fig. 4) was the reason for FDA to develop and introduce the PAT and QbD initiatives (2). The PAT initiative has prompted the installation of additional in-process control units in the manufacturing departments for optimizing the quality (6,7). Interestingly, the PAT initiative did not affect with the same visibility the

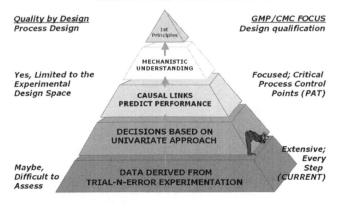

Product and Process Quality Knowledge: Science-Risk Based cGMP's

FIGURE 4 Knowledge pyramid. *Source*: Courtesy of Dr. A. Hussain, FDA.

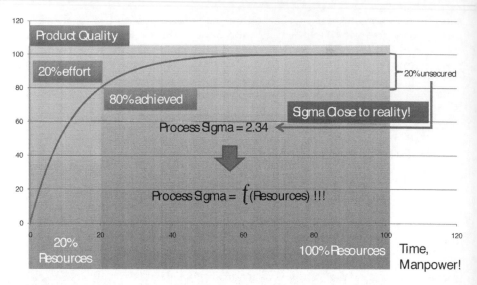

FIGURE 5 "Learning," resp. "Optimization" profile concerning the quality of a product. *Source*: From Ref. 1.

pharmaceutical R&D departments with their task to build-in and not to test-in the quality, but to implement QbD according to ICH Q8 (8).

It is known that the quality $Q(\mu, t)$ is a function of resources μ and time t. $Q(\mu, t)$ can be expressed in general (1) as an exponential asymptotic function as follows:

$$Q(\mu, t) = Q_{opt}(1 - e^{-\mu t}) \tag{1}$$

With Q_{opt} = optimal quality for $t \rightarrow \infty$, μ = amount of means, that is, tools, resources, etc. Depending on μ and time t, the "learning" resp. "optimization" process shows in the beginning a fast increase and then levels off. For this reason, the so-called "20%/80%" rule became very popular in the pharmaceutical industry. The idea of the 20%/80% rule consists in obtaining 80% of the performance (optimal quality) at only 20% of time and resources invested. In other words, this rule means in practice that one person takes simultaneous care of five projects, dedicating 20% of time and resources per project. Figure 5 shows that the resulting quality of the product corresponds to a sigma value of ~2.3, which is very close to the reported one (2). Even if the parameter μt is increased by a factor of 5, that is, one person dedicates 100% of the time per project, a six-sigma value cannot be obtained (1). Thus, new means need to be identified to achieve a six-sigma quality for the dosage forms already in clinical phase I.

F-CAD, A New Concept for Designing and Testing of Solid Dosage Forms "In Silico"

F-CAD (1,2,9), developed by CINCAP GmbH, consists of unique software modules (Fig. 6) and is conceptually different in design to the existing "expert systems" that can be purchased in the market. The core module is based, among other, on the concept of cellular automata. This concept is based on a "first-principle"

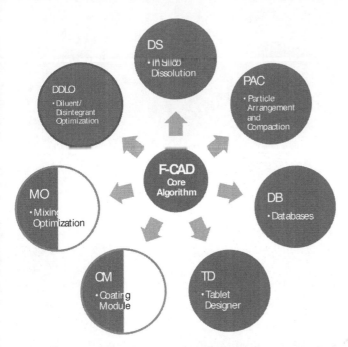

FIGURE 6 F-CAD software modules: the semifilled circles indicate that this module has been complemented with discrete element methods. *Source*: From Ref. 1.

approach and permits a straightforward calculation of the drug release profile of the formulation. The F-CAD cellular automata software module is not identical with the software applied by other groups (10–14), but is based on similar assumptions. The F-CAD core module allows to calculate dissolution profiles of the drug substance as a function of the composition and of the physicochemical properties of the components in a formulation (solubility of the drug substance, solubility, swellability, effect of the particle size distribution of the drug substance, and the excipients, etc.). F-CAD also takes into account the shape (Fig. 7) of the tablet and its influence on the dissolution profile (1).

With this concept, it is also possible to calculate percolation thresholds, which play an important role in the design and the functionality of the formulation of solid dosage forms (9,15–17).

It is important to keep in mind that in this early phase of development only a minimum amount of drug substance is needed for the determination of its physicochemical properties. The physicochemical properties of the functional excipients are usually known.

The potential of F-CAD is as follows:

- Search for an optimal and robust formulation for the market with a minimum amount of drug substance, that is, already in an early phase of development
- Define the desired dissolution profile of the drug substance
- Explore the whole design space in a minimum of time

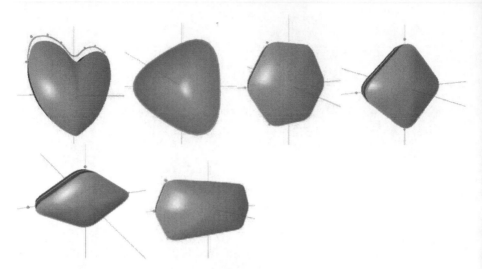

FIGURE 7 Different tablet shapes created by the "Tablet Designer" software module, which may influence the dissolution profile. *Source*: From Ref. 1.

- Define the necessary specifications of the drug substance and the excipients on a scientific base such as particle size distribution etc.
- Establish a sensitivity analysis of the chosen dosage form concerning changes in the formulation (amount of excipient, change of other parameters such as particle size, etc.)
- Search for root cause in case of OoS (out-of-specification) problems
- Check for equivalence in case of exchange of an excipient by the same type having, for example, a different size distribution
- Generate a feasibility study for the project including a sensitivity analysis to assure the robustness of the formulation
- Save time and money by improving quality and shortening time to market
- Establish intellectual property rights by providing results for systems before experimental confirmation
- Effectuate only a minimum of laboratory experiments to confirm the results of the suggested formulations by F-CAD
- Monitor in silico the dissolution progress of your desired formulation at any time point elapsed (Figs. 8 and 9).

Practical Requirements for the Application of F-CAD

- Knowledge of the solubility of the drug substance in the solvents used for measuring the dissolution rate of the desired dosage form
- Knowledge of the intrinsic dissolution rate of the drug substance
- Knowledge of the true density of the drug substance
- Knowledge of the excipients, which are chemically compatible with the drug substance
- Knowledge of the physicochemical properties of the excipients, in case that excipients are used, which have special properties and are not well known

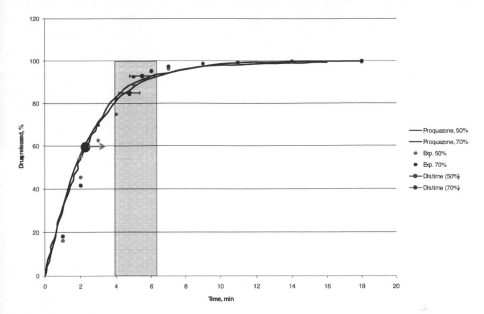

FIGURE 8   Dissolution profile of a tablet. F-CAD marks in addition to the specific time point, when the water molecules have reached the geometric center point of the tablet, that is, "center time," indicated by blue circle (laboratory data taken from the PhD thesis of Johannes von Orelli (5), mean experimental disintegration time is depicted by the gray region).

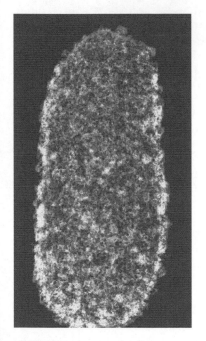

FIGURE 9   Screenshot of the computer-generated matrix-type formulation, which contains a swelling excipient (light-gray to white) after, for example, time $t^* = 100$ seconds.

- Dissolution profile of the drug substance in a standard hard gelatin capsule and standard tablet formulation in different buffer systems such as pH 1.2, pH 4.5, and pH 6.8.

Knowledge Related to the Goals of the Application of F-CAD

- Knowledge of the *desired dissolution profile* of the marketed dosage form, for example, immediate release, controlled release, etc., in case of a new formulation or in case of developing a generic
- Search for *dissolution profiles* of the marketed tablet dosage form in different buffer media *being identical* to the dissolution profile of the early hard gelatin capsule formulation

Some Important Additional Comments Related to F-CAD

It is important to realize that for the application of F-CAD it is not needed to know the chemical formula of the drug substance and its therapeutical application. F-CAD is capable to calculate from scratch formulations, which give already a good estimate of the properties of the solid dosage form. The standard or reference formulations mentioned above have the function to increase the precision of the calculation, that is, to "fine-tune" and "calibrate" such calculations. Thus, it is possible to take care of the type of dissolution measurement equipment such as USP methods 1 and 2, the effect of the ionic strength of the dissolution media, and to explore the design space with a higher precision. In this respect, the quality of the explored formulations is related to the quality of the reference ones.

The main goal of F-CAD is to calculate a robust formulation, which shows the desired dissolution profile of the drug substance at the sample times t_i with the cumulative amount of drug dissolved $y_d * (t_i)$. The subsequent formulation manufactured in the laboratory according to the proposed calculated, that is, predicted formulation will lead the experimentally verified dissolution profile $y_v(t_i)$. In the ideal case, the sum of squares $SSQ = \sum_{i=1}^{n} [y_d * (t_i) - y_v(t_i)]^2$ is a minimum. The values $y_d * (t_i)$ correspond to the F-CAD calculated, that is, predicted values and the values $y_v(t_i)$ are the results of the laboratory experiments to confirm the F-CAD calculated values with $i = 1 \ldots n$ sample times. The value of SSQ/n is in fact a measurement of the precision of the calculated formulation.

It is evident that the precision SSQ/n of the calculated formulations is, in reality, a function of the "distance" from the reference formulations. According to the law of error propagation, the precision suffers if the distance is larger. That is the reason why an interpolation procedure yields better results than an extrapolation. The distance Δ of the calculated formulation consisting of the excipient concentrations x_{pj} in the design space from existing laboratory reference laboratory formulations with the excipients x_{rj} can be calculated as follows (n = number of components):

$$\Delta = \sqrt{\sum_{j=1}^{n} (x_{pj} - x_{rj})^2} \tag{2}$$

In this context, the process used for manufacturing the reference laboratory formulations and for the F-CAD calculated formulation was not changed, for example, in both cases a direct compression process was applied. In case of a quantitative and/or qualitative change of an excipients of the calculated formulation with respect to the reference formulation such a distance Δ can be also calculated formally. In case of keeping the same excipients, the quantity x_j of the excipient j was changed in the calculated formulation. In case that a new excipient k was added and the excipient j was replaced, the quantity x_j becomes zero in the new calculated formulation. However, it is important to realize that this new excipient, that is, this variable, is missing in the reference formulation and its contribution may have a strong influence on the properties of the calculated formulation. As a consequence, it is not possible at all to give an estimate of the precision of the quality of the calculated formulation. This comment is also true in the case of a change of the manufacturing process compared to the reference formulation. In both cases, an important change in the properties of the formulation can be considered as the result of entering into a new, not yet explored, design space, which is different from the previous one.

The proof of concept of the application of F-CAD is described in detail in Ref. (1). It is evident that F-CAD can also be applied for drug delivery systems with more than one drug substance, which represents a special challenge (18). In addition, the application of F-CAD is not limited to classical solid dosage forms but can be extended, for example, to matrix-type nanostructured microparticles (Fig. 9) for pulmonary administration (19,20).

The aircraft industry has used similar approaches to design and test in silico aircraft prototypes. In this context, the aircraft manufacturers could realize savings of up to 90% while improving quality (21).

VES FOR TRAINING, SCALE-UP, AND MANUFACTURING REALITY
F-CAD and VES
It is possible to combine F-CAD, that is, the in silico design and testing of solid dosage forms with the concept of VES (22). The software modules in Figure 6, which are represented by semifilled circles indicate that the concept of the core module has been complemented by dedicated discrete element software models, which allow to calculate, analyze, and visualize important pharmaceutical processes such as pan coating (Fig. 10).

The focus of F-CAD is the formulation of a solid dosage form, which depends on the composition, on the manufacturing method, and on the testing tools such as the determination of the dissolution profile of the drug substance in a certain solvent. F-CAD can be used also as a training tool for a better understanding of the behavior of a formulation. In fact, it is possible to calculate whether and how a change in the granule size distribution will affect the dissolution profile of the drug substance. It is not possible to calculate the disintegration time, but it is possible to calculate the time when the water molecules have reached the center of the tablet volume. This event prevails the disintegration time in case of a disintegrating tablet (Fig. 8).

F-CAD can be combined with the concept of VES, which can include any type of equipment, that is, not only equipment for manufacturing but also for testing. The VES for the determination of the drug dissolution profile combined with F-CAD is of special interest as the calibration methods for the validation of the dissolution test equipment can be included. In fact, any physical test method such as friabilators (Fig. 11) can be simulated.

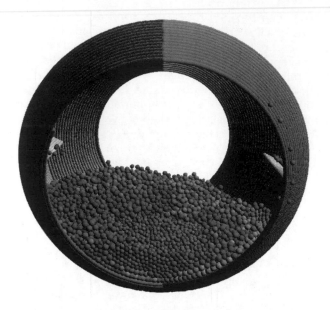

FIGURE 10 Snapshot view of the movement of spherical particles in a drum. Using discrete element methods, it is possible to analyze the effects of the bowl geometry, etc. on the formation of "dead" zones and general mixing quality. *Source*: From Ref. 1.

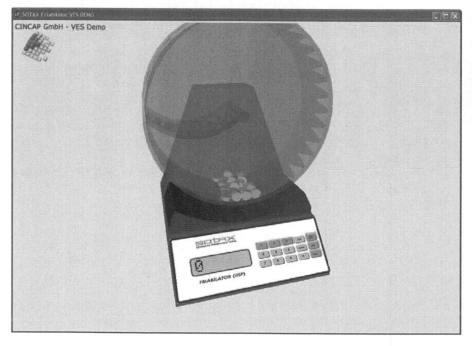

FIGURE 11 Friabilator as a VES (study made for SOTAX AG, CH-4123 Allschwil/Switzerland). *Abbreviation*: VES, virtual equipment simulator.

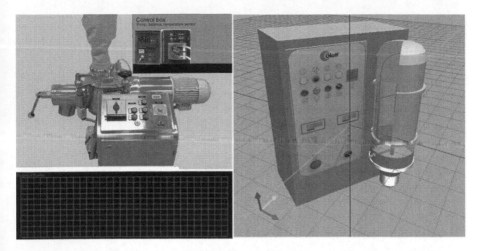

FIGURE 12 Simulators of high-shear mixer/granulator (*left side*) and fluidized-bed equipment. *Source*: From Ref. 22.

As shown in Figure 12, any equipment, not only a friabilator, can be developed also for 3D virtual application (screen shots of a high-shear mixer and a table-top fluidized-bed processor).

Concerning the task of scale-up, the main goal is to develop VES software modules that are capable of performing the tasks of typical unit operations in pharmaceutical technology such as wet agglomeration and drying of granules in a fluidized-bed laboratory, pilot plant, and manufacturing scale equipment. Such VES can be designed as 3D or as 2D replicates, which is often sufficient (Fig. 13).

It is evident that such VES developments are not restricted to fluidized-bed equipment but can involve equipment for coating tablets (Fig. 10), high-shear mixers, etc. In fact, the application of VES is not limited to equipment of pharmaceutical technology, but can include equipment of pharmaceutical analytical laboratories, such as high-performance liquid chromatography (HPLC) simulators, for the development and training of test methods using different solvent gradients.

VES is a science-based tool and goes beyond classical e-manufacturing tools to optimize the cycle time, assigning manufacturing equipment for efficient use, etc. VES takes into account the underlying physical laws. Thus, VES can be used in addition as a training tool for the better understanding of pharmaceutical unit operations. It can be also helpful for writing down standard operation procedures. The following chapter shows an example of a VES representing a fluidized-bed granulator.

VES AS A TOOL FOR LABORATORY STAFF TRAINING OR FOR UNIVERSITY STUDENTS

The regulatory agencies require a sufficient training of laboratory staff for a current good manufacturing practice (cGMP) conform manufacturing of medicinal products. In case of large-scale equipment, human errors in manufacturing batches lead to expensive losses. Thus, VES is a tool to train the specialist operating an important manufacturing equipment. In fact, VES has the similar

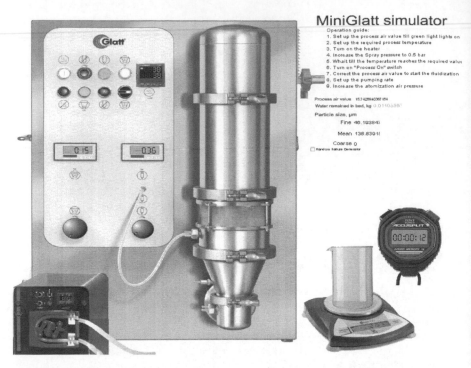

FIGURE 13 Screenshot of the 2D VES for MiniGlatt table-top processor. *Abbreviation*: VES, virtual equipment simulator.

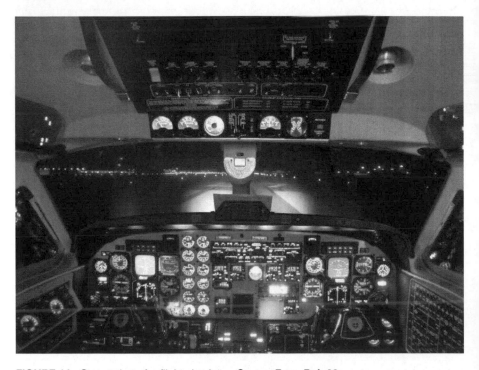

FIGURE 14 Screenshot of a flight simulator. *Source*: From Ref. 22.

task of a flight simulator (Fig. 14) for training pilots. It is important to keep in mind that VES is exactly describing the behavior of the equipment, and thus it is possible to simulate potential "crash" situations to explore technological limits.

It is evident that VES also has a great potential as a training tool in academic environments, which may not have the means to buy and use large-scale equipment. For educational purposes it is suggested to use VES in parallel with a small-scale equipment such as a "MiniGlatt fluidized-bed table-top processor" (Fig. 13), which the student can be first trained in silico and subsequently verify and confirm the results in a laboratory experiment using a minimum of material. The application of such VES fluidized-bed equipment for student training is described in detail as follows.

The physical laws governing the fluidized-bed drying process are well known and need to be taken into account such as the thermodynamic laws concerning the drying process (Mollier diagram, see Fig. 15) and the physical law to keep the particles fluidized.

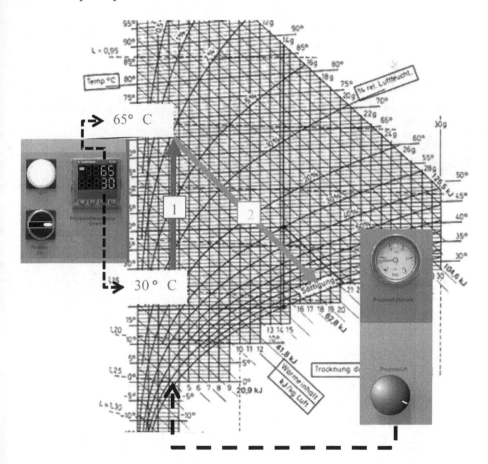

FIGURE 15 Mollier chart as backbone for calculating the process parameters and the output results. [Process 1—heating from 30°C up to 65°C; process 2—evaporation (drying) at constant enthalpy; *dashed lines* indicates parameter transfer from VES control panel to calculation model (air-throughput, temperature).]

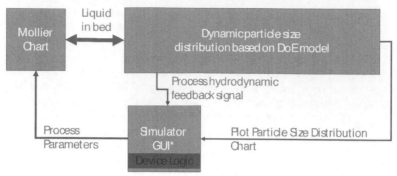

*GUI: Graphical User Interface

FIGURE 16 Internal mathematical model for the calculation of the resulting granule size distribution of a model placebo formulation as a function of the process parameter settings. *Source*: From Ref. 22.

To take into account effects related to the equipment type, its size, construction, which includes effects of energy losses, etc., it is necessary to carry out real laboratory experiments based on an experimental factorial design with a standard formulation. Such a design of experiments has as a goal to calibrate the model used for VES and to adjust it to reality connecting input and output data (Fig. 16).

As an output data, the granule size distribution after successfully applying the virtual fluidized-bed granulator/dryer is generated. In order to obtain such a result, it is also necessary, as in a real experiment, to calibrate the pump used to add a granulating liquid to the primary particles, as described in the virtual experiment using a VES (22):

Description of the Task for the Student

1. *General goal:* Student has to granulate a starting powder mix (mean diameter = 140 μm, placebo composition: 20% w/w cornstarch, 76% w/w lactose monohydrate) to obtain a mean granule size of ~300 μm. This mean granule size distribution is achieved, if the binder concentration (PVP) has reached ~4% (w/w) in the formulation. The binder solution has a concentration of 5% (w/w).
2. *Preparatory tasks and reasoning:* Pump calibration; estimation of residence time; calculating amount of binder required; study the fluidization regimes; calculate required drying time; proper response to a given critical situation (e.g., air conditioning failure).
3. *Given process constants etc.:*
   a. Air source: 20%RH, 25°C;
   b. Assumed exhaust air saturation is constant: 85% (can be changed);
   c. *Special task:* establish pressure (bar) to air throughput (m^3/hr) calibration curve;
4. *Process parameters calculation by VES:*
   a. Mollier chart → water removal capacity of process air, product temperature

   b. Heat and mass balance → pumping rate, residence time, drying time
   c. Special task: select spray pressure from support resources
5. *Start experiment with VES:*
   a. Be aware to set 0.5 bar spray pressure prior to start fluidization (prevents clogging of a nozzle).
   b. Check the dynamics of particles growth.
   c. When product has reached required particle size distribution, switch to drying (stop pumping).
   d. Continue drying until required product residual moisture content is reached
   e. Stop the process by turning the process knob to "off" position.
   f. Print report.
   g. Include a complete record of all events and user interactions during process in report.
   h. There is a possibility to "play back" the recorded process.
   i. Assumed exhaust air saturation is constant: 85% (can be changed).
   j. Special task: establish pressure (bar) to air throughput (m^3/hr) calibration curve.
6. *Advanced training to cover critical situations:*
   It is possible to switch on the in-built generator of a critical situation, which generates at random times technical problems such as:
   a. Air conditioning failure
   b. Pump failure
   c. Sudden clogging of filters
   d. Temperature sensor failure
   The student must properly react to a failure and try to continue operation if possible.
7. *Advanced training based on acquired knowledge with VES:*
   Student repeats experiments with the goal to optimize following points:
   a. Shorter residence time
   b. Lower energy consumption
   c. Better conditions for thermolabile products
8. *Goals, which can be achieved with VES training:*
   a. Possibility of real personalized individual training
   b. Identifying weaknesses and improving operator's skills
   c. Identifying weaknesses of the equipment
   d. Identifying weaknesses of the formulation
   e. Testing existing SOPs and developing new SOPs
   f. In case that a *large-scale VES* is available: testing scale-up problems involved with a new formulation
9. *General benefits of the application of VES for the pharmaceutical company and for the equipment manufacturer:*
   a. Reducing human errors during the manufacturing process
   b. Better process understanding leading to a higher product quality
   c. Tailor-made VES taking into account specific on-site equipment
   d. Better understanding of site-to-site, resp. lab-to-lab differences
   e. Facilitated troubleshooting with equipment vendor leading to shorter repair times
   f. Before buying new equipment, test it with VES, if available
   g. VES as a tool for optimized operation for the pharmaceutical company and as a development tool for the equipment manufacturer.

VES can be used as an educational tool leading to a better process understanding fulfilling the requirements of PAT and QbD initiatives (8).

IMPLEMENTATION OF VES AS A TOOL FOR FACILITATING SCALE-UP EXERCISES

What is the difference between the application of VES in case of a small- and a large-scale equipment?

In case of a small-scale equipment like the table-top fluidized-bed processor described in chapter 2.2, it is possible to make a number of laboratory experiments according to a design of experiments (DoE, see also Fig. 16) to explore the limits and capabilities of the process equipment. In case of a large-scale equipment it would become extremely expensive to manufacture trial batches to explore the manufacturing limits of the equipment. Thus, the concept to model large-scale equipment needs to be modified as follows:

A. In order to develop a VES for large-scale equipment, *scale-down experiments* of selected existing formulations need to be carried out in a laboratory. Thus, formulation-specific "transfer results" can be obtained.
B. The collection of the existing batch records for a selected formulation needs to be fully exploited.
C. The combination of the experimental results from the small-scale VES combined with the results of A and B will lead to the implementation of the corresponding large-scale VES.

The authors of this chapter are convinced that the behavior of large-scale laboratory equipment can be translated 1:1 to a corresponding VES, taking into an account the results of earlier batch records and settings. As it could be shown with the PhD thesis of Lars Rehoric (23), the existing batch records of the results of pharmaceuticals manufactured with certain equipment represent a wealth of knowledge, which has not yet been fully exploited. VES is also able to take into an account the site-to-site specific differences of the equipment, such as differences in the construction, which influences the heat capacity of the equipment. The details of the method to develop and implement a large-scale VES depend on the specific manufacturing equipment involved. In case, a high-shear mixer/granulator and a subsequent fluidized-bed dryer are used, the following procedure is recommended:

– Analysis of the equipment used for the scale-up process, that is, the laboratory-scale high-shear mixer/granulator, laboratory-scale fluidized-bed dryer, medium- and large-sized high-shear mixer/granulator, medium- and large-scale fluidized-bed dryer.
– Development of the corresponding VES for the equivalent small- and large-scale equipment based on the physicochemical laws involved for the construction of the VES internal mathematical model (Fig. 16 in case of the fluidized-bed equipment).
– Study of the batch records of existing formulations A, B, C manufactured with the large-scale equipment.
– Extraction of the relevant data from the batch records *for preparing scale-down laboratory experiments* of the formulations A, B, and C.
– Study of batch-to-batch variability of the formulations A, B, and C.

- Identification of the relevant *scale-down*, respectively, *scale-up factors* for the specific formulations A, B, and C taking into account batch-to-batch variability of the specific formulations.
- Determination of the *internal transfer coefficients* for the corresponding small- and large-scale VES for the specific formulations A, B, and C.
- Identification of formulation specific and general internal scale-up transfer coefficients of VES.
- Validation of the *virtual scale-up process* using small- and large-scale VES on the basis of formulations D, E, and F, which have been manufactured on small-scale laboratory equipment *with the following steps*: in silico production of three registration batches for the formulations D, E, and F and comparison with the subsequent real batches.

The combined application of F-CAD and small- and large-scale VES has the potential to facilitate substantially scale-up exercise and to minimize risks. These new tools have the capacity to save money and improve simultaneously product quality and to reduce time to market (24).

CONCLUSIONS

Pharmaceutical solid dosage forms are complex systems consisting of the drug substance and functional auxiliary substances, which interact in a complex manner as a function of the environment. The confirmation of the in silico results by laboratory experiments is very promising. The authors of this chapter are convinced that the replacement of laboratory experiments by in silico experiments is not limited to the design of classical solid dosage forms (Fig. 17).

In addition, for companies developing and manufacturing pharmaceutical equipment, the test of new equipment using a VES approach is very rewarding. In addition, the specific VES will replace the technical manual for the new equipment and the laboratory staff can be first trained with the VES. The maintenance of the new equipment will become easier as VES will improve the communication between the equipment vendor and the customer. Thus, the root cause finding of the problem involved with the equipment will become easier and problems may be resolved together with the laboratory staff on site.

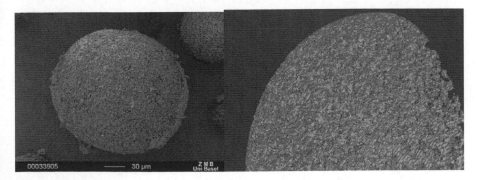

FIGURE 17   Real and computer-generated nanostructured micropellet. *Source*: Laboratory data from the PhD thesis of Matthias Plitzko (20).

In future, it should be also possible to use such concepts not only by the aircraft and pharmaceutical industry but also in other areas, where the engineering plays an important role such as in the area of nanotechnology, for example, for the development of novel photovoltaic devices or devices for quantum communication.

The proof of concept obtained with F-CAD in the area of dosage form design and testing (1) leads to the conclusion that the pharmaceutical virtual R&D approach can be extended to pharmaceutical manufacturing boosting quality and saving money.

Companies applying this new approach will have an important competitive advantage. To be successful in this approach it is not sufficient to buy such software. The important point is a close cooperation between the software provider who needs to have an experience in the area of pharmaceutical technology and who needs to take into account the industrial in-house scientific expertise.

ACKNOWLEDGMENTS

The authors want to thank the persons, companies, and institutions, which allowed to develop, test, and validate F-CAD as well as VES for solid dosage forms including in silico processes such as the coating of tablets. Respecting confidentiality agreements, only publically available laboratory data are cited in this chapter. In this context, the authors acknowledge the respective institutions and persons involved.

REFERENCES

1. Leuenberger M, Leuenberger N, Puchkov M. Implementing virtual R&D reality in industry: *in silico* design and testing of solid dosage forms. Swiss Pharma 2009; 31:18–24.
2. Leuenberger H, Puchkov M. Invited Presentation: How will the quality by design initiative affect formulation development and manufacturing? R.P. Scherrer Workshop, Frankfurt am Main, June 19, 2008.
3. Leuenberger H, Lanz M. Pharmaceutical powder technology—from art to science: the challenge of FDA's PAT initiative. Adv Powder Technol 2005; 16:3–25.
4. Lanz M. Pharmaceutical Powder Technology: Towards a Science Based Understanding of the Behavior of Powder Systems (PhD thesis). Basel, Switzerland: University of Basel, Faculty of Science, 2006.
5. von Orelli JC. Search for Technological Reasons to Develop a Capsule or a Tablet Formulation (PhD thesis). Basel, Switzerland: University of Basel, Faculty of Science, 2005.
6. Maurer L, Leuenberger H. Application of near infrared spectroscopy in the full-scale manufacturing of pharmaceutical solid dosage forms. Pharm Ind 2009; 71:672–678.
7. Maurer L, Leuenberger H. Terahertz pulsed imaging and near infrared imaging to monitor the coating process of pharmaceutical tablets. Int J Pharm 2009; 370:8–16.
8. ICH Q8 Pharmaceutical Development. Available at: http://www.emea.europa.eu/pdfs/human/ich/16706804en.pdf.
9. Puchkov M. Swiss Pharma Science Day 2008, Pharmaceutical Technology Lecture: Reasons and advantages of *in silico* approach in design of robust formulations. Swiss Pharma 2008; 30(Nr. 10/08):10.
10. Barat A, Ruskin JH, Crane M. Probabilistic models for drug dissolution part 1. Review of Monte Carlo and stochastic cellular automata approaches, simulation, modelling. Pract Theory 2006; 14:843–856, 857–873.
11. Bertrand N, Leclair G, Hildgen P. Modeling drug release from bioerodible microspheres using a cellular automaton. Int J Pharm 2007; 343:196–207.

12. Laaksonen TJ, Laaksonen HM, Hirvonen JT, et al. Cellular automata model for drug release from binary matrix and reservoir polymeric devices. Biomaterials 2009; 30:1978–1987.
13. Laaksonen H, Hirvonen J, Laaksonen T. Cellular automata model for swelling—controlled drug release. Int J Pharm 2009; 380:25–32.
14. Yu R, Chen H, Chen T, et al. Modeling and simulation of drug release from multi-layer biodegradable polymer microstructure in three dimensions, simulation, modelling. Pract Theory 2008; 16:15–25.
15. Leuenberger H, Bonny JD, Kolb M. Percolation effects in matrix-type controlled drug release systems. Int J Pharm 1995; 115:217–224.
16. Leuenberger H. The application of percolation theory in powder technology (invited review). Adv Powder Technol 1999; 10:323–353.
17. Krausbauer E, Puchkov M, Betz G, et al. Rational estimation of the optimum amount of non-fibrous disintegrant applying percolation theory for binary fast disintegrating formulation. J Pharm Sci 2008; 97:529–541.
18. Simon F. The trouble with making combination drugs. Nat Rev Drug Discov 2006; 5:881–882.
19. Leuenberger H. Spray freeze drying—the process of choice for low water soluble Drugs? J Nanopart Res 2002; 4:111–119.
20. Plitzko M. Gefriertrocknung in der Wirbelschicht: Möglichkeiten und Grenzen für die Anwendung in der Pharmazie (PhD thesis). Basel, Switzerland: University of Basel, Faculty of Science, 2006.
21. Boieng 777. Available at: http://www.cds.caltech.edu/conferences/1997/vecs/tutorial/Examples/Cases/777.htm.
22. Leuenberger H, Puchkov M. Invited Presentation: Virtual Equipment Simulators in pharmaceutical production – a novel tool for continuous education and personnel training. Manupharma Summit 2007, Marcus Eavens Seminar, Monte Carlo, Monaco, March 28–30, 2007.
23. Rehorik-Valer Farfan L. Ganzheitliche systemische Qualitätsbetrachtung in der Produktion fester Arzneiformen: ein praxisorientiertes Vorgehensmodell anhand einer Synthese der Methoden Prozesssimulation und multivariate Datenanalyse (PhD thesis). Basel, Switzerland: University of Basel, Faculty of Science, 2006.
24. Leuenberger H, Leuenberger MN, Puchkov M. Right first time: computer-aided scale-up for manufacturing solid dosage forms with a shorter time to market. Swiss Pharma 2010; 32:3–13.

Appendix A: Relevant FDA Guidance for Industry—Internet link addresses

- SUPAC-IR: Immediate Release Solid Oral Dosage Forms Scale-Up and Postapproval Changes: Chemistry, Manufacturing, and Controls, *In Vitro* Dissolution Testing, and *In Vivo* Bioequivalence Documentation.
  http://www.fda.gov/downloads/Drugs/
  GuidanceComplianceRegulatoryInformation/Guidances/UCM070636.pdf
- SUPAC-MR: Modified Release Solid Oral Dosage Forms. Scale-Up and Postapproval Changes: Chemistry, Manufacturing, and Controls; In Vitro Dissolution Testing and In Vivo Bioequivalence Documentation.
  http://www.fda.gov/downloads/Drugs/
  GuidanceComplianceRegulatoryInformation/Guidances/UCM070640.pdf
- SUPAC-IR/MR: Immediate Release and Modified Release Solid Oral Dosage Forms Manufacturing Equipment Addendum.
  http://www.fda.gov/downloads/Drugs/
  GuidanceComplianceRegulatoryInformation/Guidances/UCM070637.pdf
- SUPAC-ER: Extended Release Oral Dosage Forms: Development, Evaluation, and Application of In Vitro/In Vivo Correlations.
  http://www.fda.gov/downloads/Drugs/
  GuidanceComplianceRegulatoryInformation/Guidances/UCM070239.pdf
- SUPAC-SS: Nonsterile Semisolid Dosage Forms. Scale-Up and Postapproval Changes: Chemistry, Manufacturing, and Controls; In Vitro Release Testing and In Vivo Bioequivalence Documentation.
  http://www.fda.gov/downloads/Drugs/
  GuidanceComplianceRegulatoryInformation/Guidances/UCM070930.pdf
- SUPAC-SS: Nonsterile Semisolid Dosage Forms Manufacturing Equipment Addendum (Draft).
  http://www.fda.gov/downloads/Drugs/
  GuidanceComplianceRegulatoryInformation/Guidances/ucm070928.pdf
- Changes to an Approved NDA or ANDA. Questions and Answers.
  http://www.fda.gov/downloads/Drugs/
  GuidanceComplianceRegulatoryInformation/Guidances/ucm122871.pdf
- Waiver of In Vivo Bioavailability and Bioequivalence Studies for Immediate-Release Solid Oral Dosage Forms Based on a Biopharmaceutics Classification System.
  http://www.fda.gov/downloads/Drugs/
  GuidanceComplianceRegulatoryInformation/Guidances/UCM070246.pdf
- Guidance for Industry: PAT—A Framework for Innovative Pharmaceutical Development, Manufacturing, and Quality Assurance, September 2004.
  http://www.fda.gov/downloads/Drugs/
  GuidanceComplianceRegulatoryInformation/Guidances/UCM070305.pdf

Appendix B: Relevant EU Guidance for Industry—Internet link addresses

- Directive 2001/20/EC of the European Parliament and of the Council of 4 April 2001 on the approximation of the laws, regulations and administrative provisions of the Member States relating to the implementation of good clinical practice in the conduct of clinical trials on medicinal products for human use.
http://www.eortc.be/Services/Doc/clinical-EU-directive-04-April-01.pdf
- Directive 2001/83/EC of the European Parliament and of the Council of 6 November 2001 on the community code relating to medicinal products for human use, as amended. http://www.edctp.org/fileadmin/documents/ethics/DIRECTIVE_200183EC_OF_THE_EUROPEAN_PARLIAMENT.pdf
- Commission Directive 2003/94/EC of 8 October 2003 laying down the principles and guidelines of good manufacturing practice in respect of medicinal products for human use and investigational medicinal products for human use. http://ec.europa.eu/health/files/eudralex/vol-1/dir_2003_94/dir_2003_94_en.pdf
- Regulation (EC) No 726/2004 of the European Parliament and of the Council of 31 March 2004 laying down Community procedures for the authorisation and supervision of medicinal products for human and veterinary use and establishing a European Medicines Agency. http://eur-lex.europa.eu/LexUriServ/LexUriServ.do?uri=OJ:L:2004:136:0001:0033:EN:PDF
- EMEA/CHMP/167068/2004—ICH Topic Q8 Pharmaceutical Development, May 2006. http://www.tga.gov.au/docs/pdf/euguide/emea/16706804en.pdf
- Commission Directive 2005/28/EC of 8 April 2005 laying down principles and detailed guidelines for good clinical practice as regards investigational medicinal products for human use, as well as the requirements for authorisation of the manufacturing or importation of such products. http://eur-lex.europa.eu/LexUriServ/LexUriServ.do?uri=OJ:L:2005:091:0013:0019:en:PDF
- EMEA/CHMP/ICH/518819/2007 ICH Topic Q 8 Annex Pharmaceutical Development, June 2009. http://www.rsihata.com/updateguidance/emea2/2009/51881907enfin.pdf
- EMEA/CHMP/ICH/265145/2009 ICH Topic Q8, Q9 and Q10 Note for Guidance on Pharmaceutical Development Quality Risk Management Pharmaceutical Quality System. Questions and Answers, June 2009. http://www.ema.europa.eu/pdfs/human/ich/26514509en.pdf

Appendix C: Relevant ICH Documents: International Conference on Harmonisation of Technical Requirements for Registration of Pharmaceuticals for Human Use—Internet link addresses

- ICH Harmonised Tripartite Guideline Q7—Good Manufacturing Practice Guide For Active Pharmaceutical Ingredients. Version dated November 2000.
  http://www.ich.org/lob/media/media433.pdf
  Current *Step 5 (Implementation)*
- ICH Harmonised Tripartite Guideline Q8 (R2)—Pharmaceutical Development, with Annex incorporated into Core Guideline. Version dated August 2009.
  http://www.ich.org/lob/media/media4986.pdf
  Current *Step 5 (Implementation)*
- ICH Harmonised Tripartite Guideline Q9—Quality Risk Management. Version dated November 2005. http://www.ich.org/lob/media/media1957.pdf
  Current *Step 5 (Implementation)*
- ICH Harmonised Tripartite Guideline Q10—Pharmaceutical Quality System. Version dated June 2008. http://www.ich.org/lob/media/media3917.pdf
  Current *Step 5 (Implementation)*
- ICH Quality Implementation Working Group on Q8, Q9 and Q10—Questions & Answers. Version dated October 29, 2009.
  http://www.ich.org/lob/media/media5783.pdf
  Current *Step 5 (Implementation)*

Index